FOUNDATIONAL ASSESSMENTS AND WELLNESS PROMOTION IN INTEGRATIVE CHIROPRACTIC AND FUNCTIONAL MEDICINE

*The art of co-creating wellness
while effectively managing
acute and chronic
health disorders and
musculoskeletal complaints*

DR. ALEX VASQUEZ

- Doctor of Osteopathic Medicine, graduate of University of North Texas Health Science Center, Texas College of Osteopathic Medicine (2010)
- Doctor of Naturopathic Medicine, graduate of Bastyr University (1999)
- Doctor of Chiropractic, graduate of Western States Chiropractic College (1996)
- Director of the Medical Board of Advisors (2011-present), Researcher and Lecturer (2004-2010), Biotics Research Corporation in Rosenberg, Texas
- Adjunct Faculty (2004-2005, 2010-present) and Forum Consultant (2003-2007), The Institute for Functional Medicine in Gig Harbor, Washington
- Adjunct Professor of Pharmacology, Program Director for Master of Science in Nutrition and Functional Medicine, University of Western States in Portland, Oregon
- Former Adjunct Professor of Orthopedics (2000) and Rheumatology (2001), Bastyr University in Kenmore, Washington
- Private practice in Seattle, Washington (2000-2001), Houston, Texas (2001-2006), Portland, Oregon (2011-present)
- Author of approximately 100 articles and letters published in *Annals of Pharmacotherapy, The Lancet, Nutritional Perspectives, BMJ—British Medical Journal, Journal of Manipulative and Physiological Therapeutics, JAMA—Journal of the American Medical Association, The Original Internist, Integrative Medicine, Holistic Primary Care, Nutritional Wellness, Dynamic Chiropractic, Alternative Therapies in Health and Medicine, JAOA—Journal of the American Osteopathic Association, Evidence-based Complementary and Alternative Medicine, Journal of Clinical Endocrinology and Metabolism,* and *Arthritis & Rheumatism*: Official Journal of the American College of Rheumatology

OPTIMALHEALTHRESEARCH.COM

Vasquez A. <u>Foundational Assessments and Wellness Promotion in Integrative Chiropractic and Functional Medicine</u>. Portland, Oregon; Integrative and Biological Medicine Research and Consulting, LLC.

The intended audiences for this book are health science students and doctorate-level clinicians. This book has been written with every intention to make it as accurate as possible, and each section has undergone peer-review by an interdisciplinary group of clinicians. In view of the possibility of human error and as well as ongoing discoveries in the biomedical sciences, neither the author nor any party associated in any way with this text warrants that this text is perfect, accurate, or complete in every way, and we disclaim responsibility for harm or loss associated with the application of the material herein. Information and treatments applicable to a specific *condition* may not be appropriate for or applicable to a specific *patient*; this is especially true for patients with multiple comorbidities and those taking pharmaceutical medications with multiple adverse effects and drug/nutrient/herb interactions. Given that this book is available on an open market, lay persons who read this material should discuss the information with a licensed healthcare provider before implementing any treatments and interventions described herein.

See website for updated information: www.OptimalHealthResearch.com

Table of Contents	Page

- Revisiting the Five-Part Nutritional Wellness Protocol: The Supplemented Paleo-Mediterranean Diet. *Nutritional Perspectives* 2011
- The clinical importance of vitamin D: a paradigm shift with implications for all healthcare providers. *Altern Ther Health Med* 2004
- Reducing Pain and Inflammation Naturally - Part 1: New Insights into Fatty Acid Biochemistry and the Influence of Diet. *Nutritional Perspectives* 2004
- Reducing Pain and Inflammation Naturally - Part 2: New Insights into Fatty Acid Supplementation and Its Effect on Eicosanoid Production and Genetic Expression. *Nutritional Perspectives* 2005
- Reducing Pain and Inflammation Naturally - Part 3: Improving overall health while safely and effectively treating musculoskeletal pain. *Nutritional Perspectives* 2005
- Reducing Pain and Inflammation Naturally - Part 4: Nutritional and Botanical Inhibition of NF-kappaB, the Major Intracellular Amplifier of the Inflammatory Cascade. A Practical Clinical Strategy Exemplifying Anti-Inflammatory Nutrigenomics. *Nutritional Perspectives* 2005
- Reducing Pain and Inflammation Naturally - Part 5: Improving neuromusculoskeletal health by optimizing immune function and reducing allergic reactions: a review of 16 treatments and a 3-step clinical approach. *Nutritional Perspectives* 2005
- Reducing Pain and Inflammation Naturally - Part 6: Nutritional and Botanical Treatments Against "Silent Infections" and Gastrointestinal Dysbiosis, Commonly Overlooked Causes of Neuromusculoskeletal Inflammation and Chronic Health Problems. *Nutritional Perspectives* 2006

Dedications: I dedicate this book to the following people in appreciation for their works, their direct and indirect support of this work, and for their contributions to the advancement of true healthcare.

- **To the students and practitioners of chiropractic and naturopathic medicine**, those who continue to learn so that they can provide the best possible care to their patients.
- **To the researchers** whose works are cited in this text.
- **To Drs Alan Gaby, Jeffrey Bland, Ronald LeFebvre, Robert Richard, and Gilbert Manso,** my most memorable and influential professors and mentors.
- **To Dr Bruce Ames**[1] and the late **Dr Roger Williams**[2], for helping us to view our individuality as biochemically unique.
- **To Dr Chester Wilk**[3,4] **and important others** for documenting and resisting the organized oppression of natural, non-pharmaceutical, non-surgical healthcare.[5,6,7]
- **To Jorge Strunz and Ardeshir Farah,** for artistic inspiration

Acknowledgments for Peer and Editorial Review: Acknowledgement here does not imply that the reviewer fully agrees with or endorses the material in this text but rather that they were willing to review specific sections of the book for clinical applicability and clarity and to make suggestions to their own level of satisfaction. Credit for improvements and refinements to this text are due in part to these reviewers; responsibility for oversights remains that of the author.

- 2012 Edition of Migraine Headaches, Hypothyroidism, and Fibromyalgia: Holly Furlong DC
- 2011 Edition of *Integrative Chiropractic Management of High Blood Pressure and Chronic Hypertension*: Barry Morgan MD, Holly Furlong DC, Kris Young DC, Erika Mennerick DC, and Bill Beakey DOM
- 2011 Edition of *Integrative Medicine and Functional Medicine for Chronic Hypertension*: Erika Mennerick DC, Holly Furlong DC, JoAnn Fawcett DC, Ileana Bourland MSOM LAc, James Bogash DC, Bill Beakey
- 2010 Edition of *Chiropractic Management of Chronic Hypertension*: Joseph Paun MS DC, Joe Brimhall DC, David Candelario OMS4 (TCOM c/o 2010), James Bogash DC, Bill Beakey DOM, Robert Richard DO
- 2009 Edition of *Chiropractic and Naturopathic Mastery of Common Clinical Disorders*: Heather Kahn MD, Robert Richard DO, James Leiber DO, David Candelario (UNT-HSC TCOM DO4)
- 2007 Edition of *Integrative Orthopedics*: Barry Morgan MD, Dennis Harris DC, Richard Brown DC (DACBI candidate), Ron Mariotti ND, Patrick Makarewich MBA, Reena Singh (SCNM ND4), Zachary Watkins DC, Charles Novak MS DC, Marnie Loomis ND, James Bogash DC, Sara Croteau DC, Kris Young DC, Joshua Levitt ND, Jack Powell III MD, Chad Kessler MD, Amy Neuzil ND
- 2006 Edition of *Integrative Rheumatology*: Amy Neuzil ND, Cathryn Harbor MD, Julian Vickers DC, Tamara Sachs MD, Bob Sager BSc MD DABFM (Clinical Instructor in the Department of Family Medicine, University of Kansas), Ron Mariotti ND, Titus Chiu (DC4), Zachary Watkins (DC4), Gilbert Manso MD, Bruce Milliman ND, William Groskopp DC, Robert Silverman DC, Matthew Breske (DC4), Dean Neary ND, Thomas Walton DC, Fraser Smith ND, Ladd Carlston DC, David Jones MD, Joshua Levitt ND
- 2004 Edition of *Integrative Orthopedics*: Peter Knight ND, Kent Littleton ND MS, Barry Morgan MD, Ron Hobbs ND, Joshua Levitt ND, John Neustadt (Bastyr ND4), Allison Gandre BS (Bastyr ND4), Peter Kimble ND, Jack Powell III MD, Chad Kessler MD, Mike Gruber MD, Deirdre O'Neill ND, Mary Webb ND, Leslie Charles ND, Amy Neuzil ND

[1] Ames BN, Elson-Schwab I, Silver EA. High-dose vitamin therapy stimulates variant enzymes with decreased coenzyme binding affinity (increased K(m)): relevance to genetic disease and polymorphisms. *Am J Clin Nutr*. 2002 Apr;75(4):616-58 http://www.ajcn.org/cgi/content/full/75/4/616
[2] Williams RJ. Biochemical Individuality: The Basis for the Genetotrophic Concept. Austin and London: University of Texas Press; 1956
[3] Wilk CA. Medicine, Monopolies, and Malice: How the Medical Establishment Tried to Destroy Chiropractic. Garden City Park: Avery, 1996
[4] Getzendanner S. Permanent injunction order against AMA. *JAMA*. 1988 Jan 1;259(1):81-2 http://optimalhealthresearch.com/archives/wilk.html
[5] Carter JP. Racketeering in Medicine: The Suppression of Alternatives. Norfolk: Hampton Roads Pub; 1993
[6] Morley J, Rosner AL, Redwood D. A case study of misrepresentation of the scientific literature: recent reviews of chiropractic. *J Altern Complement Med*. 2001 Feb;7(1):65-78
[7] Terrett AG. Misuse of the literature by medical authors in discussing spinal manipulative therapy injury. *J Manipulative Physiol Ther*. 1995 May;18(4):203-10

Format and Layout: The format and layout of this book is designed to efficiently take the reader though the clinically relevant spectrum of considerations for each condition that is detailed. Important topics are given their own section within each chapter, while other less important or less common conditions are only described briefly in terms of the four "clinical essentials" of 1) definition/pathophysiology, 2) clinical presentation, 3) assessment/diagnosis, and 4) treatment/management. Each expanded section which details the more important/common conditions maintains a consistent format, taking the reader through the spectrum of primary clinical considerations: definition/pathophysiology, clinical presentations, differential diagnoses, assessments (physical examination, laboratory, imaging), complications, management, and treatment. As my books have progressed, I am increasingly using an article-by-article review format (especially in the sections on management and treatment) so that readers have more direct access to the information so as to understand and *incorporate* more deeply what the research actually states; the goal and general approach here is to use a *representative sampling* of the research literature.

References and Citations: Citations to articles, abstracts, texts, and personal communications are footnoted throughout the text to provide supporting information and to provide interested readers the resources to find additional information. Many of the cited articles are available on-line for free, and when possible I have included the website addresses so that readers can access the complete article.

Peer-review and Quality Control: Peer-review is essential to help ensure accuracy and clinical applicability of health-related information. Consistent with the importance of our goals, I have employed several "checks and balances" to increase the accuracy and applicability of the information within my textbooks:
- Reliance upon authoritative references: Nearly all important statements are referenced to peer-reviewed biomedical journals or authoritative texts, such as *The Merck Manual* and *Current Medical Diagnosis and Treatment*. Each citation is provided by a footnote at the bottom of each page so that readers will know quickly and easily exactly from where the information was obtained.
- Extensive cross-referencing: Readers will notice, if not be overwhelmed by, the number of references and citations. Many important statements have several references. Many references (especially textbooks) are referenced several times even on the same page. The purpose of this extensive referencing is three-fold: 1) to guide you to additional information, 2) to help me (as writer) stay organized, and 3) to help you and me (the practicing physicians) employ this information with confidence.
- Periodic revision: All of my books will be updated and revised on an *as-needed* basis. New information is added; superfluous information removed. Inspired by the popular text *Current Medical Diagnosis and Treatment* which is updated every year, I want my books to be accurate, timely, and in pace with the ever-growing literature on natural medicine. Any significant errors that are discovered will be posted at OptimalHealthResearch.com/updates; please check this page periodically to ensure that you are working with the most accurate information of which I am aware.
- Peer-review: The peer-review process for my books takes several forms. First, colleagues and students are invited to review new and revised sections of the text before publication; every section of the book that you are holding has been independently reviewed by health science students and/or practicing clinicians from various backgrounds: allopathic, chiropractic, osteopathic, naturopathic. Second, you - the reader - are invited to provide feedback about the information in the book, typographical errors, syntax, case reports, new research, etc. If your ideas truly change the nature of the material, I will be glad to acknowledge you in the text (with your permission, of course). If your contribution is hugely significant, such as reviewing three or more chapters or helping in some important way, I will be glad to not only acknowledge you, but to also send you the next edition at a discount or courtesy when your ideas take effect. Third, I keep abreast of new literature by constantly perusing new research and advancements in the health sciences. Having been successful in three separate doctoral programs in the health sciences, I have learned not only to master large amounts of material but to also separate and integrate different viewpoints as appropriate. I also "field test" my protocols with patients in the various clinical arenas in which I work and also with professionals and academicians via presentations and

critical dialogue. By implementing these quality control steps, I hope to create a useful text and advance our professions and our practices by improving the quality of care that we deliver to our patients.

How to Use This Book Safely and Most Effectively: Ideally, these books should be read cover-to-cover within a context of coursework that is supervised by an experienced professor. For post-graduate professionals, they might consider forming a local "book club" and meeting for weekly or monthly discussions to check their understandings and share their clinical experiences to refine the application of clinical knowledge, perceptions, and skills. Virtual groups and internet forums—specifically the forum hosted by the Institute for Functional Medicine at www.FunctionalMedicine.org—can provide access to an assembly of international professional peers wherein sharing of clinical questions and experiences are synergistic. Throughout this book, references are amply provided and are often footnoted with hyperlinks providing full-text access. This book is intended for licensed doctorate-level healthcare professionals with graduate and post-graduate training.

Notice: The intention and scope of this text are to provide doctorate-level clinicians with useful information and a familiarity with available research and resources pertinent to the management of patients in an integrative primary care setting. Specifically, the information in this book is intended to be used by licensed healthcare professionals who have received hands-on clinical training and supervision at accredited health science colleges. Additionally, information in this book should be used in conjunction with other resources, texts, and in combination with the clinician's best judgment and intention to "*first, do no harm*" and second to provide effective healthcare. Information and treatments applicable to a specific *condition* may not be appropriate for or applicable to a specific *patient* in your office; this is especially true for patients with multiple comorbidities and those taking pharmaceutical medications with multiple adverse effects and drug/nutrient/herb interactions. In my books and articles, I describe treatments—manual, dietary, nutritional, botanical, pharmacologic, and occasionally surgical—and their research support for the clinical condition being discussed; each practitioner must determine appropriateness of these treatments for his/her individual patient and with consideration of the doctor's scope of practice, education, training, skill, and—occasionally—the appropriateness of "off label" use of medications and treatments. This book has been carefully written and checked for accuracy by the author and professional colleagues. However, in view of the possibility of human error and new discoveries in the biomedical sciences, neither the author nor any party associated in any way with this text warrants that this text is perfect, accurate, or complete in every way, and we disclaim responsibility for harm or loss associated with the application of the material herein. With all conditions/treatments described herein, each physician must be sure to consider the balance between what is best for the patient and the physician's own level of ability, expertise, and experience. When in doubt, or if the physician is not a specialist in the treatment of a given severe condition, referral is appropriate. These notes are written with the routine "outpatient" in mind and are not tailored to severely injured patients or "playing field" or "emergency response" situations; consult your First Aid and Emergency Response texts and course materials for appropriate information. These notes represent the author's perspective based on academic education, experience, and post-graduate continuing education and are not inclusive of every fact that a clinician may need to know. This is not an "entry level" book except when used in an academic setting with a knowledgeable professor who can explain the concepts, tests, physical exam procedures, and treatments; this book requires a certain level of knowledge from the reader and familiarity with clinical concepts, laboratory assessments, and physical examination procedures.

Updates, Corrections, and Newsletter: When and if omissions, errata, and the need for important updates become clear, I will post these at the website: OptimalHealthResearch.com/updates.html. A reader might access this page periodically to ensure staying informed of any corrections that might have clinical relevance. This book consists not only of the text in the printed pages you are holding, but also the footnotes and any updates at the website. Be alerted to new integrative clinical research and updates to this textbook by signing-up for the free newsletter at www.OptimalHealthResearch.com/newsletter.html.

Language, Semantics, and Perspective: As a diligent student who previously aspired to be an English professor, I have written this text with great (though inevitably imperfect) attention to detail. Individual words were chosen with care. I confess to knowing, pushing, and creatively breaking several rules of grammar and punctuation. With regard to the he/she and him/her debacle of the English language, I've mixed singular and plural pronouns for the sake of being efficient and so that the images remain gender-neutral to the extent reasonable. The subtitle *The art of creating wellness while effectively managing acute and chronic musculoskeletal/health disorders* was chosen to emphasize the intentional creation of wellness rather than a limited focus on disease treatment and symptom suppression. For the 2009 printing of *Chiropractic and Naturopathic Mastery of Common Clinical Disorders*, this subtitle was slightly modified from "creating" to "co-creating" to emphasize the **team effort** required between physician and patient. *Managing* was chosen to emphasize the importance of treating-monitoring-referring-reassessing, rather than merely *treating*. *Disorders* was chosen to reflect the fact that a distinguishing characteristic of *life* is the ability to habitually create *organized structure* and *higher order* from chaos and *disorder*. For example, plants organize the randomly moving molecules of air and water into the organized structure of biomolecules which eventually take shape as plant structure—fiber, leaves, flowers, petals. Similarly, the human body creates organized structure of increased complexity from consumed plants and other foods; molecules ingested and inhaled from the environment are organized into specific biochemicals and tissue structures with distinct characteristics and definite functions. Injury and disease *result in* or *result from* a lack of order, hence my use of the word "disorders" to characterize human illness and disease. A motor vehicle accident that results in bodily injury, for example, is an example of an external chaotic force, which, when imparted upon human body tissues, results in a disruption (disorder) of the normal structure and organization that previously defined and characterized the now-damaged tissues of the body. Likewise, an autoimmune disease process that results in tissue destruction is an *anti-evolutionary* process that takes molecules of higher complexity and reverts them to simpler, fragmented, and non-functional forms. From the perspective of "health" as *organized structure and meaningful function* and "disease" as *the reversion to chaos, destruction of structure, and the loss of function*, the task of healthcare providers is essentially to restore order, and to acutely reduce and proactively prevent/eliminate clinical-biochemical-biomechanical-emotional chaos insofar as it adversely affects the patient's life experience as an individual and our collective experience as an interdependent society. What is required of clinicians then is the ability first to create conceptual order from what appears to be chaotic phenomena, and then second to materialize that conceptual order into our physical world; this is our task, and no small task it is.

Integrity and Creativity: I have endeavored to accurately represent the facts as they have been presented in texts and research, and to specifically resist any temptation to embellish or misrepresent data as others have done.[8,9] Conversely, I have not endeavored to make this book appeal to the "average" student or reader; my goal is to write and teach to the students at the top of the class, thereby affirming them and pulling the other students forward and upward. While I offer *explanations*, I intentionally resist *simplifications*, except when one simplification might facilitate the comprehension of a more complex phenomenon, or when such a simplification might facilitate the conveyance of information from clinician to patient. I have allowed this text to be unique in format, content, and style, so that the personality of this text can be contrasted with that of the instructor and reader, thus enabling the learner to at least benefit from an intentionally different – and intentionally honest – perspective and approach. Students using this text with the guidance of a qualified professor will benefit from the experience of "two teachers" rather than just one.

Linearity, Nonlinearity, Redundancy, Asynchronicity: Although the overall flow of the text is highly linear and sequential, occasionally I place a conclusion before its introduction for the sake of foreshadowing and therefore for preparing the reader for what is to come. The purpose of this is not simply one of preparation for the sake of allowing the reader to know what is already lying ahead on the path, but more to begin

---

[8] **Vasquez A**. Zinc treatment for reduction of hyperplasia of prostate. *Townsend Letter for Doctors and Patients* 1996; January: 100
[9] Broad W, Wade N. *Betrayers of the Truth: Fraud and Deceit in the Halls of Science*. New York: Simon and Schuster; 1982

creating new "shelf space" in the reader's intellectual-neuronal "library" so that when the new—particularly if *neoparadigmatic*—information is encountered, a space will already exist for it; it other words: the intent is to make learning easier. Likewise, for the sake of *information retention*—or what is better understood as synaptogenesis—important points are presented more than once, either identically or variantly. Given that "*No one ever reads the same book twice*"[10] (because the "person who starts" the reading of a meaningful book is changed into the "person who finishes" the reading of that book (assuming proper intentionality and application of one's "self"), the person reading these words might consider a second glace after the first.

The Functional Medicine Matrix (version presented in 2003): In the 2009 edition of *Chiropractic and Naturopathic Mastery of Common Clinical Disorders*, I reintroduced the Functional Medicine Matrix that I originally diagramed for the Institute for Functional Medicine (IFM) in 2003; the diagram used is updated from the original, and readers should appreciate that IFM has changed the Matrix since this version was made. My perspective is that functional medicine, naturopathic medicine, and *authentic* holistic medicine share much in common in their fundamental models of health and disease. The functional medicine matrix—designed and owned by the Institute for Functional Medicine (FunctionalMedicine.org)—is unique to the discipline of functional medicine and provides a conceptual framework for understanding the complexity of health and disease.

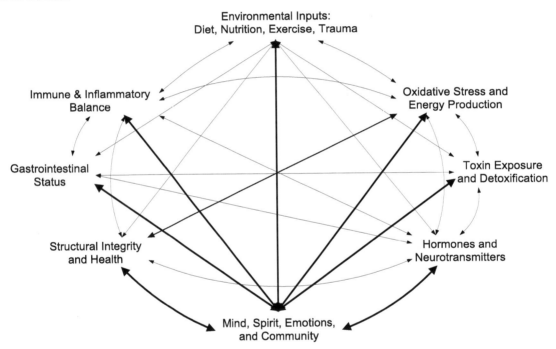

2003 Version of the Functional Medicine Matrix: Updated from the original diagram by Vasquez in 2003 for the Institute for Functional Medicine (IFM).

Distinguishing "Integrative Medicine" from "Functional Medicine"—the author's perspective[11]: The distinction of integrative medicine from functional medicine is that of *quantity* from *quality*. Integrative medicine can be understood as a quantitative extension of other already-existing healthcare models, to which additional perspectives and treatments are added; in this way, various conceptual models are "integrated" and used together in a more holistic and comprehensive approach. In contrast, functional medicine is a distinct model of health and disease that has developed an identity beyond mere integration of various models and treatments. Functional medicine is qualitatively distinct in its viewpoint of disease causation and treatment by the unique combination of emphases placed on ❶ patient-centered care (in

---

[10] Davies R. *Reading and Writing*. Salt Lake City: University of Utah Press; 1992, page 23
[11] Dr Vasquez's perspective: I have trained in functional medicine since 1994, first as a student of Jeffrey Bland PhD *et al* and later as Forum Consultant and Faculty (2003 – present in 2011) for the Institute of Functional Medicine, and I wrote three chapters in *Textbook of Functional Medicine* published by Institute of Functional Medicine. My opinions here are not necessarily currently representative of the Institute of Functional Medicine in this context.

contrast to the disease-centered care of allopathic medicine and most osteopathic medicine), ❷ detailed appreciation of the importance of the web-like interconnected nature of various organ systems[12] and psychological, physiological, and pathological processes (to a greater extent than allopathic, osteopathic, chiropractic and naturopathic medicine), ❸ its rigorous evidence-based standards, and ❹ its willingness to eagerly-yet-appropriately include *all* therapeutic options, ranging from (for example) surgical to meditative, dietary to pharmaceutical, manipulative to botanical, and antidysbiotic to psychological. In short, functional medicine can be described as an ***antiparadigmatic patient-centered discipline***, hence its therapeutic flexibility, broad applicability, and enhanced efficacy; it is antiparadigmatic due to its lack of adherence to a specific and limited set of tools (most professional disciplines are quite limited in their expertise and scope) and due to the emphasis placed on patient-centered healthcare, which first and always foremost seeks to determine the most efficient path for patient empowerment and healing.

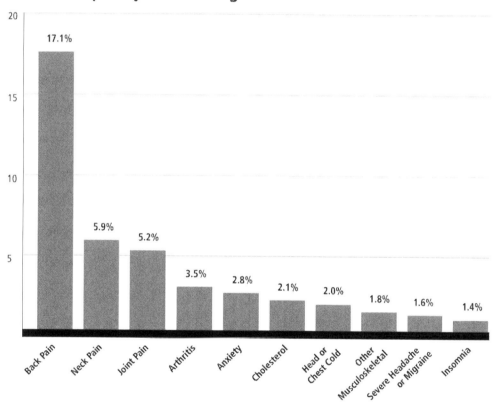

Diseases/Conditions for Which CAM Is Most Frequently Used Among Adults - 2007

Source: Barnes PM, Bloom B, Nahin R. *CDC National Health Statistics Report #12.* Complementary and Alternative Medicine Use Among Adults and Children: United States, 2007. December 2008.

Health problems for which patients most often seek so-called CAM treatment: Illustration from National Center for Complementary and Alternative Medicine, NIH, DHHS (http://nccam.nih.gov/news/camstats/2007/graphics.htm).

The following table provides a listing—in order of percentage—of the most common conditions seen in a general family practice of medicine, with hypertension and diabetes mellitus—two conditions highly amenable to integrative therapeutics—clearly dominating the clinical landscape.

---

[12] **Vasquez A**. Web-like Interconnections of Physiological Factors. *Integrative Medicine: A Clinician's Journal* 2006, April/May, 32-37

The Most Common Diagnoses in the Practice of General/Family Medicine

Top diagnoses	Notes and comments
1. Hypertension	5.9% of family medicine diagnoses; nearly 11 million patient visits per year.
2. Diabetes mellitus	4.1% of family medicine diagnoses; more than 7.6 million patient visits per year.
3. Acute upper respiratory infection	3.2% of family medicine diagnoses; more than 10 million patient visits per year. Most of these are caused by viral infections for which there is no direct medical treatment.
4. Sinusitis	2.5% of family medicine diagnoses; more than 10 million patient visits per year.
5. Acute pharyngitis	2.3% of family medicine diagnoses; more than 4 million patient visits per year.
6. Otitis media	2.3% of family medicine diagnoses; > 4 million patient visits per year.
7. Bronchitis	1.9% of family medicine diagnoses; > 3 million patient visits per year.
8. Back problems	1.8% of family medicine diagnoses; > 3 million patient visits per year. This is a diverse group of conditions ranging from post-traumatic to benign to developmental problems such as scoliosis. Note that back pain is listed separately below.
9. Hyperlipidemia	1.7% of family medicine diagnoses; > 3 million patient visits per year. This mostly includes the lifestyle-generated dyslipidemia epidemic, with comparably fewer cases of genotropic disorders requiring pharmacotherapy.
10. Urinary tract disorders	1.6% of family medicine diagnoses; almost 3 million patient visits per year. This can include a diverse group of problems ranging from simple and self-limited urinary tract infections to sexually transmitted diseases.
11. Allergic rhinitis	1.2% of family medicine diagnoses; > 2 million patient visits per year. A general approach to allergy treatment is included in this text.
12. Back pain	1.2% of family medicine diagnoses; > 2 million patient visits per year.
13. Abdominal or pelvic symptoms	1.1% of family medicine diagnoses; > 2 million patient visits per year. This can include a wide range of diagnoses ranging from appendicitis to dysmenorrhea. Due to the breadth and complexity, these are not covered in this text.
14. Joint pain	1.1% of family medicine diagnoses; > 2 million patient visits per year.
15. Depression or anxiety	1.1% of family medicine diagnoses; > 2 million patient visits per year.
16. Asthma	1.1% of family medicine diagnoses; almost 2 million patient visits per year. An approach to allergy treatment is included in this text, with a section on asthma.
17. Chest pain or shortness of breath	1.1% of family medicine diagnoses; almost 2 million patient visits per year. Some of these are benign musculoskeletal pain or gastroesophageal reflux while others turn out to be life-threatening conditions such as myocardial infarction, pneumothorax, pneumonia, or—rarely—aortic dissection. These are not directly covered in this text.
18. Soft tissue problems	1% of family medicine diagnoses; 1.8 million patient visits per year.
19. Acute bronchitis and bronchiolitis	1% of family medicine diagnoses; 1.8 million patient visits per year. These include bacterial and viral infections, ranging from mild to life-threatening, especially in patients with cardiopulmonary disease.
20. Skin problems	1% of family medicine diagnoses; 1.8 million patient visits per year.
21. Tendonitis	1% of family medicine diagnoses; 1.7 million patient visits per year.

Data from *Essentials of Family Medicine, 5th edition* edited by Sloane PD, Slatt LM, Ebell MH, Jacques LB, Smith MA published by Lippincott Williams & Wilkins (April 1, 2007)

Bon Voyage: All artists and scientists—regardless of genre—grapple with the divergent goals of *perfecting* their work and *presenting* their work; the former is impossible, while the latter is the only means by which the effort can create the desired effect in the world, whether that is pleasure, progress, or both. At some point, we must all agree that it is "good enough" and that it contains the essence of what needs to be communicated. While neither this nor any future edition of this book is likely to be "perfect", I am content with the literature reviewed, presented, and the new conclusions and implications which are described—many for the first time ever—in this text. Particularly for *Integrative Rheumatology* and *Chiropractic and Naturopathic Mastery*, each chapter aims to achieve a paradigm shift which distances us further from the simplistic pharmacocentric model and toward one which authentically empowers both practitioners and patients. With time, I will make future editions more complete and perhaps less polemical—but not less passionate. I hope you are able to implement these conclusions and research findings *into your own life* and into the treatment plans for your patients. In short time, I believe that we will see many of these concepts more broadly implemented. Hopefully this work's value and veracity will promote patients' vitality via the vigilant and virtuous clinicians viewing this volume. To the more attentive and thoroughgoing reader, more is revealed.

Authentic learning is life integration

"Ultimately, no one can extract from things—*books included*—more than he already knows. What one has no access to through experience, one has no ear for."

Friedrich Nietzsche [translated by RJ Hollingdale]. *Ecce Homo: How One Becomes What One Is*. New York & London: Penguin Books; 1979, page 70

Thank you, and I wish you and your patients the best of success and health.

Alex Vasquez, D.C., N.D., D.O.
April 30, 2012

Work as love

"You work that you may keep pace with the earth and the soul of the earth.
For to be idle is to become a stranger unto the seasons, and to step out of life's procession. ...
Work is love made visible."

Kahlil Gibran (1883-1930). The Prophet. Publisher Alfred A. Knopf, 1973

Newsletter & Updates

Be alerted to new integrative clinical research and updates to this textbook by signing-up for the free newsletter, sent several times per year as needed.
Join at:
www.OptimalHealthResearch.com/newsletter.html

Examples of commonly used abbreviations:

- **25-OH-D** = serum 25-hydroxy-vitamin D(3)
- **ACEi** = angiotensin-2 converting enzyme inhibitor
- **Alpha-blocker** = alpha-adrenergic antagonist
- **ARB** = angiotensin-2 receptor blocker/antagonist
- **ARF** = acute renal failure
- **BB** = beta blocker or beta-adrenergic antagonist
- **BMP** = basic metabolic panel, includes serum Na, K, Cl, CO2, BUN, creatinine, and glucose
- **BP** = blood pressure, **HBP** = high blood pressure
- **BUN** = blood urea nitrogen
- **C&S** = culture and sensitivity
- **CAD** = coronary artery disease
- **CBC** = complete blood count
- **CCB** = calcium channel blocker/antagonist
- **CE** = cardiac enzymes, generally including creatine kinase (CK), creatine kinase myocardial band (CKMB), and troponin-1, with the latter being the most specific serologic marker for acute myocardial injury; for the evaluation of acute MI, these are generally tested 2-3 times at 6-hour intervals with ECG performed at least as often.
- **CHF** = congestive heart failure
- **CHO** = carbohydrate
- **CK** = creatine kinase, historically named creatine phosphokinase (CPK)
- **CKD** = chronic kidney disease, generally stratified into five stages based on GFR of roughly <90, 90-60, 60-30, 30-15, and >15, respectively
- **CMP** = comprehensive metabolic panel, also called a chemistry panel, includes the BMP along with markers of hepatic status albumin, protein, ALT, AST, may also include alkaline phosphatase and rarely GGT; panels vary per laboratory and hospital.
- **CNS** = central nervous system
- **COPD** = chronic obstructive pulmonary disease
- **CRF, CRI** = chronic renal failure/insufficiency
- **CRP** = c-reactive protein, **hsCRP** = high-sensitivity c-reactive protein
- **CT** = computed tomography
- **CVD** = cardiovascular disease
- **CXR** = chest X-ray
- **DM** = diabetes mellitus
- **ECG** or **EKG** = electrocardiograph
- **Echo** = echocardiography
- **GFR** = glomerular filtration rate
- **HDL** = high density lipoprotein cholesterol
- **HTN** = hypertension
- **Ig** = immune globulin = antibodies of the G, A, M, E, or D classes.
- **IHD** = ischemic heart disease
- **IV** = intravenous
- **MCV** = mean cell volume
- **MI** = myocardial infarction
- **MRI** = magnetic resonance imaging, **MRI** = magnetic resonance angiography
- **PRN** = from the Latin "pro re nata" meaning "on occasion" or "when necessary"
- **PTH** = parathyroid hormone, **iPTH** = intact parathyroid hormone
- **PVD** = peripheral vascular disease
- **RA** = rheumatoid arthritis
- **RAD** = reactive airway disease, similar to asthma
- **SLE** = systemic lupus erythematosus
- **TRIG(s)** = serum triglycerides
- **UA** = urinalysis
- **US** = ultrasound

Dosing shorthand (mostly Latin abbreviations): q = each; qd = each day; bid = twice daily; tid = thrice daily; qid = four times per day; po = per os = by mouth; prn = as needed.

Chapter 1:
Review of Clinical Assessments and Concepts

Clinical Assessments and Concepts:

This review is included for students and for graduates desiring a concise overview of basic and advanced clinical concepts. Many clinical pearls are included.

Reviewed herein are the three essential components of patient assessment: history, physical examination, and laboratory assessment. Additional concepts and perspectives are provided that will help facilitate risk management and optimal patient care.

<u>Topics:</u>

- Moving past disease- and drug-centered medicine toward patient-centered health optimization: the goal is *wellness*
- Acute Care and Musculoskeletal Care as Opportunities for Health Optimization
- **Clinical Assessments**
  - History taking & physical examination
  - Orthopedic/musculoskeletal examination: Concepts and goals
  - Neurologic assessment: Review
  - Laboratory assessments: General considerations of commonly used tests
    i. *Routine tests*: Chemistry/metabolic panel, lipid panel, CBC, 25(OH)-vitamin D, ferritin, thyroid stimulating hormone, CRP, ESR,
    ii. *Rheumatology/inflammation*: ANA (antinuclear antibodies), ANCA (antineutrophilic cytoplasmic antibodies), RF (rheumatoid factor), CCP (cyclic citrullinated protein antibodies), complement proteins, HLA-B27
    iii. *Functional assessments*: Lactulose-mannitol assay, comprehensive stool analysis and comprehensive parasitology
- **High-Risk Pain Patients**
- **Clinical Concepts**
  - Not all injury-related problems are injury-related problems
  - Safe patient + safe treatment = safe outcome
  - Four clues to underlying problems
  - Special considerations in the evaluation of children
  - No errors allowed: Differences between primary healthcare and spectator sports
  - "Disease treatment" is different from "patient management"
  - Clinical practice involves much more than "diagnosis and treatment"
  - Risk management: A note especially to students and recent licensees
- **Musculoskeletal Emergencies**
  - Acute compartment syndrome
  - Acute red eye, including acute iritis and scleritis
  - Atlantoaxial subluxation and instability
  - Cauda equina syndrome
  - Giant cell arteritis, temporal arteritis
  - Myelopathy, spinal cord compression
  - Neuropsychiatric lupus
  - Osteomyelitis
  - Septic arthritis, acute nontraumatic monoarthritis
- **Brief Overview of Integrative Healthcare Disciplines**
  - Chiropractic
  - Naturopathic Medicine
  - Osteopathic Medicine
  - Functional Medicine

Moving past "disease and drug"-centered medicine toward patient-centered health optimization: the goal is *wellness*

Written for students and experienced clinicians, this chapter introduces and reviews many new and common terms, procedures, and concepts relevant to the management of patients with musculoskeletal disorders. Especially for students, the reading of this chapter is essential to understanding the extensive material in this book and will facilitate the clinical assessment and management of patients with various clinical presentations.

Healthcare is currently in a time of significant fluctuation and is ready for changes in the balance of power and the paradigms which direct our therapeutic interventions. For nearly a century, allopathic medicine has hailed itself as "the gold standard", and other professions have either submitted to or been crushed by their ongoing political/scientific manipulations and their continual proclamation of intellectual and therapeutic superiority[1,2,3,4,5,6,7,8,9,10,11,12,13] despite 180,000-220,000 iatrogenic *medically-induced* deaths per year (500-600 iatrogenic deaths per day)[14,15] and consistent documentation that most medical/allopathic physicians are unable to provide accurate musculoskeletal diagnoses due to pervasive inadequacies in medical training.[16,17,18,19] Increasing disenchantment with allopathic *heroic medicine* and its adverse outcomes of inefficacy, exorbitant expenses, and unnecessary death are fostering change, such that allopathic medicine has been dethroned as the leading paradigm among American patients, who spend the majority of their discretionary healthcare dollars on consultations and treatments provided by "alternative" healthcare providers.[20,21] With the ever-increasing utilization of chiropractic, naturopathic, and osteopathic medical services, we must see that our paradigms and interventions keep pace with the evolving research literature and our increasing professional responsibilities so that we can deliver the highest possible quality of care.

> **Medical iatrogenesis kills 493 Americans per day**
>
> "Recent estimates suggest that each year more than 1 million patients are injured while in the hospital and approximately 180,000 die because of these injuries. Furthermore, drug-related morbidity and mortality are common and are estimated to cost more than $136 billion a year."
>
> Holland EG, Degruy FV. Drug-induced disorders. *Am Fam Physician*. 1997;56(7):1781-8, 1791-2

While we all readily acknowledge the importance of emergency care for emergency situations, those of us who advocate and practice a more complete approach to healthcare and life readily see the shortcomings of a limited and mechanical approach to healthcare, and we aspire to do more than simply fix problems. The implementation of *multidimensional* (i.e., *comprehensive* and *multifaceted*) treatment plans that address many aspects

---

1 Wilk CA. <u>Medicine, Monopolies, and Malice: How the Medical Establishment Tried to Destroy Chiropractic</u>. Garden City Park: Avery, 1996
2 Getzendanner S. Permanent injunction order against AMA. *JAMA*. 1988 Jan 1;259(1):81-2 http://optimalhealthresearch.com/archives/wilk.html
3 Carter JP. <u>Racketeering in Medicine: The Suppression of Alternatives</u>. Norfolk: Hampton Roads Pub; 1993
4 Morley J, Rosner AL, Redwood D. A case study of misrepresentation of the scientific literature: recent reviews of chiropractic. *J Altern Complement Med*. 2001 Feb;7:65-78
5 Terrett AG. Misuse of the literature by medical authors in discussing spinal manipulative therapy injury. *J Manipulative Physiol Ther*. 1995;18(4):203-10
6 National Alliance of Professional Psychology Providers. AMA Seeks To Control and Restrict Psychologist's Scope of Practice. www.nappp.org/scope.pdf Accessed Nov 2006
7 "In an effort to marshal the medical community's resources against the growing threat of expanding scope of practice for allied health professionals, the AMA has formed a national partnership to confront such initiatives nationwide… The committee will use $25,000..." Daly R, American Psychiatric Association. AMA Forms Coalition to Thwart Non-M.D. Practice Expansion. *Psychiatric News* 2006 March; 41: 17 http://pn.psychiatryonline.org/cgi/content/full/41/5/17-a?eaf Accessed November 25, 2006
8 Spivak JL. <u>The Medical Trust Unmasked</u>. Louis S. Siegfried Publishers; New York: 1961
9 Trever W. <u>In the Public Interest</u>. Los Angeles; Scriptures Unlimited; 1972. This is probably the most authoritative documentation of the illegal actions of the AMA up to 1972; contains numerous photocopies of actual AMA documents and minutes of official meetings with overt intentionality of destroying Americans' healthcare options so that the AMA and related organizations would have a monopoly in national healthcare.
10 Wenban AB. Inappropriate use of the title 'chiropractor' and term 'chiropractic manipulation' in the peer-reviewed biomedical literature. *Chiropr Osteopat*. 2006;14:16 http://chiroandosteo.com/content/14/1/16
11 Orme-Johnson DW, Herron RE. An innovative approach to reducing medical care utilization and expenditures. *Am J Manag Care*. 1997 Jan;3:135-44 http://www.ajmc.com/Article.cfm?Menu=1&ID=2154
12 van der Steen WI, Ho VK. Drugs versus diets: disillusions with Dutch health care. *Acta Biotheor*. 2001;49(2):125-40
13 Texas Medical Association. Physicians Ask Court to Protect Patients From Illegal Chiropractic Activities. http://www.texmed.org/Template.aspx?id=5259 Accessed Feb 2007
14 Starfield B. Is US health really the best in the world? *JAMA*. 2000 Jul 26;284(4):483-5
15 "Recent estimates suggest that each year more than 1 million patients are injured while in the hospital and approximately 180,000 die because of these injuries. Furthermore, drug-related morbidity and mortality are common and are estimated to cost more than $136 billion a year." Holland EG, Degruy FV. Drug-induced disorders. *Am Fam Physician*. 1997;56(7):1781-8, 1791-2
16 Freedman KB, Bernstein J. The adequacy of medical school education in musculoskeletal medicine. *J Bone Joint Surg Am*. 1998;80(10):1421-7
17 Freedman KB, Bernstein J. Educational deficiencies in musculoskeletal medicine. *J Bone Joint Surg Am*. 2002;84-A(4):604-8
18 Matzkin E, Smith ME, Freccero CD, Richardson AB. Adequacy of education in musculoskeletal medicine. *J Bone Joint Surg Am*. 2005;87-A(2):310-4
19 Schmale GA. More evidence of educational inadequacies in musculoskeletal medicine. *Clin Orthop Relat Res*. 2005 Aug;(437):251-9
20 "...Americans made an estimated 425 million visits to providers of unconventional therapy. This number exceeds the number of visits to all U.S. primary care physicians (388 million)." Eisenberg DM, Kessler RC, Foster C, Norlock FE, Calkins DR, Delbanco TL. Unconventional medicine in the United States. Prevalence, costs, and patterns of use. *N Engl J Med*. 1993 Jan 28;328(4):246-52
21 "Estimated expenditures for alternative medicine professional services increased 45.2% between 1990 and 1997 and were conservatively estimated at $21.2 billion in 1997, with at least $12.2 billion paid out-of-pocket. This exceeds the 1997 out-of-pocket expenditures for all US hospitalizations." Eisenberg DM, Davis RB, Ettner SL, Appel S, Wilkey S, Van Rompay M, Kessler RC. Trends in alternative medicine use in the United States, 1990-1997: results of a follow-up national survey. *JAMA*. 1998 Nov 11;280(18):1569-75

of pathophysiologic phenomena is a huge step forward in creating improved health and preventing future illness in the patients who seek our professional assistance. However, even complete multidimensional treatment plans still fall short of the goal of creating wellness, if for no other reasons than 1) they are still disease- and problem-oriented, rather than health-oriented, 2) they are prescribed from outside ("The doctor told me to do it.") rather than originating internally and spontaneously by the patient's own direction and affirmation ("I *do* this because I *am* this."), and, finally and most

Ever-increasing popularity of nonallopathic medicine

"...Americans made an estimated 425 million visits to providers of unconventional therapy. This number exceeds the number of visits to all U.S. primary care physicians (388 million)."

Eisenberg DM, et al. Unconventional medicine in the United States. Prevalence, costs, and patterns of use. *N Engl J Med* 1993;328:246-52

difficult to relay, 3) they are mechanistic rather than organic, they can do no better than the sum of their parts, they flow exclusively from the mind ("do") and not also from the body-soul ("am"). The art of creating wellness takes time to understand, longer to implement clinically, and even longer to apply to one's own life. Wellness is a state of being rather than a checklist of activities in a "preventive health program." The subtle differences that distinguish "wellness" from any "program" or "prescription" are the differences between *leading* versus *following* and *flowing* versus *performing*. **Wellness is multidimensional self-actualization, full integration of one's life—present, past, and future; physical, mental, emotional, spiritual, biochemical—one's shadow[22], work[23], feelings, thoughts, and goals into a cohesive living whole – "a wheel rolling from its own center."[24]**

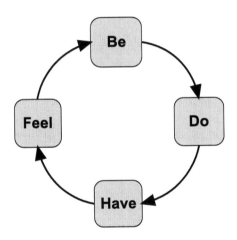

---

[22] Robert Bly. The Human Shadow. Sound Horizons 1991 [ISBN: 1879323001] and Bly R. A Little Book on the Human Shadow. [ISBN: 0062548476]
[23] Rick Jarow. Creating the Work You Love: Courage, Commitment and Career; Inner Traditions Intl Ltd; (December 1995) [ISBN: 0892815426]
[24] Walter Kaufmann (Translator), Friedrich Wilhelm Nietzsche. Thus Spoke Zarathustra: A Book for None and All. Penguin USA; 1978, page 27

Acute Care and Musculoskeletal Care: Opportunities for Health Optimization

Clinicians should appreciate that every patient encounter is an opportunity for comprehensive care, disease prevention, and health optimization. This is true whether the presenting complaint is acne, psoriasis, a respiratory infection, or musculoskeletal pain. Given the relatively high frequency of musculoskeletal complaints in clinical practice in general and chiropractic and osteopathic practices in particular, the following section will emphasize the clinical presentation of musculoskeletal complaints as an underappreciated opportunity for wellness care.

Since **approximately 1 of every 7 (14% of total) visits to a primary healthcare provider is for the treatment of musculoskeletal pain or dysfunction**[25], every healthcare provider needs to have 1) knowledge of important concepts related to musculoskeletal medicine, 2) the ability to recognize urgent and emergency conditions, 3) the ability to competently perform orthopedic examination procedures and interpret laboratory assessments, and 4) the knowledge and ability to design and implement effective treatment plans and to coordinate patient management.

In pharmacosurgical allopathic medicine, the goal of musculoskeletal treatment is to address the patient's injury or disorder by alleviating pain with the use of drugs, preventing further injury, and returning the patient to his/her previous status and activities. The most commonly employed interventions are 1) rest and "watchful waiting", 2) non-steroidal anti-inflammatory drugs (NSAIDS) and cyclooxygenase-2-inhibitors (COX-2 inhibitors, or "coxibs"), and 3) surgery. The more action-oriented approaches used by many chiropractic, naturopathic, and osteopathic physicians differs from the allopathic approach because, although avoidance of and "rest" from damaging activities is reasonable and valuable, too much rest without an emphasis on active preventive rehabilitation ❶ encourages patient passivity and ❷ the assumption of the sick role, and it ❸ fails to actively promote tissue healing and ❹ fails to address the underlying proprioceptive deficits that are common in patients with chronic musculoskeletal pain and recurrent injuries.[26,27,28] **NSAIDs are considered "first line" therapy for musculoskeletal disorders by allopaths** despite the data showing that "**There is no evidence that widely used NSAIDs have any long-term benefit on osteoarthritis.**"[29] What is worse than this lack of efficacy is the evidence showing that NSAIDs *exacerbate* musculoskeletal disease (rather than *cure* it). **NSAIDs are known to inhibit cartilage formation and to promote bone necrosis and joint degradation with long-term use**[30,31,32,33] and **NSAIDs are responsible for more than 16,000 gastrohemorrhagic deaths and 100,000 hospitalizations each year.**[34] The "coxibs" were supposed to provide anti-inflammatory benefits with an enhanced safety profile, but the gastrocentric focus of the drug developers failed to appreciate

> **Allopathic medicine has been sold to the public under the banner of "scientific" from a time when this was not the case**
>
> "…only about 15% of medical interventions are supported by solid scientific evidence…"
>
> Smith R. Where is the wisdom...? The poverty of medical evidence. *BMJ.* 1991 Oct 5;303:798-9

that COX-2 is necessary for the formation of prostacyclin, a prostaglandin created from arachidonic acid via COX-2 that plays an important role in vasodilation and antithrombosis; not surprisingly therefore, use of COX-2-inhibiting drugs has consistently been associated with increased risk for adverse cardiovascular effects including

[25] American College of Rheumatology Ad Hoc Committee on Clinical Guidelines. Guidelines for the initial evaluation of the adult patient with acute musculoskeletal symptoms. *Arthritis Rheum.* 1996 Jan;39(1):1-8 See also: **Vasquez A.** Musculoskeletal disorders and iron overload disease: comment on the American College of Rheumatology guidelines. *Arthritis Rheum* 1996;39: 1767-8

[26] McPartland JM, Brodeur RR, Hallgren RC. Chronic neck pain, standing balance, and suboccipital muscle atrophy--a pilot study. *J Manipulative Physiol Ther* 1997;20:24-9

[27] Bullock-Saxton JE, Janda V, Bullock MI. Reflex activation of gluteal muscles in walking. An approach to restoration of muscle function for patients with low-back pain. *Spine* 1993 May;18(6):704-8

[28] Sinaki M, Brey RH, Hughes CA, Larson DR, Kaufman KR. Significant reduction in risk of falls and back pain in osteoporotic-kyphotic women through a Spinal Proprioceptive Extension Exercise Dynamic (SPEED) program. *Mayo Clin Proc.* 2005 Jul;80(7):849-55

[29] Beers MH, Berkow R (eds). The Merck Manual. 17th Edition. Whitehouse Station; Merck Research Laboratories 1999 page 451

[30] "At…concentrations comparable to those… in the synovial fluid of patients treated with the drug, several NSAIDs suppress proteoglycan synthesis… These NSAID-related effects on chondrocyte metabolism … are much more profound in osteoarthritic cartilage than in normal cartilage, due to enhanced uptake of NSAIDs by the osteoarthritic cartilage." Brandt KD. Effects of nonsteroidal anti-inflammatory drugs on chondrocyte metabolism in vitro and in vivo. *Am J Med.* 1987 Nov 20; 83(5A): 29-34

[31] "The case of a young healthy man, who developed avascular necrosis of head of femur after prolonged administration of indomethacin, is reported here." Prathapkumar KR, Smith I, Attara GA. Indomethacin induced avascular necrosis of head of femur. *Postgrad Med J.* 2000 Sep; 76(899): 574-5

[32] "This highly significant association between NSAID use and acetabular destruction gives cause for concern, not least because of the difficulty in achieving satisfactory hip replacements in patients with severely damaged acetabula." Newman NM, Ling RS. Acetabular bone destruction related to non-steroidal anti-inflammatory drugs. *Lancet.* 1985 Jul 6; 2(8445): 11-4

[33] Vidal y Plana RR, Bizzarri D, Rovati AL. Articular cartilage pharmacology: I. In vitro studies on glucosamine and non steroidal antiinflammatory drugs. *Pharmacol Res Commun.* 1978 Jun;10(6):557-69

[34] Singh G. Recent considerations in nonsteroidal anti-inflammatory drug gastropathy. *Am J Med.* 1998;105(1B):31S-38S

myocardial infarction, unstable angina, cardiac thrombus, resuscitated cardiac arrest, sudden or unexplained death, ischemic stroke, and transient ischemic attacks.[35] Additionally, the use of a COX-2 inhibiting treatment in patients who overconsume arachidonic acid (i.e., most people in America and other industrialized nations[36]) would be expected to shunt bioavailable arachidonate into the formation of leukotrienes, a group of inflammatory mediators now known to contribute directly to atherogenesis.[37] Thus, the outcome was entirely predictable: overuse of COX-2 inhibitors should have been expected to create a catastrophe of iatrogenic cardiovascular death, and this is exactly what was allowed to occur—clearly indicating independent but synergistic failures on the part of pharmaceutical companies, the FDA, and the medical profession.[38,39,40,41] According to statements by David J. Graham, MD, MPH, (Associate Director for Science, Office of Drug Safety, FDA) in 2005, an estimated 139,000 Americans who took Vioxx suffered serious complications including stroke or myocardial infarction; between 26,000 and 55,000 Americans died as a result of their doctors' prescribing Vioxx.[42] Additionally, the surgical procedures employed by allopaths for the treatment of musculoskeletal pain do not consistently show evidence of efficacy, safety, or cost-effectiveness. Arthroscopic surgery for osteoarthritis of the knee, for example, costs thousands of dollars to each individual and billions of dollars to the American healthcare system but is no more effective than placebo.[43,44,45] In a review which also noted that only 15% of medical procedures are supported by literature references and that only 1% of such references are deemed scientifically valid, Rosner[46] showed that the risks of serious injury (i.e., cauda equina syndrome or vertebral artery dissection) associated with spinal manipulation are *"400 times lower* than the death rates observed from gastrointestinal bleeding due to the use of nonsteroidal anti-inflammatory drugs and *700 times lower* than the overall mortality rate for spinal surgery."

In chiropractic, osteopathic, and naturopathic medicine, the goal and means of musculoskeletal treatment is to address the patient's injury or disorder by simultaneously alleviating pain with the use of natural, noninvasive, low-cost, and low-risk interventions while improving the patient's overall health, preventing future health problems, and "upgrading" the patient's overall paradigm of health maintenance and disease prevention from one that is passive and reactive to one that is empowered and pro-active. Commonly employed therapeutics include spinal manipulation[47,48,49], exercise[50] and the use of nutritional supplements and botanical medicines[51,52] which have been demonstrated in peer-reviewed clinical trials to be safe and effective for the alleviation of musculoskeletal pain. More specifically, chiropractic and naturopathic physicians are particularly well-versed in the clinical utilization of such treatments as niacinamide[53], glucosamine and chondroitin sulfates[54], vitamin D[55],

[35] Mukherjee D, Nissen SE, Topol EJ. Risk of cardiovascular events associated with selective COX-2 inhibitors. *JAMA*. 2001 Aug 22-29;286(8):954-9

[36] Seaman DR. The diet-induced proinflammatory state: a cause of chronic pain and other degenerative diseases? *J Manipulative Physiol Ther*. 2002;25(3):168-79

[37] Dwyer JH, Allayee H, Dwyer KM, Fan J, Wu H, Mar R, Lusis AJ, Mehrabian M. Arachidonate 5-lipoxygenase promoter genotype, dietary arachidonic acid, and atherosclerosis. *N Engl J Med*. 2004 Jan 1;350(1):29-37

[38] Topol EJ. Arthritis medicines and cardiovascular events--"house of coxibs". *JAMA*. 2005 Jan 19;293(3):366-8. Epub 2004 Dec 28

[39] Ray WA, Griffin MR, Stein CM. Cardiovascular toxicity of valdecoxib. *N Engl J Med*. 2004 Dec 23;351(26):2767. Epub 2004 Dec 17

[40] Topol EJ. Failing the public health--rofecoxib, Merck, and the FDA. *N Engl J Med*. 2004 Oct 21;351(17):1707-9

[41] Horton R. Vioxx, the implosion of Merck, and aftershocks at the FDA. *Lancet*. 2004 Dec 4-10;364(9450):1995-6

[42] David J. Graham, MD, MPH, (Associate Director for Science, Office of Drug Safety, US FDA) estimated that 139,000 Americans who took Vioxx suffered serious side effects; he estimated that the drug killed between 26,000 and 55,000 people. http://www.commondreams.org/views05/0223-35.htm http://www.fda.gov/cder/drug/infopage/vioxx/vioxxgraham.pdf Accessed November 25, 2006

[43] Gina Kolata. A Knee Surgery for Arthritis Is Called Sham. *The New York Times*, July 11, 2002

[44] Moseley JB, O'Malley K, Petersen NJ, Menke TJ, Brody BA, Kuykendall DH, Hollingsworth JC, Ashton CM, Wray NP. A controlled trial of arthroscopic surgery for osteoarthritis of the knee. *N Engl J Med*. 2002;347:81-8

[45] Bernstein J, Quach T. A perspective on the study of Moseley et al: questioning the value of arthroscopic knee surgery for osteoarthritis. *Cleve Clin J Med*. 2003;70(5):401, 405-6, 408-10

[46] Rosner AL. Evidence-based clinical guidelines for the management of acute low-back pain: response to the guidelines prepared for the Australian Medical Health and Research Council. *J Manipulative Physiol Ther*. 2001;24(3):214-20

[47] Manga P, Angus D, Papadopoulos C, et al. The Effectiveness and Cost-Effectiveness of Chiropractic Management of Low-Back Pain. Richmond Hill, Ontario: Kenilworth Publishing; 1993

[48] Meade TW, Dyer S, Browne W, Townsend J, Frank AO. Low-back pain of mechanical origin: randomised comparison of chiropractic and hospital outpatient treatment. *BMJ*. 1990;300(6737):1431-7

[49] Meade TW, Dyer S, Browne W, Frank AO. Randomised comparison of chiropractic and hospital outpatient management for low-back pain: results from extended follow up. *BMJ*. 1995;311(7001):349-5

[50] Harold Elrick, MD. Exercise is Medicine. *The Physician and Sportsmedicine* - Volume 24 - No. 2 - February 1996

[51] **Vasquez A**. Revisiting the Five-Part Nutritional Wellness Protocol: The Supplemented Paleo-Mediterranean Diet. *Nutritional Perspectives* 2011 January http://optimalhealthresearch.com/part8.html

[52] **Vasquez A**. Reducing pain and inflammation naturally - Part 3: Improving overall health while safely and effectively treating musculoskeletal pain. *Nutritional Perspectives* 2005; 28: 34-38, 40-42 http://optimalhealthresearch.com/part3.html

[53] Kaufman W. Niacinamide therapy for joint mobility. Therapeutic reversal of a common clinical manifestation of the "normal" aging process. *Conn State Med J* 1953;17:584-591

[54] Reginster JY, Deroisy R, Rovati LC, Lee RL, Lejeune E, Bruyere O, Giacovelli G, Henrotin Y, Dacre JE, Gossett C. Long-term effects of glucosamine sulphate on osteoarthritis progression: a randomised, placebo-controlled clinical trial. *Lancet*. 2001;357(9252):251-6

[55] **Vasquez A**, Manso G, Cannell J. The clinical importance of vitamin D: a paradigm shift with implications for all healthcare providers. *Altern Ther Health Med* 2004;10:28-36 http://optimalhealthresearch.com/monograph04.html

vitamin B-12[56], balanced and complete fatty acid therapy[57,58], anti-inflammatory diets[59,60,61], proteolytic/pancreatic enzymes[62], and botanical medicines such as *Boswellia*[63], *Harpagophytum*[64], *Uncaria*, and willow bark[65,66]—each of these interventions has been validated in peer-reviewed research for safety and effectiveness.[67] Furthermore, from the perspective of integrative chiropractic and naturopathic medicine, aiming for such a limited accomplishment as mere "returning the patient to previous status and activities" would be considered substandard, since the patient's overall health was neither addressed nor improved and since returning the patient to his/her previous status and activities would be a direct invitation for the problem to recur indefinitely. Chiropractic and naturopathic physicians appreciate that, especially regarding chronic health problems, any treatment plan that allows the patient to resume his/her previous lifestyle is by definition doomed to fail because a return to the patient's previous lifestyle and activities that allowed the onset of the disease/disorder in the first place will most certainly result in the perpetuation and recurrence of the illness or disorder. **Stated more directly: for *healing* to truly be effective, the comprehensive treatment plan must generally result in a permanent and profound change in the patient's lifestyle and emotional climate, which are the primary modifiable determinants of either health or disease.**

---

[56] Mauro GL, Martorana U, Cataldo P, Brancato G, Letizia G. Vitamin B12 in low back pain: a randomised, double-blind, placebo-controlled study. *Eur Rev Med Pharmacol Sci.* 2000 May-Jun;4(3):53-8

[57] **Vasquez A**. Reducing Pain and Inflammation Naturally. Part 1: New Insights into Fatty Acid Biochemistry and the Influence of Diet. *Nutritional Perspectives* 2004; Oct: 5, 7-10,12,14 http://optimalhealthresearch.com/part1.html

[58] **Vasquez A**. Reducing Pain and Inflammation Naturally. Part 2: New Insights into Fatty Acid Supplementation and Its Effect on Eicosanoid Production and Genetic Expression. *Nutritional Perspectives* 2005; January: 5-16 http://optimalhealthresearch.com/part2.html

[59] Seaman DR. The diet-induced proinflammatory state: a cause of chronic pain and other degenerative diseases? *J Manipulative Physiol Ther.* 2002 Mar-Apr;25(3):168-7

[60] **Vasquez A**. *Integrative Orthopedics. Second Edition 2007.* http://optimalhealthresearch.com/orthopedics.html

[61] **Vasquez A**. Reducing Pain and Inflammation Naturally. Part 1: New Insights into Fatty Acid Biochemistry and the Influence of Diet. *Nutritional Perspectives* 2004; October: 5, 7-10, 12, 14 http://optimalhealthresearch.com/part1.html

[62] Trickett P. Proteolytic enzymes in treatment of athletic injuries. *Appl Ther.* 1964;30:647-52

[63] Kimmatkar N, Thawani V, Hingorani L, Khiyani R. Efficacy and tolerability of Boswellia serrata extract in treatment of osteoarthritis of knee--a randomized double blind placebo controlled trial. *Phytomedicine.* 2003 Jan;10(1):3-7

[64] Chrubasik S, Junck H, Breitschwerdt H, Conradt C, Zappe H. Effectiveness of Harpagophytum extract WS 1531 in the treatment of exacerbation of low-back pain: a randomized, placebo-controlled, double-blind study. *Eur J Anaesthesiol* 1999 Feb;16(2):118-29

[65] Chrubasik S, Eisenberg E, Balan E, Weinberger T, Luzzati R, Conradt C. Treatment of low-back pain exacerbations with willow bark extract: a randomized double-blind study. *Am J Med.* 2000;109:9-14

[66] **Vasquez A**, Muanza DN. Comment: Evaluation of Presence of Aspirin-Related Warnings with Willow Bark. *Ann Pharmacotherapy* 2005 Oct;39(10):1763

[67] **Vasquez A**. Reducing pain and inflammation naturally. Part 3: Improving overall health while safely and effectively treating musculoskeletal pain. *Nutritional Perspectives* 2005;28:34-42 http://optimalhealthresearch.com/part3.html

Clinical Assessments

The clinical assessments reviewed in the following sections are history-taking, orthopedic/musculoskeletal, and neurologic examinations, and commonly used laboratory tests. **History taking is the art of conducting an *informative* and *collaborative* patient interview.**

The role of the doctor during the interview process is not merely that of a data-collecting machine, spewing out questions and receiving responses. Patient interviews can be a creative, enjoyable, comforting opportunity to build rapport and to establish meaningful connection with another human being. Patients are not simply people with health problems – they are first and foremost our fellow human beings, not so dissimilar from ourselves perhaps, and always full of complexity. Our task is not to fully understand their complexity nor to solve all of their mysteries, but rather to help orchestrate these dynamics into a coordinated if not unified direction that promotes health and healing.

Beyond its diagnostic value, the interview process also provides a key opportunity to gain insight into the patient's psychoepistimology—the patient's operating system for interacting with data and the world and internalizing and metabolizing external inputs in such a way as to merge these with internal experiences (i.e., emotions, feelings, preferences, responses). Epistemology is the branch of philosophy concerned with the nature and scope of knowledge. Per Rand[68], psychoepistimology is a person's "method of awareness"; a person's psychoepistimology creates a "corollary view of existence" and in turn, "A man's method of using his consciousness determines his method of survival." By understanding how the patient views him/herself in the world, understanding his/her goals, and—in essence—what "drives" the patient and what "makes him/her tick", clinicians can shape the nuances of the conversation and the treatment plan to promote the desired cognitive-conceptual-behavioral changes in behavior that are prerequisite for the attainment of optimized health outcomes.

History & Assessment

History of the primary complaint: "D.O.P.P. Q.R.S.T."
- Description/location
- Onset
- Provocation: exacerbates
- Palliation: alleviates
- Quality
- Radiation of pain
- Severity
- Timing

Associated complaints
- Additional manifestations
- Concomitant diseases

Review of systems
- Head-to-toe inventory of health status, associated health problems, and complications

Past health history
- Surgeries
- Hospitalizations
- Traumas
- Vaccinations and medications
- Successful and failed treatments for the current complaint(s)

Family health history
- Genotropic illnesses and predispositions
- Lifestyle patterns
- Emotional expectations

Social history
- Hobbies, work, exposures
- Relationships and emotional experiences
- Interpersonal support
- Malpractice litigation

Health Habits
- Diet: appropriate intake of protein, fruits, vegetables, fats, sugars
- Sleep
- Stress management
- Exercise / Sedentary Lifestyle
- Spirituality / Centeredness
- Caffeine and tobacco
- Ethanol and recreational drugs

Medication and supplements
- Reason, doses, duration, cost
- Side-effects
- Interactions

Responsibility and Compliance
- Ability and willingness to comply with prescribed treatment plan and to incorporate the necessary diet-exercise-relationship-emotional-lifestyle modifications
- *Internal* versus *external* locus of control

---

[68] Rand A. For the New Intellectual. New York; Signet:1961, 16

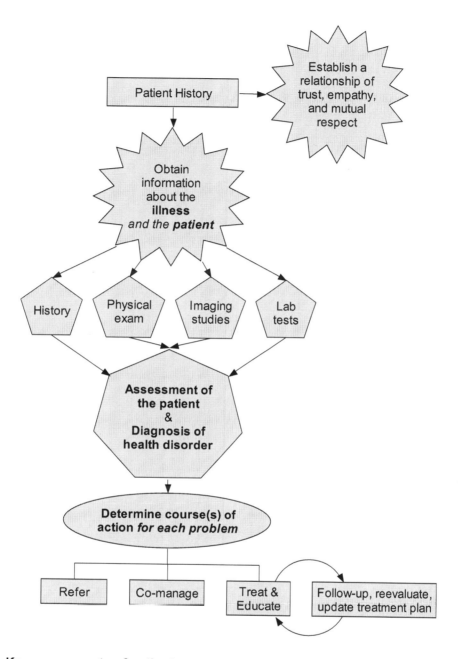

Key components of patient assessment and management: Patient assessment and management is an on-going process that begins with the initial history taken at the first clinical encounter and continues through the physical examination and laboratory assessments and thereafter by monitoring the patient's implementation of and response to the treatment plan. The plan is complete when the desired outcome of health optimization is achieved and sustained.

Components of a Complete Patient History: "D.O.P.P. Q.R.S.T."

Category	Patient history questions and implications
Description, Location: Always start with open-ended questions	• *What is it like for you?* • *What do you experience?* • *What are you feeling?* • *Where is the pain/sensation/problem)?* • Ask about specifics: **Pain, numbness, weakness, tingling**, fatigue, recent or chronic infections, burning, aching, dull, sharp, cramping, stretching, pins and needles, weakness, changes in function (i.e., bowel and bladder continence).
Onset	• *When did it begin? Have you ever had anything like this before?* • *Was there a specific event associated with the onset of the problem, such as an injury or an illness, or did the problem start gradually or insidiously?* • *How has it changed over time?* • *Prior injuries to site?* • *Why are you seeking care for this now (rather than last week or last month)?* • *What has changed? How is the pain/problem developing over time—getting worse or getting better?*
Palliation	• *How have you tried treating it? Does anything make it go away?* • *What makes it better? What relieves the pain?* • Ask about prior and current treatments, radiographs, medications, supplements (herbs, vitamins, minerals), injections, surgery, massage, manipulation, counseling. • Knowing response/resistance to previous treatments can provide clinical insight.
Provocation	• *Are your symptoms constant, or does the problem come and go?* • *What makes it worse? What makes the pain worse?* • *When during the day/week/month/year are your symptoms the worst?*
Quality	• *Can you describe the pain to me?* • *What does it feel like?* • *What do you experience?* • Get a clear understanding of the type of sensation(s): stabbing, shooting pain, pins and needles, sharp pain, electric sensation, numbness, burning, aching, throbbing, weakness, tingling, gel phenomenon (stiffness worsened by inactivity), dizziness, confusion, fatigue, shortness of breath.
Radiation	• *Does the pain stay localized or does it move to your arm/leg/head/face?* • *Do you feel pain in other areas of your body?*
Severity	• *How bad is it? How would you rate it on a scale of one to ten if one were almost no pain and ten was the worst pain you could imagine?* Use the validated VAS—visual analog scale—to quantify the level of pain and impairment. • *Does this problem prevent you from engaging in your daily activities, such as work, exercise, or hobbies?* This is a very important question for determining functional impairment and internal consistency; if the patient is "too injured to work" yet is still able to fully participate in recreational activities that are physically challenging, then malingering is likely.
Timing	• *When do you notice this problem?* • *Is it constant, or does it come and go? Where are you when you notice it the most?* • *Is it worse in the morning, or worse in the evening?* • *Does anyone else in your [home/office/worksite] have this same problem?* • *What times of the day or what days of the week is it the worst?*

Components of a Complete Patient History: "D.O.P.P. Q.R.S.T."—*continued*

Category	Patient history questions and implications
Associated manifestations and constitutional symptoms	• *Have you noticed any other problems associated with this problem?* • ***Fatigue?*** • ***Fever?*** • ***Weight loss?*** *Weight gain?* • *Night sweats?* • ***Diarrhea? Constipation?*** • ***Weakness?*** • *Nausea?* • *Bowel or bladder difficulties or changes? Difficulty with sexual function?* These could be related to hormonal imbalances, drug side-effects, relationship problems, nutritional deficiencies, nerve compression, and/or depression. • *Change in sensation near your anus/genitals?* Cauda equina syndrome is an important consideration in patients with low-back pain. • *Loss of appetite?* • *Difficulty sleeping?* • *Skin rash or change in pigmentation?*
ROS: review of systems	• <u>General constitution</u>: fatigue, malaise, fever, chills, weight gain/loss… • *"Now we are going to conduct a head-to-toe inventory just to make sure that we have covered everything."* • <u>Head</u>: headaches, head pain, pressure inside head, difficulty concentrating, difficulty remembering, mental function • <u>Ears:</u> ringing in ears, dizziness, hearing loss, hypersensitivity to noise, ear pain, discharge from ear, pressure in ears • <u>Eyes</u>: eye pain, loss of vision or decreased vision or ability to focus, redness or irritation, seeing flashing lights or spots, double vision • <u>Nose</u>: sinus problems, chronically stuffy nose, difficulty smelling things, nose bleeds, change or decrease in sense of smell or taste • <u>Mouth</u>, teeth, TMJ, pain or sores in mouth, difficulty chewing, sensitive teeth, bleeding gums, pain in jaw joint, change or decrease in sense of taste • <u>Neck:</u> pain at the base of skull, pain in neck, stiffness • <u>Throat:</u> difficulty swallowing, pain in throat, feeling like things get stuck in throat, change in voice, difficulty getting air or food in or out • <u>Chest and breasts</u>: any chest pain, difficult breathing, wheezing, coughing, pain, lumps, or discharge from nipple • <u>Shoulders:</u> pain or aching in your shoulders, restricted motion or stiffness • <u>Arms, elbows, hands</u>: pain or problems with your arms, elbows, hands, …in the joints or the muscles…, numbness, tingling, weakness, swelling, changes in fingernails, cold hands? • <u>Stomach, abdomen, pelvis, genitals, urinary tract, rectum,</u> : pain in stomach or abdomen, difficulty with digestion, gas, bloating, regurgitation, ulcer, any problems lower down in your abdomen—near your lower intestines? Pain, lumps, swelling, difficulty passing stool, pain or itching near your anus, genitalia; any genital pain, burning, discharge, redness, irritation, sexual dysfunction or impotence, loss of bowel or bladder control? Diarrhea or constipation? How often do you have a bowel movement? • <u>Hips, legs, knees, ankles, feet</u>: numbness, weakness, pain or tingling in the hips, knees, ankles, or feet; pain in calves with walking, swelling of ankles, cold feet • *Is there anything else that you think I should know in order to help you?*

Components of a Complete Patient History: "D.O.P.P. Q.R.S.T." —continued

Category	Patient history questions and implications

Medical history	• *Are you taking any **medications**? What medications have you taken in the past few years?* Finding out that your new patient recently discontinued his 20-year regimen of valproic acid, lithium, and risperidone may significantly change your interpretation of the clinical interview
	• *Have you been **treated for any medical conditions** or health problems?*
	• *Have you ever been **hospitalized**?*
	• *Have you ever had **surgery**?*
	• *Have you ever been **diagnosed with any health problems** such as high blood pressure or diabetes?*
	• Investigate for specific problems in the past health history that would be a major oversight to miss:
	   o Current or past diseases: Cancer, Diabetes, Mental illness
	   o Hypertension or high cholesterol
	   o Medications, especially corticosteroids
	   o Surgeries & Hospitalizations
	   o Infections, Immune disorders
	   o Trauma or previous injuries

Social history	• **Work**—*What do you do for work? Are you exposed to chemicals or fumes at your workplace?* • **Hobbies**—*What do you do for recreation or hobbies? Are you exposed to chemicals or fumes at home or with your hobbies (e.g., painting, gardening)?* • **Eat**—*Tell me about your breakfast, lunch, dinner, snacks... Do you consume foods or drinks that contain aspartame* (linked to increased incidence of brain tumors[69]) *or carrageenan* (possibly linked to increased risk of breast cancer and inflammatory bowel disease[70,71])? • **Exercise**—*What do you do for exercise or physical activity?* • **Drink**—*Do you **drink alcohol**? Coffee/caffeine? Water?* • **Drugs**—*Do you use recreational **drugs**? **Now or in the past?*** • **Smoke**—*Do you **smoke**?* • **Sex**—*Are you **sexually active**? If so, do you practice safer sex practices? For all women: Is there any chance you could be pregnant right now? A "yes" reply may contraindicate radiographic assessment and the use of certain nutrients, botanicals, and/or drugs.* • **Emotional support** • **Family contact and relationships**
Family health history	• *Does anyone in your family have any health problems, especially your parents and siblings?* • *Do you have any children? Do they have any health problems?* • *Do any diseases "run in the family" such as cancer, diabetes, arthritis, heart disease?*
Additional questions	• *Do you have any other information for me? Is there anything that I did not ask?* • *What is your opinion as to why you are having this health problem?* • *Are you in litigation for your illness or injuries?*

---

[69] "In the past two decades brain tumor rates have risen in several industrialized countries, including the United States... Compared to other environmental factors putatively linked to brain tumors, the artificial sweetener aspartame is a promising candidate to explain the recent increase in incidence and degree of malignancy of brain tumors." Olney JW, Farber NB, Spitznagel E, Robins LN. Increasing brain tumor rates: is there a link to aspartame? *J Neuropathol Exp Neurol* 1996 Nov;55(11):1115-23

[70] Tobacman JK. Review of harmful gastrointestinal effects of carrageenan in animal experiments. *Environ Health Perspect.* 2001 Oct;109(10):983-94

[71] "However, the gum carrageenan which is comprised of linked, sulfated galactose residues has potent biological activity and undergoes acid hydrolysis to poligeenan, an acknowledged carcinogen." Tobacman JK, Wallace RB, Zimmerman MB. Consumption of carrageenan and other water-soluble polymers used as food additives and incidence of mammary carcinoma. *Med Hypotheses.* 2001 May;56(5):589-98

<u>Physical Examination</u>

<u>Goals and purpose of the orthopedic/musculoskeletal examination</u>:
1. **To establish an accurate diagnosis (or diagnoses),**
2. **To assess the patient's functional status and current condition,**
3. **To assess for concomitant and/or underlying and preexisting problems,**
4. **To rule out emergency situations**

- *Example*: If your patient presents with low back and leg pain, and you determine that his fall off a horse resulted in ischial bursitis, have you also excluded a lumbar compression fracture? You can send the patient home with anti-inflammatory treatments and icepacks for the bursitis; but if you missed the spinal fracture, your patient could suffer neurologic injury resultant from your "failure to diagnose." **Don't assume that the patient has only one problem until you have proven with your history and examination that other likely problems do not exist.**

<u>Functional assessment</u>: When working with patients with acute injuries and systemic diseases, **take a wider view of the patient than simply diagnosing the problem.**
- *Will she be able to return to work?*
- *Will he be able to drive home safely?*
- *Will she need help with activities of daily living?*
- *Is there an occult disease, infection, malignancy, or toxic exposure that is causing these problems?*
- *Is this an acute presentation of a new problem, or an acute exacerbation of a chronic problem?*

<u>Neurologic examination</u>: One of the most important areas to assess when a patient presents with a musculoskeletal complaint is the neurologic system, especially if the complaint is related to a recent traumatic injury. Blood circulation is essential for life; but lack of circulation is only a major consideration in a small number of injuries, and it is usually readily apparent when severe because the problem will become acute quickly. Nerve injuries, however, can be subtle. All patients with spine (neck, thoracic, low back) pain must be questioned thoroughly for evidence of neurologic compromise. **Neurologic insults—such as cauda equina syndrome and transverse myelitis—can be painless**, can progress rapidly, and can lead to permanent functional disability from muscle weakness or paralysis. **Every patient with pain, weakness, or recent trauma must be evaluated for neurologic deficits before the patient is treated and released from care.** Neurologic examinations are briefly reviewed in the pages that follow; citations can be used for sources of additional information.

<u>Resources for students on neurologic assessment</u>:
- Goldberg S. <u>The Four-Minute Neurologic Exam</u>. Medmaster http://www.medmaster.net/
- http://www.neuroexam.com/neuroexam/ Information and free videos of a neurologic exam.
- http://rad.usuhs.mil/rad/eye_simulator/eyesimulator.html Excellent interactive simulation of assessment of extraocular muscles in a neurologic examination.
- http://emedicine.medscape.com/article/1147993-overview Excellent review, noteworthy for its description of a "+5" level of reflex grading denoting sustained clonus.

Orthopedic Musculoskeletal Examination: Concepts and Goals

Orthopedic tests are detailed or reviewed in each respective chapter of *Integrative Orthopedics*[72] (i.e., shoulder exams are in the chapter on shoulders, knee exams in the chapter on knees). This section reviews the concepts and goals that provide the rationale for performing these tests. **Orthopedic tests are designed to place particular types of stress on specific body tissues.** Types of stress include tension/distraction, compression/pressure, shear force, vibration, friction, and percussion. Each type of stress is applied to elicit specific information about the exact tissue or structure that is being tested. *If you understand the reason for the type of stress that you are applying, and you are aware of the tissue/structure that you are testing, then you will find it much easier to perform the dozens of tests that are required in clinical practice.* If you understand the "how" and the "why" then you won't be overwhelmed with named tests that otherwise appear illogical or superfluous.

> **Types of stress applied during the physical examination for specific purposes**
>
> - **Tension, traction**: To provoke pain from injured/compromised tissues: tendons, muscles, ligaments, and nerves
> - **Compression, pressure**: To provoke pain from inflamed tissues; also used to assess for swelling and fluid accumulation in subcutaneous tissue, bursa, and joint spaces such as the knee
> - **Shearing force**: To test the integrity of ligaments and intervertebral discs
> - **Vibration (using ultrasound or 128 Hz tuning fork)**: To assess vibration sense (neurologic: peripheral nerves and dorsal columns) and screen for broken bones (orthopedic)
> - **Friction, grinding**: To elicit pain from injured tissues (cross-fiber friction) and articular surfaces (grinding tests)
> - **Percussion, over bone and discs**: To assess for bone fractures, bone infections, and acute disc injuries
> - **Percussion, over peripheral nerves**: To assess hypesthesia/tingling suggesting reduced threshold for depolarization secondary to nerve irritation or compression, i.e., Tinel's sign
> - **Fulcrum tests**: To assess for bone fractures: commonly the doctor's arm or a firm object is placed centrally under the bone in question and increasingly firm downward stress is applied to both ends of the bone to test for occult fracture
> - **Torque, twisting**: To test joint integrity (restriction or laxity) or for occult bone fracture (particularly of the digits)

The tests that are described in *Integrative Orthopedics* meet at least one of the following two criteria: 1) it is a common test that all doctors know and which is needed for the sake of communication and for passing academic and licensing examinations, or 2) it is going to be a useful test in clinical practice.

Always remember that abnormalities found during the physical examination—particularly the neurologic examination—are often indicative of an underlying *nonmusculoskeletal* problem that must be identified or—at the very least—considered and then excluded by additional testing. For example, a patient **shoulder pain** and neurologic deficits found during the neuromusculoskeletal portion of your examination could have a **herniated cervical disc** as the underlying cause; but the cause could also be **syringomyelia**, or an **apical lung tumor** that is invading local bone and destroying the nerves of the brachial plexus.[73] As a clinician, the successful management and treatment of your patients depends in large part on the following: ❶ **knowledge**: your ability to conceptualize broadly and to consider many *functional* and *pathologic* causes of your patient's complaints, ❷ **tact**: the efficiency and accuracy with which you assess, accept, and exclude the various differential diagnoses into your final working diagnosis from which your treatment, management, referral, and co-management decisions are made, ❸ **art**: your ability to create the changes in your patient's outlook, lifestyle, biochemistry, biomechanics/anatomy, and physiology to effect the desired outcome.

Neurologic Assessment

Clinical neurology is a complex area of study. However, for most doctors, knowledge of clinical neurology hinges on answering three questions:

- **Is this patient's presentation normal or abnormal?**
- **If it is abnormal, does it indicate a specific disease or lesion?**
- **Does this condition require referral to a specialist or emergency care?**

---

[72] **Vasquez A**. Integrative Orthopedics: Concepts, Algorithms, and Therapeutics. www.OptimalHealthResearch.com
[73] "Pancoast tumor has long been implicated as a cause of brachial plexopathy...The possibility of Pancoast lesion should be considered not only in the presence of brachial plexopathy, but also when C8 or T1 radiculopathy is found." Vargo MM, Flood KM. Pancoast tumor presenting as cervical radiculopathy. *Arch Phys Med Rehabil*. 1990 Jul;71(8):606-9

Every clinician needs thorough training in anatomy and clinical neurology to be competent in the management of patients, because even common problems such as "pain" and "fatigue" and "headache" may herald devastating neurologic illness that must be assessed accurately and managed skillfully. While a complete review of clinical neurology is beyond the scope of this text, the following section provides a basic review of the clinical essentials. Clinicians needing an refresher course in clinical neurology are encouraged to read the concise reviews by Goldberg.[74,75]

Reliable indicators of organic neurologic disease: These cannot be feigned and must be assumed to reveal organic neurologic illness that **must be evaluated by a neurologist**:
- **Significant asymmetry of pupillary light reflex,**
- **Ocular divergence,**
- **Papilledema,**
- **Marked nystagmus,**
- **Muscle atrophy and fasciculation,**
- **Muscle weakness with neurologic deficit**; upper motor neuron lesions (UMNL) indicate a central nervous system (CNS) lesion and need to be fully evaluated by a specialist; the need for referral is less necessary in cases of peripheral neuropathy of known cause.

Purpose of Neurologic Examination and *Principle of Neurologic Localization*:
The purpose of the neurologic examination is to qualify ("yes" or "no") the presence of a neurologic deficit, and — if present—to localize the lesion so that it can be further assessed with the proper laboratory, imaging, electrodiagnostic, or biopsy techniques. The following 9-point summary of localized lesions does not supplant independent studies of neurology and neuroanatomy but is useful for a quick clinically-relevant review:
1. **Cerebral cortex and internal capsule**: Neurologic deficit depends on location of lesion but is typically a combination of sensory/motor deficit and impaired higher neurologic function such as comprehension (superior temporal gyrus) or socially appropriate behavior (frontal lobe, ventral frontal gyri).
2. **Basal ganglia and striatal system**: Athetosis (lentiform nucleus: putamen and globus pallidus), (hemi)ballism (subthalamic nucleus), chorea (putamen), akinesia, bradykinesia, hypokinesia (lack of nigrostriatal dopamine).
3. **Cerebellum**: Ataxia, awkward clumsy execution of *intentional* motions; may have nystagmus, hypotonia.
4. **Brainstem**: Cranial nerve deficit(s) with contralateral distal sensory and/or UMN motor deficits.
5. **Spinal cord**: Cranial nerves and higher cortical functions are intact; lesion can be a combination of sensory and motor (UMN and LMN) deficits and the pattern distal to lesion may be a complete or incomplete pattern of sensory and motor deficits on one or both sides of body depending on area of spinal cord affected.
6. **Nerve root**: Segmental unilateral motor deficit; dermatomal distribution pain or sensory disturbance.
7. **Peripheral nerve**: Localized combination of sensory and motor deficits; may be bilateral or unilateral.
8. **Neuromuscular junction**: Painless weakness and "fatigable weakness": weakness that *worsens* with repeated testing; typically involves cranial nerves first in myasthenia gravis; also consider Lambert-Eaton Syndrome (LES: autoimmune neuromuscular junction disorder associated with occult malignancy; contrasts with myasthenia gravis in that in LES strength *increases* with repeated testing).
9. **Muscle disease**: Painless weakness, typically involving proximal hip/shoulder muscles first; test for elevated serum aldolase and (phospho)creatine kinase.

---

[74] Goldberg S. Clinical Neuroanatomy Made Ridiculously Simple. Miami, Medimaster, Inc, 1990. Now in a third edition with interactive CD.
[75] Goldberg S. The Four-Minute Neurologic Exam. Miami, Medimaster, Inc, 1992

Clinical assessments of neurologic function and structures

Cortex	Cerebellum
• <u>Orientation</u>: Person, place, time, situation. • <u>Mood and cooperation</u> • <u>Level of consciousness</u>: Alert, lethargic, stupor, coma (indirect assessment of reticular system in brainstem) • <u>Memory</u>: Remember objects or numbers; *recent memory is most commonly affected by brain lesions: What day of the month is it? How did you get here?* • <u>Mentation</u>: *Count backward from 100 by 7's.* • <u>Spelling</u>: *Spell the word "hand" backwards.* • <u>Stereognosis</u>: Identify by touch a familiar object such as a key or coin. • <u>Hoffman's reflex</u>: Doctor rapidly extends distal joint of patient's middle finger and watches for patient's hand to perform grasp reflex; this test is performed for motor tract lesions involving the cerebral cortex, cerebellum, and upper motor neurons of the spinal cord. • <u>Pronator drift</u>: Supinated hands and arms outstretched forward for 30 seconds; doctor taps on palms; falling of hands and arms into pronation suggests UMNL. • <u>Babinski reflex</u>: Scraping the bottom of the foot results in splaying and flexing of the toes and extension (dorsiflexion) of the big toe; normal in infants.	• <u>Gait</u> (lesion: ataxia) • <u>Heel-to-toe walk</u> • <u>Tandem gait</u> • <u>Hand flip, foot tap</u> (lesion: dysdiadochokinesia) • <u>Finger-to-nose</u>: Patient reaches out to doctor's finger, then patient touches patient nose, then back to new location of doctor's finger. • <u>Heel-to-shin</u>: Slide heel along shin. • <u>Walk in circle around chair</u> • <u>Move eyes in a rapid "figure 8"</u>: Technique for provoking latent nystagmus • <u>Rhomberg's test</u>: Patient stands with feet close together and eyes closed; tests proprioception (peripheral nerves, dorsal columns, spinocerebellar tracts); vision (eyes open tests optic righting reflex) and coordinated motor activity (cerebellum).

Several of the above '"cerebral" deficits may also result from intoxicative, nutritional, or metabolic disorders rather than an organic irreversible physical lesion. Likewise "cerebellar" deficits may also result from lesion of the brainstem tracts/nuclei and cerebellar peduncles, rather than the cerebellum itself.

Brainstem and Cranial Nerves	Spinal Cord, Roots, Nerves

1. Olfactory: **smell**
• Smell: Test with strong and common odors such as coffee; do not use ammonia or other irritants which are perceived via trigeminal nerve (cranial nerve 5)
• This is a worthwhile test in patients with recent head trauma (direct or indirect) such as from motor vehicle accidents (MVA); any violent motion of the head may result in injury to the olfactory fibers passing through the cribiform plate; patients may have associated anosmia or altered sense of flavor; frontal lobe disorders such as altered social behavior may be noted in lesioned patients
2. Ophthalmic: **reading, peripheral vision, fundoscopic**
• Snellen chart for far vision, Rosenbaum card for near vision
• Peripheral vision
• Fundoscopic examination
3. Oculomotor: **move eyes and constrict pupils**
• Eye motion in cardinal fields of gaze
• Pupil contraction to light
• Pupil contraction to accommodation
4. Trochlear: **motor to superior oblique**
• Look "down and in" toward nose
5. Trigeminal: **bite, sensory to face and eyes**
• Bite (motor to muscles of mastication)
• Feel (sensory to face, eyes, and tongue)
6. Abducens: **motor to lateral rectus**
• Looks laterally to the ear
7. Facial: **face muscles and taste to anterior tongue**
• Furrow forehead, close eyes forcefully, smile and frown
• Taste to anterior tongue
8. Vestibulocochlear: **hearing and balance**
• Hearing, Rinne-Weber tests[76]
• Balance: observe gait and Romberg test
9. Glossopharyngeal: **swallowing, and gag reflex**
• Swallow
• Gag reflex (sensory component)
10. Vagus: **motor to palate**
• Say "ahh" to raise uvula
• Gag reflex (motor component)
11. Spinal accessory: **motor to SCM and trapezius**
• Raise your shoulders (against resistance)
• Turn your head (against resistance)
12. Hypoglossal: **motor to tongue**
• Stick out tongue to front
	Motor and reflex
	• Strength: Specific muscles are tested and rated 0-5
	• Plantar (Babinski) reflex: Signifies UMNL
	• Abdominal reflexes: "Present" or "absent" (not rated 0-4); superficial reflexes are lost (rather than hyperactive) with UMNL
	   ○ Upper abdominal: T8-10
	   ○ Lower abdominal: T10-12
	• Anal reflex: Cauda equina and sacral nerve roots
	• Reflexes: Rate 0-4; asymmetric reflexes are more significant than finding absent or hyperactive (+3) reflexes; +4 reflex with sustained clonus is almost always pathologic and requires neurologist referral. Deep tendon reflexes with main spinal root levels are as follows:
	   ○ Biceps: C5
	   ○ Brachioradialis: C6
	   ○ Triceps: C7
	   ○ Patellar: L3-L4
	   ○ Hamstring: L5
	   ○ Achilles: S1
	Sensory
	• Light touch
	• Two-point discrimination
	• Vibration (use 128 Hz tuning fork)
	• Joint position sense and proprioception (eyes closed, locate position of joint)
	• Sharp and dull
	• Hot and cold
	• Sensory loss mapping (if deficits are found)
	• Romberg (peripheral nerves, dorsal columns, vestibular, cerebellar)
	• Nerve root tension tests such as straight leg raising
	• **Subjective pain and discomfort can be indicated on pain diagrams and VAS (visual analog scale) as shown on the following page**

---

[76] "The Rinne and Weber tuning fork tests are the most important tools in distinguishing between conductive and sensorineural hearing loss." Ruckenstein MJ. Hearing loss. A plan for individualized management. *Postgrad Med.* 1995 Oct;98(4):197-200, 203, 206

Deep tendon reflexes are summarized below and on the following page. Hyperreflexia is noted with upper motor neuron lesions (UMNL) in the cortex, subcortical nuclei, brainstem, or corticospinal tracts of the spinal cord, whereas hyporeflexia can result from lesions of lower motor neurons (LMNL) in spinal cord, peripheral nerves, as well as from sensory/afferent defects including diabetic neuropathy, vitamin B-12 deficiency, and Guillain-Barre disorder. Muscle strength should always be "five over five" to be considered normal, whereas in the testing of reflexes, symmetry/asymmetry is generally more important than the grade of response (except with sustained clonus). **Asymmetry of reflex or strength (especially when seen together) is never normal and requires clinical correlation and investigation.** Reflexes and strength are evaluated as follows in the following table.

Deep tendon reflexes	Muscle strength
+5 Hyperreflexia with sustained clonus: Sustained clonus strongly suggests UMNL and requires investigation; most textbooks use a 0-4 scale, yet this 0-5 scale facilitates clear communication of observed lesions.[77]	5/5 Normal: Full strength: able to withstand gravity and full resistance.
+4 Marked hyperreflexia: Up to 4 beats of unsustained clonus may be normal[78]; suggests UMNL but may be caused by medications, electrolyte disturbances, etc.	4/5 Partial strength: Able to withstand gravity and partial resistance.
+3 Hyperreflexia: More than normal.	3/5 Partial strength: Only able to resist gravity.
+2 Normal: Neither hyporeflexia nor hyperreflexia.	2/5 Partial strength: Able to contract muscle but unable to resist gravity.
+1 Hyporeflexia: Less than normal	1/5 Slight flicker of muscle contraction: Does not result in joint movement.
0 No reflex: Requires clinical correlation for lesion of sensory receptors, peripheral nerve, spinal cord, anterior horn, or neuromuscular junction; this is a common finding in normal individuals.	0/5 No clinically detectable contraction: Correlate with lesion of peripheral nerve, cord, cerebrum, anterior horn, or neuromuscular junction.

[77] Oommen K, edited by Berman SA, et al. Neurological History and Physical Examination. Last Updated: October 4, 2006. *eMedicine* http://www.emedicine.com/neuro/topic632.htm
[78] "…three to four beats of clonus can be elicited at the ankles in some normal individuals." Waxman SG. Clinical Neuroanatomy 25th Edition. McGraw Hill Medical, New York, 2003, p 325

Patients can be asked to <u>localize</u> and <u>describe</u> their pain/discomfort on drawings such as these.
Examples of descriptions:

- Numb
- Hypersensitive
- Tingling

- Shooting pain
- Electrical pain
- Stabbing pain

- Burning pain
- Dull ache
- Muscle weakness

FRONT OF BODY   BACK OF BODY

On the lines below, indicate which pain/discomfort you are referring to and then quantify it by placing an "X" on the line.

Location of pain:_____

No pain at all   Worst pain imaginable

Location of pain:_____

No pain at all   Worst pain imaginable

Laboratory Assessments: General Considerations of Commonly Used Tests

"The laboratory evaluation of patients with rheumatic disease is often informative but rarely definitive."[79]

Laboratory tests are immensely important in evaluating patients with musculoskeletal pain, as these tests allow the clinician to 1) assess for infection (e.g., subacute osteomyelitis), 2) quantify the degree of inflammation (i.e., with CRP or ESR), 3) assess or exclude other disease processes that may be the cause of pain or dysfunction, and 4) assess for concomitant diseases (e.g., septic arthritis complicating rheumatoid arthritis). Additionally, 5) these tests open the door to more complete patient care and holistic management of the whole person because they allow for a more comprehensive and complete understanding of the patient's underlying physiology. **The recommended routine is to use the following panel of tests when assessing patients with musculoskeletal pain: 1) CBC, 2) CRP, 3) chemistry/metabolic panel, and preferably also 4) ferritin, 5) 25(OH)-vitamin D, and 6) thyroid assessment, minimally including TSH** and optimally including free T4, total T3, reverse T3 and anti-thyroid antibodies. The use of a screening evaluation on a routine basis helps identify patients with occult diseases and also allows for more comprehensive management of the patient's overall health. Other tests are indicated in specific situations. *Orthopedics* relies heavily upon physical examination and imaging, whereas *Rheumatology* relies more heavily upon laboratory analysis. In Orthopedics, laboratory tests are used mainly for the purposes of discovering or excluding rheumatic and systemic diseases. In Rheumatology, lab tests are used to specifically identify the type of illness, quantify the severity of the condition, and to assess for concomitant illnesses and complications.

Essential Tests: These Tests are <u>Required</u> for <u>Basic</u> Patient Assessment

Test	Purpose	Clinical application
CRP (or ESR)	Screening for **infection**, **inflammation**, and possibly **cancer**; if inflammation is present, then these tests allow for a generalized quantification of severity.	**Useful in all new patients** for helping to differentiate systemic/inflammatory disorders from those which are noninflammatory and mechanical. Also very helpful as a general "barometer" of health since higher values correlate with increased risk for diabetes mellitus and cardiovascular disease; thus this test helps bridge the gap between acute care and wellness promotion.
CBC	Screening for **anemia**, **infection**, certain cancers (namely **leukemia**).	Useful in any patient with **nontraumatic musculoskeletal pain** or **systemic manifestations**, especially **fever or weight loss**; occasionally detects occult B-12 and folate deficiencies.
Chemistry panel	Screening for **diabetes**, **liver disease**, **kidney failure**, bone lesions (alkaline phosphatase), **electrolyte disturbances**, adrenal insufficiency (hyponatremia with hyperkalemia), **hyperparathyroidism, hypercalcemia.**	Use this panel in any patient with **nontraumatic musculoskeletal pain** or **systemic manifestations**; all patients with **hypertension, diabetes**, or who use **medications** that cause **hepatotoxicity, nephrotoxicity**, etc.
Thyroid assessments	Hypothyroidism is a common problem and is an often overlooked cause of musculoskeletal pain.[80]	This is a reasonable test panel for any patient with fatigue, cold extremities, depression, "arthritis", muscle pain, hypercholesterolemia, or other manifestations of hypothyroidism.

---

[79] Klippel JH (ed). <u>Primer on the Rheumatic Diseases. 11th Edition</u>. Atlanta: Arthritis Foundation. 1997 page 94
[80] "Hypothyroidism is frequently accompanied by musculoskeletal manifestations ranging from myalgias and arthralgias to true myopathy and arthritis." McLean RM, Podell DN. Bone and joint manifestations of hypothyroidism. *Semin Arthritis Rheum.* 1995 Feb;24(4):282-90

<u>Overview of Important Tests</u>: Common Components of Routine Evaluation

Test	Purpose	Clinical Application
Ferritin *For more details on the treatment of iron overload and iron deficiency, see the guidelines on the website.*[81]	Important for assessing for **iron overload** (e.g., hemochromatoic polyarthropathy), and **iron deficiency** (e.g., low back pain due to colon cancer metastasis). Ferritin values less than 20 in adults (e.g., iron deficiency) or greater than 200 in women and 300 in men (e.g., iron overload) necessitate evaluation and effective treatment.	*Ferritin is the ideal test for both iron overload and iron deficiency.* All patients should be screened for hemochromatosis and other hereditary forms of iron overload regardless of age, gender, or ethnicity.[82] Iron deficiency—particularly in adults—may be the first clue to gastric/colon cancer and generally necessitates referral to gastroenterologist.
Serum 25-hydroxy-vitamin D, 25(OH)D	**Vitamin D deficiency is a common cause of musculoskeletal pain and inflammation**[83,84], and vitamin D deficiency is a significant risk factor for cancer and other serious health problems.[85,86,87]	Measurement of serum 25(OH) vitamin D (or empiric treatment with 2,000 – 4,000 IU vitamin D3 per day for adults) is indicated in patients with chronic musculoskeletal pain.[88,89] Optimal vitamin D status correlates with serum 25(OH)D levels of 50 – 100 ng/mL.[90]
Antinuclear antibodies (ANA)	Sensitive (but not specific) for the detection of several autoimmune diseases, especially systemic lupus erythematosus (SLE).	This test is particularly valuable for assessing patients with polyarthropathy, facial rash, and/or fatigue.
Rheumatoid factor (RF)	The primary value of this test is in supporting a diagnosis of rheumatoid arthritis; specificity is low.	RF may be positive in normal health, iron overload, chronic infections, hepatitis, sarcoidosis, and bacterial endocarditis.
Cyclic citrullinated protein (CCP) antibodies	Cyclic citrullinated protein (CCP) antibodies are currently the single best laboratory test for rheumatoid arthritis (RA) and have largely replaced RF.	Citrullinated protein antibodies are rapidly becoming *the test* for diagnosing and confirming RA; used with RF for highly specific "conjugate seropositivity."
Lactulose-mannitol assay	Assesses for malabsorption and excess intestinal permeability—"leaky gut."	Diagnostic test for intestinal damage; excellent nonspecific screening test for pathology or pathophysiology such as celiac and Crohns.
Comprehensive parasitology, stool analysis	Identification and quantification of intestinal yeast, bacteria, and other microbes.	Extremely valuable test when working with patients with chronic fatigue syndromes, fibromyalgia, or autoimmunity; see chapter 4 of *Integrative Rheumatology*.

[81] Excerpt from **Vasquez A**. Integrative Rheumatology on iron overload http://optimalhealthresearch.com/hemochromatosis.html
[82] **Vasquez A**. Musculoskeletal disorders and iron overload disease: comment on the American College of Rheumatology guidelines for the initial evaluation of the adult patient with acute musculoskeletal symptoms. *Arthritis Rheum* 1996;39: 1767-8 http://optimalhealthresearch.com/hemochromatosis.html
[83] Masood H, Narang AP, Bhat IA, Shah GN. Persistent limb pain and raised serum alkaline phosphatase the earliest markers of subclinical hypovitaminosis D in Kashmir. *Indian J Physiol Pharmacol.* 1989 Oct-Dec;33(4):259-61
[84] Al Faraj S, Al Mutairi K. Vitamin D deficiency and chronic low back pain in Saudi Arabia. *Spine.* 2003 Jan 15;28(2):177-9
[85] Grant WB. An estimate of premature cancer mortality in the U.S. due to inadequate doses of solar ultraviolet-B radiation. *Cancer.* 2002;94(6):1867-75
[86] Zittermannn A. Vitamin D in preventive medicine: are we ignoring the evidence? *Br J Nutr.* 2003 May;89(5):552-72
[87] Holick MF. Vitamin D: importance in the prevention of cancers, type 1 diabetes, heart disease, and osteoporosis. *Am J Clin Nutr.* 2004;79(3):362-71
[88] Plotnikoff GA, Quigley JM. Prevalence of severe hypovitaminosis D in patients with persistent, nonspecific musculoskeletal pain. *Mayo Clin Proc.* 2003 Dec;78(12):1463-70
[89] Al Faraj S, Al Mutairi K. Vitamin D deficiency and chronic low back pain in Saudi Arabia. *Spine.* 2003 Jan 15;28(2):177-9
[90] **Vasquez A**, Manso G, Cannell J. The Clinical Importance of Vitamin D (Cholecalciferol): A Paradigm Shift with Implications for All Healthcare Providers. *Alternative Therapies in Health and Medicine* 2004;10:28-37 and *Integrative Medicine* 2004;3:44-54 http://optimalhealthresearch.com/cholecalciferol.html

Chemistry/metabolic panel	
Overview and interpretation:	▪ Accurate interpretation requires knowledge and pattern-recognition by the doctor to translate numbers into differential diagnoses that are correlated with the clinical presentation, examination, and imaging findings to arrive at probable diagnoses. ▪ Variation exists in the components and ranges offered by different laboratories.
Advantages:	▪ Inexpensive and easy to perform—venipuncture + serum separator tube. ▪ Provides a quick screen for diabetes, hepatitis, renal insufficiency, suggestions of alcohol abuse, hyperparathyroidism, electrolyte imbalances, etc.

Limitation and considerations:	▪ Individual tests and the most common clinical considerations for low and high values are listed in the following section. These values and considerations are provided with the routine adult outpatient in mind and are not inclusive of every possible differential diagnosis and therapeutic consideration. Consult your laboratory texts and reference manuals as needed per patient.
	▪ Abnormal laboratory results are always due to one of four problems:
	  1. Technical error: Error with the laboratory analysis, improper patient identification correlating with the sample, alteration of the sample before delivery to the laboratory (e.g., too much time, too much heat, lysis of cells). Given the importance of laboratory accuracy and the life-and-death decisions that are based upon such reports, this type of error is inexcusable, however, it does occur, occasionally producing results that defy physiologic possibility or which contradict the clinical picture. Repeating the test is appropriate. *Example*: Hypercalcemia (elevated serum calcium) may be reported in error by the laboratory due to problems with the analyzing machinery.
	  2. Drug effect: An otherwise healthy patient may develop a laboratory abnormality due to a drug effect. *Example*: Hypercalcemia can be secondary to the effect of a calcium-sparing diuretic, such as hydrochlorothiazide (HCTZ).
	  3. Pathology: The patient has a diagnosable disease causing the laboratory abnormality. *Example*: Hypercalcemia can be secondary to a parathyroid adenoma which secretes abnormally high amounts of parathyroid hormone; hypercalcemia can also be a presentation of malignancy such as breast cancer or prostate cancer, or from a granulomatous disease such as sarcoidosis.
	  4. Physiologic abnormality: The patient has a physiologic abnormality causing the laboratory abnormality. *Example*: Hypercalcemia can be secondary to excess intake of vitamin D. In practice, hypercalcemia from hypervitaminosis D is very rare because vitamin D has a wide safety margin; but for the sake of this discussion, vitamin D toxicity will be listed as a possible cause of hypercalcemia.

Comments:	▪ All abnormalities require follow-up—repeat test within 2-4 weeks as part of routine follow-up along with additional investigation and clinical re-assessment. Extraordinary abnormalities and those with life-threatening implications should of course be retested immediately; often, the laboratory will hold the blood sample for 7 days and the repeat analysis can be performed on the same blood sample to exclude technical error. ▪ Many ill patients (such as those with chronic fatigue syndrome, fibromyalgia, etc) will have normal results with the metabolic panel and other basic routine laboratory assessments. Therefore, normal results do not ensure that the patient is healthy nor without life-threatening illness. ▪ Generally, laboratory tests are performed in the morning under fasting conditions; such is the standard but is not necessarily required depending on the nature of the test, convenience, and the clinical situation.

Practical overview of common abnormalities on the chemistry/metabolic panel —*continued*

Low values—considerations	Analyte[91]	High values—considerations
Technical error due to faulty processing of sample (i.e., hemolysis); insulinoma, exogenous insulin administration (test serum C-peptide), overdose of anti-hyperglycemic drugs, hypopituitarism and adrenal insufficiency.	**Glucose**: 65-99 mg/dL *Clinical pearl*: *Fasting glucose levels can miss mild type-2 diabetes mellitus; a better test for long-term glucose status is hemoglobin A1c.*	Postprandial sample, diabetes mellitus type-1 or type-2, Cushing disease or syndrome, acromegally, pheochromocytoma, glucagonoma, hyperthyroidism. If glucose is >300 mg/dL and patient is unstable (e.g., tachypnic or stuporous), evaluate for diabetic ketoacidosis or hyperosmolar state. Optimal fasting serum glucose is in the range of 70-75 up to 85 mg/dL, since levels >85 mg/dL have been associated with increased mortality.
Hyponatremia is potentially fatal and is also a cause of permanent neurologic injury (e.g., pontine myelinolysis). Clinicians should be particularly concerned when the sodium level drops below 125 mmol/L. Symptomatic hyponatremia is worthy of treatment in hospital setting; mild cases due to a recent event such as excess diaphoresis (e.g., prolonged sweating and exercise) or excess fluid intake (e.g., beer potomania [i.e., binge drinking], overhydration with unmineralized water) might be managed with sodium replacement and water restriction. Older patients, patients with pulmonary disease, and patients taking certain drugs such as serotonin-reuptake inhibitors may develop a chronic and relatively benign mild hyponatremia associated with "reset osmostat syndrome." Sodium levels can be altered downward by conditions that introduce osmotically active substances into the serum, such as immunoglobulins (e.g., multiple myeloma), hyperglycemia, and hypertriglyceridemia; corrective equations are available for such situations. For additional information see on-line reviews by Goh[92] and Decaux and Musch.[93]	**Sodium**: 136 to 144 mEq/L (mmol/L)	Hypernatremia in outpatients is rare; assess for drug effect and dehydration with hemoconcentration. Some clinicians will determine the free water deficit, while others will treat with oral or IV hydration with plain water or half-normal saline, respectively. Electrolyte abnormalities—particularly involving sodium—should generally be corrected slowly and with close supervision.

---

[91] The reference range for this table and some provisional information was derived from Medline Plus provided by the U.S. Department of Health and Human Services and National Institutes of Health. http://www.nlm.nih.gov/medlineplus/ency/article/003468.htm Accessed June 28, 2011. However, the majority of the information in this table comes from the author's (Dr Vasquez's) clinical training and experience. Editorial and peer reviews were provided by colleagues Barry Morgan MD (emergency medicine), Holly Furlong DC, Kris Young DC, Erika Mennerick DC, and Bill Beakey DOM of Professional Co-op Services, Inc. professionalco-op.com.

[92] Goh KP. Management of hyponatremia. *Am Fam Physician*. 2004;69:2387-94 http://www.aafp.org/afp/2004/0515/p2387.html Accessed June 2011.

[93] Decaux G, Musch W. Clinical laboratory evaluation of the syndrome of inappropriate secretion of antidiuretic hormone. *Clin J Am Soc Nephrol*. 2008 Jul;3(4):1175-84 http://cjasn.asnjournals.org/content/3/4/1175.full.pdf Accessed June 29, 2011.

Practical overview of common abnormalities on the chemistry/metabolic panel—*continued*

Low values—*considerations*	*Analyte*	*High values*—*considerations*
Hypokalemia can cause fatal cardiac arrhythmias and needs to be taken seriously. Replacement is generally via oral administration of potassium-rich foods, juices, or supplements such as potassium citrate (best option) or potassium chloride (KCl, inexpensive and therefore commonly used in medical settings even though KCl is clearly not optimal therapy due to the acidifying effect of the chloride anion). Recalcitrant hypokalemia is often a sign of magnesium depletion.[94] Causes of hypokalemia include diarrhea, vomiting, diuretics, Cushing disease/syndrome, dietary insufficiency, overhydration with mineral-free fluids, hyperaldosteronism and renal artery stenosis. Acute metabolic acidosis should cause relative or absolute elevations in serum K; the finding of normal or low serum K in a patient with acidosis (e.g., diabetic ketoacidosis) indicates (severe) potassium depletion.	**Potassium**: 3.6 to 5.2 mEq/L (mmol/L)	**Hyperkalemia is defined as a potassium level greater than 5.5 mmol/L. Severe hyperkalemia (>7 mmol/L) can be fatal and needs to be taken seriously.** In severe hyperkalemia, treatment and emergency management should be implemented before a complete evaluation and differential diagnosis are performed.[95] ❶ Ensure that blood sample was not hemolyzed. Repeat test if patient is stable and time allows. ❷ If hyperkalemia is severe or patient is symptomatic or has electrocardiographic changes, treat hyperkalemia with intravenous calcium, beta-adrenergic agonists (e.g., albuterol), bicarbonate, insulin and glucose; magnesium sulfate may also help alleviate arrhythmias; oral sodium polystyrene sulfonate (SPS, also known as Kayexalate) is a frequently used potassium-binding agent. ❸ DDX includes adrenal insufficiency, potassium-sparing diuretics, ACE-inhibitors and ARBs, NSAIDs, rhabdomyolysis, renal failure, massive cell necrosis such as with tumor lysis syndrome.
Evaluate hypocalcemia clinically with Chvostek's sign (~30% sensitive) and Trousseau sign (~90% sensitive) which may also be present in hypomagnesemia; evaluate clinically for arrhythmia, muscle spasm/hypertonicity, and hyperreflexia. Measure serum albumin and perform equation for "corrected calcium" if albumin is low. DDX includes renal failure, hypoparathyroidism, malabsorption, and drug effect (e.g., rarely a loop diuretic such as furosemide). Chronic mild hypocalcemia is treated with oral vitamin D and calcium supplementation; subacute symptomatic hypocalcemia can be treated with intravenous calcium gluconate especially if cardiac arrhythmias are present.	**Calcium**: 8.6 to 10.2 mg/dL	Outpatient hypercalcemia is potentially serious and needs to be evaluated in a stepwise manner: ❶ repeat the test to rule out lab error unless you are confident in the performance of the laboratory and stability of the submitted sample, ❷ review drug list for adverse effect, such as from hydrochlorothiazide (HCTZ) or rarely from excess cholecalciferol intake, ❸ test intact parathyroid hormone (iPTH) to evaluate for hyperparathyroidism, ❹ evaluate for possible granulomatous disease such as sarcoidosis, tuberculosis, Crohns disease, and possible leukemia or lymphoma, ❺ consider metabolic bone disease such as Paget disease of bone or metastatic bone disease, ❻ evaluate for cancer, ❼ test urine calcium for familial hypocalciuric hypercalcemia, ❽ refer to specialist such as internist or endocrinologist if hypercalcemia persists and answer is not forthcoming.

Corrected calcium (cCa) equations: Used when both serum calcium and albumin are low
American units: cCa (mg/dL) = serum Ca (mg/dL) + 0.8 (4.0 - serum albumin [g/dL])
International units: cCa (mmol/L) = measured total Ca (mmol/L) + 0.02 (40 - serum albumin [g/L])

---

[94] "Herein is reviewed literature suggesting that magnesium deficiency exacerbates potassium wasting by increasing distal potassium secretion." Huang CL, Kuo E. Mechanism of hypokalemia in magnesium deficiency. *J Am Soc Nephrol*. 2007;18:2649-52 jasn.asnjournals.org/content/18/10/2649

[95] "If the hyperkalemia is severe (potassium >7.0 mEq/L) or if the patient is symptomatic, begin treatment before diagnostic investigation of the underlying cause." Garth D. Hyperkalemia in emergency medicine treatment and management. *Medscape Reference* http://emedicine.medscape.com/article/766479-treatment#a1126 Accessed June 2011

Practical overview of common abnormalities on the chemistry/metabolic panel —*continued*

Low values—considerations	Analyte	High values—considerations
Clinically meaningful hypochloremia is rare among outpatients. Hypochloremic metabolic alkalosis is commonly seen after persistent vomiting. Consider syndrome of inappropriate diuretic hormone (SIADH) secretion, cardiopulmonary disease, and adrenal insufficiency.	**Chloride**: 97 to 111 mmol/L	Hyperchloremia in outpatients is rare; assess for drug effect and dehydration with hemoconcentration; assess for acid-base disturbance, especially acidosis.
Reduced CO2 correlates with hyperventilation; consider acid-base disturbance, salicylate overdose, asthma. Slight decrements in healthy outpatients are probably due to anxious hyperventilation at time of venipuncture.	**CO2 (carbon dioxide)**: 20 - 30 mmol/L	Elevated CO2 can suggest cardiopulmonary compromise and/or acid-base disturbance; assess clinically. Slight elevations in otherwise healthy outpatients are probably due to breath-holding at time of venipuncture.
Reduced total protein with normal albumin suggests hypogammaglobulinemia; evaluate for nephrotic syndrome, liver disease, protein deficiency and malabsorption/enteropathy, immunosuppressive syndromes and consider intravenous gammaglobulin therapy.	**Total protein (albumin + globulins)**: 6.3 - 8.0 g/dL	Elevated total protein with normal albumin suggests hypergammaglobulinemia, such as due to infection or plasma cell dyscrasia (e.g., multiple myeloma and Waldenstrom's disease). Evaluate within the clinical context; order serum protein electrophoresis if cause remains elusive, especially if patient has immune complex disease, neuropathy, or nephropathy.
Assess for liver disease, nephrotic syndrome, protein deficiency, malabsorption (consider celiac disease).	**Albumin**: 3.9 - 5.0 g/dL	Assess for dehydration/hemoconcentration.
Loss of hepatic mass due to cirrhosis, possible pyridoxine deficiency.	**ALT (alanine aminotransferase)**: 10 - 40 IU/L	Hepatocellular liver injury due to chemical toxicity, viral hepatitis, hemochromatosis, metastatic or infectious disease, muscle injury. ALT is preferentially elevated over AST in viral hepatitis.
Loss of hepatic mass due to cirrhosis, possible pyridoxine deficiency.	**AST (aspartate aminotransferase)**: 10 - 40 IU/L	Hepatocellular liver injury due to chemical toxicity, viral hepatitis, hemochromatosis, metastatic or infectious liver disease, myocardial infarct, muscle injury. AST is preferentially elevated over ALT in alcoholic hepatitis and rhabdomyolysis.
Consider zinc deficiency, malnutrition.	**Alkaline phosphatase**: 44 - 147 IU/L	Metabolic bone disease, metastatic bone disease, vitamin D deficiency, congestive liver disease. Test isoenzymes to differentiate bone versus hepatic origin if cause of elevation remains unclear.

Practical overview of common abnormalities on the chemistry/metabolic panel —*continued*

Low values—considerations	*Analyte*	*High values—considerations*
Low values are rare but might be noted with severe chronic anemia.	**Total bilirubin**: 0.2 to 1.5 mg/dL Direct (conjugated) bilirubin: 0 to 0.3 mg/dL Indirect (unconjugated) bilirubin: Determined by subtracting the *direct* from the *total* bilirubin.	Indirect/unconjugated bilirubin is elevated with hemolysis (e.g., hemolytic anemia) and impaired enzymatic conjugation (e.g., Gilbert's syndrome) or both (e.g., neonates). Direct/conjugated bilirubin has been enzymatically conjugated with glucuronic acid but is blocked from hepatobiliary excretion; consider performing liver and gall bladder sonogram (or CT or MRI) to evaluate for causes of biliary obstruction in addition to a careful abdominal exam. In patients with advanced liver disease, perform the Model for End-Stage Liver Disease (MELD) score and/or the MELD-Na score to predict 3-month mortality.[96] Fluoridated water inhibits glucuronidation in some patients with Gilbert's syndrome; biochemical improvement follows avoidance of fluoridated water.[97]
Liver disease, nephrotic syndrome, protein deficiency and malabsorption. **BUN-to-creatinine ratio (normal = 10)** >10-20: Renal underperfusion, post-renal obstruction <10: Suggests intrinsic renal disease	**BUN (blood urea nitrogen)**: 7 to 20 mg/dL	Consider renal underperfusion (e.g., due to heart failure, GI bleeding, renal artery stenosis, dehydration), intrinsic renal failure, post-renal urinary tract obstruction. When renal disease is initially considered, order a urinalysis with microscopic analysis—see following section on urinalysis (UA).
Sarcopenia (insufficient muscle mass), protein deficiency and malabsorption. **Methods for estimating creatinine clearance, glomerular filtration rate (GFR)** 1. Modification of Diet in Renal Disease (MDRD) equation*, 2. 24-hour urine creatinine measurement, 3. Serum cystatin-C measurement, 4. Cockcroft-Gault equation (below): $$GFR = \frac{(140 - age\ years) \times wt\ kg \times (0.85\ if\ female)}{72 \times serum\ creatinine\ in\ mg/dL}$$ Clinical pearls for managing the chronic kidney disease (CKD) patient with declining renal function: • When the GFR ≤ 60 (CKD stage 3): Modify dosages or withdraw certain drugs. Treat the causative problem and/or begin specialist co-management. • When the GFR ≤ 30 (CKD stage 4): The patient needs to consult a nephrologist. • When the GFR ≤ 15 (CKD stage 5): The patient needs a transplant or dialysis. *National Institute of Diabetes and Digestive and Kidney Diseases (NIDDK). GFR MDRD Calculator for Adults (Conventional units). Accessed June 2011 nkdep.nih.gov/professionals/gfr_calculators/idms_con.htm	**Creatinine**: 0.8 to 1.3 mg/dL	Excess dietary protein, creatine supplementation, renal hypoperfusion; the most important consideration is intrinsic renal failure. Creatinine production (from arginine and creatine) is proportional to muscle mass. A rise in creatinine does not become evident until renal function (measured by glomerular filtration rate [GFR]) has fallen by approximately 50%. Creatinine levels indicative of impaired renal function to such an extent that modifications in diet, medications, and co-management become relevant are 1.4 mg/dL in women and 1.5 mg/dL in men. In the evaluation of renal function, the patient's age is a crucial determinant of how the serum creatinine is interpreted for the estimation of renal function (via GFR—see the Cockcroft-Gault equation). Cystatin C is more sensitive than are singular or conjugate interpretations of BUN and creatinine. If drug-induced nephritis is suspected, test urine eosinophils.

---

[96] MELD calculations are best performed electronically, such as with http://www.mayoclinic.org/meld/mayomodel8.html or other medical calculator.
[97] Lee J. Gilbert's disease and fluoride intake. *Fluoride* 1983; 16: 139-45

Chapter 1: Review of Clinical Assessments and Concepts

Cystatin C	

Overview and interpretation:	• Cystatin C is gaining acceptance as studies confirm and define its usefulness, especially as an early, sensitive marker for chronic kidney disease. Concentrations of cystatin C are not affected by gender, age, or race, and cystatin C is not affected by most drugs (prednisone increases; cyclosporine decreases), infections, diet, or inflammation.[98]
	• Produced at a constant rate by all nucleated cells.
	• Freely filtered by the glomerulus.
	• Elevated in: renal disorders.
	    ○ Cystatin C rises more rapidly than creatinine (Cr) in early renal impairment.
	    ○ Good predictor of the severity of ATN (acute tubular necrosis).
	    ○ The cystatin C concentration is an independent risk factor for heart failure, mortality, CVD and non-CVD outcomes in older adults and appears to provide a better measure of risk assessment than the serum Cr concentration.

Advantages:	• More accurate assessment of renal function than creatinine-based assessments. • Can be used to accurately assess renal function when creatinine-based assessments suggest impending renal impairment inconsistent with clinical presentation.
Limitations:	• Cost is approximately US $80. • False "non-renal" elevations may occur with cancer and/or rheumatic disease.

Presentation: 40yo male presenting for follow-up on abnormal renal function assessment—use of cystatin C to confirm normal kidney function: This apperantly healthy and athletic 40yo man displays consistently elevated creatinine and an estimated glomerular filtration rate (eGFR) that is close enough at 62 to warrant concern. Clinicians must appreciate that eGFR <60 is consistent with stage 3 chronic kidney disease (CKD) which warrants monitoring and which often necessitates changes in drug dosing (e.g., to avoid metformin-induced lactic acidosis) and diet (e.g., to avoid hyperkalemia).

Date and Time Collected	Date Entered	Date and Time Reported	Physician Name	NPI	Physician ID
12/07/11 11:10	12/08/11	12/13/11 04:07ET	VASQUEZ , A		

Tests Ordered
Comp. Metabolic Panel (14); FSH+TestT+LH+DHEA S+Prog+E2...; Chlamydia pneumoniae(IgG/M); Venipuncture

TESTS	RESULT	FLAG	UNITS	REFERENCE INTERVAL	LAB
Comp. Metabolic Panel (14)					
Glucose, Serum	89		mg/dL	65 - 99	01
BUN	18		mg/dL	6 - 24	01
Creatinine, Serum	**1.41**	**High**	mg/dL	0.76 - 1.27	01
eGFR If NonAfricn Am	62		mL/min/1.73	>59	
eGFR If Africn Am	72		mL/min/1.73	>59	

    Note: A persistent eGFR <60 mL/min/1.73 m2 (3 months or more) may indicate chronic kidney disease. An eGFR >59 mL/min/1.73 m2 with an elevated urine protein also may indicate chronic kidney disease. Calculated using CKD-EPI formula.

BUN/Creatinine Ratio	13			9 - 20	

In this situation, cystatin C was performed and confirmed normal renal function despite persistently elevated creatinine, which is probably attrlbutable to this patient's athleticism and muscle mass.[99]

Date and Time Collected	Date Entered	Date and Time Reported	Physician Name	NPI	Physician ID
12/07/11 11:10	12/12/11	12/15/11 07:14ET	VASQUEZ , A		

Tests Ordered
Cystatin C; Written Authorization

TESTS	RESULT	FLAG	UNITS	REFERENCE INTERVAL	LAB
Cystatin C	0.71		mg/L	0.53 - 0.95	01

[98] http://labtestsonline.org/understanding/analytes/cystatin-c/tab/test Accessed April 2012
[99] Thank you, Bill Beakey DOM of Professional Co-op Services, Inc. professionalco-op.com for provision of these laboratory services.

OptimalHealthResearch.com   FOUNDATIONAL ASSESSMENTS & WELLNESS PROMOTION   27

Presentation: 69yo female presenting for routine outpatient health assessment with no acute complaints: Review the following labs and outline your treatment plan before reading the discussion below.

PATIENT NAME	PATIENT ID	ROOM NUMBER	AGE	SEX	PHYSICIAN
			69 Y 1941	F	Vasque-?

REQUISITION NO	ACCESSION NO	ID.NO.	COLLECTION DATE & TIME	LOG-IN-DATE	REPORT DATE & TIME
			09/22/10 08:00 AM	09/22/10 06:37 PM	09/23/10 03:36AM

NOTES:
PT FASTING

TEST	RESULTS OUT OF RANGE	RESULTS WITHIN RANGE	UNITS	EXPECTED RANGE	LAB
BASIC METABOLIC PROFILE					
GLUCOSE		98	MG/DL	65-100	
BUN		19	MG/DL	8-25	
CREATININE		1.2	MG/DL	0.6-1.3	
EGFR AFRICAN AMER.	54		ML/MIN/1.73	>60	
EGFR NON-AFRICAN AMER.	45		ML/MIN/1.73	>60	
SODIUM		136	MEQ/L	133-146	
POTASSIUM	8.5		MEQ/L	3.5-5.3	

RESULTS RECHECKED AND VERIFIED
NOTE: NO VISIBLE HEMOLYSIS OBSERVED.

CHLORIDE		100	MEQ/L	97-110	
CARBON DIOXIDE		27	MEQ/L	18-30	
CALCIUM		10.0	MG/DL	8.5-10.5	
LIPID PANEL					
CHOLESTEROL		193	MG/DL	<200	
TRIGLYCERIDES		129	MG/DL	<150	
HDL CHOLESTEROL		52	MG/DL	>39	
CALCULATED LDL CHOL	115		MG/DL	<100	
RISK RATIO LDL/HDL		2.22	RATIO	<3.22	
HEMOGLOBIN A1C	7.0		%	4.0-5.6	

AMERICAN DIABETES ASSOCIATION GUIDELINES FOR HGB A1C:
GLYCEMIC GOAL IN DIABETES . . . . <7.0%
DIAGNOSIS OF DIABETES . . . . >/=6.5%
    CONFIRMED ON REPEAT ANALYSIS OR
    WITH APPROPRIATE SYMPTOMS.
INCREASED RISK FOR DIABETES 5.7-6.4%

TSH	10.5		UIU/ML	0.3-5.1	

PERFORMING LAB(S) LEGEND:

> Chemistry/metabolic panels should be performed on all new patients prior to the initiation of treatment and periodically on all established patients to monitor for disease emergence, disease progression, and response to treatment
>
> Treating this diabetic patient with a potassium-rich diet emphasizing low-carbohydrate fruits and vegetables would exacerbate her already life-threatening hyperkalemia. Note also that her hypothyroidism would be expected to contribute to her obesity which is exacerbating her diabetes and that (somewhat theoretically since we don't have her vital signs here) hypothyroid bradycardia could also reduce renal perfusion and contribute to her low GFR and hyperkalemia.

Assessments and plan: ❶ Life-threatening hyperkalemia: The clinician must focus on the emergency issue(s). Many books quote a potassium of 6 mEq/L as a panic value; note that the laboratory already excluded technical error and checked for hemolysis, which are the two most common causes of spurious hyperkalemia. This patient should be called at home and advised to immediately seek transportation by a secondary driver (e.g., taxi, ambulance, friend, neighbor, or relative) to the nearest hospital. If the patient is demented or otherwise incompetent, the clinician should contact the patient's caretaker or call directly for an ambulance. Attention must be given to the reliability of the driver, the urgency of the situation, and the speed by which the driver can get the patient to the hospital; failure by the clinician to ensure proper patient care—which in this case and most situations is best ensured by enrolling the ambulance service—could easily result in medicolegal complications. Hospital treatment for hyperkalemia will include assessment for electrocardiographic changes and treatment of hyperkalemia with intravenous calcium to stabilize cardioelectroconductivity, beta-adrenergic agonists, bicarbonate, diuretics, insulin and glucose; magnesium may also help alleviate arrhythmias; oral sodium polystyrene sulfonate (Kayexalate) is a potassium-binding agent. ❷ Diabetes mellitus: Notice that this patient's fasting glucose level is "normal" and yet the patient is clearly diabetic per the hemoglobin A1c value >6.5%. This patient needs a comprehensive nutritional plan for diabetes management. Promoting dependence on drugs at this early point should be considered inappropriate. ❸ Hypothyroidism: The TSH >10 indicates primary hypothyroidism by any standard; in all probability, unless major contraindications exist (of which very few exist), this patient should be started on a thyroid hormone combination as discussed in the section on thyroid assessment. ❹ Renal insufficiency: This patient has stage-3 chronic kidney disease and should begin a renoprotective and renorestorative program—beyond the basics of hypertension and hyperglycemia control—as discussed in *Chiropractic and Naturopathic Mastery of Common Clinical Disorders*. Use of ACE-inhibitor or ARB is contraindicated due to hyperkalemia. ❺ Dyslipidemia: The elevated LDL cholesterol and triglycerides should both be below 100 mg/dL. Diet is key, followed by fatty acid therapy, niacin, berberine.

Lipid panel:	
Overview and interpretation:	<ul><li>"High cholesterol" was a buzz phrase many years ago indicating an unfavorable lipid profile causally associated with accelerated atherogenesis and the resultant CVD in its myriad forms. The next step was to identify low-density lipoprotein (LDL) cholesterol as the most obvious kingpin of vascular villains. Advances over the past decade include:<ol><li>Appreciation that other non-lipid molecules such as homocysteine and c-reactive protein are important contributors to the atherogenic process,</li><li>Renewed interest in the beneficial effects of high-density lipoprotein (HDL) cholesterol in mediating vasculoprotection, and</li><li>Additional appreciation that the "non-standard" lipid mediators such as very-low-density lipoprotein (VLDL), β-VLDL, intermediate-density lipoprotein (IDL) cholesterol and lipoprotein-a (Lp-a) are also clinically important. For the sake of this introductory section on the basics of laboratory interpretation, the discussion will be limited to the components of the standard lipid panel; additional tests and details are provided in the disease-specific chapters on metabolic and inflammatory disorders.</li></ol></li></ul>

Lipids: Goals	*Clinical notes:*
Total cholesterol: < 200 mg/dL	<ul><li>Higher cholesterol levels correlate with increased risk for CVD. Except in very rare cases of genotropic disease, the vast majority of humans should be able to achieve a total cholesterol <200 mg/dL via nutritional optimization, exercise, and proper endocrine (especially thyroid) status. The so-called "statin" drugs which block HMG-CoA reductase (3-hydroxy-3-methyl-glutaryl-CoA reductase, the rate-limiting enzyme for the endogenous production of cholesterol) would and should be *orphan drugs*. Reducing serum levels of insulin—the primary inducer of HMG-CoA reductase—is the most rational means by which to reduce total cholesterol levels. Thyroid hormone downregulates HMG-CoA reductase; this explains the well-established association of hypothyroidism with dyslipidemia and hypercholesterolemia.</li></ul>
LDL: <100 mg/dL	<ul><li>O'Keefe and Cordain and colleagues[100] have noted that optimal LDL is 50-70 mg/dl and that lower is better and is physiologically normal for humans who eat appropriate diets and who are physically active.</li></ul>
HDL: >50-60 mg/dL	<ul><li>Per the American Heart Association[101], "An HDL of 60 mg/dL and above is considered protective against heart disease." Of note, a recent report linked accumulation of persistent organic pollutants (POP) with elevated HDL levels.[102]</li></ul>
Triglycerides: <100 mg/dL	<ul><li>Elevated serum triglycerides—except in rare cases of genotropic disease—are indicators of dietary carbohydrate excess and/or alcohol excess and/or insulin resistance. Hypertriglyceridemia is associated with increased CVD risk, higher body mass index (BMI), vitamin D deficiency, and increased risks of breast cancer and prostate cancer. Extreme hypertriglyceridemia (500 mg/dL or more) can cause pancreatitis; administration of omega-3 fatty acids from fish oil is protective.</li></ul>
Advantages	<ul><li>Allows for the monitoring of established cardiovascular risk factors and a surrogate marker for dietary compliance and lifestyle optimization.</li></ul>
Limitations:	<ul><li>Other non-lipid risk factors should also be monitored and optimized.</li></ul>
Comments:	<ul><li>Important panel for overall patient management and disease prevention.</li></ul>

[100] O'Keefe JH Jr, Cordain L, Harris WH, Moe RM, Vogel R. Optimal low-density lipoprotein is 50 to 70 mg/dl: lower is better and physiologically normal. *J Am Coll Cardiol.* 2004 Jun 2;43(11):2142-6

[101] American Heart Association. heart.org/HEARTORG/Conditions/What-Your-Cholesterol-Levels-Mean_UCM_305562_Article.jsp Accessed June 2011

[102] "However, unlike the findings with p,p'-DDE, after the initial decrease of HDL-cholesterol from the 1st to 2nd quartile, HDL-cholesterol increased from the 2nd to 4th quartile of these PCBs." Lee DH, Steffes MW, Sjödin A, Jones RS, Needham LL, Jacobs DR Jr. Low dose organochlorine pesticides and polychlorinated biphenyls predict obesity, dyslipidemia, and insulin resistance among people free of diabetes. *PLoS One.* 2011 Jan 26;6(1):e15977

CBC: complete blood count

Overview and interpretation:

This test measures numbers and indices of white and red blood cells and platelets. A routine "CBC with differential" is affordable, practical, and thus preferred for the vast majority of situations (step 1); the next step when the clinical picture remains unclear is—generally—to order a peripheral blood smear (step 2) before proceeding to a hematologist referral (step 3). Additional tests—more components of step 2—are listed below per topic. If all three blood cell populations are reduced (pancytopenia) consider nutritional anemia, hypersplenism (especially secondary to hepatic cirrhosis), autoimmunity (especially systemic lupus erythematosus), or bone marrow disorder such as myelofibrosis or aplastic anemia.

- WBC (white blood cells): The three most commonly encountered disorders that cause an abnormal WBC count are ❶ bone marrow suppression (causing low WBC count) and conditions associated with elevated WBC count including ❷ leukemia/lymphoma and ❸ response to infection. An elevated WBC count suggests the possibility of infection (especially bacterial infection) or leukemia/lymphoma and therefore requires the clinician's attention. However, relying on the WBC count for the assessment of serious infection is potentially misleading, particularly since, for example, it is elevated in less than 50% of patients with acute and chronic musculoskeletal infections; per Shaw et al[103] "Therefore, it [the WBC count] is helpful when it is high, but potentially misleading when it is normal." Clinicians can gain additional information by assessing percentage and quantitative indices of neutrophils, lymphocytes, and eosinophils, elevations of which may suggest bacterial infections, viral infections, or allergic or parasitic conditions, respectively. Primary care clinicians may also choose to perform lymphocyte immunophenotyping by flow cytometry in patients with unexplained lymphocytosis prior to hematologist consult.

  - Neutropenia: Severe suppression of WBC count resulting in neutropenia can occur in liver disease, viral infections (including but not limited to HIV), autoimmune disorders, bone marrow infiltration/failure, and toxin/alcohol exposure. For severe neutropenia, hospitalization, isolation precautions; prophylactic antibiotics, and marrow-stimulating agents are often indicated. Neutropenia is defined by an absolute neutrophil count (ANC) less than 1500 neutrophilic cells per mm3. Neutropenia is most commonly due to use of anti-cancer cytotoxic agents; other drugs that can cause neutropenia include anticonvulsants (e.g., carbamazepine, valproic acid, diphenylhydantoin), thyroid inhibitors (carbimazole, methimazole, propylthiouracil), antibacterial drugs (penicillins, cephalosporins, sulfonamides, chloramphenicol, vancomycin, trimethoprim-sulfamethoxazole), antipsychotic drugs (clozapine), antiarrhythmics (procainamide), antirheumatic drugs (penicillamine, gold salts, hydroxychloroquine), and NSAIDs.[104] The ANC is calculated with "segs" (segmented neutrophils) and "bands" (band neutrophils) reported on CBC with differential: ANC = Total WBC x (% Segs + % Bands).

> **Absolute neutrophil count (ANC) = Total WBC x (% "Segs" + % "Bands")**
> - Normal value: ≥ 1500 cells/mm3,
> - Mild neutropenia: 1000-1500/mm3,
> - Moderate neutropenia: 500-1000/mm3,
> - Severe neutropenia: ≤ 500/mm3; hospitalization is generally advised

---

[103] Shaw BA, Gerardi JA, Hennrikus WL. How to avoid orthopedic pitfalls in children. *Patient Care* 1999; Feb 28: 95-116

[104] Tefferi A, Hanson CA, Inwards DJ. How to interpret and pursue an abnormal complete blood cell count in adults. *Mayo Clin Proc.* 2005 Jul;80(7):923-36 www.mayoclinicproceedings.com/content/80/7/923.long This article serves as the main review for this section on CBC interpretation.

CBC: complete blood count—*continued*

Overview and interpretation —continued:	- RBC (red blood cells and associated indices): Since polycythemia is relatively rare, in most situations the clinician is looking for anemia, most often related to the categories in the subsections that follow this paragraph. The first step is to classify the anemia based on the mean corpuscular volume (MCV) as microcytic (MCV, <80 fL), normocytic (MCV, 80-95 fL), or macrocytic (MCV, >95 fL)—details on following page.
	 - Clinical notes on the most common anemias:
	  o Nutritional deficiency of B-12 or folate: My approach is to critique the mean corpuscular volume (MCV) and to interpret MCV values greater than 90 with an increased suspicion for folate and/or B-12 deficiency. Clinical experience has shown that MCV values greater than 95 correlate with increased homocysteine levels, and a clinical response (improvement in mood, energy, and a reduction in MCV) is commonly seen following three months of nutritional supplementation. Deficiency of vitamin B-12 can easily be treated with oral administration of 2,000 mcg per day of vitamin B-12.[105] I generally use 5 mg (rarely up to 20 mg) per day of oral folate for the treatment of probable or documented folic acid deficiency; this is safe for most patients, excluding those on antiepileptic drugs.[106] Vitamin B-12 and folic acid *function together* and should be *administered together*. Cyanocobalamin should be avoided due to the cyanide.
	  o Iron deficiency (confirmed with assessment of serum ferritin): While inadequate intake, malabsorption, or menstrual bleeding may cause iron deficiency, **adult patients with iron deficiency are at higher probability for gastrointestinal pathology and should therefore be evaluated with endoscopy or other comprehensive assessment** *beyond fecal occult-blood testing* **to rule out gastrointestinal disease.**[107,108] **The standard of care for all healthcare professionals is that adult patients with inexplicable iron deficiency are referred for gastroenterscopic evaluation to assess for occult gastrointestinal pathology; the major concerns are gastric/colon carcinoma, but malabsorptive conditions and bleeding noncancerous polyps are also worthy of diagnosis.** Iron supplementation should be administered and can reasonably be withheld during acute viral and bacterial infections as it promotes bacterial and viral replication and pathogenicity.
	  o The anemia of chronic disease: Generally associated with a corresponding disease history such as long-term RA or renal insufficiency and often associated with increased ESR, CRP, and ferritin. **Do not assume that an anemic patient has iron deficiency until proven with measurement of serum ferritin.** Anemia of chronic kidney disease (CKD) is associated with reduced renal production of erythropoietin, thereby resulting in understimulation of bone marrow.
	  o Anemia caused by hemolysis or splenic sequestration: Autoimmune hemolytic anemia most commonly occurs in patients with systemic lupus erythematosus (SLE). Pancytopenia—reduced numbers of RBC, WBC, and platelets—is seen with chronic liver disease that has progressed to cirrhosis and has resulted in hemolysis and splenic sequestration of blood cells; such patients are at risk for esophageal varices, encephalopathy, and ascites with spontaneous bacterial peritonitis and should be screened and treated appropriately.

---

[105] Kuzminski AM, et al. Effective treatment of cobalamin deficiency with oral cobalamin. *Blood* 1998 Aug 15;92(4):1191-8

[106] "PGA administered in doses up to 1,000 mg orally a day… The folate was well absorbed, as reflected by marked increases in the serum and erythrocyte folate concentrations… There was no evidence of clinical or laboratory toxicity at these high doses of folate." Boss GR, Ragsdale RA, Zettner A, Seegmiller JE. Failure of folic acid (pteroylglutamic acid) to affect hyperuricemia. *J Lab Clin Med* 1980 Nov;96(5):783-9

[107] Rockey DC, Cello JP. Evaluation of the gastrointestinal tract in patients with iron-deficiency anemia. *N Engl J Med.* 1993;329(23):1691-5

[108] "Endoscopy revealed a clinically important lesion in 23 (12%) of 186 patients. … CONCLUSIONS: Endoscopy yields important findings in premenopausal women with iron deficiency anemia, which should not be attributed solely to menstrual blood loss." Bini EJ, Micale PL, Weinshel EH. Evaluation of the gastrointestinal tract in premenopausal women with iron deficiency anemia. *Am J Med.* 1998 Oct;105(4):281-6

Anemia—the most common considerations in outpatient practice: Always assess patient for tachycardia, hypovolemia, orthostasis, and adequate perfusion; always test serum ferritin during the initial evaluation then perform peripheral blood smear (PBS) if diagnosis remains unclear

- Microcytic anemia:
  - Iron deficiency anemia (IDA)—Test serum ferritin. The confirmation of iron deficiency in adults generally requires gastroenterologic consultation to assess for occult gastrointestinal blood loss; this is especially true for all men and post-menopausal women but also applies to premenopausal women.* Testing for celiac disease and hematuria is advised.**
  - Thalassemia—Check for polycythemia, test Hgb electrophoresis; because the diagnosis of the various thalassemias can be complex, consider consulting a hematologist,
  - Anemia of chronic disease (ACD)—Assess patient, inflammatory markers, and renal function. The most common causes of ACD are temporal (giant cell) arteritis and polymyalgia rheumatica, rheumatoid arthritis, chronic infection, Hodgkin lymphoma, renal cell carcinoma, myelofibrosis, and Castleman disease (a noncancerous lymphoproliferative disorder).
- Normocytic anemia:
  - Nutritional anemia: Iron deficiency and vitamin B-12 deficiency can both cause normocytic anemia.
  - Bleeding—Assess patient for tachycardia, hypovolemia, and shock; consider transfusion and/or volume repletion as needed. Assess serum ferritin and the reticulocyte count.
  - Chronic renal failure (CRF): Anemia associated with elevated BUN and creatinine.
  - Hypersplenism: Assess for chronic hepatitis and cirrhosis. Cirrhotic patients are at increased risk for gastroesophageal hemorrhage and ascites with spontaneous bacterial peritonitis.
  - Hemolysis: Expect to see elevated reticulocytes (chronic) and lactate dehydrogenase (acute); expect high indirect bilirubin and low serum haptoglobin with intravascular hemolysis; assess for autoimmunity (ANA, direct Coombs test [direct antiglobulin test]), glucose-6-phosphate dehydrogenase (G6PD) deficiency, drug-induced hemolysis, and other causes as case warrants.
  - Bone marrow disorder: Correlate lab findings with patient presentation; consult hematologist if solution is not forthcoming.
- Macrocytosis:
  - Induced by toxins, drugs, alcohol—Assess per patient history and other findings; the most notorious offenders are hydroxyurea, zidovudine, and alcohol.
  - Vitamin B-12 and/or folate deficiency: Consider testing serum methylmalonate and homocysteine followed by empiric supplementation with B-12 at 2,000 or more micrograms per day and folate at 1-5 milligrams per day; determine cause of problem and strongly consider autoimmune gastritis, bacterial overgrowth, celiac disease. Test serum ferritin because nutritional deficiencies commonly occur together. Administration of vitamin B-12 is advised in all patients suspected of having B-12 deficiency.*** Regarding the clinical presentation of vitamin B-12 deficiency, clinicians should remember the adage that one-third of patients will present with anemia, one-third with peripheral neuropathy, and one-third with central neurologic problems such as depression, psychosis, and/or other disturbances of mood, memory, or personality. Failure to diagnose and treat vitamin B-12 deficiency in a timely manner will result in permanent neurologic damage.
  - Hypothyroidism: Measure TSH and free T4 at a minimum; assess basal body temperature, and speed of Achilles reflex return.

* "A gastrointestinal source of chronic blood loss was identified in a substantial proportion of premenopausal women with iron deficiency anemia." Green BT, Rockey DC. Gastrointestinal endoscopic evaluation of premenopausal women with iron deficiency anemia. *J Clin Gastroenterol*. 2004 Feb;38(2):104-9
** Goddard AF, James MW, McIntyre AS, Scott BB; on behalf of the British Society of Gastroenterology. Guidelines for the management of iron deficiency anaemia. *Gut*. 2011 Jun 6. [Epub ahead of print]
http://www.epocrates.com/dacc/1106/irondefbmj1106.pdf
*** "Thus, therapeutic trials of Cbl are warranted when clinical findings consistent with Cbl deficiency are present..." Solomon LR. Cobalamin-responsive disorders in the ambulatory care setting: unreliability of cobalamin, methylmalonic acid, and homocysteine testing. *Blood*. 2005 Feb 1;105(3):978-85
http://bloodjournal.hematologylibrary.org/content/105/3/978.full.pdf

CBC: complete blood count—*continued*	
Overview and interpretation —continued:	▪ <u>Platelets</u>: Elevated platelet count (thrombocytosis) can be due to malignant primary thrombocytosis, iron-deficiency anemia, hemolysis, asplenia, and reactive thrombocytosis due to cancer, infection, or chronic inflammation. Low platelet count (thrombocytopenia, fewer than 150,000 platelets per microliter) increases risk for spontaneous bleeding and can—rarely but importantly—be associated with serious and potentially life-threatening disorders such as thrombotic thrombocytopenic purpura/hemolytic uremic syndrome (TTP/HUS) and disseminated intravascular coagulation (DIC). In relatively asymptomatic and nonacute outpatients, the most common causes of thrombocytopenia are hypersplenism due to liver cirrhosis, idiopathic thrombocytopenic purpura (ITP), and drug reaction, most notoriously secondary to trimethoprim-sulfamethoxazole ("Bactrim"), cardiac medications (e.g., quinidine, procainamide, thiazide diuretics), antirheumatic drugs (gold salts [rarely used these days]), and heparin. Heparin-induced thrombocytopenia (HIT, type-2) is potentially fatal and requires immediate cessation of heparin administration. Patients with unexplained persistent thrombocytopenia should be tested for HIV, autoimmunity (ANA), and lymphoproliferative disorders (PBS, immunophenotyping, serum protein electrophoresis and serum immunofixation). Isolated mild to moderate thrombocytopenia (75,000 – 150,000 platelets per microliter) during pregnancy generally is considered nonpathologic.
Advantages:	▪ The **CBC with differential** is inexpensive and easy to perform and is appropriate for asymptomatic patients. The "CBC with diff" is an appropriate first test for patients who are symptomatic (e.g., fatigue, fever) or have an ongoing history of health problems. In certain healthcare settings where cost containment is a major priority, CBC *without* differential is commonly ordered; however, in outpatient private practice, the additional expenditure of $2 for the CBC *with* differential is the preferred evaluation. It provides a quick screen for anemia, leukemia, infection, and for provisional evidence of B-12/folate and iron deficiencies. The CBC can also identify more complex conditions such as pancytopenia and thereby promote comprehensive patient management; for example, pancytopenia may unmask hepatic cirrhosis which may necessitate use of nadolol for prophylaxis against gastroesophageal variceal hemorrhage as well as use of prophylactic antibiotics against spontaneous bacterial peritonitis. ▪ The **peripheral blood smear (PBS)** is used to further evaluate leukocytosis, anemias, and other abnormalities. In the investigation of persistent leukocytosis, the PBS is of limited value and therefore, while the PBS should certainly be performed, it is generally followed by **immunophenotyping by flow cytometry** if not a direct referral to a hematologist. An excellent review by Tefferi et al[109] concluded, "In general, it is prudent to perform a PBS in most instances of abnormal CBC, along with basic tests that are dictated by the type of CBC abnormalities. The latter may include, for example, serum ferritin in patients with microcytic anemia or lymphocyte immunophenotyping by flow cytometry in patients with lymphocytosis..."
Limitations:	▪ WBC count may be normal even in patients with serious infections. ▪ RBC indices may be normal in people with severe iron deficiency. ○ **Dr Vasquez's experience**—*Many outpatients with no evidence of anemia on the CBC will be grossly iron deficient with ferritin values less than 6 mcg/L, clearly indicating iron deficiency. Nonanemic iron deficiency contributes to fatigue, depression, and attention deficit.*
Comments:	▪ The **CBC** is a foundational part of the assessment for all new patients. Generally, "CBC *with* differential" should be ordered.

[109] Tefferi A, Hanson CA, Inwards DJ. How to interpret and pursue an abnormal complete blood cell count in adults. *Mayo Clin Proc* 2005;80(7):923-3

Presentation: Classic iron insufficiency in a healthy 32yo athletic female: This limited laboratory report is from a 32yo athletic female whose primary complaint is that of "less endurance than expected" given her healthy lifestyle and frequent participation in physical exercise of various types such as running, biking, hiking, and kayaking. Her TSH is on the low end of normal consistent with her taking 17 mcg daily of liothyroinine (T3); note however that the total T3 level remains on the low end of the normal range, suggesting that she may benefit from additional T3 supplementation. The RBC parameters Hgb and Hct are on the low end of the normal range consistent with recent menstruation; the response of the bone marrow to recent blood loss is noted with the RDW being toward the high end of normal, refecting increased marrow production of reticulocytes. Ferritin is suboptimal at 25 ng/mL, given that the optimal range is approximately 40-70 ng/mL.[110] Altough various iron supplements are available on the market and high-iron foods such as beef and blackstrap molasis can be used, typical treatment is with iron 18 mg per day often provided as ferrous sulfate 90 mg; note that 5 mg ferrous sulfate = 1 mg elemental iron. Other forms of iron such as ferrous aspartate may be better tolerated. Daily iron supplementation for 2-3 months should elevate the ferritin level and improve the feeling of energy not simply by ❶ improving oxygen delivery to tissues but also by ❷ improving function of the electron transport chain where iron is a required cofactor, ❸ improving the conversion of thyroid hormone (T4) into the active form of T3, and by ❹ improving the production of dopamine and norepinephrine, since iron is a required cofactor for the enzyme tyrosine hydroxylase which converts the amino acid tyrosine into L-DOPA which is converted to dopamine and then partially to norepinephrine. Given that this patient menstruates monthly and has no significant medical history and—specifically—no gastrointestinal complaints; the probability is high that her state of iron insufficiency is due to physiologic blood loss; however, a case could be made for endoscopic evaluation[111], and in the event that the patient suffered from an diagnosed intestinal lesion such as colon cancer, the practitioner who did not refer for gastroenterologic evaluation would be challenged to produce effective medicolegal defense. Guidelines[112] published in 2011 support testing for celiac disease, *H. pylori* infection, and hematuria while reserving endoscopy in premenopausal women to those aged 50 years or older, or with symptoms of gastrointestinal disease, or those with a strong family history of colorectal cancer.

Reported: 07/07/2011 / 06:02 CDT

Test Name	In Range	Out Of Range	Reference Range
TSH, 3RD GENERATION	0.54		mIU/L
	Reference Range		
	> or = 20 Years 0.40-4.50		
	Pregnancy Ranges		
	First trimester 0.20-4.70		
	Second trimester 0.30-4.10		
	Third trimester 0.40-2.70		
T3, TOTAL	97		76-181 ng/dL
CBC (INCLUDES DIFF/PLT)			
WHITE BLOOD CELL COUNT	7.1		3.8-10.8 Thousand/uL
RED BLOOD CELL COUNT	4.28		3.80-5.10 Million/uL
HEMOGLOBIN	12.1		11.7-15.5 g/dL
HEMATOCRIT	36.2		35.0-45.0 %
MCV	84.5		80.0-100.0 fL
MCH	28.4		27.0-33.0 pg
MCHC	33.6		32.0-36.0 g/dL
RDW	14.8		11.0-15.0 %
PLATELET COUNT	248		140-400 Thousand/uL
ABSOLUTE NEUTROPHILS	3586		1500-7800 cells/uL
ABSOLUTE LYMPHOCYTES	2854		850-3900 cells/uL
ABSOLUTE MONOCYTES	525		200-950 cells/uL
ABSOLUTE EOSINOPHILS	107		15-500 cells/uL
ABSOLUTE BASOPHILS	28		0-200 cells/uL
NEUTROPHILS	50.5		%
LYMPHOCYTES	40.2		%
MONOCYTES	7.4		%
EOSINOPHILS	1.5		%
BASOPHILS	0.4		%
FERRITIN	25		10-154 ng/mL

[110] See excerpt from Vasquez A. *Integrative Rheumatology*. http://optimalhealthresearch.com/hemochromatosis.html
[111] "A gastrointestinal source of chronic blood loss was identified in a substantial proportion of premenopausal women with iron deficiency anemia." Green BT, Rockey DC. Gastrointestinal endoscopic evaluation of premenopausal women with iron deficiency anemia. *J Clin Gastroenterol*. 2004 Feb;38(2):104-9
[112] Goddard AF, James MW, McIntyre AS, Scott BB; on behalf of the British Society of Gastroenterology. Guidelines for the management of iron deficiency anaemia. *Gut*. 2011 Jun 6. [Epub ahead of print] http://www.epocrates.com/dacc/1106/irondefbmj1106.pdf

Presentation: Vitamin B-12 deficiency without hematologic abnormality—report and discussion: This elderly patient shows no signs of anemia; note also that the MCV is perfectly normal. Given that the psychiatric literature supports a minimal serum vitamin B-12 level of 600 pg/ml, the advocation by medical reference laboratories of a lower "normal" limit of 200 pg/ml is scientifically absurd and ethically indefensible; this is yet another example of the importance of clinicians' knowledge of the literature overriding the laboratory's reference range. The consistent documentation of the rapid reversibility of severe neuropsychiatric illness with vitamin B-12 therapy as the only intervention[113,114] provides additional justification for empiric vitamin B-12 administration in patients with clinical symptoms consistent with vitamin B-12 deficiency regardless of hematologic and serologic findings.[115] Vitamin B-12 deficiency is very serious because it can lead to permanent brain damage, resulting in personality changes, memory impairment, and overt psychotic disorders, including catatonia; mechanisms of neurologic injury may include homocysteine toxicity, autoimmune neuronal demyelinization, and axonal degeneration and nerve-sheath demyelination especially in the median forebrain bundle area.[116]

HEMATOLOGY

----- CBC - WBC STUDIES -----

Procedure:	WBC 10E3
Reference:	[4.50-11.00]
Units:	/CMM
07DEC06 0926 THU	7.32

----- CBC - RBC STUDIES -----

Procedure:	RBC 10E6	HEMOGLOBIN	HEMATOCRIT	MCV	MCH	MCHC	RDW-CV
Reference:	[4.50-5.90]	[13.5-17.5]	[41.0-53.0]	[80.0-94.0]	[27.0-31.0]	[32.0-36.0]	[11.0-16.0]
Units:	/CMM	G/DL	%	FL	PG	%	%
07DEC06 0926 THU	5.16	15.7	46.3	89.7	30.4	33.9	14.1

----- CBC - PLATELET STUDIES -----

Procedure:	PLATELET 10E3	MPV
Reference:	[150-500]	[9.0-13.0]
Units:	/CMM	FL
07DEC06 0926 THU	308	11.2

CHEMISTRY PROFILES

----- ROUTINE CHEMISTRY PROFILES -----

Procedure:	SODIUM	POTASSIUM	CHLORIDE	CO2	GLUCOSE	BUN	CREATININE	CALCIUM
Reference:	[133-145]	[3.5-5.3]	[100-110]	[22.0-29.0]	[70-110]	[5-25]	[0.5-1.4]	[8.3-10.3]
Units:	MMOL/L	MEQ/L	MMOL/L	MMOL/L	MG/DL	MG/DL	MG/DL	MG/DL
07DEC06 0926 THU	137	4.3	101	27.0	90	16	0.9	9.9

Procedure:	ANION GAP	OSMOLARITY	BUN/CREAT
Reference:	[6-14]	[272-305]	
Units:	MEQ/L	MOSM/K	MG/DL
07DEC06 0926 THU	13	275	17.8

SPECIAL CHEMISTRY

----- CHEMISTRY SPECIAL/MISCELLANEOUS -----

Procedure:	FOLATE	VITAMIN B-12
Reference:	[2.0-18.0]	[193-982]
Units:	NG/ML	PG/ML
07DEC06 0926 THU	14.7	182 L

---

[113] Berry N, Sagar R, Tripathi BM. Catatonia and other psychiatric symptoms with vitamin B12 deficiency. *Acta Psychiatr Scand*. 2003 ;108(2):156-9
[114] Newbold HL. Vitamin B-12: placebo or neglected therapeutic tool? *Med Hypotheses*. 1989 Mar;28(3):155-64
[115] Solomon LR. Cobalamin-responsive disorders in the ambulatory care setting: unreliability of cobalamin, methylmalonic acid, and homocysteine testing. *Blood*. 2005 Feb 1;105(3):978-85
[116] Catalano G, Catalano MC, Rosenberg EI, Embi PJ, Embi CS. Catatonia. Another neuropsychiatric presentation of vitamin B12 deficiency? *Psychosomatics*. 1998 Sep-Oct;39(5):456-60 http://psy.psychiatryonline.org/cgi/reprint/39/5/456

Consequences of vitamin B-12 deficiency:

Initially the manifestations are mild and reversible, but over time they become more severe and strongly refractory to treatment to the point that permanent damage (particularly in the CNS) is anticipated:

- "Bipolar disorder"—a condition indistinguishable from a bipolar disorder,
- Organic brain syndrome, delirium, confusion, poor memory, impaired cognition,
- Dementia and erroneous diagnosis of "Alzheimer's disease",
- Mood disorders, depression, catatonia, paranoia, paranoid psychosis, violent behavior,
- Peripheral neuropathy, "combined degeneration" of anterior and posterior columns of the spinal cord,
- As a result of the above problems, patients who are mismanaged by doctors unknowledgeable about basic nutrition often suffer directly from these effects but also suffer from the medical management from these problems. Mood disorders and psychosis may result from B-12 deficiency, and the medical management of mood disorders and psychosis includes medicalization, electroconvulsive therapy (ECT), and institutionalization.

The medical profession's failure to train its students and doctors in nutrition is widely and consistently documented; given that such a profession-wide policy can do nothing other than result in patient harm and/or drug dependency under the guise of "healthcare", it is—borrowing a phrase from Nietzsche—"the highest of all conceivable corruptions."

- Nutritional deficiencies and the medical paradigm (*J Clin Endocrinol Metab* 2003 Nov): "But public health measures in the first half of the 20th century eradicated the most extreme of the vitamin deficiencies in the industrialized nations, and the physician's actual experience of [obvious] deficiency disease dropped to near zero. Perhaps as a result, the medical profession's approach to nutrition today is still dominated by the external agent paradigm, as witnessed in the national campaigns for cholesterol, saturated fat, and salt. Those who think more seriously in terms of the continuing importance of deficiency per se are often derogated or relegated to the quackery fringe. The result, at the very least, is inattention to the real deficiencies that may masquerade as other disorders, or that may simply be ignored altogether."
- Failure of surgical treatment for low-back pain caused by vitamin D deficiency (*J Am Board Fam Med* 2009 Jan): The author of this case series describes six cases of chronic debilitating back pain—three of which "required surgery"—which were greatly relieved or completely cured by correction of vitamin D deficiency. The author notes, "Chronic low back pain and failed back surgery may improve with repletion of vitamin D from a state of deficiency/insufficiency to sufficiency. Vitamin D insufficiency is common; repletion of vitamin D to normal levels in patients who have chronic low back pain or have had failed back surgery may improve quality of life or, in some cases, result in complete resolution of symptoms."

That nutritional deficiencies can cause mood disorders and mental disease is well-known; in contrast to what patients actually need, the general allopathic approach to these clinical presentations is founded upon the administration of drugs, followed by ECT, institutionalization, and psychosurgery and—lately, instead of scalpel-induced brain damage—radiofrequency heating (thermocapsulotomy) or gamma radiation (radiosurgery, gammacapsulotomy) for the destruction of brain structures, and the surgical implantation of brain electrostimulators. Meanwhile, thousands of these psychiatrically-labeled patients simply need nutritional supplementation. Minor exceptions noted, the medical profession as a whole chooses to remain blind to the value of nutrition so that the pharmacosurgical paradigm can remain dominant by continuing to *appear* omnipotent. The dual illusions that are maintained are "Drugs and surgery are the answers to all major health problems" and "If no drug exists for a condition, then it is idiopathic and no curative treatment is available."

As an example, type-2 diabetes mellitus (T2DM) has burgeoned into an epidemic under the dominance of the allopathic disease model, and patients are told that the condition is genetic, progressive and incurable; a review published in the May 2011 issue of *Journal of the American Osteopathic Association* admonished physicians to (mis)educate their patients as follows, with Dr Vasquez's comments in brackets: "Be absolutely clear that T2DM is a lifelong disease [false statement] that will require lifelong treatment [false statement fostering dependency]. Success in controlling the disease and preventing future complications will depend on the patient and physician working together [creation of dependency under the guise of "working together"]. There is often a fatalistic attitude in patients with T2DM [perhaps because they have been lied to and disempowered], so it is important to establish a relationship that on one hand offers hope [creating the illusion of hope while enforcing drug dependency] and on the other does not suggest that the disease will be cured [although the diseases is generally curable with appropriate nutritional intervention]. Be up front with the patient from the first visit and make it clear that T2DM is a chronic illness [enforce drug dependency starting a the first visit]…" This babble

Nutritional deficiency, diet-responsive disorders, and the allopathic medical paradigm: Review and commentary with emphases on diabetes mellitus and vitamins D and B-12	

was published in a peer-reviewed medical journal despite clear multi-decade evidence showing that T2DM is reversible with nutritional intervention. Recent examples of the safety and efficacy of diet intervention for T2DM are provided here with many more examples and details in *Nutritional, Integrative and Functional Medicine Mastery of Common Clinical Disorders*.

- T2DM is rapidly reversible with diet (*Diabetologia* 2011 Jun): "Normalization of both beta cell function and hepatic insulin sensitivity in type 2 diabetes was achieved by dietary energy restriction alone. This was associated with decreased pancreatic and liver triacylglycerol stores. **The abnormalities underlying type 2 diabetes are reversible by reducing dietary energy intake**."
- Diet therapy effective, safe, and is at least as effective as injected insulin for reducing chronic hyperglycemia in T2DM (*Nutr Metab* 2009 May): "The number of patients on sulfonylureas decreased from 7 at baseline to 2 at 6 months. No patient required inpatient care or insulin therapy. In summary, the 30%-carbohydrate diet over 6 months led to a remarkable reduction in HbA1c levels, even among outpatients with severe type 2 diabetes, without any insulin therapy, hospital care or increase in sulfonylureas. **The effectiveness of the [low-carbohydrate] diet may be comparable to that of insulin therapy**."

Ironically (or not), the first-line drug for T2DM—metformin—causes vitamin B-12 (cobalamin, Cbl) deficiency and exacerbation of the often debilitating peripheral neuropathy of T2DM which is often treated with the drugs gabapentin/Neurontin or pregabalin/Lyrica, which exacerbates obesity and T2DM, thereby promoting a vicious cycle.

- Pregabalin/Lyrica and gabapentin/Neurontin promote fat-weight gain, thereby exacerbating T2DM (*Prescrire Int* 2005 Dec): "Pregabalin, like gabapentin, can lead to weight gain and peripheral edema especially in elderly patients."
- Metformin causes vitamin B-12 deficiency and exacerbates diabetic peripheral neuropathy (*Diabetes Care* 2010 Jan): "Metformin-treated patients had depressed Cbl levels and elevated fasting MMA and Hcy levels. Clinical and electrophysiological measures identified more severe peripheral neuropathy in these patients; the cumulative metformin dose correlated strongly with these clinical and paraclinical group differences. CONCLUSIONS: Metformin exposure may be an iatrogenic cause for exacerbation of peripheral neuropathy in patients with type 2 diabetes."
- Vitamin B-12 deficiency secondary to metformin prescription (*Rev Assoc Med Bras* 2011 Jan): "The present findings suggest a high prevalence of vitamin B12 deficiency in metformin-treated diabetic patients [n=144]. Older patients, patients in long term treatment with metformin and low vitamin B12 intake are probably more prone to this deficiency."
- Metformin-induced vitamin B12 deficiency presenting as a peripheral neuropathy (*South Med J* 2010 Mar): "Chronic metformin use results in vitamin B12 deficiency in 30% of patients. ... **Vitamin B12 deficiency, which may present without anemia and as a peripheral neuropathy, is often misdiagnosed as diabetic neuropathy, although the clinical findings are usually different. Failure to diagnose the cause of the neuropathy will result in progression of central and/or peripheral neuronal damage which can be arrested but not reversed with vitamin B12 replacement**."
- Low vitamin B-12 status correlates with expedited brain atrophy (*Neurology* 2008 Sep): "The decrease in brain volume was greater among those with lower vitamin B(12) and holoTC levels and higher plasma tHcy and MMA levels at baseline. ... Using the upper (for the vitamins) or lower tertile (for the metabolites) as reference in logistic regression analysis and adjusting for the above covariates, vitamin B(12) in the bottom tertile (<308 pmol/L) was associated with increased rate of brain volume loss (odds ratio 6.17, 95% CI 1.25-30.47)."

Consequences for the clinician:
Given that the evidence in favor of early and empiric treatment for possible vitamin B-12 deficiency is stronger than evidence in favor of allowing vitamin B-12 deficiency or dependency to persist with potentially catastrophic outcomes, no scientific argument can be made in favor of failing to diagnose and treat vitamin B-12 deficiency/dependency. However, since, in general, the allopathic and osteopathic medical professions have failed to educate their students and doctors about nutrition, these professions have established ignorance as their defense and therefore no standard of care exists for the treatment or failure of treatment of chronic nutritional deficiencies. Ethically, the results are failure to achieve beneficence via failure to diagnose and treat, and the widespread implementation of malfeasance via diagnostic/therapeutic failure complicated by the unnecessary expenses and adverse effects of drugs/surgeries/interventions used in place of nutritional

supplementation. The enforcement of a standard of care is meaningless when nutritional incompetence is the standard. Fortunately for patients, the biomedical literature uses increasingly strong language in favor of mandating standards for nutritional evaluation and treatment:

- Nutritional deficiencies and the medical paradigm (*J Clin Endocrinol Metab* 2003 Nov): "J. Cannell (submitted for publication) has written that measures such as this editorial will not change the situation, and that only tort litigation will work. One can only hope that he is wrong. Either way, something needs to change"
- Physicians should routinely use vitamin supplementation as treatment for patients (*JAMA* 2002 Jun): "Physicians should make specific efforts to ensure that patients are taking vitamins they should..."
- Testing and treating for vitamin D deficiency among patients with chronic nonspecific musculoskeletal pain should be the standard of care (*Mayo Clin Proc* 2003 Dec): "Because osteomalacia is a known cause of persistent, nonspecific musculoskeletal pain, screening all outpatients with such pain for hypovitaminosis D should be standard practice in clinical care."
- Testing and treating for vitamin D deficiency among patients with chronic low-back pain should be the standard of care (*Spine* 2003 Jan): "Screening for vitamin D deficiency and treatment with supplements should be mandatory in this setting."

Citations for this section:
1. Catalano G, Catalano MC, Rosenberg EI, Embi PJ, Embi CS. Catatonia. Another neuropsychiatric presentation of vitamin B12 deficiency? *Psychosomatics*. 1998 Sep-Oct;39(5):456-60
2. Newbold HL. Vitamin B-12: placebo or neglected therapeutic tool? *Med Hypotheses*. 1989 Mar;28(3):155-64
3. Solomon LR. Cobalamin-responsive disorders in the ambulatory care setting: unreliability of cobalamin, methylmalonic acid, and homocysteine testing. *Blood*. 2005 Feb 1;105(3):978-85
4. Christmas D, Eljamel MS, Butler S, et al. Long term outcome of thermal anterior capsulotomy for chronic, treatment refractory depression. *J Neurol Neurosurg Psychiatry*. 2011 Jun;82(6):594-600
5. Malone DA Jr. Use of deep brain stimulation in treatment-resistant depression. *Cleve Clin J Med*. 2010 Jul;77 Suppl 3:S77-80
6. Heaney RP. Vitamin D, nutritional deficiency, and the medical paradigm. *J Clin Endocrinol Metab*. 2003;88:5107-8
7. Schwalfenberg G. Improvement of chronic back pain or failed back surgery with vitamin D repletion: a case series. *J Am Board Fam Med*. 2009 Jan-Feb;22(1):69-74
8. Gavin JR 3rd, Freeman JS, Shubrook JH Jr, Lavernia F. Type 2 diabetes mellitus: practical approaches for primary care physicians. *J Am Osteopath Assoc*. 2011 May;111(5 Suppl 4):S3-S12
9. Lim EL, Hollingsworth KG, Aribisala BS, et al. Reversal of type 2 diabetes: normalisation of beta cell function in association with decreased pancreas and liver triacylglycerol. *Diabetologia*. 2011 Jun 9. Published on-line.
10. Haimoto H, Sasakabe T, Wakai K, Umegaki H. Effects of a low-carbohydrate diet on glycemic control in outpatients with severe type 2 diabetes. *Nutr Metab* 2009:6;21
11. Gabapentin/Neurontin causes "Gains of up to 15 kg (33lbs) during 3 months of treatment." http://pacmedweightloss.com/docs/medications_that_cause_weight_gain.pdf Accessed July 2011.
12. Vogiatzoglou A, Refsum H, Johnston C, Smith SM, Bradley KM, de Jager C, Budge MM, Smith AD. Vitamin B12 status and rate of brain volume loss in community-dwelling elderly. *Neurology*. 2008 Sep 9;71(11):826-32
13. Wile DJ, Toth C. Association of metformin, elevated homocysteine, and methylmalonic acid levels and clinically worsened diabetic peripheral neuropathy. *Diabetes Care*. 2010 Jan;33(1):156-61
14. Nervo M, Lubini A, Raimundo FV, Faulhaber GA, Leite C, Fischer LM, Furlanetto TW. Vitamin B12 in metformin-treated diabetic patients: a cross-sectional study in Brazil. *Rev Assoc Med Bras*. 2011 Jan-Feb;57(1):46-9
15. Bell DS. Metformin-induced vitamin B12 deficiency presenting as a peripheral neuropathy. *South Med J*. 2010 Mar;103(3):265-7
16. [No authors listed] Pregabalin: new drug. Very similar to gabapentin. *Prescrire Int*. 2005 Dec;14(80):203-6
17. Fletcher RH, Fairfield KM. Harvard Medical School. Vitamins for chronic disease prevention in adults: clinical applications. *JAMA*. 2002;287:3127-9
18. Plotnikoff GA, Quigley JM. Prevalence of severe hypovitaminosis D in patients with persistent, nonspecific musculoskeletal pain. *Mayo Clin Proc*. 2003;78:1463-70
19. Al Faraj S, Al Mutairi K. Vitamin D deficiency and chronic low back pain in Saudi Arabia. *Spine* 2003 ;28:177-9

UA: Urinalysis	

Overview and interpretation:	▪ <u>Collection</u>: Unless catheterized, patients are advised to pass approximately one-third of their available urine into the toilet, then pass approximately the middle-third of their urine into the specimen container. Use of an antiseptic to clean the urethral meatus was once advocated to avoid/reduce specimen contamination, but this step is ineffective and therefore unnecessary because contamination rates remain similar at 32% and 29% whether or not, respectively, urethral meatus cleansing is performed.[117]
	
	▪ <u>Analysis</u>: Analysis should be performed on fresh urine, preferably within 1-2 hours; in outpatient clinical practice this two-hour timeframe is consistently possible only if the clinician performs in-office dipstick analysis (and perhaps microscopic visualization). Samples that cannot be analyzed within 1-2 hours or those which are destined for a reference laboratory should be refrigerated. Dipstick UA can be performed in office and is simple, inexpensive, and—when performed and interpreted with a modicum of competence—sufficiently accurate. Per Klatt[118], "The color change occurring on each segment of the strip is compared to a color chart to obtain results. However, a careless doctor, nurse, or assistant is entirely capable of misreading or misinterpreting the results." Urine samples can be sent to a reference laboratory for more accurate chemical analysis as well as microscopic analysis, culture and sensitivity. Whether infection is clinically suspected or not, clinicians might chose to order "UA with reflex to microscopy and culture" to ensure that urine samples are appropriately processed if the laboratory finds suspicion of UTI upon dipstick analysis.
	
	▪ <u>Scope of this review</u>: The purpose of this brief review is to concisely refresh clinicians' appreciation of the components of the routine urinalysis, one that is generally performed in-office with a dipstick reagent stick or that is performed by a reference laboratory. This is not an exhaustive review, and microscopic findings have not been detailed here because most clinicians do not perform microscopy in their offices; additional details on UA and microscopic assessment is available in articles such as the excellent review by Simerville, Maxted, and Pahira published in *American Family Physician* 2005 and available on-line at http://www.aafp.org/afp/2005/0315/p1153.html as of July 2011.
	
	▪ <u>Components of routine urinalysis</u>:
	   o <u>Visual inspection</u>: Urine should be clear with a color ranging from faint yellow (well hydrated, dilute urine) to bright yellow (especially with B-vitamin supplementation). An amber-brown hue might be due to dehydration or a pathologic process resulting in myoglobinuria (i.e., rhabdomyolysis) or the presence of bile pigments (i.e., biliary tract obstruction). A red color to urine suggests hematuria, recent beet consumption, or use of certain drugs or food dyes; the antibiotic rifampin/rifampicin is notorious for adding a red-orange color to the urine (and to a lesser extent to sweat and tears). The urine of patients with porphyria cutanea tarda will be red-brown in natural light and pink-red in fluorescent light.[119] Cloudy urine is due to pyruia (infection), proteinuria, or precipitated phosphate crystals in alkaline urine.
	   o <u>Strong odor</u>: Odiferous or malodorous urine suggests infection, recent ingestion of foods such as asparagus or nutritional supplements such as lipoic acid, certain medications, concentrated urine due to dehydration or underperfusion of the kidneys.
	   o <u>Specific gravity</u>: Specific gravity is a measure of solute concentration and thus is proportional to urine osmolality; as such it reflects renal perfusion, hydration, and the ability of the kidneys to perform their critical function of concentrating filtrate. Dilute urine has a specific gravity <1.010 and is seen with adequate/excessive hydration, diuretic use, diabetes insipidus, adrenal insufficiency, hyperaldosteronism, and impaired renal

[117] Simerville JA, Maxted WC, Pahira JJ. Urinalysis: a comprehensive review. *Am Fam Physician.* 2005 Mar 15;71(6):1153-62 http://www.aafp.org/afp/2005/0315/p1153.html
[118] Klatt EC. WebPath. Savannah, Georgia, USA. http://library.med.utah.edu/WebPath/tutorial/urine/urine.html Accessed July 1, 2011
[119] Rich MW. Porphyria cutanea tarda. Don't forget to look at the urine. *Postgrad Med.* 1999 Apr;105(4):208-10, 213-4

function (i.e., failure of the kidneys to concentrate urine). Concentrated urine has a specific gravity >1.020 and correlates with dehydration, renal artery stenosis, hypoperfusion/shock, glucosuria, and syndrome of inappropriate anti-diuretic hormone secretion (SIADH), which is often associated with hyponatremia.

- o pH: Urine pH may range from 4.5 (very acidic) to as high as 8.5 (very alkaline). Urine pH correlates with serum pH except in patients with renal tubular acidosis (RTA type-1, a condition associated with chronically alkaline urine). Therefore, urine pH can be used to screen for various conditions of systemic alkalosis and acidosis. The Western diet—also called the standard American diet or S.A.D.—causes mild diet-induced metabolic acidosis[120] which promotes degenerative diseases; in contrast, a diet rich in fruits and vegetables such as the Paleo-Mediterranean diet[121] promotes mild systemic and urinary alkalinization.[122] From a wellness perspective, urine pH should be 7.5 up to 8.0 because urinary alkalinization facilitates xenobiotic excretion[123], promotes urinary retention of minerals such as potassium, magnesium, and calcium, and causes a reduction in serum cortisol.[124] Urine pH—like urine sodium:potassium ratio—can be used as a marker of compliance for intake of fruits, vegetables, and alkalinizing supplements such as potassium citrate. For some patients (mostly female), urine alkalinization may encourage urinary tract infection, especially if gastrointestinal dysbiosis[125] is present; in such situations, the often causative GI dysbiosis should be treated, and consistent or transient urinary acidification can be achieved with oral ascorbic acid. Urea-splitting bacteria can cause the urine to be alkaline, and such bacteria can also promote development of magnesium-ammonium phosphate crystals and so-called staghorn nephrolithiasis. Acidic urine promotes development of uric acid nephrolithiasis; therapeutic urinary alkalinization such as by use of supplemental potassium citrate or an alkalinizing diet is preventive and therapeutic. On this topic, Cicerello et al[126] wrote, "In conclusion urinary alkalization with maintaining continuously high urinary pH values, could be the treatment of choice for stone dissolution and prevention of uric acid stones."
- o Bilirubin in urine: If present, bilirubin in urine is of the direct/conjugated fraction (rather than indirect/unconjugated, which is nonhydrosoluble) and indicates the need to evaluate for biliary tract obstruction.
- o Urobilinogen: Urobilinogen is (direct) bilirubin that has been conjugated in the liver, passed through the biliary system into the intestine, partially metabolized by bacteria, then reabsorbed via the portal circulation and filtered by the kidney. Elevated urobilinogen is associated with liver disease and hemolytic diseases.
- o Glucose: Glucose is found in the urine when the serum glucose exceeds approximately 190 mg/dL and overwhelms the reabsorptive capacity of the proximal tubule. Glucose in the urine is presumptive evidence supporting the diagnosis of diabetes mellitus. Rare non-diabetic causes of glucosuria/glycosuria include liver disease, pancreatic disease, and Fanconi's syndrome (characterized by a failure of the proximal renal tubules to reabsorb glucose, amino acids, uric acid, phosphate and bicarbonate).

---

[120] "The modern Western-type diet is deficient in fruits and vegetables and contains excessive animal products, generating the accumulation of non-metabolizable anions and a lifespan state of overlooked metabolic acidosis, whose magnitude increases progressively with aging due to the physiological decline in kidney function." Adeva MM, Souto G. Diet-induced metabolic acidosis. *Clin Nutr.* 2011 Aug;30(4):416-21. Epub 2011 Apr 9.

[121] **Vasquez A**. Revisiting the Five-Part Nutritional Wellness Protocol: The Supplemented Paleo-Mediterranean Diet. *Nutritional Perspectives* 2011 January This article is available at http://optimalhealthresearch.com/part8.html and is also included in this textbook.

[122] Cordain L, Eaton SB, Sebastian A, Mann N, Lindeberg S, Watkins BA, O'Keefe JH, Brand-Miller J. Origins and evolution of the Western diet: health implications for the 21st century. *Am J Clin Nutr.* 2005 Feb;81(2):341-54

[123] Proudfoot AT, Krenzelok EP, Vale JA. Position Paper on urine alkalinization. *J Toxicol Clin Toxicol.* 2004;42(1):1-26

[124] Maurer M, Riesen W, Muser J, Hulter HN, Krapf R. Neutralization of Western diet inhibits bone resorption independently of K intake and reduces cortisol secretion in humans. *Am J Physiol Renal Physiol.* 2003 Jan;284(1):F32-40

[125] **Vasquez A**. Reducing Pain and Inflammation Naturally - Part 6: Nutritional and Botanical Treatments Against "Silent Infections" and Gastrointestinal Dysbiosis, Commonly Overlooked Causes of Neuromusculoskeletal Inflammation and Chronic Health Problems. *Nutritional Perspectives* 2006; January. For a more extensive review, see the most recent edition of Integrative Rheumatology: http://optimalhealthresearch.com/rheumatology.html

[126] Cicerello E, Merlo F, Maccatrozzo L. Urinary alkalization for the treatment of uric acid nephrolithiasis. *Arch Ital Urol Androl.* 2010 Sep;82(3):145-8

UA: Urinalysis

- ○ <u>Ketones</u>: UA dipsticks detect acetic acid; other products of fatty acid metabolism found in urine include acetone and beta-hydroxybutyric acid. Ketonuria indicates either metabolic disturbance such as diabetes mellitus or normal physiology in the fasting or lipolytic state. Many clinicians—particularly medical students and physicians[note 127]—have been taught to view ketonuria as synonymous with ketoacidosis; this is obviously inaccurate since lipolysis and the resulting ketonuria are normal *and quite desirable* physiologic states. Ketonuria can be measured with ketone-specific dipsticks as a marker of weight-loss efficacy and compliance with diet and exercise programs.
- ○ <u>Protein</u>: Urine should not contain measurable protein on routine urinalysis. Any finding of protein in the urine—even a "trace" amount—requires follow-up; specifically, the test should be repeated within 2-4 weeks and consistently positive results require more detailed testing including serum BUN and creatinine. Urine protein can also be measured in 24-hour urine collections and should not exceed 150 mg/day; greater than this amount is diagnostic of proteinuria, while ≥ 3.5 gm/day is consistent with nephrotic syndrome, mandating a much more comprehensive *and urgent* patient evaluation. Testing for "protein" with a routine urinalysis will not detect all forms of clinically relevant proteinuria; specifically and classically, routine UA is insensitive for the microalbuminuria of diabetes mellitus (detected with the urinary albumin:creatinine ratio) and also the Bence-Jones proteinuria seen with multiple myeloma.

Evaluation of persistent proteinuria
1. Comprehensive evaluation of patient history, physical exam, and overall clinical impression,
2. Measurement of serum BUN, creatinine, albumin, and lipids; consider measuring cystatin c,
3. Microscopic examination of urinary sediment,
4. Assessment for conditions that commonly cause proteinuria, especially hypertension (sphygmomanometry), diabetes (hemoglobin A1c), autoimmune conditions (screen with ANA);
5. Measurement of 24-hour urinary creatinine excretion (or spot urinary albumin-creatinine ratio),
6. Urinary protein electrophoresis,
7. If the above measures are pathoetiologically unfruitful, refer to an internist or nephrologist.

---

[127] One of the arguments most commonly leveled against the ketogenic diet—in particular the Atkins diet—is that the induction of ketosis, as measured by ketonuria, is a potentially problematic state that should be avoided. This is an example of selective medical ignorance since mild ketosis is physiologically normal is clinically advantageous for weight loss and seizure control. In our osteopathic medical school, one lecturer advised our student body of 170 that ketosis was evidence of the "danger from diet therapies." On the contrary, given that most of my medical school professors were obese, they should have more carefully considered the benefits of rational dietary therapy, including low-carbohydrate versions of the Paleo-Mediterranean diet (described in this text) which can produce mild ketosis en route to alleviating diabetes mellitus and hypertension. Examples of selective medical ignorance and bias against low-carbohydrate ketogenic diets abound from allopathic institutions. "One diet that has raised safety concerns among the scientific community is the low-carbohydrate, high-protein diet." Tapper-Gardzina Y, Cotugna N, Vickery CE. Should you recommend a low-carb, high-protein diet? *Nurse Pract.* 2002 Apr;27(4):52-3, 55-6, 58-9. "High Protein / Low Carb (Carbohydrate) Diets. Long term, these fad diets can be harmful. Many of the health claims about these diets are not based on scientific proof. Low carb diets are still just that – a diet. Most people find maintaining a low carb diet difficult if not impossible long term. Even if weight is lost, 90% of fad dieters gain all or most of the weight back in five years." Ohio State University. http://medicalcenter.osu.edu/PatientEd/Materials/PDFDocs/nut-diet/nut-other/high-pro.pdf Accessed July 2011.

Overview and interpretation:	○ <u>Nitrite</u>: Urinary nit<u>ri</u>te is most often the result of bacterial action on excreted urinary nit<u>ra</u>te; students and clinicians can remember this by recalling that nit<u>ra</u>te is consumed in foods via the <u>a</u>limentary tract, while nit<u>ri</u>te in the urine generally indicates urinary tract <u>i</u>nfection (UTI). A small amount of nitrate is naturally present in some foods, including tap water, beer, some cheese products, cured meats and bacon. Additional environmental sources of nitrate include the nitrates that are intentionally added to foods as preservatives, those which are contaminants from nitrate-containing fertilizers, and those which are present in our polluted environment from pesticides and the manufacture of rubber and latex. Not all bacteria can convert nitrate to nitrite; generally, this reaction indicates the presence of Gram-negative rods such as *Escherichia coli*, the causative agent in the vast majority of UTIs in both men and women. Much less commonly, Gram-positive bacteria may also cause nitrite-positive UTI. A negative urine nitrite does not exclude UTI as it may be due to either a low-nitrate diet, diuretic use, or infection with bacteria that are incapable of reducing nitrate to nitrite. **UTI management** Finding evidence of a UTI requires the clinician to determine the nature of that UTI—urethritis, prostatitis/vaginitis, cystitis, pyelonephritis—and to evaluate the severity of the infection in the context of the patient's age and comorbidities. ○ <u>Leukocyte esterase</u>: Leukocyte esterase—as its name suggests—is an enzyme produced by white blood cells and is therefore associated with urinary tract infection. Up to five minutes is required for the enzyme to fully react with the dipstick reagent. Obviously, a positive dipstick leukocyte esterase does not itself distinguish between benign infectious cystitis and life-threatening pyelonephritis. ○ <u>Red blood cells (RBC)</u>: On a dipstick urinalysis (in contrast to a legitimate microscopic exam), "RBC" are reported not because of the presence of cells but because of the peroxidase activity of erythrocytes, which is also noted with myoglobinuria or hemoglobinuria. Thus, a dipstick analysis "positive for RBC" could indicate legitimate hematuria, or the presence of hemoglobin or myoglobin such as from marked intravascular hemolysis or rhabdomyolysis, respectively. Red blood cells in urine are not "normal" per se, but are not necessarily pathologic. Microhematuria can be induced by many benign events, including sexual intercourse, exercise, and sample contamination from menstruation. Conversely, pathologic causes of hematuria include urinary tract infections, glomerulonephritis, IgA nephropathy, and nephrolithiasis; overt hematuria is often the first sign of renal or bladder carcinoma. Thus, when consistently present over 2-3 samples, overt or microscopic hematuria—just like any degree of proteinuria—always requires the clinician's attention. **Overt hematuria and cancer** "Up to 20 percent of patients with gross hematuria have urinary tract malignancy; a full work-up with cystoscopy and upper-tract imaging is indicated in patients with this condition." Simerville JA, Maxted WC, Pahira JJ. Urinalysis: a comprehensive review. *Am Fam Physician*. 2005 Mar 15;71(6):1153-62 aafp.org/afp/2005/0315/p1153.html
Advantages:	▪ Allows point-of-care testing and thereby facilitates assessment and treatment.
Limitations:	▪ Noted above, e.g., insensitivity to microalbuminuria and mild Bence-Jones proteinuria
Comments:	▪ For additional information, please see any of several excellent clinically-oriented reviews such as Simerville JA, Maxted WC, Pahira JJ. Urinalysis: a comprehensive review. *Am Fam Physician* 2005 Mar http://www.aafp.org/afp/2005/0315/p1153.html

Presentation: Routine lab evaluation in an asymptomatic elderly female—part 1: Whereas a healthy young adult might be treated nonpharmacologically such as with fluid loading and cranberry juice for a routine UTI, clinicians should appreciate several nuances of this case that add to the complexity of appropriate management. This female patient presented for a routine annual examination. Note the patient's date of birth and the date of examination in the lower right-hand corner of the report. Because of the patient's advanced age, additional considerations are warranted. This patient was also noted to be vitamin D deficient and diabetic at the time of the exam—how does this change the overall management? Clinicians must appreciate that elderly patients are less likely to mount a symptomatic and febrile response to advanced urinary tract infections; therefore consideration to the possiblity of pyelonephritis (life-threatening) in contrast to a simple cystitis (benign) must be considered. If the patient has dementia or clinically significant forgetfulness (both of which are easily tested during the office visit), compliance with treatment is much less likely, particularly if the patient does not have access to home nursing and/or does not have a spouse, relative, friend or neighbor who can aid with the supervision of care. Urinary tract infections tend to be more aggressive in elderly patients, especially those who are diabetic, especially those with micronutrient deficiencies.

Questions:
1. What additional assessments are warranted?
2. Would fluid-loading and use of cranberry juice be appropriate treatment for this patient's UTI?
3. What follow-up is recommended?

```
URINALYSIS              01/06/10
                        11:21
U COLOR                 YELLOW
U CLARITY               CLOUDY**
U GLUCOSE               NEGATIVE
U BILE                  NEGATIVE
U KETONES               NEGATIVE
U SPEC GRAVITY          1.012
U BLOOD                 NEGATIVE
U PH                    6.0
                        (NOTE06)
U PROTEIN QUAL          20**
U UROBILINOGEN          0.2
U NITRITE               NEGATIVE
U LEUK ESTERASE         MODERATE**
U WBC                   53*H
U WBCC                  RARE**
U RBC                   5*H
U SQUAM EPITH           13
U HYALINE CAST          2
U MUCOUS                RARE
(NOTE06)
URINE SAMPLES SUBMITTED FOR TESTING MORE THAN 2 HOURS AFTER COLLECTION MAY
YIELD UNRELIABLE RESULTS WHICH INCLUDE INCREASED pH, INCREASED CRYSTAL
FORMATION AND BACTERIAL CONTENT, AND DEGRADATION OF CELLULAR ELEMENTS.
- - - - - - - - - - - - - - - - - - - - - - - - - - - - - - - - - - - - - - - -
                          BDATE: 03/20/1926 SEX: F RACE:
                          13:59 01/29/10
```

Answers:
1. Assessments: Clinical examination must include cardiac auscultatory exam, careful pulmonary auscultation for basilar crackles, dlstal extremity examination for edema and peripheral vascular disease, assessment for tenderness of the flanks, abdomen, and back. Vital signs are assessed: ❶ temperature, ❷ pulse, ❸ blood pressure, ❹ respiratory rate, and ❺ pain. A chemistry panel, CBC with differential, and CRP or ESR should be performed. The urinalysis is sent for microbial culture and sensitivity. Review patient's current drug regimen. If WBC casts were noted on the microscopic exam, then suspected pyelonephritis would warrant hospitalization.
2. Treatments: Fluid-loading would not be appropriate in an elderly patient who might have cardiopulmonary failure, renal insufficiency, or plasma electrolyte imbalance. Cranberry juice is not universally effective and is generally used for UTIs in younger patients who have evidence of *E coli* infection as evidenced by positive urinary nitrite; because this patient's nitrite is negative, a more likely probability exists that the UTI is due to Gram-positive bacteria and thus cranberry juice is less likely to be effective. A clinician could reasonably label this a complicated UTI due to the patient's advanced age and diabetes; thus, either an extended course of Bactrim DS (po b.i.d. for 7-10 days), or Ciprofloxacin (250-500 mg po b.i.d. for 3 days), or Nitrofurantoin (50-100 mg po q6h x7 days or 100 mg ER po q12h x7 days; give w/ food) would be considered. Drug choice depends on patient's tolerance, recent exposure, renal status, drugs, and results of culture and sensitivity.
3. Follow-up: Review laboratory results as soon as possible; if this visit is occurring at the end of the week, the lab should be alerted to phone the clinician with results over the weekend because concomitant leukocytosis or severe acute phase response (suggesting possible pyelonephritis or urosepsis) would change the management on an urgent basis. Patient should return to the office within 24-48 hours for reassessment and repeat UA. Patient is advised to return to office or go to hospital if symptoms develop— especially fever, chills, dizziness, or persistent nausea.

Presentation: Routine laboratory evaluation in an asymptomatic elderly female—part 2: Readers should review the lab report in the left side of the page before reading the discussion on the right side of the page. *Write the appropriate interpretation and intervention before looking at the answers in the column on the right.* Normal ranges were not provided with the original report.

```
CBC                   01/06/10
                      11:21
WBC  10E3             7.50
NRBC %               0.0
NRBC  10E3           0.00
RBC  10E6            4.08*L
HGB                 11.7*L
HCT                 35.1*L
MCV                 86.0
MCH                 28.7
MCHC                33.3
RDW-CV              13.7
RDW-SD              43.1
PLATELET 10E3        175
MPV                 12.3
------------------------------------
CHEM PANEL           01/06/10
                     11:21
SODIUM               140
POTASSIUM            4.2
CHLORIDE             102
CO2 VENOUS           27.0
GLUCOSE             248*H
BUN                  22
SER CREATININE       1.2
CALCIUM              9.5
GLOBULIN             3.2
TOTAL PROTEIN        7.3
ALBUMIN TOT          4.1
BILI TOTAL           0.5
ALKALINE PHOSPHA     63
SGOT (AST)           15
CHOLESTEROL          186
                   (NOTE01)
TRIGLYCERIDES        122
SGPT (ALT)           11
ANION GAP            11
OSMOLRTY CALC        291
BUN/CREAT            18.3
ALB/GLOB RATIO       1.30
HDL                  31
                   (NOTE02)
LDL CALC            131*H
                   (NOTE03)
(NOTE01)
BORDERLINE HIGH RISK = 200-239
HIGH RISK = 240 AND ABOVE.
(NOTE02)
12-16 HR FASTING:
(NOTE03)
NORMAL = LESS THAN 130 MG/DL
130-159 BORDERLINE/HIGH RISK
>/= 160 HIGH RISK
------------------------------------
CHEM SPECIAL         01/06/10
                     11:21
HEMOGLOBIN A1C       7.6*H
                   (NOTE04)
25-OHD TOTAL         29
------------------------------------
BDATE: 03/20/1926 SEX: F
13:59 01/29/10 FROM E585
```

This patient is anemic. The anemia is not of a severity that would be expected to cause cardiopulmonary/perfusion deficits, but the patient should be assessed, particularly if he/she has history of heart failure or lung disease such as emphysema. The MCV is not elevated, nor is it low. This could be due to combined B-12/folate and iron deficiencies; the patient should be tested and treated appropriately. Assuming that the ferritin is low, what is the next mandatory step in the management of this patient? [Answer: Treat the iron deficiency with iron supplementation but be sure to refer the patient for gastrointestinal endoscopy because of the increased probability of intestinal lesion, especially colon cancer.]

This patient is diagnosed with diabetes mellitus because the glucose is above 200. Cardioprotective measures must be implemented, ophthalmologist eye exam initiated, and foot exam performed. An integrative anti-diabetes plan[128] should be implemented.

Clinicians must appreciate the importance of the MDRD equation in this case. The answer is provided below. Perform the Cockcroft-Gault equation on paper (with use of a calculator if necessary), then perform the MDRD equation. Does this change the management of this patient's UTI? Does this change the overall management of this patient? [Answer: This patient has renal insufficiency (GFR 48-55 if African-American and 42-45 if "other race") and therefore some drugs are now contraindicated. Patient is at increased risk of hyperkalemia, especially if taking ACEi or ARB medications. The wise clinician would consider referral to an internist or nephrologist in order to ensure that the patient receives proper monitoring; for example, if the diabetes and renal insufficiency progress, the patient may require dialysis and—possibly—renal transplant, although transplant is unlikely in a patient of this advanced age.][Note 129]

Triglycerides and LDL are higher than optimal. Diet therapy and combination fatty acid supplementation (described later in this text) is indicated. Berberine might be considered as an adjunct.

HgbA1c greater than 6.5% diagnoses diabetes mellitus.

The vitamin D level is low and should be supported with oral administration of 2,000 - 10,000 IU/d and retested at 2-6 months. Serum calcium should be tested after 2-4 weeks of therapy—sooner if the patient is taking a calcium-sparing drug such as hydrochlorothiazide—and again at about 6 and 12 months.

[128] Vasquez A. *Chiropractic and Naturopathic Mastery of Common Clinical Disorders*. http://optimalhealthresearch.com/clinical_mastery.html
[129] Review of this case by Dr Barry Morgan (MD, emergency medicine) is acknowledged and appreciated.

Presentation: 45yo HLA-B27+ woman with recurrent UTIs and a 7-year history of ankylosing spondylitis treated with anti-TNF drugs: Positive urine culture and positive stool culture demonstrating bacteria (*Escherichia coli* and *Klebsiella pneumoniae*) known to share molecular mimicry and cross-reactivity with HLA-B27: The Gram-negative bacterium *E. coli* produces a protein named "hypothetical protein 168" (Protein Identification Resource [PIR] data bank access code #jp0612) which shares the amino acid sequence "**RRYLE**" with HLA-B27, which contains the sequence "EWL**RRYLE**IGKETLQRVDP."[130] Per the same citation, *Klebsiella pneumoniae*'s protein (PIR s01840) nitrogenase (reductase) molybdenum-iron protein NifN contains the sequence "EWLRR." This amino acid homology confers validation to the phenomenon of molecular mimicry and thus that immune system components such as immunoglobulins and activated T-cells can cross-react between microbial peptides and human tissue antigens.[131] This patient was treated with the combination pharmaceutical antibiotic trimethoprim and sulfamethoxazole commonly referred to as "Bactrim DS" in addition to dietary optimization, hormonal optimization, and nutritional supplementation. Antimicrobial treatment with amoxicillin-clavulanate would have been reasonable, too, except for this patient's prior allergic reaction to the drug.

```
Urine Culture, Routine
  Urine Culture, Routine          Final Report
  Result 1
      Escherichia coli
      50,000-100,000 colony forming units per mL
  Antimicrobial Susceptibility
        ***** S = Susceptible; I = Intermediate; R = Resistant *****
                   P = Positive; N = Negative
        MICS are expressed in micrograms per mL
```

Antibiotic	RSLT#1
Amoxicillin/Clavulanic Acid	S
Ampicillin	S
Cefazolin	S
Cefepime	S
Ceftriaxone	S
Cefuroxime	S
Cephalothin	I
Ciprofloxacin	R
ESBL	N
Ertapenem	S
Gentamicin	S
Imipenem	S
Levofloxacin	R
Nitrofurantoin	S
Piperacillin	S
Tetracycline	S
Tobramycin	S
Trimethoprim/Sulfa	S

Comprehensive Stool Analysis / Parasitology x3

BACTERIOLOGY CULTURE		
Expected/Beneficial flora	**Commensal (Imbalanced) flora**	**Dysbiotic flora**
4+ Bacteroides fragilis group	3+ Alpha hemolytic strep	3+ Klebsiella pneumoniae ssp pneumoniae
3+ Bifidobacterium spp.		
4+ Escherichia coli		
3+ Lactobacillus spp.		
NG Enterococcus spp.		
2+ Clostridium spp.		
NG = No Growth		

PRESCRIPTIVE AGENTS			
	Resistant	**Intermediate**	**Susceptible**
Amoxicillin-Clavulanic Acid			S
Ampicillin	R		
Cefazolin			S
Ceftazidime			S
Ciprofloxacin			S
Trimeth-sulfa			S

Susceptible results imply that an infection due to the bacteria may be appropriately treated when the recommended dosage of the tested antimicrobial agent is used.
Intermediate results imply that response rates may be lower than for susceptible bacteria when the tested antimicrobial agent is used.
Resistant results imply that the bacteria will not be inhibited by normal dosage levels of the tested antimicrobial agent.

[130] Scofield RH, Warren WL, Koelsch G, Harley JB. A hypothesis for the HLA-B27 immune dysregulation in spondyloarthropathy: contributions from enteric organisms, B27 structure, peptides bound by B27, and convergent evolution. *Proc Natl Acad Sci U S A*. 1993 Oct 15;90(20):9330-4
[131] Rashid T, Ebringer A. Ankylosing spondylitis is linked to Klebsiella--the evidence. *Clin Rheumatol*. 2007 Jun;26(6):858-64

CRP: C-reactive protein	
Overview and interpretation:	▪ CRP is a protein made by the liver in response to the immunologic activation characteristic of infectious and inflammatory conditions. Generally, any tissue injury or inflammatory process especially that involves the immune system's increased production of IL-6 will result in increased production of CRP.[132] High sensitivity CRP (hsCRP) is preferred over regular CRP due to its greater sensitivity and use in assessing cardiovascular risk. ▪ Elevated values are seen with: <ul><li>Infections: Bacterial, fungal, parasitic, viral diseases; some patients with dysbiosis[133] will have mildly-moderately elevated CRP,</li><li>Inflammatory bowel disease: Crohn's disease and ulcerative colitis (higher in CD than UC),</li><li>Autoimmune disease: Rheumatoid arthritis, polymyalgia rheumatica, giant cell arteritis, polyarteritis nodosa, (not always SLE),</li><li>Acute myocardial infarction or other tissue ischemia</li><li>Organ transplant rejection: Renal, (not cardiac),</li><li>Trauma: Burns, surgery,</li><li>Obesity: Leads to modest elevations in CRP.</li></ul>
Advantages:	▪ This is an excellent screening test for differentiating "serious problems" (e.g., inflammatory and infectious arthropathy) from "benign problems" such as osteoarthritis. ▪ Since higher values of CRP are a well-recognized risk factor for cardiovascular disease, screening "musculoskeletal patients" with hsCRP provides data for cardiovascular risk assessment and a more comprehensive and holistic treatment approach, thus bridging the gap between acute care and preventive care.
Limitations:	▪ Elevations in CRP are completely nonspecific, requiring clinical investigation to determine the underlying cause of the immune activation. ▪ CRP may be normal in some patients with severe systemic diseases (such as lupus or cancer), and therefore a normal CRP does not entirely exclude the presence of significant illness.
Comments:	▪ Writing in *The New England Journal of Medicine*, authors Gabay and Kushner[134] note that measurements of plasma or serum **C-reactive protein can help differentiate inflammatory from non-inflammatory conditions and are useful in managing the patient's disease, since "the concentration often reflects the response to and the need for therapeutic intervention."** Additionally, they note, "Most normal subjects have plasma C-reactive protein concentrations of 2 mg per liter or less, but some have concentrations as high as 10 mg per liter." Deodhar[135] noted that **"Any clinical disease characterized by tissue injury and/or inflammation is accompanied by significant elevation of serum CRP..."** and that **CRP should replace ESR as a method of laboratory evaluation.** Deodhar also noted that **some patients with severe SLE will have normal CRP levels.**

---

[132] Deodhar SD. C-reactive protein: the best laboratory indicator available for monitoring disease activity. *Cleve Clin J Med* 1989 Mar-Apr;56(2):126-30

[133] See chapter 4 of *Integrative Rheumatology* and Vasquez A. Reducing Pain and Inflammation Naturally. Part 6: Nutritional and Botanical Treatments Against "Silent Infections" and Gastrointestinal Dysbiosis, Commonly Overlooked Causes of Neuromusculoskeletal Inflammation and Chronic Health Problems. *Nutr Perspect* 2006; Jan http://optimalhealthresearch.com/part6

[134] Gabay C, Kushner I. Acute-phase proteins and other systemic responses to inflammation. *N Engl J Med*. 1999 Feb 11;340(6):448-54

[135] Deodhar SD. C-reactive protein: the best laboratory indicator available for monitoring disease activity. *Cleve Clin J Med* 1989 Mar-Apr;56(2):126-30

Presentation: Elevated hsCRP (high-sensitivity c-reactive protein) in a male patient with metabolic syndrome and rheumatoid arthritis—response to treatment protocol in *Integrative Rheumatology*: This 52-year-old male patient presented with a 4-year history of rheumatoid arthritis which was unresponsive to prednisone and anti-TNF (tumor necrosis factor alpha) drugs, ie, "biologics." As expected, the prednisone exacerbated the patient's insulin resistance and hypertension; the drug failed to produce an anti-inflammatory benefit for this patient. At a cost of several thousand dollars per treatment, the anti-TNF "biologic" drugs failed to provide any benefit. At the intial visit in July 2005, the hsCRP level was 124 mg/L (normal range 0-3 mg/L), as shown in these lab results.

DATE OF SPECIMEN	TIME	DATE RECEIVED	DATE REPORTED	TIME		Houston		TX	77036-0000
7/08/2005	16:19	7/08/2005	7/11/2005	7:38	419	ACCOUNT NUMBER:	42407150		

TEST	RESULT	LIMITS	LAB
C-Reactive Protein, Cardiac			
> C-Reactive Protein, Cardiac	124.00H mg/L	0.00 - 3.00	HD
	Relative Risk for Future Cardiovascular Event		
	Low	<1.00	
	Average	1.00 - 3.00	
	High	>3.00	

The patient was treated with the protocol outlined in Chapter 4 of *Integrative Rheumatology*.[136] Stool testing showed *Citrobacter freundii* (renamed *Citrobacter rodentium*) which was addressed with botanical medicines; the insufficiency dysbiosis was also corrected per the five-part protocol. Slightly low testosterone and slightly elevated estradiol was optimized with a pharmaceutical aromatase inhibitor (Arimidex) given twice weekly. The five-part nutritional wellness protocol (supplemented Paleo-Mediterranean diet [SPMD]) was implemented.[137]

Comprehensive Parasitology, stool, x2

MICROBIOLOGY

Bacteriology Culture

Beneficial flora		Imbalances		Dysbiotic flora	
Bifidobacter	0+	Gamma strep	1+	Citrobacter freundii	1+
E. coli	2+	Enterobacter sp.	1+		
Lactobacillus	0+				

Mycology (Yeast) Culture

Normal flora	Dysbiotic flora
No yeast isolated	

PARASITOLOGY

	Sample 1		Sample 2
No	Ova or Parasites	No	Ova or Parasites

No anti-inflammatory drugs or botanicals were used. Within five weeks of treatment, the patient's hsCRP dropped from 124 mg/L to 7.58 mg/L—a reduction of approximately 95%—far superior to any previoius response to corticosteroid and biologic drugs. Patient experienced significant alleviation of pain and improved mobility.

8/17/2005	11:06	8/18/2005	8/18/2005	12:32	738	ACCOUNT NUMBER:	42407150		

TEST	RESULT	LIMITS	LAB
C-Reactive Protein, Cardiac			
C-Reactive Protein, Cardiac	7.58H mg/L	0.00 - 3.00	HD

---

[136] Vasquez A. *Integrative Rheumatology*. http://optimalhealthresearch.com/textbooks/rheumatology.html
[137] Vasquez A. Revisiting the Five-Part Nutritional Wellness Protocol. *Nutritional Perspectives* 2011 January http://optimalhealthresearch.com/spmd

ESR: erythrocyte sedimentation rate	
Overview and interpretation:	<ul><li>Values may be elevated even when no pathology is present because ESR increases with anemia and with age.</li><li>Much more sensitive than WBC count when screening for infection.[138]</li><li>May be normal in about 10% of patients who have pathology such as **giant cell arteritis** and **polymyalgia rheumatica** (conditions where it is generally the only lab abnormality, besides anemia); may also be normal in several other diseases.</li><li>**May be normal in patients with septic arthritis and patients with crystal-induced arthritis: joint aspiration for synovial fluid analysis is indicated if septic arthritis is suspected.**[139]</li><li>Increased with age, anemia, inflammation; higher in women than men. Age-adjusted normal ranges: any value over 25 is considered high in young people, or 40 in elderly women.</li><li>Age-related adjustments for men and women are as follows:<ol><li>Men: age divided by 2</li><li>Women: (age + 10) divided by 2</li></ol></li></ul>
Advantages:	<ul><li>Inexpensive and easy to perform—use the same lavender-topped tube that you use for CBC.</li><li>Provides a quick screen for infection, inflammation, and multiple myeloma—the most common primary bone tumor in adults.</li><li>In patients with elevated levels, ESR can be used to monitor progression of disease and response to treatment.[140] However, a negative/normal test result does not exclude the presence of significant disease; some noteworthy examples include the following: 1) elderly—due to diminished ability to mount an inflammatory response, 2) patients taking anti-inflammatory drugs and immunosuppressants, 3) a significant proportion of patients with lupus will have normal ESR despite aggressive disease, and 4) some cancer patients with clinically significant tumor burden will not show signs of systemic inflammation.</li><li>**ESR may be more reliable than CRP for multiple myeloma.**[141]</li></ul>
Limitations:	<ul><li>ESR may be normal in a subset of patients with clinically significant infection or inflammation.</li><li>Values are elevated in the elderly and patients with anemia and are thus not necessarily indicative of disease in these populations.</li></ul>
Comments:	<ul><li>**This test is generally considered *outdated* and has been replaced in most circumstances by CRP for the evaluation of inflammation and infection.**</li><li>**The only time I use this test clinically is when I am highly suspicious of inflammation and the CRP is normal. Further, this test may be preferred when assessing for temporal arteritis and for multiple myeloma, two conditions which are classically associated with elevated ESR.**</li></ul>

---

[138] Shaw BA, Gerardi JA, Hennrikus WL. How to avoid orthopedic pitfalls in children. *Patient Care* 1999; Feb 28: 95-116
[139] Klippel JH (ed). Primer on the Rheumatic Diseases. 11th Edition. Atlanta: Arthritis Foundation. 1997 page 94
[140] Shojania K. Rheumatology: 2. What laboratory tests are needed? *CMAJ*. 2000 Apr 18;162(8):1157-63 http://www.cmaj.ca/cgi/content/full/162/8/1157
[141] "We conclude that ESR, a simple and easily performed marker, was found to be an independent prognostic factor for survival in patients with multiple myeloma." Alexandrakis MG, Passam FH, Ganotakis ES, Sfiridaki K, Xilouri I, Perisinakis K, Kyriakou DS. The clinical and prognostic significance of erythrocyte sedimentation rate (ESR), serum interleukin-6 (IL-6) and acute phase protein levels in multiple myeloma. *Clin Lab Haematol*. 2003;25:41-6

Ferritin	
Overview and interpretation:	▪ Ferritin levels are directly proportional to body iron stores, except in patients with inflammation, infection, hepatitis, or cancer. Therefore, measuring ferritin allows assessment for iron deficiency (a cause of fatigue, or early manifestation of GI cancer) and allows for assessment of iron overload (as a cause of joint pain and arthropathy). This test should be performed in all African Americans[142,143], white men over age 30 years[144], diabetics[145], and patients with peripheral arthropathy[146], and exercise-associated joint pain[147,148] The research also justifies testing children[149], women[150], young adults[151] and the general asymptomatic public.[152] ▪ <u>Low ferritin = iron deficiency</u> ▪ <u>High ferritin = iron overload, cancer, inflammation, infection, and/or hepatitis (viral, alcoholic, or toxic)</u>
Advantages:	▪ Reliable screening test for iron overload when used in conjunction with patient assessment and evidence (e.g., normal CRP) of no infection or acute phase response. ▪ This is the blood test of choice for iron deficiency *and* iron overload.
Limitations:	▪ Iron-deficient patients with an acute phase response may have a falsely normal level of ferritin since ferritin is an acute phase reactant and will be elevated *disproportionate to iron status* during inflammation. ▪ Elevations of ferritin (i.e., >200 mcg/L in women and >300 mcg/L in men) need to be retested along with CRP (to rule out false elevation due to excessive inflammation) before making the presumptive diagnosis of iron overload. **In the absence of significant inflammation, ferritin values >200 mcg/L in women and >300 mcg/L in men indicate iron overload and the need for treatment regardless of the absence of symptoms or end-stage complications.**[153]
Comments:	▪ Note that since ferritin is an acute-phase reactant, a high level of serum ferritin by itself does not allow differentiation between iron overload, infection, and the inflammation associated with tissue injury or metastatic disease. Ferritin must be evaluated within the context of the patient's clinical condition and the assessment of at least one other marker for inflammation such as CRP. If the patient is not acutely ill or has not recently suffered tissue injury (e.g., myocardial infarction) and the CRP is normal, then an elevated ferritin value indicates iron overload until proven otherwise with diagnostic phlebotomy, which is safer and less expensive than liver biopsy or MRI. Transferrin saturation can also be measured when the interpretation of ferritin is unclear. By itself, serum iron is unreliable.

[142] Barton JC, Edwards CQ, Bertoli LF, Shroyer TW, Hudson SL. Iron overload in African Americans. *Am J Med.* 1995 Dec;99(6):616-23

[143] Wurapa RK, Gordeuk VR, Brittenham GM, et al. Primary iron overload in African Americans. *Am J Med.* 1996;101(1):9-18

[144] Baer DM, Simons JL, et al. Hemochromatosis screening in asymptomatic ambulatory men 30 years of age and older. *Am J Med.* 1995 May;98:464-8

[145] Phelps G, Chapman I, Hall P, Braund W, Mackinnon M. Prevalence of genetic haemochromatosis among diabetic patients. *Lancet* 1989; 2: 233-4

[146] Olynyk J, Hall P, Ahern M, KwiatekR, MackinnonM. Screening for hemochromatosis in a rheumatology clinic. *Aust NZ J Med* 1994; 24: 22-5

[147] McCurdie I, Perry JD. Haemochromatosis and exercise related joint pains. *BMJ.* 1999 Feb 13;318(7181):449-5

[148] "RESULTS: Our findings indicate a high prevalence of HFE gene mutations in this population (49.2%) compared with sedentary controls (33.5%). No association was detected in the athletes between mutations and blood iron markers. CONCLUSIONS: The findings support the need to assess regularly iron stores in elite endurance athletes." Chicharro JL, Hoyos J, Gomez-Gallego F, et al. Mutations in the hereditary haemochromatosis gene HFE in professional endurance athletes. *Br J Sports Med.* 2004 Aug;38(4):418-21. Erratum in: *Br J Sports Med.* 2004 Dec;38(6):793 http://bjsm.bmjjournals.com/cgi/content/full/38/4/418 Accessed September 12, 2005

[149] Kaikov Y, Wadsworth LD, Hassall E, Dimmick JE, Rogers PCJ. Primary hemochromatosis in children: report of three newly diagnosed cases and review of the pediatric literature. *Pediatrics* 1992; 90: 37-42

[150] Edwards CQ, Kushner JP. Screening for hemochromatosis. *N Engl J Med* 1993; 328: 1616-20

[151] Gushusrt TP, Triest WE. Diagnosis and management of precirrhotic hemochromatosis. *W Virginia Med J* 1990; 86: 91-5

[152] Balan V, et al. Screening for hemochromatosis: a cost-effectiveness study based on 12, 258 patients. *Gastroenterology* 1994; 107: 453-9

[153] **Barton JC, McDonnell SM, Adams PC, Brissot P, Powell LW, Edwards CQ, Cook JD, Kowdley KV. Management of hemochromatosis. Hemochromatosis Management Working Group.** *Ann Intern Med.* **1998 Dec 1;129(11):932-9—one of the best papers ever written on this topic.**

Ferritin—*Interpretation of serum levels*

Ferritin	Categorization and management
≥ 800 mcg/L	<u>Practically diagnostic of iron overload</u>[154]: Repeat tests; rule out inflammation or occult pathology. Initiate phlebotomy and consider liver biopsy or MRI.
≥ 300 mcg/L	<u>Probable iron overload</u>[155]: Repeat tests; rule out inflammation or occult pathology. In men, initiate phlebotomy and consider liver biopsy or MRI.[156]
≥ 200 mcg/L	*In women*: <u>Suggestive of iron overload</u>[157]: Repeat tests, rule out inflammation or occult pathology. In women, initiate phlebotomy and consider liver biopsy or MRI.[158] *In men*: <u>High-normal *unhealthy* iron status with increased risk of myocardial infarction</u>[159]: Rule out inflammation or occult pathology. No follow-up is mandated, yet blood donation and/or abstention from dietary iron are recommended preventative healthcare measures.
≥ 160 mcg/L	*In women*: <u>Abnormal iron status</u>[160]: Repeat tests, rule out inflammation or occult pathology. Consider phlebotomy and liver biopsy or MRI.
≥80-120 mcg/L	<u>High-normal unhealthy iron status</u>[161,162]: No follow-up is mandated; blood donation and abstention from dietary iron are suggested preventative healthcare measures. A subset of patients with restless leg syndrome (RLS, a condition also causally associated with intestinal bacterial overgrowth dysbiosis) have impaired transport of iron into the brain and therefore require slightly elevated ferritin/iron levels (up to 120) to enhance cerebral iron uptake.
40-70 mcg/L	**<u>Optimal iron status for most people</u>**[163,164]
< 20 mcg/L	<u>Iron deficiency</u>: Search for occult gastrointestinal blood loss with endoscopy or imaging assessments in adults; refer to gastroenterologist.[165,166]

Ferritin is an acute-phase reactant, which means that its production is increased during the acute phase of inflammatory and/or infectious disorders. Therefore the numeric value and hence its clinical meaning can be interpreted only within a context that also includes assessment of the patient's inflammatory status, which is best assessed with either ESR or CRP. If CRP/ESR is high, then the physician might assume that the ferritin value is "falsely elevated"—disproportionately elevated with respect to body iron stores. *Common clinical examples requiring use and skillful interpretation of ferritin*:

- **Elderly or arthritic patient with iron deficiency despite normal serum ferritin**: An elderly patient with normal ferritin and elevated CRP/ESR is probably iron deficient; retesting of ferritin and measurement of transferrin saturation and CBC should be performed promptly. If iron deficiency is confirmed or cannot be excluded, referral for endoscopic examination must be implemented. In a patient with known inflammatory arthropathy, the ferritin may appear normal even though the patient is iron deficient and in need of supplementation and endoscopy.
- **Non-anemic iron deficiency**: A middle-aged patient (commonly a premenopausal woman) presents with fatigue and during the course of evaluation is found to have a normal CBC. **Do not let a normal CBC prevent you from assessing ferritin; many of these patients are completely iron deficient with ferritin values of 2-6 mcg/L and are in need of iron replacement as well as evaluation for celiac disease,** *H. pylori* **infection, hematuria, and—as is often warranted—gastrointestinal bleeding/lesions.**

[154] Milman N, Albeck MJ. Distinction between homozygous and heterozygous subjects with hemochromatosis using iron status markers and receiver operating characteristic (ROC) analysis. *Eur J Clin Biochem* 1995; 33: 95-8. See also Milman N. Iron status markers in hereditary hemochromatosis: distinction between individuals being homozygous and heterozygous for the hemochromatosis allele. *Eur J Haematol* 1991;47:292-8

[155] Olynyk JK, Bacon BR. Hereditary hemochromatosis: detecting and correcting iron overload. *Postgrad Med* 1994;96: 151-65

[156] "Therapeutic phlebotomy is used to remove excess iron and maintain low normal body iron stores, … initiated in men with serum ferritin levels of 300 microg/L or more and in women with serum ferritin levels of 200 microg/L or more, regardless of the presence or absence of symptoms." Barton JC, McDonnell SM, Adams PC, Brissot P, Powell LW, Edwards CQ, Cook JD, Kowdley KV. Management of hemochromatosis. Hemochromatosis Management Working Group. *Ann Intern Med*. 1998 Dec 1;129(11):932-9

[157] Barton JC, Edwards CQ, Bertoli LF, Shroyer TW, Hudson SL. Iron overload in African Americans. *Am J Med* 1995; 99: 616-23

[158] Barton JC, McDonnell SM, Adams PC, et al. Management of hemochromatosis. *Ann Intern Med*. 1998 Dec 1;129(11):932-9

[159] Salonen JT, Nyyssonen K, Korpela H,et al. High stored iron levels are associated with excess risk of myocardial infarction in eastern Finnish men. *Circulation* 1992; 86: 803-11

[160] Nicoll D. Therapeutic drug monitoring and laboratory reference ranges. In: Tierney LM, McPhee SJ, Papadakis MA. *Current Medical Diagnosis and Treatment 1996 (35th Edition)*. Stamford: Appleton and Lange, 1996: 1442

[161] Lauffer, RB. *Iron and Your Heart*. New York: St. Martin's Press, 1991: 79-8, 83-88, 162

[162] Sullivan JL. Iron and the sex difference in heart disease risk. *Lancet*. 1981 Jun 13;1(8233):1293-4

[163] Lauffer, RB. *Iron and Your Heart*. New York: St. Martin's Press, 1991: 79-8, 83-88, 162

[164] **Vasquez A**. High body iron stores: causes, effects, diagnosis, and treatment. *Nutritional Perspectives* 1994; 17: 13, 15-7, 19, 21, 28 and **Vasquez A**. Men's Health: Iron in men: why men store this nutrient in their bodies and the harm that it does. *MEN Magazine* 1997; Jan:11,21-23 vix.com/menmag/alexiron.htm

[165] Rockey DC, Cello JP. Evaluation of the gastrointestinal tract in patients with iron-deficiency anemia. *N Engl J Med*. 1993;329(23):1691-5

[166] "Endoscopy revealed a clinically important lesion in 23 (12%) of 186 patients. … CONCLUSIONS: Endoscopy yields important findings in premenopausal women with iron deficiency anemia, which should not be attributed solely to menstrual blood loss." Bini EJ, Micale PL, Weinshel EH. Evaluation of the gastrointestinal tract in premenopausal women with iron deficiency anemia. *Am J Med*. 1998 Oct;105(4):281-6

Arthritis & Rheumatism

Official Journal of the American College of Rheumatology

VOLUME 39   OCTOBER 1996   NO. 10

1767   1768

Musculoskeletal disorders and iron overload disease: comment on the American College of Rheumatology guidelines for the initial evaluation of the adult patient with acute musculoskeletal symptoms

To the Editor:

The recent clinical guidelines for the initial evaluation of the adult patient with acute musculoskeletal symptoms, proposed by the American College of Rheumatology (1), provide useful information and a good review for clinicians. However, there is one important omission in these guidelines. Nowhere in the guidelines is hemochromatosis mentioned. Such a prevalent and potentially life-threatening disease certainly deserves to be considered in the evaluation of patients with musculoskeletal disorders.

Hereditary hemochromatosis is now thought to be the most common genetic disorder in the white population (2). Approximately 1 in 250 persons is homozygous for this disorder and will develop the characteristic clinical manifestations such as diabetes, cardiomyopathy, liver disease, endocrine dysfunction, and, most notable for this discussion, arthropathy or other musculoskeletal disorders (2). Although hereditary iron overload disorders have traditionally been thought of as occurring exclusively in whites, recent research by Barton et al (3) indicates that approximately 1 in 67 African-Americans is affected by an etiologically distinct and severe form of iron overload. Hereditary iron overload disorders have been detected in persons of every ethnic background.

Arthropathy affects up to 80% of iron-overloaded patients and is often the only manifestation of this disease (4). Joint pain is a common and early symptom of iron overload, and "bone pain" has also been described as a common initial complaint (5). Clinically and radiographically, hemochromatoic arthropathy can resemble osteoarthritis, calcium pyrophosphate dihydrate deposition disease, pseudogout, rheumatoid arthritis, ankylosing spondylitis, or generalized osteopenia with osteoporotic fractures (4,6,7). Since iron overload can cause such a wide array of musculoskeletal manifestations and because definitive clinical differentiation of iron overload from other arthropathies is very difficult, patients with peripheral arthropathy should be screened for iron overload. Indeed, recent research by Olynyk et al (8) indicates that the prevalence of iron overload is 5 times higher in patients with peripheral arthropathy than in the general population. Therefore, screening of patients with peripheral arthropathy for the possible presence of iron overload is justified.

Thus, since iron overload affects such a large portion of the population and arthropathy is a common manifestation of this disorder, patients with musculoskeletal symptoms should be screened for iron overload (4,8). The current literature suggests that everyone should be screened for iron overload even if there are no symptoms (8–10).

Alex Vasquez, DC
Seattle, WA

1. American College of Rheumatology Ad Hoc Committee on Clinical Guidelines: Guidelines for the initial evaluation of the adult patient with acute musculoskeletal symptoms. Arthritis Rheum 39:1–8, 1996
2. Olynyk JK, Bacon BR: Hereditary hemochromatosis: detecting and correcting iron overload. Postgrad Med 96:151–165, 1994
3. Barton JC, Edwards CQ, Bertoli LF, Shroyer TW, Hudson SL: Iron overload in African Americans. Am J Med 99:616–623, 1995
4. Faraawi R, Harth M, Kertesz A, Bell D: Arthritis in hemochromatosis. J Rheumatol 20:448–452, 1993
5. Adams PC, Kertesz AE, Valberg LS: Clinical presentation of hemochromatosis: a changing scene. Am J Med 90:445–449, 1991
6. Bywaters EGL, Hamilton EBD, Williams R: The spine in idiopathic hemochromatosis. Ann Rheum Dis 30:453–465, 1971
7. Eyres KS, McCloskey EV, Fern ED, Rogers S, Beneton M, Aaron JE, Kanis JA: Osteoporotic fractures: an unusual presentation of hemochromatosis. Bone 13:431–433, 1992
8. Olynyk J, Hall P, Ahern M, Kwiatek R, Mackinnon M: Screening for hemochromatosis in a rheumatology clinic. Aust N Z J Med 24:22–25, 1994
9. Baer DM, Simmons JL, Staples RL, Runmore GJ, Morton CJ: Hemochromatosis screening in asymptomatic ambulatory men 30 years of age and older. Am J Med 98:464–468, 1995
10. Adams PC, Gregor JC, Kertesz AE, Valberg LS: Screening blood donors for hereditary hemochromatosis: decision analysis model based on a 30-year database. Gastroenterology 109:177–188, 1995

Vasquez A. Musculoskeletal disorders and iron overload disease: comment on the American College of Rheumatology guidelines for the initial evaluation of the adult patient with acute musculoskeletal symptoms. *Arthritis Rheum.* 1996 Oct;39(10):1767-8 http://www.ncbi.nlm.nih.gov/pubmed/8843875

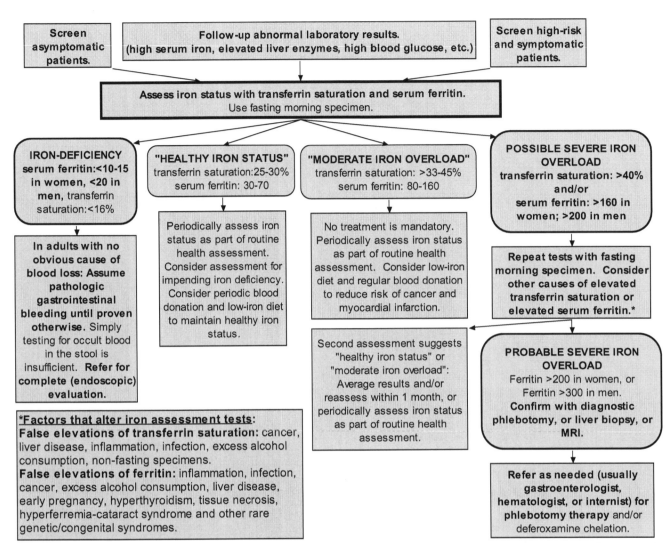

Algorithm for the comprehensive management of iron status: The above flow-chart delineates the management of high-moderate-healthy-low iron status.

Basic treatments for severe iron overload:

- **Iron-removal therapy is mandatory:** Phlebotomy therapy is generally performed weekly or twice-weekly; deferoxamine chelation is reserved for patients who do not withstand phlebotomy (due to cardiomyopathy, severe anemia, or hypoproteinemia) or may be used concurrently with phlebotomy in some patients. Periodically assess hematologic and iron indexes. Continue with weekly iron removal therapy until patient reaches mild iron-deficiency anemia, then decrease frequency and continue phlebotomy as needed (e.g., 4 times per year).
- **Laboratory tests and physical examination:** Assess general physical condition and hepatic, cardiac, endocrine, and general health status.
- **Confirm diagnosis:** Liver biopsy ("gold standard") or diagnostic phlebotomy; perhaps MRI.
- **Assess liver status:** Liver biopsy ("gold standard") or perhaps MRI. Cirrhosis indicates increased risk of hepatocellular carcinoma and reduced life expectancy. Consider liver ultrasound, serum liver enzyme measurement, and serum alpha-fetoprotein to screen for hepatocellular carcinoma every 6 months. Hepatoma surveillance is mandatory in cirrhotic patients.
- **Implement dietary modifications and nutritional therapies:** Avoid iron supplements, multivitamin supplements with iron, iron-fortified foods, liver, beef, pork, alcohol, and excess vitamin C. Ensure adequate protein intake to replace protein lost during phlebotomy. Diet modifications are not substitutes for iron removal therapy. Consider antioxidant therapy.
- **Screen all blood relatives of patients with primary iron overload**. *Mandatory!*
- **Monitor patient condition, and compliance** with lifelong phlebotomy therapy
- **Assess and address psychoemotional issues/concerns**

25(OH)D: serum 25(OH) vitamin D	
Overview and interpretation:	<ul><li>**Vitamin D deficiency is a common cause of musculoskeletal pain**[167,168,169], and vitamin D deficiency is a significant risk factor for cancer and other serious health problems.[170,171,172]</li><li>Measurement of serum 25(OH) vitamin D (or empiric treatment with 2,000 – 10,000 IU vitamin D3 per day for adults) is indicated in patients with chronic musculoskeletal pain, particularly low-back pain.[173] Optimal vitamin D status correlates with serum 25(OH)D levels of 50 – 100 ng/mL (125 - 250 nmol/L)—see our review article for more details[174]; levels greater than 100 ng/mL are unnecessary and increase the risk of hypercalcemia.</li></ul> 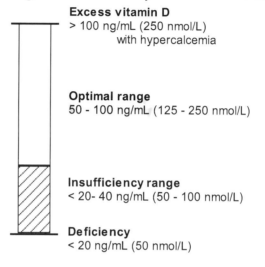 **Excess vitamin D** > 100 ng/mL (250 nmol/L) with hypercalcemia **Optimal range** 50 - 100 ng/mL (125 - 250 nmol/L) **Insufficiency range** < 20- 40 ng/mL (50 - 100 nmol/L) **Deficiency** < 20 ng/mL (50 nmol/L) **<u>Interpretation of serum 25(OH) vitamin D levels</u>**. Modified from Vasquez et al, *Alternative Therapies in Health and Medicine* 2004 and Vasquez A. <u>*Musculoskeletal Pain: Expanded Clinical Strategies*</u> (Institute for Functional Medicine) 2008.
Advantages:	<ul><li>Accurate assessment of vitamin D status.</li></ul>
Limitations:	<ul><li>Patients with certain granulomatous conditions such as sarcoidosis or Crohn's disease and patients taking certain drugs such as thiazide diuretics (hydrochlorothiazide) can develop hypercalcemia due to "vitamin D hypersensitivity" or drug side effects—these patients require frequent monitoring of serum calcium while taking vitamin D supplements.</li></ul>
Comments:	<ul><li>**Routine measurement and/or empiric treatment with vitamin D3 needs to become a routine component of patient care.**[175]</li><li>Periodic assessment of 25(OH)D and serum calcium are required to ensure effectiveness and safety of treatment, respectively.</li></ul>

[167] Masood H, Narang AP, Bhat IA, Shah GN. Persistent limb pain and raised serum alkaline phosphatase the earliest markers of subclinical hypovitaminosis D in Kashmir. *Indian J Physiol Pharmacol*. 1989 Oct-Dec;33(4):259-61

[168] Al Faraj S, Al Mutairi K. Vitamin D deficiency and chronic low back pain in Saudi Arabia. *Spine*. 2003 Jan 15;28(2):177-9

[169] Plotnikoff GA, Quigley JM. Prevalence of severe hypovitaminosis D in patients with persistent, nonspecific musculoskeletal pain. *Mayo Clin Proc*. 2003 Dec;78(12):1463-70

[170] Grant WB. An estimate of premature cancer mortality in the U.S. due to inadequate doses of solar ultraviolet-B radiation. *Cancer* 2002;94(6):1867-75

[171] Zittermannn A. Vitamin D in preventive medicine: are we ignoring the evidence? *Br J Nutr*. 2003 May;89(5):552-72

[172] Holick MF. Vitamin D: importance in the prevention of cancers, type 1 diabetes, heart disease, and osteoporosis. *Am J Clin Nutr*. 2004;79(3):362-71

[173] Al Faraj S, Al Mutairi K. Vitamin D deficiency and chronic low back pain in Saudi Arabia. *Spine*. 2003 Jan 15;28(2):177-9

[174] **Vasquez A, Manso G, Cannell J. The Clinical Importance of Vitamin D (Cholecalciferol): A Paradigm Shift with Implications for All Healthcare Providers.** *Alternative Therapies in Health and Medicine* **2004; 10: 28-37** http://optimalhealthresearch.com/cholecalciferol.html

[175] Heaney RP. Vitamin D, nutritional deficiency, and the medical paradigm. *J Clin Endocrinol Metab*. 2003;88:5107-8 http://jcem.endojournals.org/cgi/content/full/88/11/5107

THE LANCET.com

May 6, 2005

Subphysiologic Doses of Vitamin D are Subtherapeutic: Comment on the Study by The Record Trial Group

Dear Editor,
Based on recently published research, it is clear that the study by The Record Trial Group [1] on vitamin D and calcium in the prevention of fractures suffered from at least four important shortcomings which negatively skewed their results.

First, and most important, the dose of vitamin D used in their study (800 IU/d) is subphysiologic and would therefore not be expected to produce a clinically meaningful effect. The physiologic requirement for vitamin D was determined scientifically in a recent study by Heaney and colleagues [2], who showed that healthy men utilize 3,000 to 5,000 IU of cholecalciferol per day, and several recent clinical trials have been published documenting the safety and effectiveness of administering vitamin D in physiologic doses of at least 4,000 IU per day.[3-5] In fact, studies have shown a dose-response relationship with vitamin D supplementation [6], and low doses (e.g., 600 IU) are clearly less effective than higher doses in the physiologic range (e.g., 4,000 IU).[5] It is important to note that the commonly used dose of vitamin D at 800 IU per day was not determined scientifically; rather this amount was determined arbitrarily before sufficient scientific methodology was available.[2,7] Given that the commonly recommended daily intake of vitamin D in the range of 200-800 IU is not sufficient for maintaining adequate serum levels of vitamin D [8], it is therefore incumbent upon modern researchers and clinicians to use doses of vitamin D that are consistent with the physiologic requirement as established in current research.

Second, the authors recognize that patient compliance in their study population was quite poor. This poor compliance obviously contributed to the purported lack of treatment efficacy.

Third, and consistent with recent data published elsewhere [8], virtually all of their patients were still vitamin D deficient at the end of one year of treatment, thereby affirming the inadequacy of the treatment dose. Vitamin D deficiency is common in industrialized nations, particularly those of northern latitudes [9-11], including the UK, where this study was performed. By modern criteria for serum vitamin D levels [12], virtually all of the patients in this study were vitamin D deficient at the beginning of the study, and the insufficient treatment dose of 800 IU/d failed to correct this deficiency even after 1 year of treatment. Given that vitamin D levels must be raised to approximately 40 ng/mL (100 nmol/L) in order to maximally reduce parathyroid hormone levels and bone resorption [13,14], supplementation that does not accomplish the goal of raising serum vitamin D levels into the optimal physiologic range cannot be considered adequate therapy.[12]

Fourth, and finally, there is reason to question the bioavailability of their vitamin D3 supplement, as the authors note that their dose-response was generally lower than that seen in other studies. Bioavailability is a prerequisite for treatment efficacy, and the elderly have higher likeliness of comorbid conditions that impair digestion and absorption of nutrients. Specifically, it is well documented that vitamin D absorption is decreased in elderly patients compared to younger controls [15,16], and this is complicated by an age-related reduction in renal calcitriol production [17,18] and intestinal vitamin D receptors [19], thereby further impairing vitamin D metabolism and calcium absorption. Since emulsification of fat soluble vitamins is required for their absorption [20], and since pre-emulsification of nutrients has been shown to increase absorption and dose-responsiveness of the fat-soluble nutrient coenzyme Q [21, 22], it seems apparent that attention to the form (not merely the dose) of nutrient supplementation is clinically important, particularly when working with elderly patients.

These shortcomings, when combined, could have lead to an additive or synergistic reduction in treatment potency that skewed their results toward a conclusion of inefficacy. In order to produce more meaningful results in clinical trials, our group published guidelines [12] recommending that future studies 1) ensure patient compliance, 2) use physiologic doses of vitamin D (e.g., 4,000 IU per day), and 3) ensure that serum levels are raised to a minimum of 40 ng/mL (100 nmol/L), since levels below this threshold are associated with increased parathyroid hormone levels, increased bone resorption, and recalcitrance to bone-building interventions.[23,24]

Alex Vasquez
Biotics Research Corporation
Rosenberg, Texas, USA 77471

Competing Interests: Dr. Vasquez is a researcher at Biotics Research Corporation, an FDA-licensed drug manufacturing facility in the USA.

References:
1. Record Trial Group. Oral vitamin D3 and calcium for secondary prevention of low-trauma fractures in elderly people (Randomised Evaluation of Calcium Or vitamin D, RECORD): a randomised placebo-controlled trial. *Lancet* (Early Online Publication), 28 April 2005
2. Heaney RP, Davies KM, Chen TC, Holick MF, Barger-Lux MJ. Human serum 25-hydroxycholecalciferol response to extended oral dosing with cholecalciferol. *Am J Clin Nutr* 2003;77:204-10
3. Vieth R, Chan PC, MacFarlane GD. Efficacy and safety of vitamin D3 intake exceeding the lowest observed adverse effect level. *Am J Clin Nutr.* 2001;73:288-94
4. Al Faraj S, Al Mutairi K. Vitamin D deficiency and chronic low back pain in Saudi Arabia. *Spine.* 2003;28:177-9
5. Vieth R, Kimball S, Hu A, Walfish PG. Randomized comparison of the effects of the vitamin D3 adequate intake versus 100 mcg (4000 IU) per day on biochemical responses and the wellbeing of patients. *Nutr J.* 2004 Jul 19;3(1):8
   http://www.nutritionj.com/content/pdf/1475-2891-3-8.pdf
6. Van den Berghe G, Van Roosbroeck D, Vanhove P, Wouters PJ, De Pourcq L, Bouillon R. Bone turnover in prolonged critical illness: effect of vitamin D. *J Clin Endocrinol Metab.* 2003;88:4623-32
7. Vieth R. Vitamin D supplementation, 25-hydroxyvitamin D concentrations, and safety. *Am J Clin Nutr.* 1999;69:842-56
   http://www.ajcn.org/cgi/reprint/69/5/842.pdf
8. Glerup H, Mikkelsen K, Poulsen L, Hass E, Overbeck S, Thomsen J, Charles P, Eriksen EF. Commonly recommended daily intake of vitamin D is not sufficient if sunlight exposure is limited. *J Intern Med.* 2000;247:260-8
9. Thomas MK, Lloyd-Jones DM, Thadhani RI, Shaw AC, Deraska DJ, Kitch BT, Vamvakas EC, Dick IM, Prince RL, Finkelstein JS. Hypovitaminosis D in medical inpatients. *N Engl J Med* 1998;338:777-83
10. Dubbelman R, Jonxis JH, Muskiet FA, Saleh AE. Age-dependent vitamin D status and vertebral condition of white women living in Curacao (The Netherlands Antilles) as compared with their counterparts in The Netherlands. *Am J Clin Nutr* 1993;58:106-9
11. Kauppinen-Makelin R, Tahtela R, Loyttyniemi E, Karkkainen J, Valimaki MJ. A high prevalence of hypovitaminosis D in Finnish medical in- and outpatients. *J Intern Med.* 2001;249:559-63
12. Vasquez A, Manso G, Cannell J. The clinical importance of vitamin D (cholecalciferol): a paradigm shift with implications for all healthcare providers. *Altern Ther Health Med.* 2004;10:28-36; quiz 37, 94
13. Kinyamu HK, Gallagher JC, Rafferty KA, Balhorn KE. Dietary calcium and vitamin D intake in elderly women: effect on serum parathyroid hormone and vitamin D metabolites. *Am J Clin Nutr* 1998;67:342-8
14. Dawson-Hughes B, Harris SS, Dallal GE. Plasma calcidiol, season, and serum parathyroid hormone concentrations in healthy elderly men and women. *Am J Clin Nutr* 1997;65:67-71
15. Harris SS, Dawson-Hughes B, Perrone GA. Plasma 25-hydroxyvitamin D responses of younger and older men to three weeks of supplementation with 1800 IU/day of vitamin D. *J Am Coll Nutr.* 1999;18:470-4
16. Barragry JM, France MW, Corless D, Gupta SP, Switala S, Boucher BJ, Cohen RD. Intestinal cholecalciferol absorption in the elderly and in younger adults. *Clin Sci Mol Med.* 1978;55:213-20
17. Tsai KS, Heath H 3rd, Kumar R, Riggs BL. Impaired vitamin D metabolism with aging in women. Possible role in pathogenesis of senile osteoporosis. *J Clin Invest.* 1984;73:1668-72
18. Gallagher JC, Riggs BL, Eisman J, Hamstra A, Arnaud SB, DeLuca HF. Intestinal calcium absorption and serum vitamin D metabolites in normal subjects and osteoporotic patients: effect of age and dietary calcium. *J Clin Invest.* 1979;64:729-36
19. Ebeling PR, Sandgren ME, DiMagno EP, Lane AW, DeLuca HF, Riggs BL. Evidence of an age-related decrease in intestinal responsiveness to vitamin D: relationship between serum 1,25-dihydroxyvitamin D3 and intestinal vitamin D receptor concentrations in normal women. *J Clin Endocrinol Metab.* 1992;75:176-82
20. Gallo-Torres HE. Obligatory role of bile for the intestinal absorption of vitamin E. *Lipids.* 1970;5:379-84
21. Bucci LR, Pillors M, Medlin R, Henderson R, Stiles JC, Robol HJ, Sparks WS. Enhanced uptake in humans of coenzyme Q10 from an emulsified form. *Third International Congress of Biomedical Gerontology*; Acapulco, Mexico: June 1989
22. Bucci LR, Pillors M, Medlin R, Klenda B, Robol H, Stiles JC, Sparks WS. Enhanced blood levels of coenzyme Q-10 from an emulsified oral form. In Faruqui SR and Ansari MS (editors). *Second Symposium on Nutrition and Chiropractic Proceedings.* April 15-16, 1989 in Davenport, Iowa
23. Stepan JJ, Burckhardt P, Hana V. The effects of three-month intravenous ibandronate on bone mineral density and bone remodeling in Klinefelter's syndrome: the influence of vitamin D deficiency and hormonal status. *Bone* 2003;33:589-596
24. Vasquez A. Health care for our bones: a practical nutritional approach to preventing osteoporosis. [letter] *J Manipulative* Physiol Ther. 2005;28:213

Citation: Vasquez A. Subphysiologic Doses of Vitamin D are Subtherapeutic: Comment on the Study by The Record Trial Group. *Lancet* 2005 published online May 6

Internet: Originally posted at http://www.thelancet.com/journals/lancet/article/PIIS0140673605630139/comments and now available at http://optimalhealthresearch.com/cholecalciferol.html

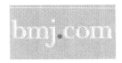

Calcium and vitamin D in preventing fractures

Data are not sufficient to show inefficacy

EDITOR—The study by Porthouse et al had two major design flaws.[1] Firstly, the dose of vitamin D (800 IU per day) is subphysiological and therefore subtherapeutic. Secondly, their use of "self report" as a measure of compliance is unreliable.

The dose of vitamin D at 800 IU daily was not determined scientifically but determined arbitrarily before sufficient scientific methodology was available.[2-4] Heaney et al determined the physiological requirement of vitamin D by showing that healthy men use 4000 IU cholecalciferol daily,[2] an amount that is safely attainable with supplementation[3] and often exceeded with exposure of the total body to equatorial sun.[4]

We provided six guidelines for interventional studies with vitamin D.[5] Dosages of vitamin D must reflect physiological requirements and natural endogenous production and should therefore be in the range of 3000-10 000 IU daily. Vitamin D supplementation must be continued for at least five to nine months. The form of vitamin D should be D_3 rather than D_2. Supplements should be assayed for potency. Effectiveness of supplementation must include measurement of serum 25-hydroxyvitamin D. Serum 25(OH)D concentrations must enter the optimal range, which is 40-65 ng/ml (100-160 nmol/l).

Since the study by Porthouse et al met only the second and third of these six criteria, their data cannot be viewed as reliable for documenting the inefficacy of vitamin D supplementation.

Alex Vasquez, *researcher*

Biotics Research Corporation, 6801 Biotics Research Drive, Rosenberg, TX 77471, USA avasquez@bioticsresearch.com

John Cannell, *president*

Vitamin D Council, 9100 San Gregorio Road, Atascadero, CA 93422, USA

Competing interests: AV is a researcher at Biotics Research Corporation, a drug manufacturing facility in the United States that has approval from the Food and Drug Administration.

References

1. Porthouse J, Cockayne S, King C, Saxon L, Steele E, Aspray T, et al. Randomised controlled trial of calcium and supplementation with cholecalciferol (vitamin D3) for prevention of fractures in primary care. *BMJ* 2005;330: 1003. (30 April.)[Abstract/Free Full Text]
2. Heaney RP, Davies KM, Chen TC, Holick MF, Barger-Lux MJ. Human serum 25-hydroxycholecalciferol response to extended oral dosing with cholecalciferol. *Am J Clin Nutr* 2003;77: 204-10.[Abstract/Free Full Text]
3. Vieth R, Chan PC, MacFarlane GD. Efficacy and safety of vitamin D3 intake exceeding the lowest observed adverse effect level. *Am J Clin Nutr* 2001;73: 288-94.[Abstract/Free Full Text]
4. Vieth R. Vitamin D supplementation, 25-hydroxyvitamin D concentrations, and safety. *Am J Clin Nutr* 1999;69: 842-56.[Abstract/Free Full Text]
5. Vasquez A, Manso G, Cannell J. The clinical importance of vitamin D (cholecalciferol): a paradigm shift with implications for all healthcare providers. *Altern Ther Health Med* 2004;10: 28-36.[ISI][Medline]

Related Article

Randomised controlled trial of calcium and supplementation with cholecalciferol (vitamin D₃) for prevention of fractures in primary care
Jill Porthouse, Sarah Cockayne, Christine King, Lucy Saxon, Elizabeth Steele, Terry Aspray, Mike Baverstock, Yvonne Birks, Jo Dumville, Roger Francis, Cynthia Iglesias, Suezann Puffer, Anne Sutcliffe, Ian Watt, and David J Torgerson
BMJ 2005 330: 1003. [Abstract] [Full Text]

Vasquez A, Cannell J. Calcium and vitamin D in preventing fractures: data are not sufficient to show inefficacy. *BMJ*. 2005 Jul 9;331(7508):108-9 http://www.ncbi.nlm.nih.gov/pubmed/16002891

Thyroid status—laboratory assessments	
Overview and interpretation:	▪ <u>Context</u>: Thyroid disorders are common in clinical practice and thus all clinicians need to have a clear understanding of the clinical presentations and laboratory assessments. Although various aspects of thyroid dysfunction, laboratory tests and clinical presentations will be reviewed here, the primary emphasis will be upon hypothyroidism, which is the most common and *unnecessarily* enigmatic of the thyroid disorders. ▪ <u>Controversy</u>: In the allopathic medical paradigm, much confusion exists regarding a common but "mysterious" and "enigmatic" condition known as hypothyroidism—low thyroid function. Its converse—**hyper**thyroidism and Graves disease—is well understood, easily diagnosed, and readily treated. Because the medical treatment for **hyper**thyroidism often leaves patients in a **hypo**thyroid state, affected patients thus transition from *clarity* (hyperthyroidism) wherein they feel ill due to the disease process into *"mystery"* (hypothyroidism) wherein they feel ill due to incomplete/inaccurate treatment. The basis for the confusion within the allopathic medical community about hypothyroidism is primarily two-fold: ❶ first, they rely on the wrong test (TSH) as the main basis for laboratory assessment, ❷ second, they use incomplete treatment (T4 without T3) which defies the known physiology of the thyroid gland, which makes at least two hormones rather than one. One might get the impression that perpetual confusion is at times the goal of the medical profession; we certainly see this with the management of hypertension, depression, diabetes mellitus, psoriasis and other inflammatory/autoimmune conditions. For people who seek clarity, it is available. ▪ <u>Basic physiology</u>: The hypothalamus produces thyrotropin-releasing hormone (TRH) which stimulates the anterior pituitary gland to make thyroid-stimulating hormone (TSH), which stimulates the thyroid gland to produce thyroxine (T4, approximately 85% of thyroid gland hormone production) and triiodothyronine (T3, approximately 15% of thyroid gland hormone production). In the periphery, the prohormone T4 is converted to active T3 by deiodinase enzymes. Stress, glucagon, and environmental toxins (halogenated phenolics, plastic monomers, flame retardants[176]) impair production of T3 and/or increase production of reverse T3, which is either inert or inhibitory to the action of T3. If the thyroid gland begins to fail, then TSH levels increase as the body attempts to stimulate production of thyroid hormones from a failing gland, which typically fails due to autoimmune attack (Hashimoto's thyroiditis); hence the association of elevated blood TSH levels with "primary hypothyroidism." Thyroid hormones have many different functions in the body, and one of the chief effects is contributing to maintenance of the basal metabolic rate, or the speed of reactions within and the temperature of the body. An insufficiency of thyroid hormone adversely effects numerous biochemical reactions and body/organ functions; hence the myriad of clinical presentations reflecting variations in biochemical and physiologic individuality. Conversely yet similarly, excess thyroid hormone (whether endogenously produced or exogenously administered) also affects numerous body systems. ▪ <u>Clinical presentation of *hyper*thyroidism</u>: The clinical pattern of thyroid excess is more narrowly-focused and thus more predictable and consistent than is the presentation of low thyroid function. The clinical manifestations of hyperthyroidism generally fall into three categories: hyper-adrenergic, hypermetabolic, and ophthalmologic/ocular. ❶ hyper-adrenergic: tachycardia, tremor, diaphoresis, insomnia and a feeling of nervousness and psychomotor agitation due to upregulation of adrenergic tone and generally some degree of relative or absolute hyperthermia; increased dopaminergic and noradrenergic tone in the brain accounts for the neuropsychiatric manifestations, such as mania, psychosis, and

[176] "All studied contaminants inhibited DI activity in a dose-response manner... This study suggests that some halogenated phenolics, including current use compounds such as plastic monomers, flame retardants and their metabolites, may disrupt thyroid hormone homeostasis through the inhibition of DI activity in vivo." Butt CM, Wang D, Stapleton HM. Halogenated Phenolic Contaminants Inhibit the In Vitro Activity of the Thyroid Regulating Deiodinases in Human Liver. *Toxicol Sci.* 2011 May 11. [Epub ahead of print]

hypersexuality, ❷ hyper-metabolic: fecal frequency often described as "diarrhea" due to expedited intestinal transit, elevated temperature, and weight loss due to increased overall metabolic rate, ❸ ophthalmologic/ocular: in chronic cases particularly of the autoimmune variety, exophthalmos develops secondary to retro-orbital connective tissue proliferation and autoimmunity directed toward the extraocular muscles; the histologic abnormalities are chiefly characterized by increased accumulation of collagen (behind the eye and within the extraocular muscles, leading to muscle weakness), accumulation of glycosaminoglycans (GAGs), and the attendant edema.

- Clinical presentation of *hypo*thyroidism: In his classic book *Biochemical Individuality*, Williams[177] noted that "a wide variation in thyroid activity exists among 'normal' human beings." Clearly, some patients do not make enough thyroid hormone to function optimally[178]; or, perhaps more precisely, they make enough thyroid hormone (T4) but do not efficiently convert it to the active form (T3) in the periphery. Further complicating the picture is that some patients make appropriate amounts of TSH, T4, and T3 but they make excess of inactive reverse T3 (rT3) which puts them into a physiologic state of hypothyroidism despite adequate glandular function. Patients may have one or more of the following: fatigue, depression, **cold hands and feet** (excluding Raynaud's syndrome, peripheral vascular disease), dry skin, menstrual irregularities, infertility, premenstrual syndrome (PMS), uterine fibroids, excess menstrual bleeding, **low basal body temperature,** weak fingernails, sleep apnea and increased need for sleep (hypersomnia), slow heart rate (relative or absolute **bradycardia**), easy weight gain and difficult weight loss (thus, predisposition to overweight and obesity), hypercholesterolemia, slow healing, decreased memory and concentration, frog-like husky voice, low libido, recurrent infections, hypertension especially diastolic hypertension, poor digestion (due to insufficient gastric production of hydrochloric acid), **delayed Achilles return** (due to delayed muscle relaxation), carotenodermia, vitamin A deficiency, and gastroesophageal acid reflux, constipation, and predisposition to small intestine bacterial overgrowth (SIBO) due to slow intestinal transit. Of these manifestations, cold hands and feet, low basal body temperature, bradycardia, and delayed Achilles return are the most specific; some very competent physicians will—following proper patient evaluation—treat with thyroid hormone based on the clinical presentation of the patient and *with proper consideration of* and *without dependency upon* laboratory findings.
- Overview of thyroid tests:
  - Thyrotropin-releasing hormone (TRH): The hypothalamus releases TRH to stimulate pituitary production of TSH. TRH is not routinely tested in clinical practice, although abnormalities of TRH secretion are noted in patients with mental "depression."
  - Thyroid-stimulating hormone (TSH: 0.4 - 5.0 mIU/L [milli-international units per liter]): TSH is the most commonly performed test for evaluating thyroid status; its frequent (over)use owes more to habit and inexpensiveness than to aspirations for clinical excellence. TSH values greater than 2 mIU/L represent a disturbance of the thyroid-pituitary axis and an increased risk for future thyroid problems[179], and the American Association of Clinical Endocrinologists states, "The target TSH level should be between 0.3 and 3.0 µIU/mL."[180] Clinical rationale is available to support implementation of a therapeutic trial of thyroid hormone treatment in patients who are clinically hypothyroid even if they are biochemically euthyroid (per TSH) provided

[177] Williams RJ. *Biochemical Individuality: The Basis for the Genetotrophic Concept*. Austin and London: University of Texas Press, 1956 page 82
[178] Broda Barnes MD, Lawrence Galton, *Hypothyroidism: The Unsuspected Illness*. Ty Crowell Co; 1976
[179] Weetman AP. Fortnightly review: Hypothyroidism: screening and subclinical disease. *BMJ: British Medical Journal* 1997;314: 1175
[180] American Association of Clinical Endocrinologists. "The target TSH level should be between 0.3 and 3.0 µIU/mL." AACE Medical Guidelines for Clinical Practice for Evaluation and Treatment of Hyperthyroidism and Hypothyroidism. 2002, 2006 Amended Version. https://www.aace.com/sites/default/files/hypo_hyper.pdf Accessed Aug 2011

Thyroid status—laboratory assessments

that treatment is implemented cautiously, in appropriately selected patients, and patients are appropriately informed.[181,182] If the clinical world were as perfect as it is portrayed in basic physiology textbooks, then a clinician might fancifully rely on TSH to perform the diagnosis *prima facie*, with reduced TSH values correlating with glandular overperformance and negative feedback suppressing TSH secretion, whilst an underperforming gland would require greater stimulation with elevated TSH levels; however, TSH has never been thus vested with infallible reliability, which explains in part why doctors need brains of their own and why better clinicians have developed the capacity for independent thought.

- Free thyroxine (free T4: 4.5 - 11.2 mcg/dL): Unbound T4 is tested to provide evidence of glandular production of thyroid hormone(s). Because T4 is the major thyroid hormone produced by the thyroid gland it serves as an excellent marker for glandular productivity but it reveals nothing about peripheral conversion of T4 to the active thyroid hormone triiodothyronine (T3); in the practice of medicine, conversion of T4 to the active T3 is assumed to reliably occur unabated despite evidence to the contrary, especially among symptomatic patients.

- Triiodothyronine (T3: 100 - 200 ng/dL[183]): In textbook-perfect physiology, T4 is converted by deiodinase enzymes type-1 and type-2 to the active thyroid hormone T3; in reality, this is only part of the story. Because T3 is the active form of the hormone responsible for the physiologic functions of thyroid physiology, a clinician desiring to assess a patient's thyroid status might reasonably ask the proper question by performing the proper test. T3 is tested as "total T3" or "free T3" in large part based on the clinician's preference; the current author prefers total T3 because it can be compared to the total level of reverse T3 (rT3) in a ratio, the optimal range of which is generally considered to be 10-14 as originally presented by McDaniel[184] and reviewed in the following pages. Patients with psychiatric depression have lower levels of T3 than do healthy controls and have been described as having "low T3 syndrome"[185]; very obviously—whether cause or effect—the low T3 levels in these patients would serve to promote and perpetuate their state of mental depression. Although the focus of this review within the subject of laboratory evaluation is not to describe the implementation of thyroid hormone treatment, clinicians should be aware that T3 administration increases hepatic production of sex hormone binding globulin (SHBG) and that therefore T3 administration can reduce cellular bioavailability of protein-bound hormones. Many authoritative and clinically-experienced sources recommend using a time-released (e.g., sustained-release) form of T3 due to its shorter half-life compared with T4. However, obtaining time-released T3 via a compounding pharmacy can be cumbersome and expensive for the patient; clearly some patients respond to once daily dosing of *non*-time-released preparations with good effects and without adverse effects. Some patients can divide the immediate-release dose into two servings per day for enhanced effect and lessened physiologic fluctuations, if necessary. Per Drugs.com[186] in August 2011, "Since liothyronine sodium (T3) is not firmly bound to serum protein, it is readily available to body tissues. The onset of activity of liothyronine sodium is rapid, occurring within a few hours. Maximum pharmacologic

[181] Skinner GR, Thomas R, Taylor M, Sellarajah M, Bolt S, Krett S, Wright A. Thyroxine should be tried in clinically hypothyroid but biochemically euthyroid patients. *BMJ: British Medical Journal* 1997 Jun 14; 314(7096): 1764

[182] McLaren EH, Kelly CJ, Pollack MA. Trial of thyroxine treatment for biochemically euthyroid patients has been approved. *BMJ* 1997; 315: 1463

[183] U.S. National Library of Medicine (NLM) and National Institutes of Health (NIH) http://www.nlm.nih.gov/medlineplus/ency/article/003687.htm Accessed August 2011

[184] McDaniel AB. Thyroid Assessment: Controversies and Conundrums. Institute for Functional Medicine 14th International Symposium. Tucson, Arizona. May 23-26, 2007

[185] "Out of 250 subjects with major psychiatric depression, 6.4% exhibited low T3 syndrome (mean serum T3 concentration 0.94 nmol/l vs normal mean serum concentration of 1.77 nmol/l)." Premachandra BN, Kabir MA, Williams IK. Low T3 syndrome in psychiatric depression. *J Endocrinol Invest.* 2006 Jun;29(6):568-72

[186] http://www.drugs.com/pro/cytomel.html Accessed August 2011.

response occurs within 2 or 3 days, providing early clinical response. The biological half-life is about 2.5 days." Very clearly, a significant portion of hypothyroid patients respond to T3 alone (either time-released, divided-dosing, or once-daily dosing) or a combination of T4 and T3 when other treatments have failed.[187,188]

  o Reverse triiodothyronine (rT3: 90 - 320 pg/mL[189]): T4 is converted by deiodinase enzymes type-1 and type-3 to the inactive thyroid hormone rT3; per a standard endocrinology textbook, "Approximately 70–80% of released T4 is converted by deiodinases to the biologically active T3, the remainder to reverse-T3 (rT3) which has no significant biological activity."[190] Clinicians must know that, "The prohormone T4 **must be converted to T3 in the body before it can exert biological effects. During periods of illness or stress, this conversion is often inhibited and can be diverted to the inactive reverse T3 (rT3) moiety.**"[191] Furthermore and very importantly, clinicians should appreciate that rT3 is not simply inactive but that it may actually impair production/utilization of normal T3; "T4-T3 and T4-rT3 conversion are provoked by different enzymes. **The <u>elevation of rT3</u> might be a cause of the observed decrease in peripheral T3 generation** in old [elderly] subjects, acting by an **<u>inhibition of the T4-T3 conversion</u>**."[192] During times of psychologic/physiologic stress and specific types of pharmacologic stress (e.g., propanolol[193] and corticosteroids), T4 metabolism is preferentially shunted away from T3 toward rT3; an anthropocentric explanation holds that by making less of the active T3 and more of the inactive rT3, the body is better able to conserve energy during times of stress by reducing overall metabolic rate, particularly resting energy expenditure and protein utilization. For example, caloric restriction and fasting result in a decrease in resting metabolic rate (RMR), and the reduced RMR persists for months after the fasting has ended and a normal diet is resumed.[194] This author (AV) terms this stress-induced impairment of thyroid hormone conversion "**metabolic hypothyroidism**" or "**functional hypothyroidism**" because the defect is in the metabolism (not the production) of thyroid hormone into its most active form; "**peripheral hypothyroidism**" might also be used to distinguish the fact that the defect is in the peripheral metabolism rather than located more centrally, within the thyroid gland itself. Because psychologic stress and certain pharmacologic exposures— as well as the thyro-metabolic stress of fasting and caloric restriction in which the counterregulatory hormone glucagon appears to trigger enhanced rT3 production— reduce T3 while simultaneously increasing rT3 levels, clinicians can appreciate that calculation of the T3/rT3 ratio will be more significantly altered (and thus a more sensitive indicator of metabolic disruption) than will be the isolated measurements of T3 or rT3 alone. Functional medicine clinicians[195] note the importance of the ratio of total T3 to reverse T3 (tT3:rT3 ratio) and consider the optimal range to be 10-14 with lower ratios indicating impaired formation or T3 and/or excess production of rT3.[196] Contrary to the previous view which held that rT3 was simply inactive, we now

[187] Bunevicius R, Kazanavicius G, Zalinkevicius R, Prange AJ Jr. Effects of thyroxine as compared with thyroxine plus triiodothyronine in patients with hypothyroidism. *N Engl J Med*. 1999 Feb 11;340(6):424-9

[188] Kelly T, Lieberman DZ. The use of triiodothyronine as an augmentation agent in treatment-resistant bipolar II and bipolar disorder NOS. *J Affect Disord*. 2009;116(3):222-6

[189] The reference range provided here for rT3 is a compilation from the laboratory reference ranges from the sample reports on the following pages, each of which is performed by either Quest Diagnostics or LabCorp, the two largest medical laboratories in the United States.

[190] Nussey S, Whitehead S. *Endocrinology: An Integrated Approach*. Oxford: BIOS Scientific Publishers; 2001. See also Box 3.29 Metabolism of thyroid hormones. http://www.ncbi.nlm.nih.gov/books/NBK28/box/A270/?report=objectonly Accessed July 2011

[191] *1998 Mosby's GenRX. Sixth Edition*. St. Louis Missouri; Mosby-Year Book, Inc., 1998

[192] Szabolcs I, Weber M, Kovács Z, Irsy G, Góth M, Halász T, Szilágyi G. The possible reason for serum 3,3'5'-(reverse) triiodothyronine increase in old people. *Acta Med Acad Sci Hung*. 1982;39(1-2):11-7

[193] "Propranolol administration (40 mg t.i.d. for a week) caused a similar rT3 elevation in old persons (n = 18) as in 12 young ones." Szabolcs I, Weber M, Kovács Z, Irsy G, Góth M, Halász T, Szilágyi G. The possible reason for serum 3,3'5'-(reverse) triiodothyronine increase in old people. *Acta Med Acad Sci Hung*. 1982;39(1-2):11-7

[194] Elliot DL, Goldberg L, Kuehl KS, Bennett WM. Sustained depression of the resting metabolic rate after massive weight loss. *Am J Clin Nutr* 1989 Jan;49(1):93-96

[195] The conclusion of this paragraph is derived from **Vasquez A**. *Musculoskeletal Pain: Expanded Clinical Strategies*. Published 2008 by The Institute for Functional Medicine. http://www.functionalmedicine.org/ifm_ecommerce/ProductDetails.aspx?ProductID=127

[196] McDaniel AB. Thyroid Assessment: Controversies and Conundrums. Institute for Functional Medicine 14th International Symposium. Tucson, Arizona. May 23-26, 2007

Thyroid status—laboratory assessments	
	appreciate that rT3 actually impairs normal thyroid hormone metabolism thus functioning as an thyrometabolic monkeywrench or "brake" on normal metabolism. Elevated rT3 levels predict mortality among critically ill patients.[197] Aberrancies in thyroid hormone levels may reflect organic disease, psychoemotional stress, or nutritional deficiency[198], and therefore such serologic abnormalities warrant consideration of underlying problems and direct treatment when possible. If no underlying cause is apparent, then a trial of thyroid hormone/hormones is reasonable in appropriately selected patients. Beyond stress reduction, allergen/gluten avoidance, and nutritional supplementation with iodine, selenium, and zinc (as indicated per patient), correction of overt, subclinical, and functional hypothyroidism generally centers on the administration of natural or synthetic thyroid hormones in the form of T4 and T3. Correction of functional hypothyroidism (relatively reduced total T3 and increased rT3) is accomplished with either time-released or twice-daily dosing of T3 *without T4* to suppress endogenous T4 conversion to T3, thereby allowing rT3 levels to fall precipitously. T3 administration allows temporary downregulation of transforming enzymes so that rT3 production is reduced following withdrawal of T3 replacement; thus, short-term and/or periodic T3 administration helps normalize or "reset" peripheral thyroid metabolism so that, following withdrawal of T3 administration, T4 can be converted to T3 without excess production of rT3. The safety and effectiveness of this approach—using T3 administration (often twice daily or in a sustained-release compounded tablet or capsule) to recalibrate peripheral thyroid hormone metabolism—has documented safety and effectiveness.[199] Alleviation of symptoms, restoration of morning body temperature to 98.6° F (oral or axillary) and other clinical objective improvements achieved by the judicious and safe administration of T3 are the criteria of success; physiologic improvement following T3 administration retrospectively confirms the diagnosis. ○ <u>Antithyroid antibodies—antithyroglobulin (anti-TG) and anti-thyroid peroxidase (anti-TPO)</u>: Autoimmune thyroiditis (also called Hashimoto's disease or chronic lymphocytic thyroiditis) or is the most common cause of overt primary hypothyroidism. The diagnosis of autoimmune thyroiditis can be made clinically (i.e., without biopsy) upon detection of elevated blood levels of antibodies against thyroglobulin (anti-thyroglobulin antibodies) and anti-thyroid peroxidase (anti-TPO) antibodies. Autoimmune thyroiditis may present asymptomatically and with normal thyroid hormone levels; classically, patients may have a slightly hyperthyroid presentation as the inflamed gland releases extra thyroid hormone before becoming atrophic and hypofunctional.
Advantages:	▪ Thyroid disorders are quite common in general practice and are often undiagnosed, undertreated, or inappropriately treated. ▪ Consistent with the principle of beneficence, patients and doctors benefit when thyroid disorders are diagnosed and treated appropriately.
Limitations:	▪ A properly interpreted TSH may overlook problems of T4 production or conversion to active T3. Additionally, in some patients, all of these tests are normal but they may have thyroid

---

[197] Peeters RP, Wouters PJ, van Toor H, Kaptein E, Visser TJ, Van den Berghe G. Serum 3,3',5'-triiodothyronine (rT3) and 3,5,3'-triiodothyronine/rT3 are prognostic markers in critically ill patients and are associated with postmortem tissue deiodinase activities. *J Clin Endocrinol Metab*. 2005 Aug;90(8):4559-65

[198] Kelly GS. Peripheral metabolism of thyroid hormones: a review. Altern Med Rev. 2000 Aug;5(4):306-33

[199] Friedman M, Miranda-Massari JR, Gonzalez MJ. Supraphysiological cyclic dosing of sustained release T3 in order to reset low basal body temperature. *P R Health Sci J*. 2006 Mar;25(1):23-9

	autoimmunity (i.e., thyroid peroxidase antibodies, anti-TPO) and should receive treatment with thyroid hormone[200] or some other corrective treatment (e.g., selenium supplementation[201,202] and a gluten-free diet[203]) to normalize thyroid status.
Comments:	▪ Comprehensive thyroid laboratory testing including ❶ TSH, ❷ free T4, ❸ total T3, ❹ rT3, ❺ antithyroid antibodies, should be evaluated alongside the ❻ heart rate, ❼ cold extremities, ❽ basal body temperature, ❾ Achilles' return rate, and ❿ overall symptoms and clinical picture. ▪ The combination of T3 and T4 (as in the prescription Liotrix/Thyrolar or Armour thyroid) appears to have similar safety to T4 alone (Levothyroxine, Synthroid) and may result in greater improvements in mood and neuropsychological function.[204] ▪ Glandular thyroid supplements and Armour thyroid generally should *not* be used in patients with thyroid autoimmunity (Hashimoto's thyroiditis) because the bovine/porcine antigens will exacerbate the anti-thyroid immune response as evidenced by increased anti-TPO antibodies.

Optimal thyroid status

Concept by Dr Vasquez: Optimal thyroid status is not defined by basic laboratory testing with TSH and free T4. It is defined *per patient* based on the levels and ratios of all major thyroid-related hormones and antibodies—in association with other hormonal, psychologic, dysbiotic, nutritional and environmental factors— that work best for that particular unique biochemically-individual patient.

Laboratory interpretation by Dr McDaniel: "Optimal hormone balance is debatable. My observations: A few "well" people and patients treated successfully with T4 and T3 seem best with:

- TSH around 0.7–0.9µIU/mL
- fT4 around 0.7–0.8ng/dL
- fT3 optimally 3.4–3.8pg/mL
- **Total T3-RT3 ratio 12 +/-2**"

McDaniel AB. Thyroid Assessment: Controversies and Conundrums. Institute for Functional Medicine Fourteenth International Symposium. Tucson, Arizona. May 23-26, 2007

---

[200] Beers MH, Berkow R (eds). The Merck Manual. 17th Edition. Whitehouse Station; Merck Research Laboratories 1999 page 96

[201] Duntas LH, Mantzou E, Koutras DA. Effects of a six month treatment with selenomethionine in patients with autoimmune thyroiditis. *Eur J Endocrinol*. 2003 Apr;148(4):389-93 http://eje-online.org/cgi/reprint/148/4/389

[202] Gartner R, Gasnier BC. Selenium in the treatment of autoimmune thyroiditis. *Biofactors*. 2003;19(3-4):165-70

[203] Sategna-Guidetti C, Volta U, Ciacci C, Usai P, Carlino A, De Franceschi L, Camera A, Pelli A, Brossa C. Prevalence of thyroid disorders in untreated adult celiac disease patients and effect of gluten withdrawal: an Italian multicenter study. *Am J Gastroenterol*. 2001 Mar;96(3):751-7

[204] "CONCLUSIONS: In patients with hypothyroidism, partial substitution of triiodothyronine for thyroxine may improve mood and neuropsychological function; this finding suggests a specific effect of the triiodothyronine normally secreted by the thyroid gland." Bunevicius R, Kazanavicius G, Zalinkevicius R, Prange AJ Jr. Effects of thyroxine as compared with thyroxine plus triiodothyronine in patients with hypothyroidism. *N Engl J Med*. 1999 Feb 11;340(6):424-9

Presentation: 38yo male under extreme psychological stress with a complaint of constantly cold extremities—testing performed in February 2010 by LabCorp: Review the following labs and outline your treatment plan before reading the discussion below.

Date and Time Collected	Date Entered	Date and Time Reported	Physician Name	NPI	Pt
02/04/10 11:41	02/04/10	02/09/10 04:0(	EBAN		190

Tests Ordered
Triiodothyronine (T3);Reverse T3;Triiodothyronine,Free,Serum

General Comments
PID: 8282293

TESTS	RESULT	FLAG	UNITS	REFERENCE INTERV
Triiodothyronine (T3)				
Triiodothyronine (T3)	57	Low	ng/dL	71-180
Reverse T3				
Reverse T3	312		pg/mL	90-350
Triiodothyronine,Free,Serum				
Triiodothyronine,Free,Serum	2.5		pg/mL	2.0-4.4

Discussion: In this case, because the T3 level is low, *prima facie* justification for administration of T3 is provided, assuming that the clinical picture is compatible and that no contraindications to treatment are present. To calculate the total T3/rT3 ratio, equilibrate the units (multiply total T3 in ng/dL x 10 to convert to pg/mL; 1 pg = 0.001 ng (1 ng = 1,000 pg); 1 dl = 100 ml). The total T3/rT3 ratio should be >10-14 (per McDaniel[205]), but in this patient's case 570/312 = 1.8. Remember, more T3 than rT3 is better; hence, the higher ratio is better. On-line calculators for this conversion have been developed[206] and surely more will be available in the future. This athletic and otherwise healthy 220-lb (100 kg) patient responded very well to T3 (liothyronine/Cytomel) with a starting dose of 150 mcg which was eventually tapered to 25 mcg and then to 12.5 mcg; in this patient's case, the initial high dose of T3 was well-tolerated because of the initially low level of T3, the elevated rT3 which appears to block T3 function, and the patient's overall excellent cardiovascular fitness. A reasonable dosage range for liothyronine/Cytomel supplementation is 12.5-50 mcg for most patients tapered to the constellation of patient tolerance, patient preference, heart rate, basal body temperature optimization to 98.6° F, suppression of TSH and T4, resolution of symptoms and objective markers, and clinician's impression and experience.

Step-by-step conversion from ng/dL to pg/mL—end result is multiply by 10 (i.e., 10x)

Original units	Convert ng to pg[207]	Convert dL to mL	Simplify the fraction
1 ng / 1 dL	1,000 pg / 1 dL	1,000 pg/ 100 mL	10 pg / 1 ml
57 ng/ 1 dL	57,000 pg / 1 dL	57,000 pg / 100 mL	570 pg / 1 mL

Contraindications to T3, liothyronine, Cytomel
Absolute contraindications:

- Anaphylaxis or severe hypersensitivity,
- Acute (current) myocardial infarction,
- Hyperthyroidism,
- Untreated adrenal insufficiency.

Relative contraindications and cautions:

- CAD, angina pectoris, or cardiac arrhythmia,
- Elderly patients—start with low dose and titrate as tolerated.

Reference: Epocrates.com August 2011

---

[205] McDaniel AB. Thyroid Assessment: Controversies and Conundrums. Institute for Functional Medicine Fourteenth International Symposium. Tucson, AZ. May 23-26, 2007
[206] http://www.stopthethyroidmadness.com/rt3-ratio/ Accessed—but not necessarily endorsed—August 2011
[207] Double-checked with http://www.unitconversion.org/weight/nanograms-to-picograms-conversion.html July 2011

Presentation: 42yo male with fatigue—testing performed by Quest Diagnostics in January 2010: Review the following labs and outline your treatment plan before reading the discussion below. Note that the "optimal ratio" provided by the laboratory in this example was performed using free T3 rather than total T3 and without converting to equal units.

```
FREE T3/REVERSE T3 RATIO
    FREE T3/REVERSE T3 RATIO                        0.93 L           1.05-1.91**
    FREE T3                             325                          230-420 pg/dL
    REVERSE T3                                       350 H           100-340*** pg/mL
            **Ratio= Free T3 in pg/dL : reverse T3 in pg/mL. Ratio for reference
            range is calculated by dividing the lower and upper end of free T3
            with the mean of reverse T3 (220 pg/mL).

            ***Observed reference range is reported for reverse T3 per client
            request.

            This test was performed using a kit that has not been approved or
            cleared by the FDA. The analytical performance characteristics of this
            test have been determined by Quest Diagnostics Nichols Institute, San
            Juan Capistrano. This test should not be used for diagnosis without
            confirmation by other medically established means.
```

Discussion: Note that if the T3 had been tested without rT3 the results would have been reported as "normal" and that a "depressed" patient so assessed would have likely been given an "antidepressant" medication and a diagnosis of depression rather than the proper treatment with T3 and a diagnosis of functional hypothyroidism. Luckily for this patient, his clinician tested rT3 and upon finding it impressively elevated treated with patient with T3 to suppress rT3 production by temporarily suppressing T4 production. The ratio calculation is provided and interpreted by the laboratory; notice that the "ideal ratio" for **total** T3/rT3 (>10) differs from that of **free** T3/rT3 (>1.05) *and that per the ratio provided by the labotatory does not equilibriate the measurement units.* This method is acceptable but is not the preferred method for determining functional thyroid status. The preferred method is the one presented by McDaniel[208] at the Institute for Functional Medicine's 14th International Symposium in 2007 wherein he advocated using total T3 (not free T3) in comparison with rT3 interpreted by an optimal ratio of 10-14.

Step-by-step conversion from pg/dL to pg/mL—end result is divide by 100 (i.e., 0.01x): Provided for the sake of completeness even though the conversion is not necessary per the laboratory interpretation provided above.

Original units	Convert dL to mL	Simplify the fraction
1 pg / 1 dL	1 pg/ 100 mL	0.01 pg/ 1 mL
325 pg/ 1 dL	325 pg / 100 mL	3.25 pg / 1 mL

---

[208] McDaniel AB. Thyroid Assessment: Controversies and Conundrums. Institute for Functional Medicine 14th International Symposium. Tucson, Arizona. May 23-26, 2007

Presentation: 31yo female with fatigue, a recent history of extreme emotional stress (death of first-degree family member), maternal history of Hashimotos thyroiditis, and a personal history of presumed gluten intolerance—testing performed in May 2010 by Quest Diagnostics: Outline your treatment plan before reading discussion.

Test Name	In Range	Out of Range	Reference Range
THYROGLOBULIN ANTIBODIES	<20		<20 IU/mL
THYROID PEROXIDASE ANTIBODIES		38 H	<35 IU/mL
T3, TOTAL	89		76-181 ng/dL
T3 UPTAKE		37 H	22-35 %
T4, FREE	1.6		0.8-1.8 ng/dL
T4 (THYROXINE), TOTAL			
T4 (THYROXINE), TOTAL	10.9		4.5-12.5 mcg/dL
FREE T4 INDEX (T7)		4.0 H	1.4-3.8
TSH, 3RD GENERATION	0.82		mIU/L

Reference Range

> or = 20 Years   0.40-4.50

Pregnancy Ranges
First trimester   0.20-4.70
Second trimester 0.30-4.10
Third trimester   0.40-2.70

Test Name	In Range	Out of Range	Reference Range
T3, FREE	318		230-420 pg/dL
T3, REVERSE		43 H	11-32 ng/dL

This test was performed using a kit that has not been approved or cleared by the FDA. The analytical performance characteristics of this test have been determined by Quest Diagnostics Nichols Institute, San Juan Capistrano. This test should not be used for diagnosis without confirmation by other medically established means.

Discussion: Note that the TSH is completely normal and thus would give the impression of normalcy and "health" if the clinician had not ordered the additional tests. Thyroid peroxidase antibodies are minimally elevated; this is consistent with thyroid autoimmunity but titers this low are of limited clinical importance. Note that the rT3 level is abnormally elevated. Note that because the units provided for total T3 (89 ng/dL) and rT3 (43 ng/dL) are identical, no unit conversion is required, thereby making the calculation of the ideal ratio (range: 10-14) very simple. In this patient's case, the ratio comes to 2.06 which is obviously significantly lower than the proposed optimal of 10-14; the patient responded well to liothyronine/Cytomel supplementation with 15 mcg/d. Patients with thyroid autoimmunity often benefit from a gluten-free diet[209] and supplementation with selenium 200 mcg/d.[210] Finally, note that the reference range for total T3 provided by this laboratory is 76-181 ng/dL which contrasts significantly from the range recommended by the US National Institutes of Health (NIH) 100 to 200 ng/dL[211]; using the NIH's reference range, this patient's T3 production is inadequate.

---

[209] "Hypothyroidism, diagnosed in 31 patients (12.9%) and nine controls (4.2%), was subclinical in 29 patients and of nonautoimmune origin in 21. ... In most patients who strictly followed a 1-yr gluten withdrawal (as confirmed by intestinal mucosa recovery), there was a normalization of subclinical hypothyroidism. The greater frequency of thyroid disease among celiac disease patients justifies a thyroid functional assessment. In distinct cases, gluten withdrawal may single-handedly reverse the abnormality." Sategna-Guidetti C, Volta U, Ciacci C, et al. Prevalence of thyroid disorders in untreated adult celiac disease patients and effect of gluten withdrawal: an Italian multicenter study. *Am J Gastroenterol.* 2001 Mar;96(3):751-7

[210] "Patients with HT assigned to Se supplementation for 3 months demonstrated significantly lower thyroid peroxidase autoantibodies (TPOab) titers (four studies, random effects weighted mean difference: −271.09, 95% confidence interval: −421.98 to −120.19, p< 10⁻⁴) and a significantly higher chance of reporting an improvement in well-being and/or mood (three studies, random effects risk ratio: 2.79, 95% confidence interval: 1.21-6.47, p= 0.016) when compared with controls. .. On the basis of the best available evidence, Se supplementation is associated with a significant decrease in TPOab titers at 3 months and with improvement in mood and/or general well-being."Toulis KA, Anastasilakis AD, Tzellos TG, Goulis DG, Kouvelas D. Selenium supplementation in the treatment of Hashimoto's thyroiditis: a systematic review and a meta-analysis. *Thyroid.* 2010 Oct;20(10):1163-73
[211] U.S. National Library of Medicine and NIH www.nlm.nih.gov/medlineplus/ency/article/003687.htm Accessed Aug 2011

Toxic metal testing—emphasis on lead and mercury	
Overview and application:	▪ Introduction: Per the US Department of Labor's Occupational Safety and Health Administration (OSHA)[212], toxic metals, including "heavy metals", are individual metals and metal compounds that negatively affect people's health. While lists of toxic metals can vary per source, OSHA names the following: arsenic, beryllium, cadmium, hexavalent chromium, lead, and mercury; of these, lead and mercury are the most commonly observed problematic toxic metals in outpatient practice. The three most important clinical concepts with regard to testing for "heavy metals" or "toxic metals" are as follows:

1. Heavy metal toxicity/accumulation is not uncommon in clinical practice: Toxic/heavy metal accumulation is clinically important due both to its frequency and its pathophysiologic consequences. An article published in *Journal of the American Medical Association (JAMA)*[213] showed that approximately 8% of [1,709 American] women had [blood mercury] concentrations higher than the US Environmental Protection Agency's recommended reference dose (5.8 µg/L), below which exposures are considered to be without adverse effects; **stated more plainly, 8% of American women have (potentially) toxic levels of mercury** *even when evaluated by the least sensitive of laboratory methods—blood mercury,* **which represents only 5% of total body mercury.** Another study, also published in *JAMA*[214], showed a positive relationship between blood lead levels and hypertension, even at blood lead levels considered within the normal range; the authors wrote, "At levels well below the current US occupational exposure limit guidelines (40 µg/dL), **blood lead level is positively associated with both systolic and diastolic blood pressure and risks of both systolic and diastolic hypertension among women aged 40 to 59 years.**"

2. The clinical presentation of heavy metal toxicity/accumulation is generally diverse and nonspecific: Clinical presentations due to or associated with toxic metal accumulation can include dyscognition, fatigue, anemia, chronic pain from myalgia or neuropathy, hypertension, autism, and immune disorders including autoimmunity and allergy. In particular, autism[215,216,217] and hypertension[218,219] are noteworthy for their consistent associations with mercury and with mercury and lead, respectively.

3. (Therefore), clinicians should test for and treat toxic metal accumulation: When problems are clinically significant and not extremely unlikely, clinicians have an obligation to test for and treat such problems for the benefit of the patient. Therefore, because toxic metal accumulation is common, clinically significant, and because it is a reversible cause of numerous symptoms, syndromes, and a contributing factor to many other diagnosable conditions (e.g., hypertension, immune disorders, mood disorders), clinicians have an obligation to consider and test for toxic metals among their patients.

▪ Additional details—mercury: Mercury is an established neurotoxin, immunotoxin, and nephrotoxin. Because pathophysiologic effects are noted even with very small doses of

---

[212] http://www.osha.gov/SLTC/metalsheavy/index.html Accessed July 2011.

[213] Schober SE, Sinks TH, Jones RL, Bolger PM, McDowell M, Osterloh J, Garrett ES, Canady RA, Dillon CF, Sun Y, Joseph CB, Mahaffey KR. Blood mercury levels in US children and women of childbearing age, 1999-2000. *JAMA* 2003;289:1667-74 http://jama.ama-assn.org/content/289/13/1667.long

[214] Nash D, Magder L, Lustberg M, Sherwin RW, Rubin RJ, Kaufmann RB, Silbergeld EK. Blood lead, blood pressure, and hypertension in perimenopausal and postmenopausal women. *JAMA*. 2003 Mar 26;289(12):1523-32. See also Muntner P, He J, Vupputuri S, Coresh J, Batuman V. Blood lead and chronic kidney disease in the general United States population: results from NHANES III. *Kidney Int*. 2003 Mar;63(3):1044-50 http://www.nature.com/ki/journal/v63/n3/pdf/4493526a.pdf

[215] Stamova B, Green PG, Tian Y, Hertz-Picciotto I, Pessah IN, Hansen R, Yang X, Teng J, Gregg JP, Ashwood P, Van de Water J, Sharp FR. Correlations between gene expression and mercury levels in blood of boys with and without autism. *Neurotox Res*. 2011;19:31-48. Epub 2009 Nov 24.

[216] "The results of the study indicated that the participants' overall ATEC scores and their scores on each of the ATEC subscales (Speech/Language, Sociability, Sensory/Cognitive Awareness, and Health/Physical/Behavior) were linearly related to urinary porphyrins associated with mercury toxicity. The results show an association between the apparent level of mercury toxicity as measured by recognized urinary porphyrin biomarkers of mercury toxicity and the magnitude of the specific hallmark features of autism as assessed by ATEC." Kern JK, Geier DA, Adams JB, Geier MR. A biomarker of mercury body-burden correlated with diagnostic domain specific clinical symptoms of autism spectrum disorder. *Biometals*. 2010 Dec;23(6):1043-51

[217] Kempuraj D, Asadi S, Zhang B, Manola A, Hogan J, Peterson E, Theoharides TC. Mercury induces inflammatory mediator release from human mast cells. *J Neuroinflammation*. 2010 Mar 11;7:20 http://www.jneuroinflammation.com/content/7/1/20

[218] Schober SE, Sinks TH, Jones RL, Bolger PM, McDowell M, Osterloh J, Garrett ES, Canady RA, Dillon CF, Sun Y, Joseph CB, Mahaffey KR. Blood mercury levels in US children and women of childbearing age, 1999-2000. *JAMA* 2003;289:1667-74 http://jama.ama-assn.org/content/289/13/1667.long

[219] Nash D, Magder L, Lustberg M, Sherwin RW, Rubin RJ, Kaufmann RB, Silbergeld EK. Blood lead, blood pressure, and hypertension in perimenopausal and postmenopausal women. *JAMA*. 2003 Mar 26;289(12):1523-32

Toxic metal testing—emphasis on lead and mercury

exposure, one could reasonably argue that no safe amount exists and therefore that any detected mercury is an indication for therapeutic intervention to remove this toxicant. According to an article by Schober et al[220] published in *JAMA—Journal of the American Medical Association* in 2003, "Approximately 8% of [1,709 American] women had [blood mercury] concentrations higher than the US Environmental Protection Agency's recommended reference dose (5.8 µg/L), below which exposures are considered to be without adverse effects." Sources of exposure include dental amalgams, vaccinations, airborne pollution, deep-water fish such as tuna, some cosmetics[221], and selected herbicides, fungicides, and germicides; recently, high-fructose corn syrup was shown to contain mercury in clinically meaningful amounts.[222] Mercury impairs catecholamine degradation and can thereby cause a clinical syndrome that can include hypertension, tremor, tachycardia, diaphoresis, and neurocognitive changes.[223] Per Shih and Gartner[224], "Mercury combines with the sulfhydryl group of S-adenosylmethionine, which is a cofactor for catecholamine-O-methyltransferase (COMT), and this inhibition of COMT allows accumulation of norepinephrine, epinephrine, and dopamine." The clinical presentation of mercury toxicity can include any of the following: diffuse erythematosus rash, dermatitis (acrodynia), anorexia, malaise, **fatigue**, **muscle pain**, proximal and/or distal muscle weakness, tremor, weight loss, **insomnia**, night sweats, burning peripheral neuropathy (axonal neuropathy), renal insufficiency/failure, **inattention**, neurocognitive compromise, personality changes, **depression**, diaphoresis, tachycardia, and **hypertension**. Mercury poisoning/accumulation can occur in humans as a result of consumption of contaminated foods—especially seafood such as shark, swordfish, king mackerel, tilefish, and albacore ("white") tuna.[225] The immunologic effects of organic and/or inorganic mercury include immunosuppression, immunostimulation, formation of antinucleolar antibodies targeting fibrillarin, and formation and deposition of immune-complexes, resulting in a syndrome called "mercury-induced autoimmunity" which can be induced by exposure of susceptible animals to mercury.[226] Mercury/"silver" amalgam dental fillings rank highly among the most significant source of mercury exposure in humans, and implantation of mercury-silver dental amalgams in susceptible animals causes chronic stimulation of the immune system with induction of systemic autoimmunity.[227] Besides being a neurotoxin with no safe exposure limit[228], mercury is known to modify/antigenize/haptenize endogenous proteins to promote autoimmunity[229], and mercury may also promote autoimmunity by contributing to a pro-inflammatory environment that awakens quiescent autoreactive immunocytes via bystander activation.[230] For example, administration of mercury

[220] Schober SE, Sinks TH, Jones RL, et al. Blood mercury levels in US children and women of childbearing age, 1999-2000. *JAMA*. 2003 Apr 2;289(13):1667-74 http://jama.ama-assn.org/content/289/13/1667.long

[221] "Most makeup manufacturers have phased out the use of mercury, but it's still added legally to some eye products as a preservative and germ-killer, said John Bailey, chief scientist with the Personal Care Products Council in Washington." Associated Press. Minnesota Bans Adding Mercury To Cosmetics. February 11, 2009. http://www.cbsnews.com/stories/2007/12/14/health/main3618048.shtml Accessed August 2011

[222] "Average daily consumption of high fructose corn syrup is about 50 grams per person in the United States. With respect to total mercury exposure, it may be necessary to account for this source of mercury in the diet of children and sensitive populations." Dufault R, LeBlanc B, Schnoll R, Cornett C, Schweitzer L, Wallinga D, Hightower J, Patrick L, Lukiw WJ. Mercury from chlor-alkali plants: measured concentrations in food product sugar. *Environ Health*. 2009 Jan 26;8:2. See also: "High fructose corn syrup has been shown to contain trace amounts of mercury as a result of some manufacturing processes, and its consumption can also lead to zinc loss." Dufault R, Schnoll R, Lukiw WJ, Leblanc B, Cornett C, Patrick L, Wallinga D, Gilbert SG, Crider R. Mercury exposure, nutritional deficiencies and metabolic disruptions may affect learning in children. *Behav Brain Funct*. 2009 Oct 27;5:44.

[223] Wössmann W, Kohl M, Grüning G, Bucsky P. Mercury intoxication presenting with hypertension and tachycardia. *Arch Dis Child*. 1999 Jun;80(6):556-7 http://www.ncbi.nlm.nih.gov/pmc/articles/PMC1717944/pdf/v080p00556.pdf

[224] Shih H, Gartner JC Jr. Weight loss, hypertension, weakness, and limb pain in an 11-year-old boy. *J Pediatr*. 2001 Apr;138(4):566-9

[225] See http://www.fda.gov/Food/FoodSafety/Product-SpecificInformation/Seafood/FoodbornePathogensContaminants/Methylmercury/ucm115662.htm for the white-washed version; see http://www.ewg.org/news/bamboozled-fish for a more accurate and complete perspective.

[226] Havarinasab S, Hultman P. Organic mercury compounds and autoimmunity. *Autoimmun Rev*. 2005;4(5):270-5 www.generationrescue.org/pdf/havarinasab.pdf Dec 2005

[227] "We hypothesize that under appropriate conditions of genetic susceptibility and adequate body burden, heavy metal exposure from dental amalgam may contribute to immunological aberrations, which could lead to overt autoimmunity." Hultman P, Johansson U, Turley SJ, Lindh U, Enestrom S, Pollard KM. Adverse immunological effects and autoimmunity induced by dental amalgam and alloy in mice. *FASEB J*. 1994 Nov;8(14):1183-90

[228] University of Calgary Faculty of Medicine. How Mercury Causes Brain Neuron Degeneration. http://commons.ucalgary.ca/mercury/ Current Aug 2011

[229] Havarinasab S, Hultman P. Organic mercury compounds and autoimmunity. *Autoimmun Rev*. 2005 Jun;4(5):270-5. www.generationrescue.org/pdf/havarinasab.pdf Dec 2005

[230] "It is therefore theoretically possible that compounds present in vaccines such as thiomersal or aluminium hydroxyde can trigger autoimmune reactions through bystander effects." Fournie GJ, Mas M, Cautain B, et al. Induction of autoimmunity through bystander effects. Lessons from immunological disorders induced by heavy metals. *J Autoimmun*. 2001 May;16(3):319-26

to "susceptible" mice induces autoimmunity via modification of the nucleolar protein *fibrillarin*[231]; noteworthy in this regard is the fact that antifibrillarin antibodies are characteristic of the human autoimmune disease scleroderma.[232] The mercury-based preservative thimerosol is a type-IV (delayed hypersensitivity) sensitizing agent[233], and recent research implicates mercury as a contributor to autism[234,235] and eczema.[236] A review and clinical report published by Bains et al[237], stated, "Eczematous eruptions may be produced through topical contact with mercury and by systemic absorption in mercury sensitive individuals. Mercury…may cause hypersensitivity leading to contact dermatitis or Coomb's Type IV hypersensitivity reactions. The typical manifestation is an urticarial or erythematous rash, and pruritus on the face and flexural aspects of limbs, followed by progression to dermatitis." Thus, this survey of the literature supports the notions that mercury toxicity—i.e., a level of mercury in human patients sufficient to cause adverse health effects—is ❶ common (e.g., 8% of American women), ❷ problematic via causation of or contribution to various health problems commonly encountered in clinical practice, ❸ diagnosable via laboratory testing followed by monitoring response to treatment, and ❹ treatable, most notably with DMSA but also to a lesser extent with potassium citrate, selenium, and phytochelatins.

- Additional details—lead: The International Agency for Research on Cancer (IARC, part of the World Health Organization [WHO]) classified lead as a "possible human carcinogen" in 1987. A 2003 review published in *British Medical Bulletin* by Järup[238] noted that lead exposure (which comes equally from air and food, particularly food served via lead-contaminated ceramics) should be avoided as much as possible because physiologic toxicity occurs with low-level exposure; "Blood levels in children should be reduced below the levels so far considered acceptable, recent data indicating that there may be neurotoxic effects of lead at lower levels of exposure than previously anticipated." Occupational exposure to lead occurs in mines, smelting plants, glass-manufacturing facilities, battery plants, and among workers who weld metals already painted with lead-containing paints; air emissions near such facilities and activities may also contaminate nonworkers. Air contamination frequently leads to water contamination, threatening wildlife and humans who are exposed to contaminated water. Children are particularly vulnerable to lead exposure due to very efficient (compared with adults) gastrointestinal absorption and a more permeable ("leaky") blood-brain barrier. Organic lead compounds such as tetramethyl lead and tetraethyl lead easily penetrate skin and blood-brain barrier of children as well as adults. Classic, large-dose, acute and subacute lead poisoning manifests as anemia, renal tubular damage, and dark blue line of lead sulphide at the gingival margin; clinicians awaiting this classic presentation prior to considering lead toxicity should fortify their knowledge of and reconsider their perspective on this topic. Other symptoms of acute lead poisoning are headache, irritability, abdominal pain and various neurologic-psychiatric symptoms generally referred to as "lead encephalopathy" characterized by sleeplessness, restlessness, confusion/dyscognition, behavioral disturbances,

[231] Nielsen JB, Hultman P. Mercury-induced autoimmunity in mice. *Environ Health Perspect.* 2002 Oct;110 Suppl 5:877-81 http://ehp.niehs.nih.gov/docs/2002/suppl-5/877-881nielsen/abstract.html

[232] "Since anti-fibrillarin antibodies are specific markers of scleroderma, the present animal model may be valuable for studies of the immunological aberrations which are likely to induce this autoimmune response." Hultman P, Enestrom S, Pollard KM, Tan EM. Anti-fibrillarin autoantibodies in mercury-treated mice. *Clin Exp Immunol.* 1989;78(3):470-7

[233] "Thimerosal is an important preservative in vaccines and ophthalmologic preparations. The substance is known to be a type IV sensitizing agent. High sensitization rates were observed in contact-allergic patients and in health care workers who had been exposed to thimerosal-preserved vaccines." Westphal GA, Schnuch A, Schulz TG, Reich K, Aberer W, Brasch J, Koch P, Wessbecher R, Szliska C, Bauer A, Hallier E. Homozygous gene deletions of the glutathione S-transferases M1 and T1 are associated with thimerosal sensitization. *Int Arch Occup Environ Health.* 2000 Aug;73(6):384-8

[234] Vojdani A, Pangborn JB, Vojdani E, Cooper EL. Infections, toxic chemicals and dietary peptides binding to lymphocyte receptors and tissue enzymes are major instigators of autoimmunity in autism. *Int J Immunopathol Pharmacol.* 2003 Sep-Dec;16(3):189-99

[235] Geier DA, Geier MR. A comparative evaluation of the effects of MMR immunization and mercury doses from thimerosal-containing childhood vaccines on the population prevalence of autism. *Med Sci Monit.* 2004 Mar;10(3):PI33-9. http://www.medscimonit.com/pub/vol_10/no_3/3986.pdf

[236] Weidinger S, Kramer U, Dunemann L, Mohrenschlager M, Ring J, Behrendt H. Body burden of mercury is associated with acute atopic eczema and total IgE in children from southern Germany. *J Allergy Clin Immunol.* 2004 Aug;114(2):457-9

[237] Bains VK, Loomba K, Loomba A, Bains R. Mercury sensitisation: review, relevance and a clinical report. *Br Dent J.* 2008 Oct 11;205(7):373-8 http://www.intolsante.com/documents/publications/-mercury-sensitisation-review-relevance-and-clinical-report-22.pdf Accessed August 2011

[238] Järup L. Hazards of heavy metal contamination. *Br Med Bull.* 2003;68:167-82

Toxic metal testing—emphasis on lead and mercury	
	particularly learning and concentration difficulties in children; more extreme manifestations can include acute psychosis and stupor. Per the previously cited review by Järup, "Individuals [chronically exposed to lead] with average blood lead levels under 3 µmol/l may show signs of peripheral nerve symptoms with reduced nerve conduction velocity and reduced dermal sensibility."
Overview and application:	▪ No universally accepted consensus exists for the most accurate testing methodology. However, from the science-based perspectives that **toxic metals have been proven to cause harm at levels previously believed to be "acceptable" and that—very importantly—toxic metals are exponentially more toxic when in combination than when present alone,** reasonable clinicians can therefore conclude that the best test for clinical use is the one that is most sensitive, along with being reasonably convenient for the patient as well as affordable. For these reasons, the current author and many other clinicians chose DMSA-provoked urine toxic metal testing. Hair and nails can also be tested for chronic exposure, as can blood which is generally only useful for recent and relatively high-level exposure. Our clinical concern in general outpatient practice is not with recent and relatively high-level exposure, and therefore blood is not necessarily optimal. Our clinical concern in general outpatient practice is with chronic low-level exposure which leads to adverse cellular effects despite the failure to "spike" the serum level into the detectable toxic range. Arguments in favor of allowing symptomatic patients to persist untreated in a state of toxic metal accumulation would be difficult to justify scientifically and ethically.
Advantages:	▪ Toxic metal accumulation is ❶ <u>sufficiently common to warrant testing in selected patients,</u> ❷ <u>problematic</u> via causation of or contribution to various health problems commonly encountered in clinical practice, ❸ <u>diagnosable</u> via laboratory testing followed by monitoring response to treatment, and ❹ <u>treatable</u>. Therefore, clinicians should establish pathways for the assessment and treatment of metal toxicity.
Limitations:	▪ Patients with toxic metal accumulation frequently have accumulation of chemical xenobiotics as well; thus testing for and treating toxicity due to metals only relieves one type of toxicity.
Comments:	▪ Clinicians should establish pathways for the assessment and treatment of toxic metal accumulation.

Presentation: Widespread musculoskeletal pain resembling fibromyalgia secondary to lead and mercury accumulation: This 54yo athletic female with healthy diet, lifestyle, and supportive relationship presented with chronic diffuse musculoskeletal pain. Health history was sigificant for decades of environmental illness/intolerance (EI) also known as multiple chemical sensitivity (MCS). Family history was positive for maternal temporal (giant cell) arteritis. Physical examination revealed numerous tender points consistent with fibromyalgia; yet the history and stool analysis with comprehensive bacteriology and parasitology were unsupportive of gastrointestinal dysbiosis, particularly of the subtype small intestine bacterial overgrowth, which is causal for fibromyalgia.[239] Laboratory investigations revealed normal results for hsCRP (high-sensitity c-reactive protein), CK (creatine kinase, a marker of muscle damage and myositis), ANA (anti-nuclear antibodies), vitamin D, calcium, phosphorus, and comprehensive thyroid evaluation. The patient was then (defensively) referred to an osteopathic internist who diagnosed fibromyalgia.

Date Completed: 10/22/2005

| Lead | 30 | < | 5 |
| Mercury | 21 | < | 3 |

Discussion: The patient, unsatisfied with the diagnosis of fibromyalgia, returned to the current author, who then performed urine heavy metal testing provoked with 10 mg per kilogram of dimercaptosuccinic acid (DMSA). Results revealed the highest levels of lead and mercury encountered in the author's practice at that time. As shown above, lead levels were 6x above the reference range and mercury levels were 7x above the reference range. The patient was commenced on DMSA 10 mg/kg/d on alternating weeks to avoid toxicity in general and bone marrow toxicity (neutropenia) in particular, selenium 800 mcg/d to promote excretion of toxic metals and to support renal and antoxidant protection, vegetable juices to provide potassium and citrate for urinary alkalinization and enhanced excretion of xenobiotics[240], and a proprietary phytochelatin (metal-binding peptides from plants[241]) concetrate to bind toxic metals in the gut and thereby promote their fecal excretion by blocking enterohepatic recycling/recirculation. The use of DMSA for children and adults is supported by peer-reviewed literature[242,243,244,245,246] and has been reviewed in more detail by this author in *Integrative Rheumatology*[247] and to a lesser extent in *Musculoskeletal Pain: Expanded Clinical Strategies*.[248] DMSA chelation is approved by the US Food and Drug Administration (FDA) for the treatment of lead toxicity in children.[249] After approximately 8 months of treatment, the patient was completely free of pain, and the clinical improvement was associated with a reduction in both lead and mercury of approximately 50% as demonstrated by follow-up laboratory testing. Testing was performed by Doctors Data. This case was published in peer-reviewed literature for continuing education credits.[250]

Date Completed: 6/30/2006

| Lead | 15 | < | 5 |
| Mercury | 8.2 | < | 4 |

[239] **Vasquez A**. Musculoskeletal Pain: Expanded Clinical Strategies. Institute for Functional Medicine. 2008
[240] Crinnion WJ. Environmental medicine, part three: long-term effects of chronic low-dose mercury exposure. *Altern Med Rev*. 2000 Jun;5(3):209-23 http://www.thorne.com/altmedrev/.fulltext/5/3/209.pdf
[241] Cobbett CS. Phytochelatins and their roles in heavy metal detoxification. *Plant Physiol*. 2000;123:825-32 plantphysiol.org/content/123/3/825
[242] Bradstreet J, Geier DA, Kartzinel JJ, Adams JB, Geier MR. A case-control study of mercury burden in children with autistic spectrum disorders. *Journal of American Physicians and Surgeons* 2003; 8: 76-79 http://www.jpands.org/vol8no3/geier.pdf
[243] Crinnion WJ. Environmental medicine, part three: long-term effects of chronic low-dose mercury exposure. *Altern Med Rev*. 2000 Jun;5(3):209-23
[244] Forman J, Moline J, Cernichiari E, Sayegh S, Torres JC, Landrigan MM, Hudson J, Adel HN, Landrigan PJ. A cluster of pediatric metallic mercury exposure cases treated with meso-2,3-dimercaptosuccinic acid (DMSA). *Environ Health Perspect*. 2000 Jun;108(6):575-7 http://ehp.niehs.nih.gov/docs/2000/108p575-577forman/abstract.html
[245] Miller AL. Dimercaptosuccinic acid (DMSA), a non-toxic, water-soluble treatment for heavy metal toxicity. *Altern Med Rev*. 1998 Jun;3(3):199-207 http://www.thorne.com/altmedrev/.fulltext/3/3/199.pdf
[246] DMSA. *Altern Med Rev*. 2000 Jun;5(3):264-7 http://thorne.com/altmedrev/.fulltext/5/3/264.pdf
[247] **Vasquez A**. Integrative Rheumatology. IBMRC 2006, 2007 and all future editions. http://optimalhealthresearch.com/rheumatology.html
[248] **Vasquez A**. Musculoskeletal Pain: Expanded Clinical Strategies. Institute for Functional Medicine. 2008
[249] "The Food and Drug Administration has recently licensed the drug DMSA (succimer) for reduction of blood lead levels >/= 45 micrograms/dl. This decision was based on the demonstrated ability of DMSA to reduce blood lead levels. An advantage of this drug is that it can be given orally." Goyer RA, Cherian MG, Jones MM, Reigart JR. Role of chelating agents for prevention, intervention, and treatment of exposures to toxic metals. *Environ Health Perspect*. 1995 Nov;103(11):1048-52 Http://ehp.niehs.nih.gov/docs/1995/103-11/meetingreport.html
[250] **Vasquez A**. Musculoskeletal Pain: Expanded Clinical Strategies. Institute for Functional Medicine. 2008

Presentation: Chronic "idiopathic" hypertension associated with lead and mercury accumulation (per DMSA-provoked urine testing): This 43yo male presents with recalcitrant stage-1 hypertension. His cardiologist prescribed drugs to "treat" (some would say "mask") his elevated blood pressure. Since hypertension always has an underlying cause, the ethical and appropriate course of action is to determine the cause of the problem rather than silencing the alarm that is alerting to an underlying dysfunction. While this case is currently in progress at the time of this writing (the patient's medical records arrived in July 2011), it does offer a model case for clinical decision-making. Clinicians should be aware that, per animal studies, the toxicity of lead and mercury are greatly enhanced when both toxins are present at the same time.

					Date Collected:	6/3/2010
Lead	8.5	<	2			
Mercury	17	<	3			

Mercury and hypertension: Mercury is an established neurotoxin, immunotoxin, and nephrotoxin. Because pathophysiologic effects are noted even with very small doses of exposure, one could reasonably argue that no safe amount exists and therefore that any detected mercury is an indication for therapeutic intervention to remove this toxicant. Sources of exposure include dental amalgams, vaccinations, airborne pollution, and fish; recently, high-fructose corn syrup was shown to contain mercury.[251] Mercury impairs catecholamine degradation and can thereby cause a clinical syndrome that can include hypertension, tremor, tachycardia, diaphoresis, and neurocognitive changes.[252] Per Shih and Gartner[253], "Mercury combines with the sulfhydryl group of S-adenosylmethionine, which is a cofactor for catecholamine-O-methyltransferase (COMT), and this inhibition of COMT allows accumulation of norepinephrine, epinephrine, and dopamine."

Lead and hypertension: In the United States, a consistent correlation has been found between body burden of lead and HTN, even when blood lead levels are well below the current US occupational exposure limit guidelines (40 microg/dl).[254] Harlan et al[255] analyzed data from the second National Health and Nutrition Examination Survey (1976-1980) and thereby found a direct relationship between blood lead levels and systolic and diastolic pressures for men and women and for white and black persons aged 12 to 74 years; they concluded, "Blood lead levels were significantly higher in younger men and women (aged 21 to 55 years) with high blood pressure, but not in older men or women (aged 56 to 74 years)." Schwartz and Stewart[256] found that blood lead was the assessment that most strongly correlated with HTN; they concluded, "Systolic blood pressure was elevated by blood lead levels as low as 5 microg/dl." Thus, clinicians might first measure blood lead levels, which do not measure total body burden but rather the lead that is mobile or *in transit* within the body and which appears to have the best correlation with HTN; the finding of normal blood lead results could then be followed with the more sensitive DMSA-provoked heavy metal testing before concluding that heavy metals are noncontributory to that particular patient's HTN. For heavy metal testing in various clinical scenarios, this author's preference is to use DMSA-provoked measurement of urine toxic metals. After a minimal test dose of DMSA (e.g., in the range of 50-100 mg) to screen for hypersensitivity, patients take oral DMSA 10 mg/kg as a single oral dose in the morning on an empty stomach after emptying the bladder and send a sample from the next urination for laboratory analysis; follow laboratory protocol if different from these instructions. Use of DMSA for lead and mercury chelation/detoxification and for diagnostic purposes is generally safe and effective[257,258,259]; detoxification procedures are reviewed in much greater detail in *Integrative Rheumatology*.[260]

---

[251] "Average daily consumption of high fructose corn syrup is about 50 grams per person in the United States. With respect to total mercury exposure, it may be necessary to account for this source of mercury in the diet of children and sensitive populations." Dufault R, LeBlanc B, Schnoll R, Cornett C, Schweitzer L, Wallinga D, Hightower J, Patrick L, Lukiw WJ. Mercury from chlor-alkali plants: measured concentrations in food product sugar. *Environ Health*. 2009 Jan 26;8:2. See also: "High fructose corn syrup has been shown to contain trace amounts of mercury as a result of some manufacturing processes, and its consumption can also lead to zinc loss." Dufault R, Schnoll R, Lukiw WJ, Leblanc B, Cornett C, Patrick L, Wallinga D, Gilbert SG, Crider R. Mercury exposure, nutritional deficiencies and metabolic disruptions may affect learning in children. *Behav Brain Funct*. 2009 Oct 27;5:44.

[252] Wössmann W, Kohl M, Grüning G, Bucsky P. Mercury intoxication presenting with hypertension and tachycardia. *Arch Dis Child*. 1999 Jun;80(6):556-7 http://www.ncbi.nlm.nih.gov/pmc/articles/PMC1717944/pdf/v080p00556.pdf

[253] Shih H, Gartner JC Jr. Weight loss, hypertension, weakness, and limb pain in an 11-year-old boy. *J Pediatr*. 2001 Apr;138(4):566-9

[254] Nash D, Magder L, Lustberg M, Sherwin RW, Rubin RJ, Kaufmann RB, Silbergeld EK. Blood lead, blood pressure, and hypertension in perimenopausal and postmenopausal women. *JAMA*. 2003 Mar 26;289(12):1523-32 http://jama.ama-assn.org/cgi/content/full/289/12/1523

[255] Harlan WR, Landis JR, Schmouder RL, Goldstein NG, Harlan LC. Blood lead and blood pressure. Relationship in the adolescent and adult US population. *JAMA*. 1985 Jan 25;253(4):530-4

[256] "Systolic blood pressure was elevated by blood lead levels as low as 5 microg/dl." Schwartz BS, Stewart WF. Different associations of blood lead, meso 2,3-dimercaptosuccinic acid (DMSA)-chelatable lead, and tibial lead levels with blood pressure in 543 former organolead manufacturing workers. *Arch Environ Health*. 2000 Mar-Apr;55(2):85-92

[257] Bradstreet J, Geier DA, Kartzinel JJ, Adams JB, Geier MR. A case-control study of mercury burden in children with autistic spectrum disorders. *Journal of American Physicians and Surgeons* 2003; 8: 76-79 http://www.jpands.org/vol8no3/geier.pdf

[258] Miller AL. Dimercaptosuccinic acid (DMSA), a non-toxic, water-soluble treatment for heavy metal toxicity. *Altern Med Rev*. 1998 Jun;3(3):199-207

[259] DMSA. *Altern Med Rev*. 2000 Jun;5(3):264-7 http://thorne.com/altmedrev/.fulltext/5/3/264.pdf

[260] **Vasquez A**. Integrative Rheumatology. IBMRC 2006, 2007 and all future editions. http://optimalhealthresearch.com/rheumatology.html

Antinuclear antibody: ANA

Overview and interpretation:	▪ **Good screening test for autoimmune conditions**: SLE, Sjogren's syndrome, and various other connective tissue diseases.
	▪ Good and "highly sensitive" for initial assessment of SLE; positive in 95-98% of SLE patients; negative result strongly suggests against diagnosis of SLE.[261] Only 2% of patients with SLE have a negative ANA test—these patients may be identified by testing with anti-RO antibodies and CH50 (complement levels).
	▪ This test measures for the presence of antibodies that react to nucleoproteins. Some labs report titers of 1:20 or 1:40 as "positive"; however, low levels of ANA are common (5-15%) in the general population. Thus, ANA is not specific for any one disease; may be positive in SLE, RA, scleroderma, Sjogren's, also seen with elderly, infected patients, cancer, and certain medications. Titers less than 1:160 should be interpreted cautiously as they may not indicate the presence of *clinical* autoimmunity.[262] **Titers greater than 1:320 are considered indicative of clinically significant autoimmunity.**
	▪ Methodologies (indirect immunofluorescence is most popular), subtypes, and patterns reported for ANA results may be irrelevant or clinically meaningful; the most common descriptors are provided in the table below.

ANA patterns and descriptions[263,264]	*Clinical correlation*
Homogeneous, diffuse nuclear staining	Nonspecific
Speckled	Least specific
Rim or **peripheral staining**	Suggests SLE and warrants assessment for anti-dsDNA, which is specific for lupus
Anti-centromere: selective staining of the centromeres of nuclei in metaphase	Highly specific for the limited scleroderma subtype associated with CREST syndrome
Nucleolar	Correlated with diffuse scleroderma (systemic sclerosis)
FANA: fluorescent ANA	The standard ANA test in the US
Anti-Sm: anti-Smith[265]	<u>Virtually diagnostic of SLE</u>: Highly specific for SLE; insensitive: positive in 20-30% of SLE patients
Anti-dsDNA: anti-double stranded DNA	<u>Virtually diagnostic of SLE</u>: Highly specific for SLE and indicative of an increased likelihood of poor prognosis with major organ involvement[266] especially active renal disease
Anti-Ro (anti-SS-A)	Correlates with SLE, Sjögren's syndrome, and neonatal SLE
Anti-La (anti-SS-B)	Sjögren's syndrome or low risk of SLE nephritis
Anti-RNP	SLE and/or mixed connective tissue disease (MCTD)
Anti-Jo-1	Specific but not sensitive for polymyositis/dermatomyositis
Antihistone	SLE and especially drug-induced SLE
Antitopoisomerase (Scl-70)	Correlates with diffuse scleroderma, especially with interstitial lung disease

---

[261] Shojania K. Rheumatology: 2. What laboratory tests are needed? *CMAJ.* 2000 Apr 18;162(8):1157-63 http://www.cmaj.ca/cgi/content/full/162/8/1157
[262] Hardin JG, Waterman J, Labson LH. Rheumatic disease: Which diagnostic tests are useful? *Patient Care* 1999; March 15: 83-102
[263] Shojania K. Rheumatology: 2. What laboratory tests are needed? *CMAJ.* 2000 Apr 18;162(8):1157-63 http://www.cmaj.ca/cgi/content/full/162/8/1157
[264] Ward MM. Laboratory testing for systemic rheumatic diseases. *Postgrad Med.* 1998 Feb;103(2):93-100.
[265] Lane SK, Gravel JW Jr. Clinical utility of common serum rheumatologic tests. *Am Fam Physician.* 2002;65:1073-80 http://www.aafp.org/afp/20020315/1073.html
[266] Shojania K. Rheumatology: 2. What laboratory tests are needed? *CMAJ.* 2000 Apr 18;162(8):1157-63 http://www.cmaj.ca/cgi/content/full/162/8/1157

Antinuclear antibody: ANA—*continued*	
Advantages:	▪ ANA has 98% sensitivity and 90% specificity for SLE in an unselected population. ▪ The negative predictive value in an unselected population is greater than 99%. ANA is therefore an excellent test for *excluding* the diagnosis of SLE.
Limitations:	▪ The positive predictive value in an unselected population is about 30%; **only 30% of unselected people with a positive result will have SLE**—this fact underscores the importance of patient selection and judicious interpretation of this test. ▪ Positive ANA is seen in patients with conditions other than SLE, including rheumatoid arthritis, Sjogren's syndrome, scleroderma, polymyositis, vasculitis, juvenile rheumatoid arthritis (JRA), and infectious diseases.
Comments:	▪ ANA is most often used to support the diagnosis of SLE in a patient with multisystemic illness and a clinical picture compatible with SLE. Nearly all patients with SLE will have positive ANA. **A positive ANA does not mean that the patient necessarily has SLE; be weary of paraneoplastic syndromes and viral hepatitis as underlying causative processes in patients with an unclear clinical picture.** ▪ I view any "positive ANA" as an indicator of poor health in general and immune dysfunction in particular. The goal, then, is to restore health. I have seen ANA show a trend toward normalization or completely normalize with effective health restoration as detailed in *Integrative Rheumatology* (chapter 4). I realize that my experience in this regard contrasts sharply with the allopathic view that serial measurements of ANA are worthless because the result never normalizes once a patient is ANA-positive[267]; I consider this evidence of the effectiveness of my integrative-functional approach and the comparable failure of the allopathic approach.

Antineutrophilic cytoplasmic antibodies: ANCA	
Overview:	▪ ANCA are autoantibodies to the cytoplasmic constituents of granulocytes and are characteristically found in vasculitic syndromes and also in (Chinese) patients with inflammatory bowel disease[268] and nearly all patients with hepatic amebiasis due to *Entamoeba histolytica.*[269] <u>Two types:</u> ▪ <u>Cytoplasmic ANCA (C-ANCA)</u>: classically seen in **Wegener's granulomatosis**; also seen in some types of glomerulonephritis and vasculitis; this test is highly sensitive and specific for these conditions. In fact, a positive C-ANCA result can replace biopsy in a patient with a clinical picture of **Wegener's granulomatosis.**[270] ▪ <u>Perinuclear ANCA (P-ANCA)</u>: considered a nonspecific finding[271] that correlates with SLE, drug induced lupus, and some types of glomerulonephritis and vasculitis. Shojania[272] stated that this test must be confirmed with antimyeloperoxidase antibodies to evaluate for Churg–Strauss syndrome, crescentic glomerulonephritis, and microscopic polyarteritis.
Advantages, limitations, and comments	▪ Not to be used as a screening test, except in patients with idiopathic vasculitis or glomerulonephritis. ▪ The fact that hepatic amebiasis due to *Entamoeba histolytica* induces production of C-ANCA antibodies in nearly 100% of infected patients may support the hypothesis that autoimmunity can be induced or exacerbated by parasitic infections.

---

[267] Shojania K. Rheumatology: 2. What laboratory tests are needed? *CMAJ.* 2000 Apr 18;162(8):1157-63 http://www.cmaj.ca/cgi/content/full/162/8/1157
[268] "Fourteen patients (73.5%) were positive, of which six (31.5%) showed a perinuclear staining pattern and eight (42%) demonstrated a cytoplasmic pattern." Sung JY, Chan KL, Hsu R, Liew CT, Lawton JW. Ulcerative colitis and antineutrophil cytoplasmic antibodies in Hong Kong Chinese. *Am J Gastroenterol.* 1993 Jun;88(6):864-9
[269] "ANCA was detected in 97.4% of amoebic sera; the pattern of staining was cytoplasmic, homogeneous, without central accentuation (C-ANCA)." Pudifin DJ, Duursma J, Gathiram V, Jackson TF. Invasive amoebiasis is associated with the development of anti-neutrophil cytoplasmic antibody. *Clin Exp Immunol.* 1994 Jul;97(1):48-5
[270] Shojania K. Rheumatology: 2. What laboratory tests are needed? *CMAJ.* 2000 Apr 18;162(8):1157-63 http://www.cmaj.ca/cgi/content/full/162/8/1157
[271] Shojania K. Rheumatology: 2. What laboratory tests are needed? *CMAJ.* 2000 Apr 18;162(8):1157-63 http://www.cmaj.ca/cgi/content/full/162/8/1157
[272] Shojania K. Rheumatology: 2. What laboratory tests are needed? *CMAJ.* 2000 Apr 18;162(8):1157-63 http://www.cmaj.ca/cgi/content/full/162/8/1157

RF: Rheumatoid Factor	
Overview and application:	▪ Rheumatoid factor—"anti-IgG antibodies"—are antibodies directed to the Fc portion of the patient's own IgG. Rheumatoid factors are anti-immunoglobulin antibodies, classically anti-IgG IgM. RF are found in low levels in most patients, and despite the "rheumatoid" name, RF is not specific for rheumatoid arthritis.[273] Current tests (latex fixation or nephelometry) detect IgM anti-immunoglobulin antibodies; however IgA-RF appears to have clinical superiority over other forms of RF because it correlates more strongly with clinical status.[274] ▪ This test is most commonly used to support the diagnosis of rheumatoid arthritis in a patient with a compelling clinical picture: peripheral polyarthritis lasting >6 weeks.[275] A negative result with a compelling clinical presentation of RA is termed "seronegative rheumatoid arthritis" by allopathic textbooks whereas a more appropriate term might be oligoarthritis, a condition described as "idiopathic" by allopathic text books despite the clear evidence that the majority of patients have one or more subsets of dysbiosis.[276] ▪ **Titers (latex fixation) of 1:160 are considered clinically significant, favoring the diagnosis of RA.**[277] However the positive predictive value is low—only 20-34% of people in an unselected population with a positive test result actually have RA.[278,279]
Advantages:	▪ Supports the diagnosis of rheumatoid arthritis: about 60-85% positive/sensitive in patients with rheumatoid arthritis (RA).[280,281] Quantitative titers of RF correlate with prognosis: a very high RF value portends a poor prognosis.
Limitations:	▪ **Positive findings are common in the following conditions: rheumatoid arthritis, viral hepatitis, Sjögren's syndrome, endocarditis, scleroderma, mycobacteria diseases, polymyositis and dermatomyositis, syphilis, systemic lupus erythematosus, old age, mixed connective tissue disease, sarcoidosis;** positive results may also been noted in: **cryoglobulinemia, parasitic infection, interstitial lung disease, asymptomatic relatives of people with autoimmune diseases.** ▪ Febrile patients with arthralgia are more likely to have endocarditis than RA.[282] ▪ Patients with iron overload present with a similar clinical picture (i.e., polyarthropathy with systemic complaints) and may have a positive RF. Thus, patients with positive RF and polyarthropathy should be tested for iron overload; use serum ferritin.[283,284]
Comments:	▪ This test should only be used to confirm the diagnosis of rheumatoid arthritis in patients with a compelling clinical picture of the disease: inflammatory peripheral polyarthropathy with systemic complaints for > 6 weeks. A negative result does not mean that the patient *does not* have rheumatoid arthritis; a positive result does not mean that the patient *does* have rheumatoid arthritis.[285] ▪ CCP (cyclic citrullinated protein) antibodies appear to be more specific and sensitive for RA and is becoming the test of choice for RA as described on the following page.

[273] Shojania K. Rheumatology: 2. What laboratory tests are needed? *CMAJ*. 2000 Apr 18;162(8):1157-63 http://www.cmaj.ca/cgi/content/full/162/8/1157
[274] Jonsson T, Valdimarsson H. What about IgA rheumatoid factor in rheumatoid arthritis? *Ann Rheum Dis*. 1998 Jan;57(1):63-4
[275] Shojania K. Rheumatology: 2. What laboratory tests are needed? *CMAJ*. 2000 Apr 18;162(8):1157-63 http://www.cmaj.ca/cgi/content/full/162/8/1157
[276] See chapter 4 of *Integrative Rheumatology* and Vasquez A. Reducing Pain and Inflammation Naturally. Part 6: Nutritional and Botanical Treatments Against "Silent Infections" and Gastrointestinal Dysbiosis, Commonly Overlooked Causes of Neuromusculoskeletal Inflammation and Chronic Health Problems. *Nutr Perspect* 2006; Jan http://optimalhealthresearch.com/part6.html
[277] Beers MH, Berkow R (eds). The Merck Manual. Seventeenth Edition. Whitehouse Station; Merck Research Laboratories 1999 Page 417
[278] Ward MM. Laboratory testing for systemic rheumatic diseases. *Postgrad Med*. 1998 Feb;103(2):93-100.
[279] Shojania K. Rheumatology: 2. What laboratory tests are needed? *CMAJ*. 2000 Apr 18;162(8):1157-63 http://www.cmaj.ca/cgi/content/full/162/8/1157
[280] Tierney ML. McPhee SJ, Papadakis MA (eds). Current Medical Diagnosis and Treatment 2002, 41ˢᵗ Edition. New York: Lange Medical, 2002 p854
[281] Shojania K. Rheumatology: 2. What laboratory tests are needed? *CMAJ*. 2000 Apr 18;162(8):1157-63 http://www.cmaj.ca/cgi/content/full/162/8/1157
[282] Klippel JH (ed). Primer on the Rheumatic Diseases. 11ᵗʰ Edition. Atlanta: Arthritis Foundation. 1997 page 96
[283] Bensen WG, Laskin CA, Little HA, Fam AG. Hemochromatoic arthropathy mimicking rheumatoid arthritis. A case with subcutaneous nodules, tenosynovitis, and bursitis. *Arthritis Rheum* 1978; 21: 844-8
[284] **Vasquez A**. Musculoskeletal disorders and iron overload disease: comment on the American College of Rheumatology guidelines for the initial evaluation of the adult patient with acute musculoskeletal symptoms. *Arthritis Rheum* 1996;39: 1767-8
[285] Shojania K. Rheumatology: 2. What laboratory tests are needed? *CMAJ*. 2000 Apr 18;162(8):1157-63 http://www.cmaj.ca/cgi/content/full/162/8/1157

CCP: Cyclic citrullinated protein antibody; Citrullinated protein antibodies (CPA); anti-CCP antibodies: anticyclic citrullinated peptide antibody	
Overview and use:	• CCP—cyclic citrullinated protein antibodies; anticitrullinated protein antibodies: this is a relatively new auto-antibody marker that shows great promise and specificity for the early diagnosis of rheumatoid arthritis (RA). The test often becomes positive/present in asymptomatic patients years before the onset of clinical manifestations of RA. • As of the first inclusion of this information in my books in December 2006, the information on anti-CCP antibodies is so new that it is not even included in most 2006-edition medical and rheumatology reference textbooks; nonetheless, doctors nationwide are already starting to use this test for the early diagnosis of RA. This may be particularly important because some research has shown that *early* and *aggressive* treatment of RA has an important impact on long-term prognosis[286]; however, the importance of early intervention is debatable.[287] • Anti-CCP antibodies are directed toward several native proteins (e.g., filaggrin, fibrinogen, and vimentin) that have become posttranslationally modified by a uncharged citrulline in contrast to the normal positively charged arginine. This "citrullination" is catalyzed by a calcium-dependent enzyme, **peptidylarginine deiminase (PAD)**. These changes in protein charge and sequence make the native protein a target of auto-antibody attack by IgG antibodies in RA.[288] However, this does not necessarily imply that citrullination of native proteins is "the cause" of RA because citrullination of native proteins can also occur *de novo* in inflamed joints, which are then further targeted for inflammatory destruction. Until more information is available, we should withhold final judgment as to the ultimate role and origin of anti-CCP antibodies and in the meanwhile view them as a very strong and sensitive association with RA that facilitates the early diagnosis of this disease.
Advantages:	• Anti-CCP antibodies have 98% specificity for RA[289] and is likely to become the future laboratory standard in the diagnosis and prognosis of RA.[290] Anti-CCP antibodies with a positive rheumatoid factor (RF) is termed "composite seropositivity" and appears to be more specific than isolated anti-CCP antibodies or RF.[291]
Limitations:	• **The best current data indicates that anti-CCP antibodies are sensitive and specific for RA[292], and clinicians should use this test to diagnose and confirm RA.**
Comments:	• Healthy people do not generally have anti-CCP antibodies. Asymptomatic patients with anti-CCP antibodies are at increased risk for clinical RA and are probably *en route* to the manifestation of clinical autoimmunity—RA, Sjogren's disease, or SLE. *Holistically intervene.* • I hypothesize that PAD may become upregulated in synovial joints exposed to allergens, xenobiotics, bacterial debris/toxins/lipopolysaccharides and that the subsequent citrullination of joint proteins may lead to an autoimmune arthropathy that persists, perhaps despite removal of the inciting immunogen. More obviously, given that PAD is calcium-dependent, it may be upregulated secondary to intracellular hypercalcinosis secondary to vitamin D deficiency, magnesium deficiency, or fatty acid imbalance.[293]

[286] "CONCLUSION: An initial 6-month cycle of intensive combination treatment that includes high-dose corticosteroids results in sustained suppression of the rate of radiologic progression in patients with early RA, independent of subsequent antirheumatic therapy." Landewe RB, et al. COBRA combination therapy in patients with early rheumatoid arthritis: long-term structural benefits of a brief intervention. *Arthritis Rheum.* 2002 Feb;46:347-56
[287] "By 5 years patients receiving early DMARDs had similar disease activity and comparable health assessment questionnaire scores to patients who received DMARDs later in their disease course." Scott DL. Evidence for early disease-modifying drugs in rheumatoid arthritis. *Arthritis Res Ther.* 2004;6(1):15-18 http://arthritis-research.com/content/6/1/15
[288] Hill J, Cairns E, Bell DA. The joy of citrulline. *J Rheumatol.* 2004 Aug;31(8):1471-3 http://www.jrheum.com/subscribers/04/08/1471.html
[289] Hill J, Cairns E, Bell DA. The joy of citrulline. *J Rheumatol.* 2004 Aug;31(8):1471-3
[290] "We conclude that, at present, the antibody response directed to citrullinated antigens has the most valuable diagnostic and prognostic potential for RA." van Boekel MA, Vossenaar ER, van den Hoogen FH, van Venrooij WJ. Autoantibody systems in rheumatoid arthritis: specificity, sensitivity and diagnostic value. *Arthritis Res.* 2002;4(2):87-93 http://arthritis-research.com/content/4/2/87
[291] "…our findings suggest that a positive anti-CCP antibody result does not necessarily exclude SLE in African American patients presenting with inflammatory arthritis. In such patients, the additional assessment of IgA-RF or IgM-RF isotypes may be of added value since composite seropositivity appears to be nearly exclusive to patients with RA." Mikuls TR, Holers VM, Parrish L, et al. Anti-cyclic citrullinated peptide antibody and rheumatoid factor isotypes in African Americans with early rheumatoid arthritis. *Arthritis Rheum.* 2006 Sep;54(9):3057-9
[292] "Serum antibodies reactive with citrullinated proteins/peptides are a very sensitive and specific marker for rheumatoid arthritis." Migliorini P, Pratesi F, Tommasi C, Anzilotti C. The immune response to citrullinated antigens in autoimmune diseases. *Autoimmun Rev.* 2005 Nov;4(8):561-4
[293] See optimalhealthresearch.com/archives/intracellular-hypercalcinosis and naturopathydigest.com/archives/2006/sep/vasquez.php for discussion

HLA-B27: Human leukocyte antigen B-27	
Overview and interpretation:	• A common (5-10% of general population) genetic marker strongly associated with seronegative* spondyloarthropathy (all of which occur more commonly in men[294]): 1. Ankylosing spondylitis (90-95% of 'whites' and 50% of 'blacks')[295] 2. Reiter's syndrome (85%) 3. Enteropathic spondyloarthropathy 4. Psoriatic spondylitis (<60%) * Recall that "seronegative" in this context implies that the *rheumatoid factor is negative*, even though *the HLA-B27 may be positive.*
Advantages: Limitations: Comments:	• *From a diagnostic perspective*: The clinical application and significance of this test is of limited value. All of the above-listed conditions are better assessed with the combination of clinical assessment and radiographs. In a patient with early and mild disease, this test may add evidence either supporting or refuting the diagnosis; but the test itself is not diagnostic of anything other than a genetic/histologic marker associated with various types of infection-induced arthropathy and autoimmunity (dysbiotic arthropathy[296]). • *From an integrative/functional medicine perspective*: This test can be of some value if the result is positive and the patient has evidence of a systemic inflammatory/autoimmune disorder since it therefore more strongly suggests that a dysbiotic locus is the cause of disease.[297] A consistent theme in the rheumatology literature is that of "molecular mimicry"—the phenomenon by which structural similarities between human and microbial structures lead to targeting of human tissues by immune responses aimed at microbial antigens. This topic is explored in considerable detail in the section on multifocal dysbiosis in *Integrative Rheumatology*. The important link between microbe-induced autoimmunity and HLA-B27 is that many dysbiotic bacteria produce an HLA-B27-like molecule that appears to trigger an immune response which then erroneously affects human tissues, leading to the clinical picture of autoimmune inflammation. Many of these HLA-B27-producing bacteria colonize the gastrointestinal and genitourinary tracts, promoting musculoskeletal inflammation via molecular mimicry and other mechanisms.[298,299] A strong and growing body of research shows that HLA-B27 is a risk factor for microbe-induced autoimmunity. "Autoimmune" patients positive for HLA-B27 are presumed to have an occult infection—especially gastrointestinal, genitourinary, or sinorespiratory—until proven otherwise. • <u>**Keep in mind that HLA-B27 itself is not a disease**</u> and therefore a "positive" result merely means that the patient has this particular human leukocyte antigen; this test is not and will never be diagnostic of a specific disease—it simply correlates with increased propensity toward dysbiotic arthropathy and suggests the need for dysbiosis testing and the (re)establishment of eubiosis.[300]

[294] "The major diseases associated with HLA-B27 (Reiter's disease, ankylosing spondylitis, acute anterior uveitis, and psoriatic arthritis) all occur much more commonly in men." James WH. Sex ratios and hormones in HLA related rheumatic diseases. *Ann Rheum Dis*. 1991 Jun;50(6):401-4

[295] Shojania K. Rheumatology: 2. What laboratory tests are needed? *CMAJ*. 2000 Apr 18;162(8):1157-63 http://www.cmaj.ca/cgi/content/full/162/8/1157

[296] See chapter 4 of *Integrative Rheumatology* and **Vasquez A**. Reducing Pain and Inflammation Naturally. Part 6: Nutritional and Botanical Treatments Against "Silent Infections" and Gastrointestinal Dysbiosis, Commonly Overlooked Causes of Neuromusculoskeletal Inflammation and Chronic Health Problems. *Nutr Perspect* 2006; Jan http://optimalhealthresearch.com/part6.html

[297] "The association between HLA-B27 and reactive arthritis (ReA) has also been well established... In a similar way, microbiological and immunological studies have revealed an association between Klebsiella pneumoniae in AS and Proteus mirabilis in RA." Ebringer A, Wilson C. HLA molecules, bacteria and autoimmunity. *J Med Microbiol*. 2000 Apr;49(4):305-11

[298] **Inman RD. Antigens, the gastrointestinal tract, and arthritis. *Rheum Dis Clin North Am*. 1991 May;17(2):309-21**

[299] **Hunter JO. Food allergy--or enterometabolic disorder? *Lancet*. 1991 Aug 24;338(8765):495-6**

[300] Dysbiotic arthropathy—joint inflammation and destruction as a result of a neuroimmune inflammatory response to microorganisms. Phrase coined by Alex Vasquez on December 15, 2005. No matching term on Medline or Google search. See chapter 4 of *Integrative Rheumatology* and **Vasquez A**. Reducing Pain and Inflammation Naturally. Part 6: Nutritional and Botanical Treatments Against "Silent Infections" and Gastrointestinal Dysbiosis, Commonly Overlooked Causes of Neuromusculoskeletal Inflammation and Chronic Health Problems. *Nutr Perspect* 2006; Jan http://optimalhealthresearch.com/part6.html

Complement C3 and C4	
Overview and interpretation:	▪ Complement proteins are consumed in the complement cascades (typically activated by immune complexes) and thus low levels of complement proteins provide indirect evidence of extensive consumption due to immune complex-mediated inflammation. **Low levels of complement are seen with immune complex disorders (such as SLE, vasculitis, mixed cryoglobulinemia, rheumatoid vasculitis, glomerulonephritis) and inherited complement deficiencies.** ▪ 10%–15% of Caucasian patients with SLE have an inherited complement deficiency.[301]
Advantages:	▪ Low complement levels provide indirect evidence of immune complex-mediated inflammation. ▪ Elevated levels of complement are seen in conditions of infection or inflammation.
Limitations:	▪ Some patients have a hereditary absence of complement proteins and thus their levels are always abnormally low; obviously the test cannot be used in these patients for monitoring inflammatory disease.

CIC: Circulating immune complexes	
Overview and interpretation:	▪ Antibodies/immunoglobulins are produced in several different "classes": IgG, IgA, IgM, IgE, IgD. IgA antibodies are produced mostly in response to mucosal infections, such as from gastrointestinal dysbiosis or overt infections. When antibodies (in the shape of the letter "Y" with 2 antigen-binding sites on one end and the immuno-reactive site on the other) combine with the target antigen (depicted here in the shape of an oval, such as a bacteria or globular protein), "immune complexes" are formed which are chain-like links of antigens and antibodies. 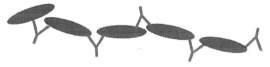 ▪ Although formed in small amounts in healthy persons, in certain disease states, immune complexes may accumulate and initiate complement-dependent injury in various organs and tissues. This activation of complement may begin a series of potentially destructive events in the host, including anaphylatoxin production, cell lysis, leukocyte stimulation, and activation of macrophages and other cells. When immune complexes become fixed to vessel walls, destruction of normal tissue can occur, as in some types of glomerulonephritis and vasculitis. Predisposed to deposition in joints, vessels, and kidneys, immune complexes contribute directly to tissue injury in several autoimmune-inflammatory diseases.[302] **Immune Complexes, (Raji Cell), Quantitative** ▪ <u>Reference Range</u>: (Enzyme immunoassay [EIA]; cost $130) ▪ <u>Normal</u>: ≤15.0 µg Eq/mL ▪ <u>Equivocal</u>: 15.1-19.9 µg Eq/mL ▪ <u>Positive</u>: ≥20.0 µg Eq/mL
Advantages:	▪ This test allows for direct quantification of immune-complex production.
Limitations:	▪ This test has only recently become available to practicing clinicians; however, it is very well supported by many publications in peer-reviewed research.[303]

[301] Shojania K. Rheumatology: 2. What laboratory tests are needed? *CMAJ*. 2000 Apr 18;162(8):1157-63 http://www.cmaj.ca/cgi/content/full/162/8/1157
[302] Jancar S, Sánchez Crespo M. Immune complex-mediated tissue injury: a multistep paradigm. *Trends Immunol*. 2005 Jan;26(1):48-55
[303] Davies KA,etal. Immune complex processing in patients with systemic lupus erythematosus. *J Clin Invest* 1992;90:2075-83 jci.org/articles/view/116090

Lactulose-mannitol assay: assessment for intestinal hyperpermeability and malabsorption	
Overview and interpretation:	▪ The lactulose-mannitol assay is a highly validated assessment for the accurate determination of small intestine permeability. This test is used to diagnose "leaky gut", which is a common problem and contributor to systemic inflammation in patients with inflammation and immune dysfunction—see chapter 4 of *Integrative Rheumatology*. Intestinal hyperpermeability reflects inflammation of and damage to the small intestine mucosa and is seen in patients with parasite infections, food allergies, celiac disease, malnutrition, bacterial infections, systemic ischemia or inflammation, ankylosing spondylitis, Crohn's disease, eczema, psoriasis, and those who consume enterotoxins such as NSAIDs and excess ethanol.[304] ▪ Elevations of **lactulose** indicate increased **paracellular** permeability caused by intestinal damage and are diagnostic of "leaky gut." *Clinical pearl*: remember that the "L" in *lactulose* rhymes with *leaky*. ▪ Decrements in **mannitol** suggest impaired **transcellular** absorption and suggest malabsorption in general and villous atrophy in particular. *Clinical pearl*: remember that the "M" in *mannitol* rhymes with *malabsorption*. ▪ Classically, in patients with damaged intestinal mucosa, we generally see a combined *increase in paracellular* permeability (measured with lactulose) and a *reduction in transcellular* transport (measured with mannitol); these divergent effects result in an increased lactulose-to-mannitol ratio.
Advantages:	▪ This test is safe and affordable for the assessment of small intestine mucosal integrity. Abnormal results—"leaky gut" and/or malabsorption—generally indicate one or more of following: 1. Malnutrition: may be due to poor intake, catabolism, or malabsorption. 2. Enterotoxins: generally NSAIDs or ethanol 3. Food allergies: including celiac disease 4. "Parasites": including yeast, bacteria, protozoa, amebas, worms, etc. [305] 5. Systemic inflammation: tissue hypoxia, trauma, recent surgery, etc. 6. Genetic predisposition toward enteropathy: check family history for IBD.
Limitations:	▪ Abnormalities and the identification of "leaky gut" are nonspecific and do not point to a specific or single diagnosis or treatment.
Comments:	▪ The value of this test is two-fold: 1) as a screening test for the above-mentioned disorders, and 2) as a method for determining the efficacy of treatment once the cause of the problem has been putatively identified and treated. ▪ This test can be used to promote compliance and to encourage the use of additional testing in patients who are otherwise prone to noncompliance or who resist other tests, such as stool testing. In other words, the clinician can gain an advantage by showing the patient an objective abnormality which then validates the need for treatment and additional testing. ▪ I only use this test on rare occasions because I more commonly either assume that a patient has leaky gut if he/she has one of the aforementioned conditions or we move directly to stool testing and comprehensive parasitology—clearly one of the most valuable tests in the management and treatment of systemic inflammation and immune dysfunction—otherwise known as "autoimmunity" and "allergy."

---

[304] Miller AL. The Pathogenesis, Clinical Implications, and Treatment of Intestinal Hyperpermeability. *Alt Med Rev* 1997:2(5):330-345 http://www.thorne.com/pdf/journal/2-5/intestinalhyperpermiability.pdf

[305] See chapter 4 of *Integrative Rheumatology* and **Vasquez A**. Reducing Pain and Inflammation Naturally. Part 6: Nutritional and Botanical Treatments Against "Silent Infections" and Gastrointestinal Dysbiosis, Commonly Overlooked Causes of Neuromusculoskeletal Inflammation and Chronic Health Problems. *Nutr Perspect* 2006; Jan http://optimalhealthresearch.com/part6.html

Presentation: Highly abnormal lactulose-mannitol ratio in a patient with idiopathic peripheral neuropathy prior to comprehensive stool analysis and parasitology showing intestinal dysbiosis: This 40-yo man presented with a multiyear history of periodic febrile exacerbations of peripheral neuropathy that would cause severe paresthesias and motor deficits. Patient had been evaluated by several board-certified medical neurologists to no avail. Laboratory, imaging, electrodiagnostic studies, and cerebrospinal fluid (CSF) analysis revealed nonspecific abnormalities that did not lead to an established diagnosis. From an integrative naturopathic and functional medicine perspective, food allergy and intestinal dysbiosis are the most obvious probable etiologies; these clinical suspicions were confirmed with laboratory testing showing increased intestinal permeability and gastrointestinal dysbiosis.

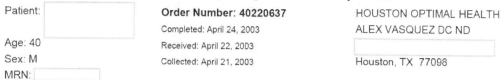

Patient:	**Order Number: 40220637**	HOUSTON OPTIMAL HEALTH
	Completed: April 24, 2003	ALEX VASQUEZ DC ND
Age: 40	Received: April 22, 2003	
Sex: M	Collected: April 21, 2003	
MRN:		Houston, TX 77098

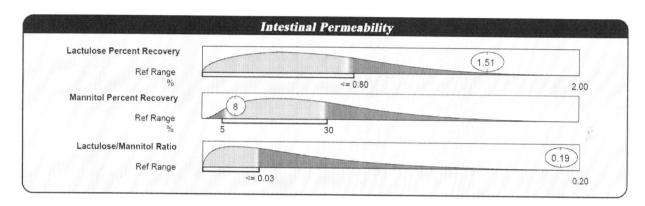

As expected, comprehensive parasitology showed intestinal dysbiosis, including insufficiency of *Lactobacillus* and presence of *Psuedomonas* and abnormal yeast species. Of particular note, *Psuedomonas aeruginosa* shows cross-reactivity with human neuronal tissues.[306,307] Eradication of the dysbiotic condition with a combination of dietary improvement, nutritional supplementation, hormonal optimization, and antimicrobial drugs and herbs lead to rapid and sustained remission of this "idiopathic peripheral neuropathy" which had defied standard medical diagnosis and treatment for many years.

Comprehensive Stool Analysis / Parasitology x3

MICROBIOLOGY

Bacteriology Culture

Beneficial flora		Imbalances		Dysbiotic flora	
Bifidobacter	4+	Haemolytic E. coli	4+	Pseudomonas sp.	4+
E. coli	4+	Gamma strep	2+		
Lactobacillus	2+				

Mycology (Yeast) Culture

Normal flora		Dysbiotic flora
Candida glabrata	1+	
Rhodotorula sp.	1+	

---

[306] Hughes LE, Bonell S, Natt RS, et al. Antibody responses to Acinetobacter spp. and Pseudomonas aeruginosa in multiple sclerosis: prospects for diagnosis using the myelin-acinetobacter-neurofilament antibody index. *Clin Diagn Lab* Immunol. 2001 Nov;8(6):1181-8 http://cvi.asm.org/content/8/6/1181.full.pdf
[307] Hughes LE, Smith PA, Bonell S, Natt RS, Wilson C, Rashid T, Amor S, Thompson EJ, Croker J, Ebringer A. Cross-reactivity between related sequences found in Acinetobacter sp., Pseudomonas aeruginosa, myelin basic protein and myelin oligodendrocyte glycoprotein in multiple sclerosis. *J Neuroimmunol*. 2003 Nov;144(1-2):105-15

Comprehensive stool analysis and comprehensive parasitology	
Overview and interpretation:	▪ **This is clearly one of the most valuable tests in clinical practice when working with patients with chronic fatigue, systemic inflammation, and autoimmunity. Second only to routine laboratory assessments such as CBC, chemistry panel, and CRP, the importance of stool testing and comprehensive parasitology assessments must be appreciated by progressive clinicians of all disciplines.** ▪ Stool testing must be performed by a specialty laboratory because the quality of testing provided by most standard "medical labs" and hospitals is completely inadequate. Initial samples should be collected on three separate occasions by the patient and each sample should be analyzed separately by the laboratory. ▪ Important qualitative and quantitative markers include the following: 1. **Beneficial bacteria (" probiotics")**: Microbiological testing should quantify and identify various beneficial bacteria, which should be present at "+4" levels on a 0-4 scale. 2. **Harmful and potentially harmful bacteria, protozoans, amebas, etc.**: Questionable or harmful microbes should be eradicated even if they are not identified as true pathogens in the paleo-classic Pasteurian/Kochian sense.[308] 3. **Yeast and mycology**: At least two tests must be performed for a complete assessment: 1) yeast culture, and 2) microscopic examination for yeast elements. Both tests are necessary because some patients—perhaps those with the most severe symptomatology and the most favorable response to anti-yeast treatment—will have a negative yeast culture and positive findings on the microscopic examination. In other words, these patients have intestinal yeast that contributes to their disease/symptomatology but which does not grow on culture despite being clearly visible with microscopy; a similar pattern (using a swab of the rectal mucosa rather than microscopy) is referred to as "negative culture with positive smear."[309] 4. **Microbial sensitivity testing**: An important component to parasitology testing is the determination of which anti-microbial agents (natural and synthetic) the microbe is sensitive to. This helps to guide and enhance the effectiveness of anti-microbial therapy. 5. **Secretory IgA**: SIgA levels are elevated in patients who are having an immune response to either food or microbial antigens.[310] Thus, in a patient with minimal dysbiosis, say for example with *Candida albicans*, an elevated sIgA can indicate that the patient is having a hypersensitivity reaction to an otherwise benign microbe—in this case, eradication of the microbe is warranted and may result in a positive clinical response. Low sIgA suggests either primary or secondary immune defect such as selective sIgA deficiency[311] or malnutrition, stress, prednisone/corticosteroids, or possibly mycotoxicosis (immunosuppression due to fungal immunotoxins). In addition to addressing any systemic causative factors, a low sIgA may be addressed with the administration of bovine colostrum, glutamine, vitamin A, and *Saccharomyces boulardii*; the following doses may be considered for use in adults with proportionately smaller doses for children: ▪ Bovine colostrum: 2.4 – 3.6 grams per day in divided doses for adults. No drug interactions are known. Side effects may include increased energy, insomnia, and

---

[308] **Vasquez A.** Reducing Pain and Inflammation Naturally. Part 6: Nutritional and Botanical Treatments Against "Silent Infections" and Gastrointestinal Dysbiosis, Commonly Overlooked Causes of Neuromusculoskeletal Inflammation and Chronic Health Problems. *Nutr Perspect* 2006; Jan http://optimalhealthresearch.com/part6.html

[309] "According to Galland, the best predictor of who will respond to anticandida medication is a negative stool culture combined with a positive smear of the rectal mucosa (for the identification of intracellular hyphal forms of the organism); however, even that test is not 100% reliable." Gaby AR. Before you order that lab test: part 2. *Townsend Letter for Doctors and Patients*. 2004; January findarticles.com/p/articles/mi_m0ISW/is_246/ai_112728028

[310] Quig DW, Higley M. Noninvasive assessment of intestinal inflammation: inflammatory bowel disease vs. irritable bowel syndrome. *Townsend Letter for Doctors and Patients* 2006;Jan:74-5

[311] "Selective IgA deficiency is the most common form of immunodeficiency. Certain select populations, including allergic individuals, patients with autoimmune and gastrointestinal tract disease and patients with recurrent upper respiratory tract illnesses, have an increased incidence of this disorder." Burks AW Jr, Steele RW. Selective IgA deficiency. *Ann Allergy*. 1986;57:3-13

Comprehensive stool analysis and comprehensive parasitology

stimulation. One study in particular used very large doses of 10 grams per day for four days in children and found no adverse effects[312]; another case report of a child involved the use of 50 grams per day for at least two weeks and showed no adverse effects.[313]

- Glutamine: 6 grams 3 times per day (18 grams per day) is a common dosage with significant literature support.
- Vitamin A: Correction of subclinical vitamin A deficiency improves mucosal integrity and increases sIgA production in humans.[314] Common doses used by integrative clinicians are in the range of 200,000 IU to 300,000 for a limited amount of time, generally 1-4 weeks; thereafter the dose is tapered. Patients are educated as to manifestations of toxicity (see the chapter on *Therapeutics* toward the end of this book) and the importance of limited duration of treatment.
- *Saccharomyces boulardii*: Common dose for adults is 250 mg thrice daily; ability of this treatment to increase sIgA levels and its anti-infective efficacy have been documented in human and animal studies.

6. **Short-chain fatty acids**: These are produced by intestinal bacteria. Quantitative excess indicates bacterial overgrowth of the intestines, while insufficiency indicates a lack of probiotics or an insufficiency of dietary substrate, i.e., soluble fiber. Abnormal patterns of individual short-chain fatty acids indicate qualitative/quantitative abnormalities in gastrointestinal microflora, particularly anaerobic bacteria that cannot be identified with routine bacterial cultures.

7. **Beta-glucuronidase**: This is an enzyme produced by several different intestinal bacteria. High levels of beta-glucuronidase in the intestinal lumen serve to nullify the benefits of detoxification (specifically glucuronidation) by cleaving the toxicant from its glucuronide conjugate. This can result in re-absorption of the toxicant through the intestinal mucosa which then re-exposes the patient to the toxin that was previously detoxified ("enterohepatic recirculation" or "enterohepatic recycling"[315]). This is an exemplary aspect of "auto-intoxication" that results in chronic fatigue and upregulation of Phase 1 detoxification systems (chapter 4 of *Integrative Rheumatology*).

8. **Lactoferrin**: The iron-binding glycoprotein lactoferrin is an inflammatory marker that helps distinguish functional disorders (i.e., IBS) from more serious diseases (i.e., IBD). Approximate values are as follows:
   - Healthy and IBS: 2 mcg/ml
   - Severe dysbiosis: up to 120 mcg/ml
   - Inactive IBD: 60-250 mcg/ml
   - Active IBD: > 400 mcg/ml.

9. **Lysozyme**: Elevated in proportion to intestinal inflammation in dysbiosis and IBD.

10. **Other markers**: Other markers of digestion, inflammation, and absorption are reported with the more comprehensive panels performed on stool samples. These tests are not always necessary, but such additional information is always helpful

---

[312] "In this double blind placebo-controlled trial, 80 children with rotavirus diarrhea were randomly assigned to receive orally either 10 g of IIBC (containing 3.6 g of antirotavirus antibodies) daily for 4 days or the same amount of a placebo preparation." Sarker SA, Casswall TH, Mahalanabis D, Alam NH, Albert MJ, Brussow H, Fuchs GJ, Hammerstrom L. Successful treatment of rotavirus diarrhea in children with immunoglobulin from immunized bovine colostrum. *Pediatr Infect Dis J.* 1998 Dec;17(12):1149-54

[313] Lactobin-R is a commercial hyperimmune bovine colostrum with some specificity for cryptosporidiosis; administration to a 4 year old child with AIDS and severe diarrhea resulted in significant clinical improvement in the diarrhea and "permanent elimination of the parasite from the gut as assessed through serial jejunal biopsy and stool specimens." Shield J, Melville C, Novelli V, Anderson G, Scheimberg I, Gibb D, Milla P. Bovine colostrum immunoglobulin concentrate for cryptosporidiosis in AIDS. *Arch Dis Child.* 1993 Oct;69(4):451-3

[314] "It can increase resistance to infection by increasing mucosal integrity, increasing surface immunoglobulin A (sIgA) and enhancing adequate neutrophil function. If infection occurs, vitamin A can act as an immune enhancer, increasing the adequacy of natural killer (NK) cells and increasing antibody production." Faisel H, Pittrof R. Vitamin A and causes of maternal mortality: association and biological plausibility. *Public Health Nutr.* 2000 Sep;3(3):321-7

[315] Parker RJ, Hirom PC, Millburn P.Enterohepatic recycling of phenolphthalein, morphine, lysergic acid diethylamide (LSD) and diphenylacetic acid in the rat. Hydrolysis of glucuronic acid conjugates in the gut lumen. *Xenobiotica.* 1980 Sep;10(9):689-70

Comprehensive stool analysis and comprehensive parasitology	
	when working with complex patients. These markers are relatively self-explanatory and/or are described on the results of the test by the laboratory.
Advantages:	▪ **Stool analysis in general and parasitology assessments in particular provide supremely valuable information in the comprehensive assessment and treatment of patients with complex illnesses such as chronic fatigue, irritable bowel syndrome, fibromyalgia, and all of the autoimmune/rheumatic diseases.**
Limitations:	▪ Tests vary in price from $250-$400. ▪ Anaerobic bacteria are difficult to culture. ▪ Specialty examinations, such as for *Helicobacter pylori* antigen and enterohemorrhagic *E. coli* cytotoxin, must be requested specifically at additional cost.
Comments:	▪ I have found stool testing to be the single most powerful diagnostic tool for helping chronically ill patients to attain improved health. Insights from stool/parasitology testing can be used to implement powerfully effective treatments. The value of this test in the treatment of patients with rheumatic disease must be appreciated and is extensively detailed in ***Integrative Rheumatology***.

Concept: Not all "Injury-related Problems" are "Injury-related Problems"

In the case of most acute injuries, the underlying problem is often the injury itself. However, the physician must conduct a thorough history and examination to assess for possible underling pathologies that cause or contribute to the problem that "appears" to be injury-related. Congenital anomalies, underlying pathology, previous injury, occult infections, and psychoemotional disorders may have been present *before* the "injury."

> **"Pediatric infections and neoplasms are notorious for masquerading as sport injuries."**
>
> "...Take the relevant history directly from the patient, and keep tumors and infections high on your list of differential diagnoses... For example, about 15% of children with leukemia present with musculoskeletal complaints..."
>
> Shaw BA, Gerardi JA, Hennrikus WL. How to avoid orthopedic pitfalls in children. *Patient Care* 1999 Feb

Just because the patient reports a problem such as pain following an injury does not mean that the injury is the *sole* cause of the pain. *Do not let a biased history lead you down the wrong path.* **In children and young adults, 5% of "sports-related" injuries are associated with preexisting infection, anomalies, or other conditions.** In adult women, "...between 9% and 20% of women with breast cancer attribute their symptoms to previous trauma to the breast. In these cases, the association of the breast mass with a traumatic event resulted in a delay in diagnosis ranging from four months to one year."[316]

A group of German physicians describe a man who presented with a soft-tissue pain following a soccer game; he was later diagnosed with a malignant tumor—synovial sarcoma.[317] Similarly, Wakeshima and Ellen[318] describe a young athletic woman who presented with chronic hip pain. The woman's history was significant for ulcerative colitis, but otherwise her radiographs were normal and her history and examination lead to a diagnosis of trochanteric bursitis. However, the patient's condition did not respond to routine treatment, and additional investigation over several months lead to a diagnosis of giant cell carcinoma. The authors concluded, "This case shows **the importance of repeat radiographic studies in patients whose joint pain does not respond or responds slowly to conservative therapy, despite initial normal findings.**"

What you expect to find and hear when taking a trauma-related history is that **1) a healthy patient** with no previous health concerns was **2) exposed to a traumatic event**, the history and consequences of which perfectly coincide with the injury you are assessing in your office, and that **3) your physical examination findings are all consistent** and lead to a specific diagnosis, which then **4) responds to your treatment.** If you find **discrepancies between the history of the injury and your physical examination findings (e.g., fever after a "sports-related" injury), if the patient appears unhealthy in disproportion to the presenting complaint, or if the patient does not respond to your treatment, then you must consider the possibility of preexisting or concomitant disease.**

When treating children, be very careful to get an accurate history—this is difficult since your two sources of information are not very reliable: parents often think that they already have the problem figured out, and so their history will be biased toward convincing you of what they think is the problem and solution; children are often not good historians and can form illogical relationships between events that can be misleading.

Astute doctors search for and rule out preexisting and underlying pathology before ascribing the problem to the "obvious cause." Always assess for consistency between the history, examination findings, and response to treatment—inconsistencies suggest the need for additional investigation.

[316] Seifert S. Medical Illness Simulating Trauma (MIST) syndrome: case reports and discussion of syndrome. *Fam Med* 1993 Apr;25(4):273-6
[317] Engel C, Kelm J, Olinger A. Blunt trauma in soccer. The initial manifestation of synovial sarcoma. [Article in German] *Zentralbl Chir* 2001 Jan;126(1):68-71
[318] Wakeshima Y, Ellen MI. Atypical hip pain origin in a young athletic woman: a case report of giant cell carcinoma. *Arch Phys Med Rehabil* 2001 Oct;82(10):1472-5

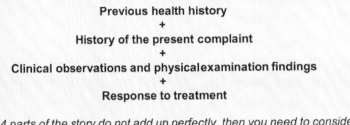

Previous health history
+
History of the present complaint
+
Clinical observations and physical examination findings
+
Response to treatment

If all 4 parts of the story do not add up perfectly, then you need to consider alternate diagnoses and take appropriate steps to ensure patient care.

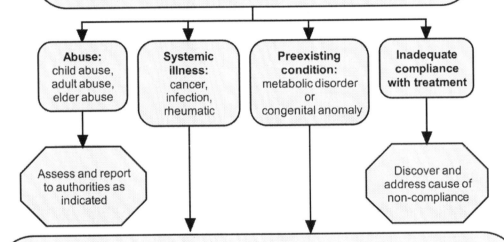

Abuse:
child abuse,
adult abuse,
elder abuse

Systemic illness:
cancer,
infection,
rheumatic

Preexisting condition:
metabolic disorder
or
congenital anomaly

Inadequate compliance with treatment

Assess and report to authorities as indicated

Discover and address cause of non-compliance

If you have a specific condition in mind, then test specifically for it. If you suspect preexisting/concomitant illness but are unsure of exact nature of the condition, gather additional information by:

1) **taking a more detailed history,**
2) **ordering lab tests:** CRP, CBC, chemistry panel, ferritin, ANA.
3) **obtaining diagnostic imaging** radiographs, bone scan, MRI, CT, US
4) **reassessing patient** within two weeks for progression of disease or crossing diagnostic threshold.
5) **referral or co-management:** if the patient does not respond to your treatment and/or you suspect an underlying serious pathology, refer the patient to another physician at least for co-management. Put your referral in writing and chart appropriately. "When in doubt, refer it out."

Clinical management: Inconsistencies between the history, exams, and response to treatment indicate the need for additional investigation and additional diagnostic considerations.

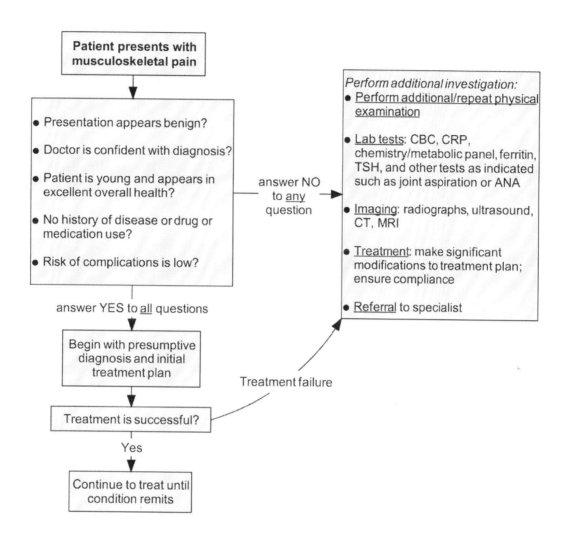

Clinical management: Inconsistencies between the history, exams, and response to treatment indicate the need for additional investigation and additional diagnostic considerations.

High-Risk Pain Patients:

When a patient has musculoskeletal pain and any of the following characteristics, radiographs should be considered as an appropriate component of comprehensive evaluation. These considerations are particularly—though not exclusively—relevant for spine and low-back pain.[319]

1. **More than 50 years of age**
2. **Physical trauma** (accident, fall, etc.)
3. **Pain at night**
4. **Back pain not relieved by lying supine**
5. **Neurologic deficits** (motor or sensory)
6. **Unexplained weight loss**
7. **Documentation or suspicion of inflammatory arthropathy**[320]
   - **Ankylosing spondylitis**
   - **Lupus**
   - **Rheumatoid arthritis**
   - **Juvenile rheumatoid arthritis**
   - **Psoriatic arthritis**
8. **Drug or alcohol abuse** (increased risk of infection, nutritional deficiencies, anesthesia)
9. **History of cancer**
10. **Intravenous drug use**
11. **Immunosuppression, due to illness (e.g., HIV) or medications (e.g., steroids or cyclosporine)**
12. **History of corticosteroid use** (causes osteoporosis and increased risk for infection)
13. **Fever above 100° F or suspicion of septic arthritis or osteomyelitis**
14. **Diabetes** (increased risk of infection, nutritional deficiencies, anesthesia)
15. **Hypertension** (abdominal aneurysm: low back pain, nausea, pulsatile abdominal mass)
16. **Recent visit for same problem and not improved**
17. **Patient seeking compensation for pain/ injury** (increased need for documentation)
18. **Skin lesion** (psoriasis, melanoma, dermatomyositis, the butterfly rash of lupus, scars from previous surgery, accident, etc.…)
19. **Deformity or immobility**
20. **Lymphadenopathy** (suggests cancer or infection)
21. **Elevated ESR/CRP** (cancer, infection, inflammatory disorder)
22. **Elevated WBC count**
23. **Elevated alkaline phosphatase** (bone lesions, metabolic bone disease, hepatopathy, vitamin D deficiency)
24. **Elevated acid phosphatase** (occasionally used to monitor prostate cancer)
25. **Positive rheumatoid factor and/or CCP—cyclic citrullinated protein antibodies**
26. **Positive HLA-B27** (propensity for inflammatory arthropathies)
27. **Serum gammopathy** (multiple myeloma is the most common primary bone tumor)
28. **"High-risk for disease"** *examples:*
   - Long-term heavy smoking of cigarettes
   - Long-term exposure to radiation
   - Obesity
29. **Strong family history of inflammatory, musculoskeletal, or malignant disease**

---

[319] Remember that metastasis often travel first from the primary site to bone, therefore bone pain may be an early manifestation of occult cancer. Most of the above are from "Table 1: The high-risk patient: clinical indications for radiography in low back pain patients." J Taylor, DC, DACBR, D Resnick, MD. Imaging decisions in the management of low back pain. Advances in Chiropractic. Mosby Year Book. 1994; 1-28

[320] Radiographs are often essential for diagnosis or to rule out complications of the disease. For example, in patients with inflammatory arthropathies such as these, spontaneous rupture of the transverse ligament (at the odontoid process) has been reported; although rare, this complication could be life-threatening if mismanaged or undiagnosed.

Concept: Safe Patient + Safe Treatment = Safe Outcome

The purpose of performing the history and physical examination on a new *or established* patient is to determine their current health status—including their mental and emotional health and their physical health, particularly as this relates to important and life-threatening possibilities such as cancer, infections, fractures, systemic diseases, and neurologic compromise. The questions that lead this investigation are: "**What is this patient's current status?**" "**Does this patient have a serious disease, neurologic injury, or are they at high risk for developing a serious complication in the near future that can be prevented with appropriate care** *now*?"

"Is this patient safe?"

* ♦ The question to ask yourself is, "Is this patient's health problem or current complaint/exacerbation a manifestation of an underlying condition that could result in a negative outcome?
* ♦ If a patient comes to you with a headache, and you neglect to find that their blood pressure is 230/130, then you missed the opportunity to help them avoid the stroke that they could have after leaving your office.
* ♦ If a patient comes to you with a complaint of low back pain, and you neglect to perform a neurologic examination to find that *the patient already has a neurologic deficit even before you treated them*, then you have lost the opportunity to defend yourself in court when the patient later claims that *your* treatment and *your* management of their case is the reason that they now have a permanent neurologic deficit.

Is your treatment safe?: Have you been perfectly clear with the patient about the risks and benefits of your treatment plan? **Have you obtained informed consent**? Have you charted **"PAR-B"** to indicate that you have discussed the **P**rocedures, **A**lternatives, **R**isks, and **B**enefits of your treatment plan? Have you been clear about the duration of treatment and the need for appropriate follow-up? If you are prescribing nutrition or botanical medicines, have you informed the patient about the duration of treatment? **Have you looked for contraindications to your otherwise brilliant treatment plan**? What about the fact that this patient was on corticosteroids for the past 15 years and only discontinued prednisone 2 months before arriving at your office? *The patient may have steroid-induced osteoporosis even though he is no longer on prednisone.* When you recommend that your patient take 100,000 IU of vitamin A to treat her throat infection, what happens when she presents to your office 8 months later with signs of vitamin A toxicity because she continued her treatment plan indefinitely

> Double-check to ensure that your patient is safe (no forthcoming complications or predictable emergencies) and that your treatment is safe (appropriate, effective, clearly communicated, and time-limited with instructions to return for office visit).

rather than using it only for 7 days as you had intended? *Be sure to put a time limit on your treatment plans.* Every treatment plan should be 1) given to the patient in legible print and clear statements, 2) be copied for the chart, 3) include "what to do if things get worse" in the event of adverse treatment effect or exacerbation of problem, and 4) include patient's responsibility for returning to office/clinic for follow-up and reassessment.

Informed consent: From a legal standpoint, doctors can only treat a patient after the patient has given *consent to treatment*. Patients can only authoritatively consent to treatment after they have been educated about the treatment—thereafter, they can provide *informed consent*. Educating the patient requires discussion (and documentation) of each of the following:

* Procedures—what may take place, what is required; duration, costs, follow-up,
* Alternatives—what options are available,
* Risks—what risks are involved,
* Benefits—what benefits can be reasonably expected,
* Questions—allow for the patient to ask questions and receive answers.

This is commonly charted as "**PARB—no questions**" or "**PARB—questions answered**" once the patient gives consent to treatment; alternatively and more humorously, this may be charted as "**PAR-B-Q**".

Concept: Four Clues to Discovering Underlying Problems

When I taught Orthopedics at Bastyr University I encouraged students to search for specific **sets of clues** when evaluating patients. These clues—often insignificant in isolation but meaningful in combination—were often the "red flags" that could help make the difference between an accurate diagnosis and a missed diagnosis. These four categories can be recalled with the mnemonic "*S.C.I.N.*" or "*S.C.I.M.*" These four areas of assessment/safety emphasis differ from the "vindicates" mnemonic which is used for differential diagnosis.

<table>
<tr><td colspan="2">Vindicates: a popular mnemonic for differential diagnosis</td></tr>
<tr><td>V</td><td>Vascular
Visceral referral</td></tr>
<tr><td>I</td><td>Infectious
Inflammatory
Immunologic</td></tr>
<tr><td>N</td><td>Neurologic
Nutritional
New growth: neoplasia or pregnancy</td></tr>
<tr><td>D</td><td>Deficiency
Degenerative</td></tr>
<tr><td>I</td><td>Iatrogenic (drug related)
Intoxication
Idiosyncratic</td></tr>
<tr><td>C</td><td>Congenital
Cardiac or circulatory</td></tr>
<tr><td>A</td><td>Allergy / Autoimmune
Abuse: drugs, alcohol, physical</td></tr>
<tr><td>T</td><td>Trauma
Toxicity</td></tr>
<tr><td>E</td><td>Endocrine
Exposure</td></tr>
<tr><td>S</td><td>Subluxation
Somatic dysfunction
Structural
Stress
Secondary gain</td></tr>
</table>

- **Systemic symptoms and signs**: Ask about systemic signs and symptoms such as fever, weight loss, lymphadenopathy, or skin rash in patients who present with pain because these "whole body" manifestations might indicate an underlying or concomitant disease that deserves attention, either independently from the musculoskeletal pain, or as a cause of the musculoskeletal pain. For example, "headache" may appear benign, whereas "headache with fever and skin rash" suggests meningitis—a medical emergency. "Low-back pain" is a common occurrence; yet "low-back pain with weight loss and fever" might suggest occult malignancy, osteomyelitis, or other systemic disease.

- **Complications:** We ask about and look for already existing complications, such as "numbness, weakness, tingling in the arms or hands, legs or feet" to rapidly screen for neurologic deficits and we follow this up with screening assessments such as "squat and rise", toe walk, heel walk, and reflexes for spinal cord and lower extremity neuromuscular integrity. Additionally, when dealing with patients with spine-related complaints or injuries, we also ask about changes or loss of function in bowel and bladder control and numbness near the anus or genitals, which may be the *only* clinical clues to cauda equina syndrome—a medical emergency. Ask about effects of the condition on ADL (activities of daily living) to attain a more comprehensive view of the condition and to ensure that the patient's story is consistent.

- **Indicators from the history**: We look for specific "red flags" and "yellow flags" such as trauma, risk factors (such as smoking, prednisone, alcohol), or a positive history of chronic infections or cancer. Nonmechanical musculoskeletal pain in a patient with a history of or high risk for cancer is highly suspicious and mandates thorough investigation.

- **Non-Mechanical pain**: Non-mechanical pain suggests a pathologic etiology rather than simple joint dysfunction. Pain at night, pain that occurs without an inciting injury, pain that is not strongly affected by motion and is not powerfully provoked by your physical examination assessments suggests the possibility of underlying disorder such as cancer, neuropathy, or infection. However, the ability to elicit an exacerbation of pain with "mechanical" maneuvers does not indicate that the pain is "mechanical" and therefore "non-pathologic." Mechanical pain can still be pathologic pain, such as the exquisite pain felt by patients with spinal fractures—they may be neurologically intact, they do have pain worse with motion, but they are not safe to manipulate, and they require appropriate treatment and referral on an urgent basis.

> Keeping these four assessment categories in mind can serve as a useful "checkpoint" to ensure that your patient is safe, and that your treatment is appropriate and therefore safe, too.

Concept: Special Considerations in the Evaluation of Children

"Pediatric infections and neoplasms are notorious for masquerading as sport injuries. ... There is only one way to avoid this trap: Take the relevant history directly from the patient, and keep tumors and infections high on your list of differential diagnoses."[321]

- **Consider the possibility of child abuse when a child presents with an injury:** As a non-naïve physician, you always have to consider the possibility of child abuse when a child presents with an injury. Be detailed in your history taking, and be sure to search for discrepancies between 1) the child's version of the incident, 2) the adult's version of the incident, and 3) what is realistic (based on your practical life experience and clinical training). As a primary care physician, you are obligated to report your *suspicion* of child abuse to law enforcement agencies and/or child protective services.
- **Children heal quickly:** This rapid healing is good as long as tissues are approximated. But if a fractured bone is displaced and not correctly replaced, then problematic malunion deformities may result *within **days***.
- **Children are more susceptible to rapidly progressing infections than are adults:** Soft tissue, joint, and bone infections need to be diagnosed expeditiously and treated aggressively.
- **Children are radiographically different from adults:** Make sure that your radiographs are interpreted by a competent radiologist with experience in the interpretation of *pediatric radiographs*. Radiographic considerations specific to children include:
  - **Epiphyseal growth plates**
  - **Secondary ossification centers**
  - **Variants in trabecular patterns and bone densities**
  - **Specific conditions that happen only in children, such as slipped capital femoral epiphysis**
  - **Congenital anomalies**
  - **Difficulty following directions with positioning** (applies to some adults, too!)
  - **Bone scans can be difficult to interpret in children:** Bone scans derive their value from the demonstration of a focal increase in uptake of radioactive isotopes, which demonstrates and localizes an area of increased metabolic activity. In adults, this increased and localized activity generally indicates pathology, especially malignant disease in bone (primary or metastatic) and recent fracture. In children, however, since their bones are already highly metabolically active due to the normal growth process, bone scans are difficult to interpret and are not highly reliable for the demonstration of focal lesions.

> Always consider the possibility of abuse, cancer, infection, or congenital anomaly as a cause of musculoskeletal pain in children, even if the injury appears to be related to injury or trauma. Strongly consider lab tests, as well as radiographs (interpreted by a pediatric radiologist). When in doubt, refer for second opinion. If you suspect abuse, you have a legal and ethical obligation to report your *suspicion*.

---

[321] Shaw BA, Gerardi JA, Hennrikus WL. How to avoid orthopedic pitfalls in children. *Patient Care* 1999; Feb 28: 95-116

Concept: Differences between Primary Healthcare and Spectator Sports

In baseball, "errors" have been defined as "a defensive mistake that allows a batter to stay at the plate or reach first base, or that advances a base runner."[322] In baseball, a few errors can make the difference between winning and losing a particular game or season. However, a few errors in a game are to be expected, and ultimately the team can start over at the next game or season and try to do better.

Healthcare, however, is not a game, and even relatively minor errors such as the doctor's forgetting to ask a particular question or perform a specific test can result in a patient's catastrophic injury or death. In healthcare, when we are dealing with serious injuries and illnesses, even a single "error" is not allowed. "Failure to diagnose" is one of the biggest reasons for malpractice claims against doctors; such judgments often result in loss of licensure and awards of hundreds of thousands of dollars. "Failure to treat" results when the patient is injured because the doctor failed to

> While your compassion for human suffering and your love of nutrition and exercise may have directed you into healthcare, your professional success and survival will depend in large part on your ability to manage the technical and defensive aspects of clinical practice.
>
> Neuromusculoskeletal disorders and autoimmune diseases are "big league" clinical problems, and they need to be taken seriously.

effectively treat the patient or when the doctor failed to provide the appropriate referral to a specialist in a timely manner. Such failures are not only capable of destroying a physician's career and forcing the liquidation of his/her possessions, but such cases can also greatly damage the integrity of whole professions, especially the naturopathic and chiropractic professions which are generally guilty until proven innocent due to the double standards imposed by those adherent to the "always right" dogma of the medical paradigm.[323] Stated differently, **if the doctor does not ask the right questions and perform the right tests, then the doctor may miss an emergency diagnosis. Missing an emergency diagnosis can result in patient death. Patient death may result in litigation, loss of license for the doctor, and irreparable harm to the profession.** The upcoming section on **Musculoskeletal Emergencies** represents *core competencies* that every clinician must keep present in his/her mind during each interaction with a patient with musculoskeletal complaints, especially patients who are elderly, on medications such as prednisone, and those with known autoimmune or immunosuppressive disorders.

Concept: "Disease Treatment" is Different from "Patient Management"

> "The key to successful intervention for orthopedic problems in a primary care practice is to know what conditions to refer and when and to whom to refer the refractory patient."[324]

Treating a problem is one thing, managing a patient is something different. "Problems" such as "low back pain" are abstract concepts, and we automatically form mental lists of treatments for problems that are irrespective of the patient who has the condition. However this list may be of only very limited applicability to the individual patient with whom you are working. Management of patients includes ❶ assessing and reassessing the differential diagnoses, ❷ monitoring compliance with treatments, including the treatments of other healthcare providers, ❸ co-treating with other healthcare providers, ❹ assessing for contraindications, ❺ monitoring patient status and effectiveness of treatments, and also ❻ the office-related tasks of charting, documentation, billing, and correspondence. The management of emergency conditions often involves transport to the nearest hospital. In some situations, the patient will be able to drive himself/herself without difficulty. In other situations, the patient should be driven by friend, family, or taxi. In the most extreme, the patient should be transported by ambulance. When in doubt about the mode of transport, do not hesitate to call 911 for an ambulance. If the taxi driver gets lost on the way to the hospital, or your patient goes into shock while being driven by a friend, the liability will come back to haunt the *doctor*, not the *friend* or the *taxi driver*.

---

[322] http://www.nocryinginbaseball.com/glossary/glossary.html Accessed November 11, 2006
[323] Micozzi MS. Double standards and double jeopardy for CAM research. *J Altern Complement Med.* 2001 Feb;7(1):13-4
[324] Brier S. Primary Care Orthopedics. St. Louis: Mosby, 1999 page ix

Concept: Clinical Practice Involves Much More than "Diagnosis and Treatment"

Emergency room and hospital-based physicians are appropriately able to focus solely on diagnosis and treatment as their primary spheres of activity and interaction with patients. However, those of us in private practice learn that *healthcare* involves much more than simply being a "good doctor." From an integrative perspective we have to go beyond diagnosis and treatment *for each health disorder* with each patient. Beyond *diagnosis* and *treatment* are *understanding* and *integration*. Orchestrating all of this into a treatment plan that the patient can actually implement requires creativity, resourcefulness, and the ability to enroll patients in the process of *redesigning*—often *rebuilding*—their lives.

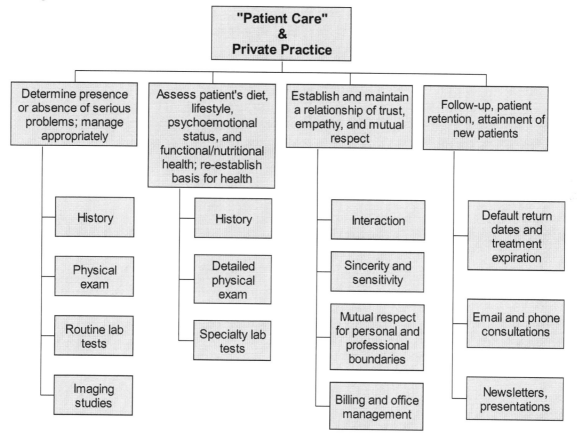

Recall that **28% of malpractice claims involve mistakes made by medical office staff**; this includes unreturned phone calls which can culminate in malpractice by way of "patient abandonment." Similarly, inability to get a timely consultation may result in sufficient "sense of harm" that a patient may decide to sue; this is a factor in 10% of malpractice cases.[325]

---

[325] James R. Hall, Ph.D., L.Psych., FABMP, FGICPP. Departments of Internal Medicine and Psychology, UNT Health Science Center at Fort Worth. "Communication and Medico-Legal Issues." October 19, 2006

Risk Management: A Note Especially to Students and Recent Licensees

Even if you are a board-certified rheumatologist and an assertive and astute clinician with years of experience, the consideration of these guidelines may help protect **you** from malpractice liability and **your patient** from harm. Practicing "good medicine" is inherently defensive and in the best interests of the patient and the doctor.

1. **Document the specifics of your treatment plan and the rationale behind it**.
2. **Do not tell your patient to discontinue their anti-rheumatic drugs unless these drugs are in your scope of practice *and* discontinuing such drugs is therapeutically appropriate.**
3. **Give your patient written instructions, and specifically delineate time parameters for the next visit to monitor for therapeutic effectiveness, adverse effects, and disease progression/regression.**
4. **Always have an internist or rheumatologist (or appropriate specialist) on-board as part of the clinical team in case the patient experiences an exacerbation and needs to be hospitalized or acutely immunosuppressed.**
5. **When working with patients that have potentially serious diseases such as most of the autoimmune diseases, you should have a back-up plan integrated into your treatment plan from day one.** You might consider having patients sign a consent form that includes language consistent with the following:
   - *"Due to the uniqueness of each disease and each individual, including his or her willingness and ability to implement the treatment plan, no guarantees of successful treatment can be offered."*
   - *"Dr.___ may not be available on a 24-hour basis at all times. If you have a serious health problem that requires immediate attention, you should call your other doctors(s), call 911, or have someone take you to the nearest hospital emergency room. If you notice an adverse effect from one of the components of your health plan, you should discontinue it then call Dr.__ and inform him/her of what occurred."*
   - *"Treatments with other physicians or healthcare providers are not necessarily to be discontinued. Please let Dr.__ know if you are being treated by other healthcare providers (physicians, counselors, therapists, etc.). Consult your prescribing doctor before discontinuing medications."*
6. **Test responsibly.**
7. **Treat responsibly.**
8. **Re-test to document effectiveness of your intervention.**
9. **When in doubt, refer the patient for co-management.** If you are working with a serious life-threatening disease, and *your plan* or *the patient's implementation of it* is unable to produce *documentable results*, then you should refer the patient for allopathic/osteopathic/specialist co-management for the sake of protecting the patient from harm and for protecting yourself from undue liability.
10. **Practice defensively.** You will thereby safeguard your patient and your livelihood.

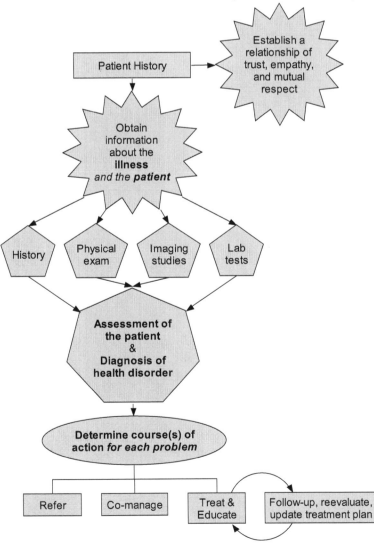

Musculoskeletal Emergencies

These are some of the "core competencies" that clinicians can never afford to miss, and these are pertinent to patients with musculoskeletal disorders, whether structural/orthopedic or metabolic/rheumatic. With these conditions, clinicians are wise to err on the side of caution— *"When in doubt, refer out"*—and implement the appropriate referral on an expedient basis. These are organized in a clinical/logical manner rather than listed alphabetically.

Neurovascular Disorders

Problem	Presentation	Assessment	Management
Neuropsychiatric lupus	<ul><li>Psychosis</li><li>Seizures</li><li>Transient ischemic attacks</li><li>Severe depression</li><li>Delirium, confusion</li></ul>	<ul><li>Neuropsychiatric manifestations with history of lupus</li></ul>	<ul><li>Emergency or prompt referral as indicated</li></ul>
Giant cell arteritis, Temporal arteritis: Considered a medical emergency since it may rapidly progress to blindness due to associated involvement of the ophthalmic artery: *"Loss of vision is the most feared manifestation and occurs quite commonly."*[326]	Presentation typically includes the following: <ul><li>Headache, scalp tenderness</li><li>Jaw claudication</li><li>Changes in vision</li><li>Systemic manifestations of rheumatic disease: fever, weight loss, muscle aches</li></ul>	<ul><li>Palpation of the temporal artery may reveal a "cord-like" artery</li><li>Elevated ESR</li><li>CBC may show anemia</li><li>Temporal artery biopsy is diagnostic</li></ul>	<ul><li>Standard medical treatment is with immediate prednisone</li><li>Implement treatment that is immediately effective or refer patient for medical treatment</li></ul>
Acute red eye: General term including acute iritis and scleritis; despite the name of this condition, redness may actually be rather minimal, and it is typically accompanied by cloudy changes in region of the iris and lens	<ul><li>Eye pain and redness</li><li>May have facial pain</li><li>May be the presenting manifestation of rheumatic disease</li></ul>	<ul><li>Red eye</li><li>Photophobia</li><li>Reduced vision</li><li>May have fixed pupil</li><li>Differential diagnosis includes acute glaucoma, bacterial/amebic/ viral conjunctivitis or keratitis, allergy, and irritation due to contact lens</li></ul>	<ul><li>"The **acute** onset of a **painful, red** eye, even in the absence of visual upset, should be regarded primarily as an ophthalmological emergency."[327]</li><li>**Granulomatous uveitis** occurs in 15% of patients with sarcoidosis and can result in bilateral blindness—this must be managed as a medically urgent condition</li></ul>

---

[326] Tierney ML. McPhee SJ, Papadakis MA (eds). <u>Current Medical Diagnosis and Treatment, 41st Edition</u>. New York: Lange Medical ; 2002. P999-1005
[327] McInnes I, Sturrock R. Rheumatological emergencies. *Practitioner*. 1994 Mar;238(1536):220-4

Neural canal compression

Problem	Presentation	Assessment	Management
Atlantoaxial instability: Excess mobility between the atlas and axis (commonly due to lesion of the dens or transverse ligament) makes the spinal cord vulnerable to compressive injury when the atlas translates anteriorly on the axis especially during cervical flexion; may progress to neurologic compromise including respiratory and somatic paralysis	• Post-traumatic neck injury • Down's syndrome • May present spontaneously (without trauma) in patients with inflammatory rheumatic disease, especially rheumatoid arthritis and ankylosing spondylitis • May have gradual or sudden onset of myelopathy: upper motor neuron lesion (UMNL) signs (e.g., spastic weakness), changes in bowel-bladder function, numbness	• Clinical suspicion is followed by lateral cervical and APOM (anteroposterior open mouth) radiographs to assess ADI (atlantodental interval) and dens • MRI should be performed in patients with suspected myelopathy • Neurologic examination of the upper and lower extremities • Do not force neck flexion; do not perform the Soto Hall test	• **Urgent neurosurgical consultation is recommended; stabilizing surgery is the best option for the prevention of neurologic catastrophes[328]** • Onset of myelopathy mandates referral to ER and/or neurosurgeon; immobilize with spine board or hard cervical collar and transport appropriately • Asymptomatic and mild increases in ADI (< 5mm) might be managed conservatively with activity restriction, exercises, and bracing/collars) • PAR discussion and referral for surgical consultation is necessary for informed consent and safe management
Myelopathy, spinal cord compression or lesion: May occur due to infection, edema, tumor, spinal fracture, stenosis, or inflammatory disease	• **Spastic weakness** • Bowel-bladder dysfunction • Numbness • Problems are distal to cord lesion	• Hyperreflexia • Rigidity • Muscle weakness • MRI (with and without contrast) should be performed in patients with suspected myelopathy; CT may also be indicated	• Obtain MRI to confirm diagnosis • Immobilize spine and transport if necessary • Acute myelopathy is a medical emergency that can result in rapid-onset paralysis
Cauda equina syndrome: Compression of the sacral nerve roots due to lumbar disc herniation **Cauda equina syndrome is a surgical emergency.**	• History of sciatic low back pain • Urinary retention, perineal numbness, and fecal incontinence are common • May have lower extremity weakness	• Assess for bladder distention • Assess anal sphincter strength with rectal exam • Lower extremity neurologic examination	• Urgent referral for CT/MRI to confirm diagnosis • If diagnosis is confirmed or strongly suspected clinically, urgent referral for surgical decompression is mandatory

---

[328] "When atlantoaxial stability is lost...it is thought that surgical stabilisation of the atlantoaxial joint is more reasonable and beneficial than conservative management. Minimal trauma of an unstable atlantoaxial joint can lead to serious neurological injury." Moon MS, Choi WT, Moon YW, Moon JL, Kim SS. Brooks' posterior stabilization surgery for atlantoaxial instability: review of 54 cases. *J Orthop Surg* (Hong Kong). 2002 Dec;10(2):160-4. http://www.josonline.org/PDF/v10i2p160.pdf

Acute peripheral nerve compression

Problem	Presentation	Assessment	Management
Acute compartment syndrome: acute onset of *potentially irreversible* muscle and/or nerve compression injury due to inflammation, swelling, or bleeding within a fascial compartment **Acute compartment syndrome is a surgical emergency.**	• Most commonly occurs in the anterior leg; may also occur in the posterior leg as well as forearm—these are the areas most notable anatomically for the investment of muscle in tight and resilient fascial sheaths • Onset generally follows strenuous exercise that leads to reactive hyperemia and secondary edema • May occur following trauma or fracture	Assess for: • Pulselessness • Palor • Painful passive stretch • Weakness • **Numbness** • Assessment and treatment should be performed on an emergency basis since irreversible nerve damage begins within 6 hours of intracompartmental hypertension	• Decompressive fasciotomy is the standard treatment for acute compartment syndrome that could result in permanent muscle necrosis and/or permanent nerve death • Acute compartment syndrome can be fatal if rhabdomyolysis precipitates renal failure[329]

Musculoskeletal infections

Problem	Presentation	Assessment	Management
Septic arthritis: intraarticular bacterial infection; complications of septic arthritis are 1) articular destruction and 2) **death in 5-10% of patients**[330] **Septic arthritis is a medical emergency**	• **Febrile** patient has **acute/subacute mono/oligo-arthritis** • Some patients may not have fever • Other possible findings: Immuno-suppression due to medications, concomitant disease (RA, DM), elderly • In some patients with concomitant disease or medications, the clinical picture can be blurred.	• **Warm, swollen, tender joint** • Clinical assessment with **immediate referral for joint aspiration**, which reveals manifestations of infection such as WBC's and bacteria • Differential diagnosis includes trauma, gout, CPPD, hemochromatosis	• **Immediate referral for joint aspiration** • **An aggressive and prolonged course of IV and oral antimicrobials** • "Immune support" such as vitamin A and glutamine and general measures to improve health and prevent recurrence
Osteomyelitis, infectious discitis: considered a medical emergency[331] **Osteomyelitis—especially vertebral osteomyelitis—is a medical emergency**	• Febrile patient with bone pain • Assess for constitutional manifestations such as weight loss, night sweats, and malaise	• Exacerbation of bone pain when stress/percussion is applied to the bone • Lab: CRP & WBC may be elevated • MRI is more sensitive than CT, bone scan, or radiography[332]	• Emergency referral for vertebral osteomyelitis, since **up to 15% of patients will develop nerve lesions or cord compression**[333] • Urgent referral for other types of osteomyelitis

[329] Paula R. Compartment Syndrome, Extremity. *eMedicine* June 22, 2006 http://www.emedicine.com/emerg/topic739.htm Accessed November 26, 2006
[330] Tierney ML. McPhee SJ, Papadakis MA. Current Medical Diagnosis and Treatment. 35th edition. Stamford: Appleton & Lange, 1996 page 759
[331] American College of Rheumatology Ad Hoc Committee on Clinical Guidelines. Guidelines for the initial evaluation of the adult patient with acute musculoskeletal symptoms. *Arthritis Rheum.* 1996;39(1):1-8
[332] Tierney ML. McPhee SJ, Papadakis MA (eds). Current Medical Diagnosis and Treatment 2002, 41st Edition. New York: Lange Medical; 2002. p 883
[333] King RW, Johnson D. Osteomyelitis. Updated July 13, 2006. *eMedicine* http://www.emedicine.com/emerg/topic349.htm Accessed Dec 24, 2006

Acute Nontraumatic Monoarthritis and Septic Arthritis

- "Acute monoarthritis is a potential medical emergency that must be investigated and treated promptly."[334]
- "Monoarthropathies should initially be investigated to exclude sepsis. ... Diagnostic joint aspiration ... should be carried out immediately."[335]
- "In acute monoarthritis, it is essential that infection of a joint be diagnosed or excluded, and this can only be done by joint aspiration and synovial fluid culture."[336]
- "Acute monoarthritis should be considered infectious until proven otherwise."[337]

Clinical presentations:

- Patient presents with acute joint pain in one joint (occasionally more than one joint may be involved).
- May or may not have fever and other systemic manifestations of infection.

> **Clinical Pearl**
>
> The primary goal of this section is to solidify your awareness of septic arthritis, its differential diagnoses, and the method and importance of assertive diagnosis and management.
>
> Septic arthritis is a medical emergency, and some authoritative textbooks report a mortality rate of 5-10%.
>
> Septic arthritis must be diagnosed urgently with joint aspiration, and it must be treated with antibiotics in order to preserve the joint and prevent spread of the infection.

Major Differential Diagnoses for Nontraumatic Monoarthritis

Problem	Presentation	Assessment & Management
Septic arthritis: intraarticular bacterial infection; complications of septic arthritis are 1) articular destruction and 2) **death in 5-10% of patients**[338]	• **Febrile** patient has **acute/subacute mono/oligo-arthritis** • **Onset over hours or days** Other possible findings: • Immuno-suppression due to medications, concomitant disease (RA, DM), elderly • Some patients may not have fever • In some patients with a previous or concomitant disease process, the clinical picture can be blurred	• **Warm, swollen, red, painful joint** • Clinical assessment with **immediate referral for <u>joint aspiration</u>**, which reveals characteristic manifestations of infection such as WBCs and bacteria • **Immediate joint aspiration** • An aggressive and prolonged course of IV and oral antimicrobials • "Immune support" and general measures to improve health and prevent recurrence **"Septic arthritis is still a life-threatening disease with a mortality of 2–5% and high morbidity."** Zacher J, Gursche A. Regional musculoskeletal conditions: 'hip' pain. *Best Practice & Research Clinical Rheumatology*. 2003 Feb;17:71-85

---

[334] Cibere J. Rheumatology: 4. Acute monoarthritis. CMAJ (*Canadian Medical Association Journal*). 2000;162(11):1577-83 www.cmaj.ca/cgi/content/full/162/11/1577 Jan 2004

[335] McInnes I, Sturrock R. Rheumatological emergencies. Practitioner. 1994 Mar;238(1536):220-4

[336] American College of Rheumatology Ad Hoc Committee on Clinical Guidelines. Guidelines for the initial evaluation of the adult patient with acute musculoskeletal symptoms. *Arthritis Rheum*. 1996 Jan;39(1):1-8

[337] Cibere J. Rheumatology: 4. Acute monoarthritis. CMAJ (*Canadian Medical Association Journal*). 2000;162(11):1577-83 www.cmaj.ca/cgi/content/full/162/11/1577 Jan 2004

[338] Tierney ML. McPhee SJ, Papadakis MA. Current Medical Diagnosis and Treatment. 35th edition. Stamford: Appleton and Lange, 1996 page 759

Major differential diagnoses for non-traumatic monoarthritis—*continued*

Problem	Presentation	Assessment & Management
Osteochondritis dissecans: A disorder of unclear etiology (trauma and/or avascular necrosis) which results in the death and subsequent fragmentation of subchondral bone[339]	▪ Primarily affects ages 10-30 years ▪ **Most common in the knees and elbows** ▪ Locking and crepitus due to intraarticular loose bodies ("joint mice") ▪ Some patients are almost asymptomatic, while others have acute pain ▪ Swelling of the affected joint	▪ Radiographs—consider to assess both knees as the condition is bilateral in 30% ▪ MRI is used to assess severity and need for surgical intervention ▪ Stable and nondisplaced lesions may be managed nonsurgically; larger and displaced fragments require surgical repair to reduce long-term complications[340]
Transient synovitis, irritable hip: Non-specific short-term inflammation and effusion of the hip joint	▪ Acute onset of painful hip and limp ▪ Decreased pain with hip in flexion and abduction ▪ Considered the most common cause of hip pain in children[341] ▪ More common in boys, age 3-6 years and generally younger than 10 years ▪ May have recent history of viral infection, and some children (1.5-10%) eventually manifest RA or AVN[342]	▪ May have slight elevation of ESR ▪ Normal WBC ▪ <u>No</u> fever; the child appears healthy ▪ "...radiography is indicated to exclude osseous pathological conditions..."[343] ▪ **Joint aspiration is indicated if septic arthritis is suspected**[344] ▪ Conservative treatment, restricted exertion and weight-bearing for several weeks
Legg-Calve-Perthe's disease: Idiopathic ischemic necrosis of the femoral head occurring in children **Avascular necrosis (AVN) of the femoral head, osteonecrosis**: Ischemic necrosis of the femoral head	Perthe's disease: ▪ 80% occur in children generally between ages of 4-9 years; more common in boys; may present with hip pain or knee pain AVN: ▪ Ages 20-40 years ▪ Unilateral hip pain ▪ May have knee pain ▪ History of trauma is common AVN associations: ▪ Steroid use, prednisone ▪ Hyperlipidemia ▪ Alcoholism ▪ Pancreatitis ▪ Hemoglobinopathies ▪ Smoking ▪ Fatty liver disease: "fat globules from the liver"[345]	▪ Limited ROM ▪ **Radiographs**; if normal and clinical suspicion is high order MRI or bone scan ▪ **Crutches** ▪ **Orthopedic referral is recommended** although not all patients will require surgery and some may be managed conservatively[346]

---

[339] Tatum R. Osteochondritis dissecans of the knee: a radiology case report. *J Manipulative Physiol Ther* 2000 Jun;23(5):347-51
[340] Browne RF, Murphy SM, Torreggiani WC, Munk PL, Marchinkow LO. Radiology for the surgeon: musculoskeletal case 30. Osteochondritis dissecans of the medial femoral condyle. *Can J Surg.* 2003;46(5):361-3 cma.ca/multimedia/staticContent/HTML/N0/l2/cjs/vol-46/issue-5/pdf/pg361.pdf
[341] Maroo S. Diagnosis of hip pain in children. *Hosp Med* 1999 Nov;60(11):788-93
[342] Souza TA. <u>Differential Diagnosis for the Chiropractor: Protocols and Algorithms</u>. Gaithersberg, Maryland: Aspen Publications. 1997 page 265
[343] Maroo S. Diagnosis of hip pain in children. *Hosp Med* 1999 Nov;60(11):788-93
[344] Maroo S. Diagnosis of hip pain in children. *Hosp Med* 1999 Nov;60(11):788-93

Major differential diagnoses for non-traumatic monoarthritis—*continued*

Problem	Presentation	Assessment & Management
<u>Gout</u>	<ul><li>**Febrile** patient has **acute/subacute mono/oligo-arthritis**</li><li>**Onset over hours or days**</li><li>"A history of discreet attacks, usually affecting one joint, that precede the onset of fixed symmetric arthritis is the major clue."[347]</li><li>May have fever, chills, tachycardia, leukocytosis—just like septic arthritis</li></ul>	<ul><li>Clinical presentation may be sufficient for DX; however septic arthritis should be excluded</li><li>Serum uric acid is generally meaningless for the diagnosis of gout since many gout patients will have normal serum uric acid</li><li>Medical treatment is rest, NSAID's, and allopurinol</li><li>Fluid loading: >3 liters per day; monitor for electrolyte imbalances and hyponatremia as needed</li><li>Integrative assessment and treatment for insulin resistance, hormonal imbalances, and nutritional deficiencies</li></ul>
CPPD: Calcium pyrophosphate dihydrate deposition disease	<ul><li>Idiopathic</li><li>May be caused by iron overload in some patients</li><li>Presentation may be acute or subacute</li></ul>	<ul><li>Medical diagnosis is by synovial biopsy</li><li>Radiographs reveal chondrocalcinosis</li><li>Allopathic treatment is NSAIDs; phytonutritional anti-inflammatory treatments may also be used (see chapter 3 of *Integrative Orthopedics/Rheumatology*)</li><li>Oral colchicine 0.5 to 1.5 mg per day prevents attacks[348]</li></ul>
<u>Hemarthrosis</u>: Generally associated with trauma, anticoagulation (i.e., coumadin), leukemia, hemophilia	<ul><li>Monoarthralgia with limited motion</li><li>May follow direct trauma</li><li>Nontraumatic hemarthrosis may be due to anticoagulation, leukemia, hemophilia</li></ul>	<ul><li>Synovial fluid analysis reveals blood</li><li>Treatment of underlying disorder; refer as indicated</li></ul>
<u>Slipped capital femoral epiphysis (SCFE)</u>: The most common cause of hip pain in adolescents[349]	<ul><li>Seen in adolescents generally 8-17 years of age</li><li>Classic presentation is a tall overweight boy with **hip pain**, knee pain, and/or a painful limp: *"Slipped femoral capital epiphysis is a developmental injury that must be considered in any adolescent who presents with hip pain."*[350]</li></ul>	<ul><li>**Radiographs** of both hips (bilateral SCFE in 40%): "<u>**AP and frog lateral views are recommended in all children over age of 9 years with hip pain.**</u>"[351]</li><li>Orthopedic referral—*"…the patient should be referred immediately to an orthopedist for surgical stabilization."* [352]</li></ul>

[345] Skinner HB, Scherger JE. Identifying structural hip and knee problems. Patient age, history, and limited examination may be all that's needed. *Postgrad Med* 1999;106(7):51-2, 55-6, 61-4

[346] Souza TA. <u>Differential Diagnosis for the Chiropractor: Protocols and Algorithms</u>. Gaithersberg, Maryland: Aspen Publications. 1997 page 263

[347] Hardin JG, Waterman J, Labson LH. Rheumatic disease: Which diagnostic tests are useful? *Patient Care* 1999; March 15: 83-102

[348] Beers MH, Berkow R (eds). <u>The Merck Manual. Seventeenth Edition</u>. Whitehouse Station; Merck Research Laboratories 1999 Page

[349] Maroo S. Diagnosis of hip pain in children. *Hosp Med* 1999 Nov;60(11):788-93

[350] O'Kane JW. Anterior hip pain. *Am Fam Physician* 1999 Oct 15;60(6):1687-96

[351] Maroo S. Diagnosis of hip pain in children. *Hosp Med* 1999 Nov;60(11):788-93

[352] O'Kane JW. Anterior hip pain. *Am Fam Physician* 1999 Oct 15;60(6):1687-96

<u>Clinical assessment</u>:
- History and orthopedic assessment of the joint
- Laboratory tests must be performed if you have a suspicion of infection

<u>History/subjective</u>:
- Acute or subacute joint pain with or without systemic manifestations and fever.
- History or may not be significant; other than the obvious risk factor of immunosuppression, septic arthritis can occur with impressive spontaneity and randomness

<u>Differential physical examination and objective findings</u>:
- **Septic arthritis**: pain and limitation of motion, swelling, redness; patient may have systemic symptoms of fever and malaise
- **Gout**: pain and limitation of motion, swelling, redness; patient may have systemic symptoms of fever and malaise
- **Pseudogout and calcium pyrophosphate dihydrate deposition disease (CPDD/CPPD)**: pain and limitation of motion, swelling, redness; patient may have systemic symptoms of fever and malaise
- **Ischemic necrosis**: pain and limitation of motion; swelling, redness and systemic symptoms are less likely.
- **Hemarthrosis**: pain and limitation of motion; often associated with trauma, use of anticoagulant medications[353], or hemophilia and other hematologic abnormalities[354]
- **Tumor**: assess with history, imaging, and biopsy if possible
- **Injury**: Meniscal injury, fracture, ligament injury; physical examination procedures are described in the chapters that follow

<u>Imaging and laboratory assessments</u>:
- **Septic arthritis**: joint aspiration; STAT CBC (for WBC count) and CRP
- **Gout**: joint aspiration; CBC (for WBC count) and CRP
- **Pseudogout and PPDD**: rule out septic arthritis with joint aspiration, CBC, and CRP; radiographs often show chondrocalcinosis
- **Ischemic necrosis**: radiographs are diagnostic
- **Hemarthrosis**: joint aspiration and assessment for underlying disease or medication, especially if the condition was not trauma-induced
- **Tumor**: assess with radiographs
- **Injury**: rule out infection; consider imaging with radiography or MRI.

<u>Establishing the diagnosis</u>:
- The aforementioned examinations and lab assessments should establish the exact diagnosis. **The priorities are 1) first exclude life-threatening illness (i.e., septic arthritis), then 2) to exclude serious injury or illness,** and finally 3) to help manage the exact problem.

<u>Complications</u>:
- **Septic arthritis can result in death 5-10% of patients. "Five to 10 percent of patients with an infected joint die, chiefly from respiratory complications of sepsis. The mortality rate is 30% for patients with polyarticular sepsis. Bony ankylosis and articular destruction commonly also occur if the treatment is delayed or inadequate."[355]** Complications vary per location, infecting organism, severity, and patient.

[353] Riley SA, Spencer GE. Destructive monarticular arthritis secondary to anticoagulant therapy. *Clin Orthop.* 1987 Oct;(223):247-51
[354] Jean-Baptiste G, De Ceulaer K. Osteoarticular disorders of haematological origin. *Baillieres Best Pract Res Clin Rheumatol.* 2000 Jun;14(2):307-23
[355] Tierney ML. McPhee SJ, Papadakis MA. <u>Current Medical Diagnosis and Treatment. 35th edition</u>. Stamford: Appleton & Lange, 1996 page 759

<u>Clinical management</u>:
- **Suspected septic arthritis requires referral for joint aspiration and antimicrobial drugs.**
- Referral if clinical outcome is unsatisfactory or if serious complications are evident.
- Treatment of other conditions that cause acute monoarthritis (such as gout and calcium pyrophosphate dihydrate deposition disease) is based on the problem and individual patient.

<u>Treatments</u>:
- <u>**Septic arthritis requires IV/oral antimicrobial drugs**</u>: Intravenous antibiotics are generally started before culture results are available. After results and culture from synovial fluid analysis have been considered, the dose, combination, and administration of antibiotics can be fine-tuned. Frequently, antibiotics are administered intravenously for at least 3-4 weeks. Surgical/endoscopic drainage/debridement and immobilization during the acute phase may also be implemented.[356]
- **Immunonutrition considerations:** Immunonutritional considerations are listed below; doses listed are for adults. Although studies have not been performed specifically in patients with bone/joint infections, general benefits derived from the use of immunonutrition are reductions in severity/frequency/duration of major infections, abbreviated hospitalization (i.e., early discharge due to expedited healing and recovery), reductions in the need for medications, significant improvements in survival, and hospital savings.[357,358,359,360,361,362,363]
  - <u>Paleo-Mediterranean diet</u>: as detailed later in this text and elsewhere[364,365]
  - <u>Vitamin and mineral supplementation</u>: anti-infective benefits shown in elderly diabetics[366]
  - <u>High-dose vitamin A</u>: Vitamin A shows potent immunosupportive benefits, and vitamin A stores are depleted by the stress of infection and injury. Consider 200,000-300,000 IU per day of retinol palmitate for 1-4 weeks, then taper; reduce dose or discontinue with onset of toxicity symptoms such as skin problems (dry skin, flaking skin, chapped or split lips, red skin rash, hair loss), joint pain, bone pain, headaches, anorexia (loss of appetite), edema (water retention, weight gain, swollen ankles, difficulty breathing), fatigue, and/or liver damage.
  - <u>Arginine</u>: Dose for adults is in the range of 5-10 grams daily

[356] Brusch JL. Septic Arthritis (Last Updated: October 18, 2005). *eMedicine*. http://www.emedicine.com/med/topic3394.htm Accessed Nov 25, 2006

[357] "To evaluate the metabolic and immune effects of dietary arginine, glutamine and omega-3 fatty acids (fish oil) supplementation, we performed a prospective study... CONCLUSIONS: The feeding of Neomune in critically injured patients was well tolerated as Traumacal and significant improvement was observed in serum protein. Shorten ICU stay and wean-off respirator day may benefit from using the immunonutrient formula." Chuntrasakul C, Siltham S, Sarasombath S, Sittapairochana C, Leowattana W, Chockvivatanavanit S, Bunnak A. Comparison of a immunonutrition formula enriched arginine, glutamine and omega-3 fatty acid, with a currently high-enriched enteral nutrition for trauma patients. *J Med Assoc Thai*. 2003 Jun;86(6):552-6

[358] "CONCLUSIONS: In conclusion, arginine-enhanced formula improves fistula rates in postoperative head and neck cancer patients and decreases length of stay." de Luis DA, Izaola O, Cuellar L, Terroba MC, Aller R. Randomized clinical trial with an enteral arginine-enhanced formula in early postsurgical head and neck cancer patients. *Eur J Clin Nutr*. 2004;58(11):1505-8

[359] "In this prospective, randomised, double-blind, placebo-controlled study, we randomly assigned 50 patients who were scheduled to undergo coronary artery bypass to receive either an oral immune-enhancing nutritional supplement containing L-arginine, omega3 polyunsaturated fatty acids, and yeast RNA (n=25), or a control (n=25) for a minimum of 5 days... Intake of an oral immune-enhancing nutritional supplement for a minimum of 5 days before surgery can improve outlook in high-risk patients who are undergoing elective cardiac surgery." Tepaske R, Velthuis H, Oudemans-van Straaten HM, Heisterkamp SH, van Deventer SJ, Ince C, Eysman L, Kesecioglu J. Effect of preoperative oral immune-enhancing nutritional supplement on patients at high risk of infection after cardiac surgery: a randomised placebo-controlled trial. *Lancet*. 2001 Sep 1;358(9283):696-701

[360] "The feeding of IMMUNE FORMULA was well tolerated and significant improvement was observed in nutritional and immunologic parameters as in other immunoenhancing diets. Further clinical trials of prospective double-blind randomized design are necessary to address the so that the necessity of using immunonutrition in critically ill patients will be clarified." Chuntrasakul C, Siltharm S, Sarasombath S, Sittapairochana C, Leowattana W, Chockvivatanavanit S, Bunnak A. Metabolic and immune effects of dietary arginine, glutamine and omega-3 fatty acids supplementation in immunocompromised patients. *J Med Assoc Thai*. 1998 May;81(5):334-43

[361] "enteral diet supplemented with arginine, dietary nucleotides, and omega-3 fatty acids (IMPACT, Sandoz Nutrition, Bern, Switzerland)" Senkal M, Mumme A, Eickhoff U, Geier B, Spath G, Wulfert D, Joosten U, Frei A, Kemen M. Early postoperative enteral immunonutrition: clinical outcome and cost-comparison analysis in surgical patients. *Crit Care Med* 1997;25(9):1489-96

[362] "supplemented diet with glutamine, arginine and omega-3-fatty acids... It was clearly established in this trial that early postoperative enteral feeding is safe in patients who have undergone major operations for gastrointestinal cancer. Supplementation of enteral nutrition with glutamine, arginine, and omega-3-fatty acids positively modulated postsurgical immunosuppressive and inflammatory responses." Wu GH, Zhang YW, Wu ZH. Modulation of postoperative immune and inflammatory response by immune-enhancing enteral diet in gastrointestinal cancer patients. *World J Gastroenterol*. 2001 Jun;7(3):357-62 http://www.wjgnet.com/1007-9327/7/357.pdf

[363] "using a formula supplemented with arginine, mRNA, and omega-3 fatty acids from fish oil (Impact)... CONCLUSIONS: Immune-enhancing enteral nutrition resulted in a significant reduction in the mortality rate and infection rate in septic patients admitted to the ICU. These reductions were greater for patients with less severe illness." Galban C, Montejo JC, Mesejo A, Marco P, Celaya S, Sanchez-Segura JM, Farre M, Bryg DJ. An immune-enhancing enteral diet reduces mortality rate and episodes of bacteremia in septic intensive care unit patients. *Crit Care Med*. 2000 Mar;28(3):643-8

[364] **Vasquez A.** A Five-Part Nutritional Protocol that Produces Consistently Positive Results. *Nutritional Wellness* 2005 September http://optimalhealthresearch.com/protocol

[365] **Vasquez A.** Implementing the Five-Part Nutritional Wellness Protocol for the Treatment of Various Health Problems. *Nutritional Wellness* 2005 November. http://optimalhealthresearch.com/protocol

[366] "CONCLUSIONS: A multivitamin and mineral supplement reduced the incidence of participant-reported infection and related absenteeism in a sample of participants with type 2 diabetes mellitus and a high prevalence of subclinical micronutrient deficiency." Barringer TA, Kirk JK, Santaniello AC, Foley KL, Michielutte R. Effect of a multivitamin and mineral supplement on infection and quality of life. A randomized, double-blind, placebo-controlled trial. *Ann Intern Med*. 2003 Mar 4;138(5):365-71 http://www.annals.org/cgi/reprint/138/5/365

- o Fatty acid supplementation: In contrast to the higher doses used to provide an anti-inflammatory effect in patients with autoimmune/inflammatory disorders, doses used for immunosupportive treatments should be kept rather modest to avoid the *relative* immunosuppression that has been controversially reported in patients treated with EPA and DHA. Reasonable doses are in the following ranges for adults: EPA+DHA: 500-1,500, and GLA: 300-500 mg.
- o Glutamine: Glutamine enhances bacterial killing by neutrophils[367], and administration of 18 grams per day in divided doses to patients in intensive care units was shown to improve survival, expedite hospital discharge, and reduce total healthcare costs.[368] Another study using glutamine 12-18 grams per day showed no benefit in overall mortality but significant benefits in terms of reduced healthcare costs (-30%) and significantly reduced need for medical interventions.[369] After administering glutamine 26 grams/d to severely burned patients, Garrel et al[370] concluded that glutamine reduced the risk of infection by 3-fold and that oral glutamine "may be a life-saving intervention" in patients with severe burns. A dose of 30 grams/d was used in a recent clinical trial showing hemodynamic benefit in patients with sickle cell anemia.[371] The highest glutamine dose that the current author is aware of is the study by Scheltinga et al[372] who used 0.57 gm/kg/day in cancer patients following chemotherapy administration; for a 220-lb-pt, this would be approximately 57 grams of glutamine per day.
- o Melatonin: 20-40 mg hs (*hora somni*—Latin: sleep time). Immunostimulatory anti-infective action of melatonin was demonstrated in a small clinical trial wherein septic newborns administered 20 mg melatonin showed significantly increased survival over nontreated controls.[373]

---

[367] Furukawa S, Saito H, Fukatsu K, Hashiguchi Y, Inaba T, Lin MT, Inoue T, Han I, Matsuda T, Muto T. Glutamine-enhanced bacterial killing by neutrophils from postoperative patients. *Nutrition* 1997;13(10):863-9. *In vitro* study.
[368] Griffiths RD, Jones C, Palmer TE. Six-month outcome of critically ill patients given glutamine-supplemented parenteral nutrition. *Nutrition* 1997;13(4):295-302
[369] "There was no mortality difference between those patients receiving glutamine-containing enteral feed and the controls. However, there was a significant reduction in the median postintervention ICU and hospital patient costs in the glutamine recipients $23 000 versus $30 900 in the control patients." Jones C, Palmer TE, Griffiths RD. Randomized clinical outcome study of critically ill patients given glutamine-supplemented enteral nutrition. *Nutrition*. 1999 Feb;15(2):108-15
[370] The glutamine dose in this study was "a total of 26 g/day" administered in four divided doses. CONCLUSION: "The results of this prospective randomized clinical trial show that enteral G reduces blood culture positivity, particularly with P. aeruginosa, in adults with severe burns and may be a life-saving intervention." Garrel D, Patenaude J, Nedelec B, et al. Decreased mortality and infectious morbidity in adult burn patients given enteral glutamine supplements: a prospective, controlled, randomized clinical trial. *Crit Care Med*. 2003 Oct;31(10):2444-9
[371] Niihara Y, Matsui NM, Shen YM, et al. L-glutamine therapy reduces endothelial adhesion of sickle red blood cells to human umbilical vein endothelial cells. *BMC Blood Disord*. 2005 Jul 25;5:4 http://www.biomedcentral.com.proxy.hsc.unt.edu/1471-2326/5/4
[372] "Subjects with hematologic malignancies in remission underwent a standard treatment of high-dose chemotherapy and total body irradiation before bone marrow transplantation. After completion of this regimen, they were randomized to receive either standard parenteral nutrition (STD, n = 10) or an isocaloric, isonitrogenous nutrient solution enriched with crystalline L-glutamine (0.57 g/kg/day, GLN, n = 10)." Scheltinga MR, Young LS, Benfell K, Bye RL, Ziegler TR, Santos AA, Antin JH, Schloerb PR, Wilmore DW. Glutamine-enriched intravenous feedings attenuate extracellular fluid expansion after a standard stress. *Ann Surg*. 1991 Oct;214(4):385-93; discussion 393-5 pubmedcentral.nih.gov/articlerender.fcgi?tool=pubmed&pubmedid=1953094 For additional review, see Ziegler TR. Glutamine supplementation in cancer patients receiving bone marrow transplantation and high dose chemotherapy. J Nutr. 2001 Sep;131(9 Suppl):2578S-84S http://jn.nutrition.org/cgi/content/full/131/9/2578S
[373] Gitto E, et al. Effects of melatonin treatment in septic newborns. *Pediatr Res*. 2001;50:756-60 pedresearch.org/cgi/content/full/50/6/756

Brief Overview of Integrative Healthcare Disciplines

Chiropractic

"Doctors of Chiropractic are physicians who consider man as an integrated being and give special attention to the physiological and biochemical aspects including structural, spinal, musculoskeletal, neurological, vascular, nutritional, emotional and environmental relationships." *American Chiropractic Association, 2004*[374]

"The human body represents the actions of three laws—spiritual, mechanical, and chemical—united as one triune. As long as there is perfect union of these three, there is health." *Daniel David Palmer, founder of the modern chiropractic profession*[375]

The basic philosophical model which is taught in many chiropractic colleges is to envision health, disease, and patient care from a conceptual model named the "triad of health" which gives its attention to the three fundamental foundations for well-being: namely, the physical/structural, mental/emotional, and biochemical/nutritional aspects of health. Revolutionary at the time of its inception in the early 1900's, this model now forms the foundation for the increasingly dominant and very popular paradigm of "holistic medicine." It remains a powerful contrast and an attractive alternative to the reductionistic allopathic approach, which generally approaches the human body as if it were simply a conglomerate of independent organ systems that have little or no functional relationship to each other.[376]

Using the state of the sciences before the year 1910, chiropractic was founded with a profound appreciation of the integrated nature of health, and the therapeutic focus was on spinal

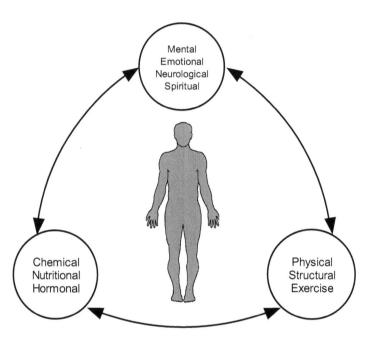

The chiropractic "triad of health"

manipulation. In describing the chiropractic model of health, DD Palmer[377] wrote, "The human body represents the actions of three laws—spiritual, mechanical, and chemical—united as one triune. As long as there is perfect union of these three, there is health." While the therapeutic focus of the profession has been spinal manipulation, from its inception the chiropractic profession has emphasized a holistic, integrative model of therapeutic intervention, health, and disease, and chiropractic was the first healthcare profession in America to specifically claim that the optimization of health requires attention to spiritual-emotional-psychological, mechanical-physical-structural, and biochemical-nutritional-hormonal-chemical considerations. Accordingly, these cornerstones are fundamental to the 2005 definition of the chiropractic profession articulated by the American Chiropractic Association[378]: "Doctors of Chiropractic are physicians who consider man as an integrated being and give special attention to the physiological and biochemical aspects including structural, spinal, musculoskeletal, neurological, vascular, nutritional, emotional, and environmental relationships."

---

[374] American Chiropractic Association. http://www.amerchiro.org/media/whatis/ Accessed March 13, 2004

[375] Palmer DD. The Science, Art, and Phiosophy, of Chiropractic. Portland, OR; Portland Printing House Company, 1910: 107

[376] Beckman JF, Fernandez CE, Coulter ID. A systems model of health care: a proposal. *J Manipulative Physiol Ther*. 1996 Mar-Apr; 19(3): 208-15

[377] Palmer DD. The Science, Art, and Phiosophy, of Chiropractic. Portland, OR; Portland Printing House Company, 1910: 107

[378] American Chiropractic Association. What is Chiropractic? http://amerchiro.org/media/whatis/ Accessed January 9, 2005

From its inception, chiropractic was a philosophy of healing that considered the entire health of the patient by addressing the interconnected aspects of our chemical-spiritual-physical being. Later, intraprofessional factions polarized between holistic and vitalistic paradigms; the latter has been presumed to be the philosophy of the entire profession by organizations such as the American Medical Association[379] that have sought to contain and eliminate chiropractic and other forms of natural healthcare[380] by falsifying research[381,382], intentionally misleading the public and manipulating politicians[383,384,385], arriving at illogical conclusions which support the medical paradigm and refute the value of manual therapies[386], and exploiting weaknesses within the profession for its own financial profitability and political advantage.[387] Intentional misrepresentation and defamation of chiropractic continues to occur today, as documented by the 2006 review by Wenban.[388]

Chiropractic Training and Clinical Benefits: In addition to the basic sciences and foundational skills of laboratory and clinical diagnosis, chiropractic physicians receive extensive training in manual physical manipulation, rehabilitation, therapeutic exercise, and clinical nutrition.

An irony exists in the observation that chiropractic education emphasizes anatomy, musculoskeletal therapeutics, and nutrition while these are the very topics that are neglected in allopathic and osteopathic education; the majority medical students and medical physicians who have graduated from allopathic and osteopathic medical schools lack competence in their knowledge of clinical anatomy and musculoskeletal medicine[389,390,391,392,393,394] as well as diet and nutrition.[395,396,397] In contrast to this replicable data showing that osteopathic and allopathic students and graduates generally fail to demonstrate competence in musculoskeletal medicine and nutrition, one study with 123 chiropractic students and 10 chiropractic doctors showed that chiropractic training in musculoskeletal medicine is significantly superior to allopathic and osteopathic musculoskeletal training.[398]

In accord with the comprehensive chiropractic training in musculoskeletal management, numerous sources of evidence demonstrate that chiropractic management of the most common spinal pain syndromes is safer and less expensive than allopathic medical treatment, particularly for the treatment of low-back pain. In

[379] American Medical Association. Report 12 of the Council on Scientific Affairs (A-97) Full Text. http://www.ama-assn.org/ama/pub/category/13638.html Accessed Sep 10, 2005

[380] Getzendanner S. Permanent injunction order against AMA. *JAMA*. 1988 Jan 1;259(1):81-2

[381] Terrett AG. Misuse of the literature by medical authors in discussing spinal manipulative therapy injury. *J Manipulative Physiol Ther*. 1995 May;18(4):203-10

[382] Morley J, Rosner AL, Redwood D. A case study of misrepresentation of the scientific literature: recent reviews of chiropractic. *J Altern Complement Med*. 2001 Feb;7(1):65-78

[383] Spivak JL. The Medical Trust Unmasked. Louis S. Siegfried Publishers; New York: 1961

[384] Trever W. In the Public Interest. Los Angeles; Scriptures Unlimited; 1972. This is probably the most authoritative documentation of the illegal actions of the AMA up to 1972; contains numerous photocopies of actual AMA documents and minutes of official meetings with overt intentionality of destroying Americans' healthcare options so that the AMA and related organizations would have a monopoly in healthcare.

[385] Wolinsky H, Brune T. The Serpent on the Staff: The Unhealthy Politics of the American Medical Association. GP Putnam and Sons, New York, 1994

[386] Mein EA, Greenman PE, McMillin DL, Richards DG, Nelson CD. Manual medicine diversity: research pitfalls and the emerging medical paradigm. *J Am Osteopath Assoc*. 2001 Aug;101(8):441-4

[387] Wilk CA. Medicine, Monopolies, and Malice: How the Medical Establishment Tried to Destroy Chiropractic. Garden City Park: Avery, 1996

[388] Wenban AB. Inappropriate use of the title 'chiropractor' and term 'chiropractic manipulation' in the peer-reviewed biomedical literature. *Chiropr Osteopat*. 2006;14:16 http://chiroandosteo.com/content/14/1/16

[389] "In summary, seventy (82 per cent) of eighty-five medical school graduates failed a valid musculoskeletal competency examination. We therefore believe that medical school preparation in musculoskeletal medicine is inadequate." Freedman KB, Bernstein J. The adequacy of medical school education in musculoskeletal medicine. *J Bone Joint Surg Am*. 1998;80(10):1421-7

[390] "CONCLUSIONS: According to the standard suggested by the program directors of internal medicine residency departments, a large majority of the examinees once again failed to demonstrate basic competency in musculoskeletal medicine on the examination. It is therefore reasonable to conclude that medical school preparation in musculoskeletal medicine is inadequate." Freedman KB, Bernstein J. Educational deficiencies in musculoskeletal medicine. *J Bone Joint Surg Am*. 2002;84-A(4):604-8

[391] Joy EA, Hala SV. Musculoskeletal Curricula in Medical Education: Filling In the Missing Pieces. *The Physician and Sportsmedicine* 2004; 32: 42-45

[392] "CONCLUSIONS: Seventy-nine percent of the participants failed the basic musculoskeletal cognitive examination. This suggests that training in musculoskeletal medicine is inadequate in both medical school and nonorthopaedic residency training programs." Matzkin E, Smith ME, Freccero CD, Richardson AB. Adequacy of education in musculoskeletal medicine. *J Bone Joint Surg Am*. 2005 Feb;87-A(2):310-4

[393] "Despite generally improved levels of competency with each year at medical school, less than 50% of fourth-year students showed competency. ... These results suggested that the curricular approach toward teaching musculoskeletal medicine at this medical school was insufficient and that competency increased when learning was reinforced during the clinical years." Schmale GA. More evidence of educational inadequacies in musculoskeletal medicine. *Clin Orthop Relat Res*. 2005 Aug;(437):251-9

[394] "RESULTS: When the minimum passing level as determined by orthopedic program directors was applied to the results of these examinations, 70.4% of graduating COM students (n=54) and 82% of allopathic graduates (n=85) failed to demonstrate basic competency in musculoskeletal medicine." Stockard AR, Allen TW. Competence levels in musculoskeletal medicine: comparison of osteopathic and allopathic medical graduates. *J Am Osteopath Assoc*. 2006 Jun;106(6):350-5

[395] "CONCLUSIONS: Internal medicine interns' perceive nutrition counseling as a priority, but lack the confidence and knowledge to effectively provide adequate nutrition education." Vetter ML, Herring SJ, Sood M, Shah NR, Kalet AL. What do resident physicians know about nutrition? An evaluation of attitudes, self-perceived proficiency and knowledge. *J Am Coll Nutr*. 2008 Apr;27(2):287-98

[396] "CONCLUSIONS: The amount of nutrition education that medical students receive continues to be inadequate." Adams KM, Kohlmeier M, Zeisel SH. Nutrition education in U.S. medical schools: latest update of a national survey. *Acad Med*. 2010 Sep;85(9):1537-42

[397] CONCLUSIONS: This survey suggests that multiple barriers exist that prevent the primary care practitioner from providing dietary counseling. A multifaceted approach will be needed to change physician counseling behavior." Kushner RF. Barriers to providing nutrition counseling by physicians: a survey of primary care practitioners. *Prev Med*. 1995 Nov;24(6):546-52

[398] Humphreys BK, Sulkowski A, McIntyre K, Kasiban M, Patrick AN. An examination of musculoskeletal cognitive competency in chiropractic interns. *J Manipulative Physiol Ther*. 2007;30(1):44-9

their extensive review of the literature, Manga et al[399] published in 1993 that chiropractic management of low-back pain is superior to allopathic medical management in terms of greater safety, greater effectiveness, and reduced cost; they concluded, "There is an overwhelming body of evidence indicating that chiropractic management of low-back pain is more cost-effective than medical management" and "There would be highly significant cost savings if more management of LBP [low-back pain] was transferred from medical physicians to chiropractors." In a randomized trial involving 741 patients, Meade et al[400] showed, "Chiropractic treatment was more effective than hospital outpatient management, mainly for patients with chronic or severe back pain... The benefit of chiropractic treatment became more evident throughout the follow up period. Secondary outcome measures also showed that chiropractic was more beneficial." A 3-year follow-up study by these same authors[401] in 1995 showed, "At three years the results confirm the findings of an earlier report that when chiropractic or hospital therapists treat patients with low-back pain as they would in day to day practice, those treated by chiropractic derive more benefit and long term satisfaction than those treated by hospitals." More recently, in 2004 Legorreta et al[402] reported that the availability of chiropractic care was associated with significant cost savings among 700,000 patients with chiropractic coverage compared to 1 million patients whose insurance coverage was limited to allopathic medical treatments. Simple extrapolation of the average savings per patient in this study ($208 annual savings associated with chiropractic coverage) to the US population (295 million citizens in 2005[403]) suggests that, if fully implemented in a nation-wide basis, America could save $61,360,000,000 (more than $61 billion per year) in annual healthcare expenses by ensuring chiropractic for all citizens in contrast to failing to provide such coverage; obviously extrapolations such as this should consider other variables, such as the relatively higher prevalence of injury and death among patients treated with drugs and surgery.[404,405] Furthermore, whether the cost savings associated with chiropractic availability are due to 1) improved overall health and reduced need for pharmacosurgical intervention, 2) greater safety and lower cost of chiropractic treatment versus pharmacosurgical treatment, and/or 3) self-selection by wellness-oriented, perhaps healthier, and higher-income patients, remains to be determined.

A literature review by Dabbs and Lauretti[406] showed that spinal manipulation is safer than the use of NSAIDs in the treatment of neck pain. Contrasting the rates of manipulation-associated cerebrovascular accidents to the dangers of medical and surgical treatments for spinal disorders, Rosner[407] noted, "These rates are 400 times lower than the death rates observed from gastrointestinal bleeding due to the use of nonsteroidal anti-inflammatory drugs and 700 times lower than the overall mortality rate for spinal surgery." Similarly, in his review of the literature comparing the safety of chiropractic manipulation in patients with low-back pain associated with lumbar disc herniation, Oliphant[408] showed that, "The apparent safety of spinal manipulation, especially when compared with other [medically] accepted treatments for [lumbar disk herniation], should stimulate its use in the conservative treatment plan of [lumbar disk herniation]."

The clinical benefits and cost-effectiveness of chiropractic management of musculoskeletal conditions is extensively documented, and that spinal manipulation generally shows superior safety to drug and surgical treatment of back and neck pain is also well established.[409,410,411,412,413,414,415] Adjunctive therapies such as post-

[399] Manga P, Angus D, Papadopoulos C, et al. The Effectiveness and Cost-Effectiveness of Chiropractic Management of Low-Back Pain. Richmond Hill, Ontario: Kenilworth Publishing; 1993
[400] Meade TW, Dyer S, Browne W, Townsend J, Frank AO. Low-back pain of mechanical origin: randomised comparison of chiropractic and hospital outpatient treatment. BMJ. 1990;300(6737):1431-7
[401] Meade TW, Dyer S, Browne W, Frank AO. Randomised comparison of chiropractic and hospital outpatient management for low-back pain: results from extended follow up. BMJ. 1995;311(7001):349-5
[402] Legorreta AP, Metz RD, Nelson CF, Ray S, Chernicoff HO, Dinubile NA. Comparative analysis of individuals with and without chiropractic coverage: patient characteristics, utilization, and costs. Arch Intern Med. 2004;164:1985-92
[403] US Census Bureau http://factfinder.census.gov/home/saff/main.html?_lang=en Accessed January 12, 2005
[404] Rosner AL. Evidence-based clinical guidelines for the management of acute low-back pain: response to the guidelines prepared for the Australian Medical Health and Research Council. J Manipulative Physiol Ther. 2001;24(3):214-20
[405] Topol EJ. Failing the public health--rofecoxib, Merck, and the FDA. N Engl J Med. 2004 Oct 21;351(17):1707-9
[406] Dabbs V, Lauretti WJ. A risk assessment of cervical manipulation vs. NSAIDs for the treatment of neck pain. J Manipulative Physiol Ther. 1995;18:530-6
[407] Rosner AL. Evidence-based clinical guidelines for the management of acute low-back pain: response to the guidelines prepared for the Australian Medical Health and Research Council. J Manipulative Physiol Ther. 2001;24(3):214-20
[408] Oliphant D. Safety of spinal manipulation in the treatment of lumbar disk herniations: a systematic review and risk assessment. J Manipulative Physiol Ther. 2004;27:197-210
[409] Dabbs V, Lauretti WJ. A risk assessment of cervical manipulation vs. NSAIDs for the treatment of neck pain. J Manipulative Physiol Ther. 1995;18:530-6
[410] Rosner AL. Evidence-based clinical guidelines for the management of acute low-back pain: response to the guidelines prepared for the Australian Medical Health and Research Council. J Manipulative Physiol Ther. 2001 Mar-Apr;24(3):214-20
[411] Oliphant D. Safety of spinal manipulation in the treatment of lumbar disk herniations: a systematic review and risk assessment. J Manipulative Physiol Ther. 2004;27:197-210
[412] Meade TW, Dyer S, Browne W, Townsend J, Frank AO. Low-back pain of mechanical origin: randomised comparison of chiropractic and hospital outpatient treatment. BMJ. 1990;300(6737):1431-7
[413] Meade TW, Dyer S, Browne W, Frank AO. Randomised comparison of chiropractic and hospital outpatient management for low-back pain: results from extended follow up. BMJ. 1995;311(7001):349-5

isometric relaxation[416] and correction of myofascial dysfunction[417] can lead to tremendous and rapid reductions in musculoskeletal pain without the hazards and expense associated with pharmaceutical drugs. Nonmusculoskeletal benefits of musculoskeletal/spinal manipulation include improved pulmonary function and/or quality of life in patients with asthma[418,419,420,421] and—according to a series of cases published by an osteopathic ophthalmologist—improvement or restoration of vision in patients with post-traumatic and acute-onset visual loss.[422,423,424,425,426,427,428,429] More research is required to quantify the potential benefits of spinal manipulation in patients with wide-ranging conditions such as epilepsy[430,431], attention-deficit hyperactivity disorder[432,433], and Parkinson's disease.[434] Given that most pharmaceutical drugs work on single biochemical pathways, spinal manipulation is discordant with the medical/drug paradigm because its effects are numerous (rather than singular) and physical and physiological (rather than biochemical). Thus, when viewed through the allopathic/pharmaceutical lens, spinal manipulation (like acupuncture and other physical modalities) "does not make sense" and will be viewed as "unscientific" simply because it is based in physiology rather than pharmacology. In this case, the fault lies with the viewer and the lens, not with the object.

Research documenting the systemic and "nonmusculoskeletal" benefits of spinal manipulation mandates that our concept of "musculoskeletal" must be expanded to appreciate that **musculoskeletal interventions benefit nonmusculoskeletal body systems and physiologic processes**. This conceptual expansion applies also to soft tissue therapeutics such as massage, which can reduce adolescent aggression[435], improve outcome in preterm infants[436], alleviate premenstrual syndrome[437], and increase serotonin and dopamine levels in patients with low-back pain.[438]

[414] Manga P, Angus D, Papadopoulos C, et al. The Effectiveness and Cost-Effectiveness of Chiropractic Management of Low-Back Pain. Richmond Hill, Ontario: Kenilworth Publishing; 1993

[415] Legorreta AP, Metz RD, Nelson CF, Ray S, Chernicoff HO, Dinubile NA. Comparative analysis of individuals with and without chiropractic coverage: patient characteristics, utilization, and costs. *Arch Intern Med.* 2004;164:1985-92

[416] Lewit K, Simons DG. Myofascial pain: relief by post-isometric relaxation. *Arch Phys Med Rehabil.* 1984;65(8):452-6

[417] Ingber RS. Iliopsoas myofascial dysfunction: a treatable cause of "failed" low-back syndrome. *Arch Phys Med Rehabil.* 1989 May;70(5):382-6

[418] Nielson NH, Bronfort G, Bendix T, Madsen F, Wecke B. Chronic asthma and chiropractic spinal manipulation: a randomized clinical trial. *Clin Exp Allergy* 1995;25:80-8

[419] Mein EA, Greenman PE, McMillin DL, Richards DG, Nelson CD. Manual medicine diversity: research pitfalls and the emerging medical paradigm. *J Am Osteopath Assoc.* 2001 Aug;101(8):441-4

[420] "There were small increases (7 to 12 liters per minute) in peak expiratory flow in the morning and the evening in both treatment groups,... Symptoms of asthma and use of beta-agonists decreased and the quality of life increased in both groups, with no significant differences between the groups." Balon J, Aker PD, Crowther ER, Danielson C, Cox PG, O'Shaughnessy D, Walker C, Goldsmith CH, Duku E, Sears MR. A comparison of active and simulated chiropractic manipulation as adjunctive treatment for childhood asthma. *N Engl J Med.* 1998 Oct 8;339(15):1013-20

[421] Bronfort G, Evans RL, Kubic P, Filkin P. Chronic pediatric asthma and chiropractic spinal manipulation: a prospective clinical series and randomized clinical pilot study. *J Manipulative Physiol Ther.* 2001 Jul-Aug;24(6):369-77

[422] Stephens D, Pollard H, Bilton D, Thomson P, Gorman F. Bilateral simultaneous optic nerve dysfunction after periorbital trauma: recovery of vision in association with chiropractic spinal manipulation therapy. *J Manipulative Physiol Ther.* 1999 Nov-Dec;22(9):615-21

[423] Stephens D, Gorman F, Bilton D. The step phenomenon in the recovery of vision with spinal manipulation: a report on two 13-yr-olds treated together. *J Manipulative Physiol Ther.* 1997;20(9):628-33

[424] Stephens D, Gorman F. The association between visual incompetence and spinal derangement: an instructive case history. *J Manipulative Physiol Ther.* 1997 Jun;20(5):343-50.

[425] Stephens D, Gorman RF. Does 'normal' vision improve with spinal manipulation? *J Manipulative Physiol Ther.* 1996 Jul-Aug;19(6):415-8

[426] Gorman RF. Monocular scotomata and spinal manipulation: the step phenomenon. *J Manipulative Physiol Ther.* 1996 Jun;19(5):344-9

[427] Gorman RF. Monocular visual loss after closed head trauma: immediate resolution associated with spinal manipulation. *J Manipulative Physiol Ther.* 1995 Jun;18(5):308-14

[428] Gorman RF. The treatment of presumptive optic nerve ischemia by spinal manipulation. *J Manipulative Physiol Ther.* 1995;18(3):172-7

[429] Gorman RF. Automated static perimetry in chiropractic. *J Manipulative Physiol Ther.* 1993 Sep;16(7):481-7

[430] Elster EL. Treatment of bipolar, seizure, and sleep disorders and migraine headaches utilizing a chiropractic technique. *J Manipulative Physiol* Ther. 2004 Mar-Apr;27(3):E5

[431] Alcantara J, Heschong R, Plaugher G, Alcantara J. Chiropractic management of a patient with subluxations, low-back pain and epileptic seizures. *J Manipulative Physiol Ther.* 1998;21(6):410-8

[432] Giesen JM, Center DB, Leach RA. An evaluation of chiropractic manipulation as a treatment of hyperactivity in children. *J Manipulative Physiol Ther.* 1989 Oct;12(5):353-63

[433] Bastecki AV, Harrison DE, Haas JW. Cervical kyphosis is a possible link to attention-deficit/hyperactivity disorder. *J Manipulative Physiol Ther.* 2004 Oct;27(8):e14

[434] Elster EL. Upper cervical chiropractic management of a patient with Parkinson's disease: a case report. *J Manipulative Physiol Ther.* 2000 Oct;23(8):573-7

[435] Diego MA, Field T, Hernandez-Reif M, Shaw JA, Rothe EM, Castellanos D, Mesner L. Aggressive adolescents benefit from massage therapy. *Adolescence* 2002 Fall;37(147):597-607

[436] Mainous RO. Infant massage as a component of developmental care: past, present, and future. *Holist Nurs Pract* 2002 Oct;16(5):1-7

[437] Hernandez-Reif M, Martinez A, Field T, Quintero O, Hart S, Burman I. Premenstrual symptoms are relieved by massage therapy. *J Psychosom Obstet Gynaecol* 2000 Mar;21(1):9-15

[438] "RESULTS: By the end of the study, the massage therapy group, as compared to the relaxation group, reported experiencing less pain, depression, anxiety and improved sleep. They also showed improved trunk and pain flexion performance, and their serotonin and dopamine levels were higher." Hernandez-Reif M, Field T, Krasnegor J, Theakston H. Lower back pain is reduced and range of motion increased after massage therapy. *Int J Neurosci* 2001;106(3-4):131-45

Spinal Manipulation: Mechanistic Considerations: Applied to either the spine or peripheral joints, high-velocity low-amplitude (HVLA) joint manipulation appears to have numerous physical and physiological effects, including but not limited to the following:

1. Releasing entrapped intraarticular menisci and synovial folds,
2. Acutely reducing intradiscal pressure, thus promoting replacement of decentralized disc material,
3. Stretching of deep periarticular muscles to break the cycle of chronic autonomous muscle contraction by lengthening the muscles and thereby releasing excessive actin-myosin binding,
4. Promoting restoration of proper kinesthesia and proprioception,
5. Promoting relaxation of paraspinal muscles by stretching facet joint capsules,
6. Promoting relaxation of paraspinal muscles via "postactivation depression", which is the temporary depletion of contractile neurotransmitters,
7. Temporarily elevating plasma beta-endorphin,
8. Temporarily enhancing phagocytic ability of neutrophils and monocytes,
9. Activation of the diffuse descending pain inhibitory system located in the periaqueductal gray matter—this is an important aspect of nociceptive inhibition by intense sensory/mechanoreceptor stimulation, which will be discussed in a following section for its relevance to neurogenic inflammation, and
10. Improving neurotransmitter balance and reducing pain (soft-tissue manipulation).[439]

While the above list of mechanisms-of-action is certainly not complete, for purposes of this paper it is sufficient for the establishment that—indeed—joint manipulation in general and spinal manipulation in particular have objective mechanistic effects that correlate with their clinical benefits. Additional details are provided in numerous published reviews and primary research[440,441,442,443,444,445,446] and by Leach[447], whose extensive description of the mechanisms of action of spinal manipulative therapy is unsurpassed. Given such a wide base of experimental and clinical support published in peer-reviewed journals and widely-available textbooks, denigrations directed toward spinal manipulation on the grounds that it is "unscientific" or "unsupported by research" are unfounded and are indicative of selective ignorance.

[439] "RESULTS: By the end of the study, the massage therapy group, as compared to the relaxation group, reported experiencing less pain, depression, anxiety and improved sleep. They also showed improved trunk and pain flexion performance, and their serotonin and dopamine levels were higher." Hernandez-Reif M, Field T, Krasnegor J, Theakston H. Lower back pain is reduced and range of motion increased after massage therapy. *Int J Neurosci* 2001;106(3-4):131-45

[440] Maigne JY, Vautravers P. Mechanism of action of spinal manipulative therapy. *Joint Bone Spine*. 2003;70(5):336-41

[441] Brennan PC, Triano JJ, McGregor M, Kokjohn K, Hondras MA, Brennan DC. Enhanced neutrophil respiratory burst as a biological marker for manipulation forces: duration of the effect and association with substance P and tumor necrosis factor. *J Manipulative Physiol Ther*. 1992 Feb;15(2):83-9

[442] Brennan PC, Kokjohn K, Kaltinger CJ, Lohr GE, Glendening C, Hondras MA, McGregor M, Triano JJ. Enhanced phagocytic cell respiratory burst induced by spinal manipulation: potential role of substance P. *J Manipulative Physiol Ther*. 1991 Sep;14(7):399-408

[443] Heikkila H, Johansson M, Wenngren BI. Effects of acupuncture, cervical manipulation and NSAID therapy on dizziness and impaired head repositioning of suspected cervical origin: a pilot study. *Man Ther*. 2000 Aug;5(3):151-7

[444] Rogers RG. The effects of spinal manipulation on cervical kinesthesia in patients with chronic neck pain: a pilot study. *J Manipulative Physiol Ther*. 1997;20(2):80-5

[445] Bergman, Peterson, Lawrence. Chiropractic Technique. New York: Churchill Livingstone 1993. An updated edition is now availabe from Mosby.

[446] Herzog WH. Mechanical and physiological responses to spinal manipulative treatments. *JNMS: J Neuromusculoskeltal System* 1995; 3: 1-9

[447] Leach RA. (ed). The Chiropractic Theories: A Textbook of Scientific Research, Fourth Edition. Baltimore: Lippincott, Williams & Wilkins, 2004

Mechanoreceptor-Mediated Inhibition of Neurogenic Inflammation: A Possible Mechanism of Action of Spinal Manipulation: Neurogenic inflammation causes catabolism of articular structures and thus promotes joint destruction[448,449], a phenomena that the current author has termed "neurogenic chondrolysis."[450] The biologic and scientific basis for this concept rests on the following sequence of events which ultimately form a self-perpetuating and multisystem cycle:

1. Using joint pain as an example, we know that acute or chronic joint injury results in the release of inflammatory mediators in local tissues as **immunogenic inflammation**.

2. Nociceptive input is received centrally and results in release of inflammatory mediators *from sensory neurons* termed **neurogenic inflammation**[451] and results in a neurologically-mediated catabolic effect in articular cartilage[452,453] termed here as **neurogenic chondrolysis**.

3. As immunogenic and neurogenic inflammation synergize to promote joint destruction, pain from degenerating joints further increases nociceptive afferent transmission to further increase neurogenic and thus immunogenic inflammation. Thus, a *positive feedback* vicious cycle of immunogenic and neurogenic inflammation promotes and perpetuates joint destruction.

4. Further complicating this *regional* cycle of neurogenic-immunogenic inflammation and tissue destruction would be any pain or inflammation *in distant parts of the body*, since pain in one part of the body can exacerbate neurogenic inflammation in another part of the body via **neurogenic switching**[454,455] and immunologic reactivity such as allergy or autoimmunity in one part of the body may be transmitted *via the nervous system* to cause immunogenic inflammation in another part of the body via **immunogenic switching**.[456]

The clinical relevance of neurogenic inflammation and immunogenic switching is that when combined they provide a means *beyond biochemistry* by which to understand how and why inflammation ❶ is *transmitted and perpetuated by the nervous system* and ❷ must be treated with a body-wide *holistic* approach.

The current author is the first to propose the concept of **mechanoreceptor-mediated inhibition of neurogenic inflammation**.[457] Since neurogenic chondrolysis is inhibited by interference with C-fiber (type IV) mediated afferent transmission[458] and since chiropractic high-velocity low-amplitude (HVLA) manipulation appears to inhibit C-fiber mediated nociception[459,460], then chiropractic-type HVLA manipulation may reduce neurogenic inflammation and may promote articular integrity by inhibiting neurogenic chondrolysis. Further, mechanoreceptor-mediated inhibition of neurogenic inflammation would, for example, help explain the benefits of spinal manipulation in the treatment of asthma[461,462,463], since asthma is known to be mediated in large part by

---

[448] Gouze-Decaris E, Philippe L, Minn A, Haouzi P, Gillet P, Netter P, Terlain B. Neurophysiological basis for neurogenic-mediated articular cartilage anabolism alteration. *Am J Physiol Regul Integr Comp Physiol*. 2001;280(1):R115-22

[449] Decaris E, Guingamp C, Chat M, Philippe L, Grillasca JP, Abid A, Minn A, Gillet P, Netter P, Terlain B. Evidence for neurogenic transmission inducing degenerative cartilage damage distant from local inflammation. *Arthritis Rheum*. 1999;42(9):1951-60

[450] Vasquez A. *Integrative Orthopedics: Exploring the Structural Aspect of the Matrix*. Applying Functional Medicine in Clinical Practice. Tampa, Florida November 29-December 4, 2004. Hosted by the Institute for Functional Medicine: www.FunctionalMedicine.org

[451] Meggs WJ.Mechanisms of allergy and chemical sensitivity. *Toxicol Ind Health*. 1999 Apr-Jun;15(3-4):331-8

[452] Gouze-Decaris E, Philippe L, Minn A, Haouzi P, Gillet P, Netter P, Terlain B. Neurophysiological basis for neurogenic-mediated articular cartilage anabolism alteration. *Am J Physiol Regul Integr Comp Physiol*. 2001;280(1):R115-22

[453] Decaris E, Guingamp C, Chat M, Philippe L, Grillasca JP, Abid A, Minn A, Gillet P, Netter P, Terlain B. Evidence for neurogenic transmission inducing degenerative cartilage damage distant from local inflammation. *Arthritis Rheum*. 1999;42(9):1951-60

[454] Meggs WJ. Neurogenic Switching: A Hypothesis for a Mechanism for Shifting the Site of Inflammation in Allergy and Chemical Sensitivity. *Environ Health Perspect* 1995; 103:54-56

[455] Meggs WJ. Mechanisms of allergy and chemical sensitivity. *Toxicol Ind Health*. 1999 Apr-Jun;15(3-4):331-8

[456] "… immunogenic switching—… In this scenario, the afferent stimulation from the cranial vasculature, which is inflamed during a migraine because of neurogenic processes, is rerouted by the CNS to produce immunogenic inflammation at the nose and sinuses." Cady RK, Schreiber CP. Sinus headache or migraine? Considerations in making a differential diagnosis. *Neurology*. 2002;58(9 Suppl 6):S10-4

[457] Vasquez A. *Integrative Orthopedics: Exploring the Structural Aspect of the Matrix*. Applying Functional Medicine in Clinical Practice. Tampa, Florida November 29-December 4, 2004. Hosted by the Institute for Functional Medicine: www.FunctionalMedicine.org

[458] Gouze-Decaris E, Philippe L, Minn A, Haouzi P, Gillet P, Netter P, Terlain B. Neurophysiological basis for neurogenic-mediated articular cartilage anabolism alteration. *Am J Physiol Regul Integr Comp Physiol*. 2001;280(1):R115-22

[459] Gillette R. A speculative argument for the coactivation of diverse somatic receptor populations by forceful chiropractic adjustments. *Man Med* 1987; 3:1-14

[460] Boal RW, Gillette RG. Central neuronal plasticity, low-back pain and spinal manipulative therapy. *J Manipulative Physiol Ther*. 2004;27(5):314-26

[461] Nielson NH, Bronfort G, Bendix T, Madsen F, Wecke B. Chronic asthma and chiropractic spinal manipulation: a randomized clinical trial. *Clin Exp Allergy* 1995;25:80-8

[462] "There were small increases (7 to 12 liters per minute) in peak expiratory flow in the morning and the evening in both treatment groups,… Symptoms of asthma and use of beta-agonists decreased and the quality of life increased in both groups, with no significant differences between the groups." Balon J, Aker PD, Crowther ER, Danielson C, Cox PG, O'Shaughnessy D, Walker C, Goldsmith CH, Duku E, Sears MR. A comparison of active and simulated chiropractic manipulation as adjunctive treatment for childhood asthma. *N Engl J Med*. 1998 Oct 8;339(15):1013-20

[463] Bronfort G, Evans RL, Kubic P, Filkin P. Chronic pediatric asthma and chiropractic spinal manipulation: a prospective clinical series and randomized clinical pilot study. *J Manipulative Physiol Ther*. 2001 Jul-Aug;24(6):369-77

neurogenic inflammation.[464,465] Thus, spinal manipulation appears to provide a means—*in addition to the use of other anti-inflammatory interventions such as diet, lifestyle and phytonutritional interventions*—by which pain and inflammation can be treated naturally, without drugs and surgery.

A science-based comprehensive protocol can be implemented against pain and inflammation by using ❶ an anti-inflammatory diet, ❷ frequent exercise, ❸ lifestyle and bodyweight optimization, ❹ nutritional supplementation, ❺ botanical supplementation[466,467], ❻ spinal manipulation (with its kinesthetic, analgesic, *directly* and *indirectly* anti-inflammatory, and *probably* piezoelectric benefits[468]), ❼ stress reduction[469,470], ❽ anti-dysbiosis protocols[471], ❾ hormonal correction ("orthoendocrinology"), and ❿ ancillary treatments such as acupuncture.[472,473] Additional details and citations for these interventions are provided in chapter 3 of *Integrative Orthopedics*[474] and chapter 4 of *Integrative Rheumatology*.[475] Pain and inflammation are self-perpetuating vicious cycles, well suited to intervention with comprehensive and multicomponent treatment plans as profiled above.

Wilk vs American Medical Association

The following two pages provide the transcript of the judgment in 1987 that supposedly ended the American Medical Association's antitrust violations and attempt to destroy the chiropractic profession.

A PDF copy of this document is available online:
http://www.optimalhealthresearch.com/archives/wilk.html

---

[464] Renz H. Neurotrophins in bronchial asthma. *Respir Res*. 2001;2(5):265-8

[465] Groneberg DA, Quarcoo D, Frossard N, Fischer A. Neurogenic mechanisms in bronchial inflammatory diseases. *Allergy*. 2004 Nov; 59(11): 1139-52

[466] Jancso N, Jancso-Gabor A, Szolcsanyi J. Direct evidence for neurogenic inflammation and its prevention by denervation and by pretreatment with capsaicin. *Br J Pharmacol*. 1967 Sep;31(1):138-51

[467] Miller MJ, Vergnolle N, McKnight W, Musah RA, Davison CA, Trentacosti AM, Thompson JH, Sandoval M, Wallace JL. Inhibition of neurogenic inflammation by the Amazonian herbal medicine sangre de grado. *J Invest Dermatol*. 2001;117(3):725-30

[468] Lipinski B. Biological significance of piezoelectricity in relation to acupuncture, Hatha Yoga, osteopathic medicine and action of air ions. *Med Hypotheses*. 1977;3(1):9-12 See also: Athenstaedt H. Pyroelectric and piezoelectric properties of vertebrates. *Ann N Y Acad Sci*. 1974;238:68-94 See also: Athenstaedt H. "Functional polarity" of the spinal cord caused by its longitudinal electric dipole moment. *Am J Physiol*. 1984;247(3 Pt 2):R482-7

[469] Lutgendorf S, Logan H, Kirchner HL, Rothrock N, Svengalis S, Iverson K, Lubaroff D. Effects of relaxation and stress on the capsaicin-induced local inflammatory response. *Psychosom Med*. 2000;62:524-34

[470] "Couples who demonstrated consistently higher levels of hostile behaviors across both their interactions healed at 60% of the rate of low-hostile couples. High-hostile couples also produced relatively larger increases in plasma IL-6 and tumor necrosis factor alpha..." Kiecolt-Glaser JK, Loving TJ, Stowell JR, Malarkey WB, Lemeshow S, Dickinson SL, Glaser R. Hostile marital interactions, proinflammatory cytokine production, and wound healing. *Arch Gen Psychiatry*. 2005 Dec;62(12):1377-84

[471] Chapter 4 of Integrative Rheumatology and Vasquez A. Reducing Pain and Inflammation Naturally. Part 6: Nutritional and Botanical Treatments Against "Silent Infections" and Gastrointestinal Dysbiosis, Commonly Overlooked Causes of Neuromusculoskeletal Inflammation and Chronic Health Problems. *Nutr Perspect* 2006; Jan http://optimalhealthresearch.com/part6.html

[472] Joos S, Brinkhaus B, Maluche C, Maupai N, Kohnen R, Kraehmer N, Hahn EG, Schuppan D. Acupuncture and moxibustion in the treatment of active Crohn's disease: a randomized controlled study. *Digestion*. 2004;69(3):131-9

[473] "These results demonstrate an unorthodox new type of neurohumoral regulatory mechanism of sensory fibres and provide a possible mode of action for the anti-inflammatory effect of counter-irritation and acupuncture." Pinter E, Szolcsanyi J. Systemic anti-inflammatory effect induced by antidromic stimulation of the dorsal roots in the rat. *Neurosci Lett*. 1996;212(1):33-6

[474] Vasquez A. *Integrative Orthopedics: Second Edition*. Fort Worth, Texas; Integrative and Biological Medicine Research and Consulting, 2007 OptimalHealthResearch.com

[475] Vasquez A. *Integrative Rheumatology: Second Edition*. Fort Worth, Texas; Integrative and Biological Medicine Research and Consulting, 2007 OptimalHealthResearch.com

Special Communication

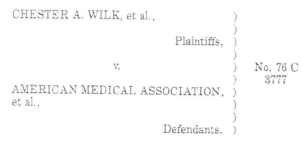

IN THE UNITED STATES DISTRICT COURT
FOR THE NORTHERN DISTRICT OF ILLINOIS
EASTERN DIVISION

CHESTER A. WILK, et al.,)	
)	
Plaintiffs,)	
)	
v.)	No. 76 C
)	3777
AMERICAN MEDICAL ASSOCIATION,)	
et al.,)	
)	
Defendants.)	

PERMANENT INJUNCTION ORDER AGAINST AMA

Susan Getzendanner, District Judge

The court conducted a lengthy trial of this case in May and June of 1987 and on August 27, 1987, issued a 101 page opinion finding that the American Medical Association ("AMA") and its members participated in a conspiracy against chiropractors in violation of the nation's antitrust laws. Thereafter an opinion dated September 25, 1987 was substituted for the August 27, 1987 opinion. The question now before the court is the form of injunctive relief that the court will order.

See also p 83.

As part of the injunctive relief to be ordered by the court against the AMA, the AMA shall be required to send a copy of this Permanent Injunction Order to each of its current members. The members of the AMA are bound by the terms of the Permanent Injunction Order if they act in concert with the AMA to violate the terms of the order. Accordingly, it is important that the AMA members understand the order and the reasons why the order has been entered.

The AMA's Boycott and Conspiracy

In the early 1960s, the AMA decided to contain and eliminate chiropractic as a profession. In 1963 the AMA's Committee on Quackery was formed. The committee worked aggressively—both overtly and covertly—to eliminate chiropractic. One of the principal means used by the AMA to achieve its goal was to make it unethical for medical physicians to professionally associate with chiropractors. Under Principle 3 of the AMA's Principles of Medical Ethics, it was unethical for a physician to associate with an "unscientific practitioner," and in 1966 the AMA's House of Delegates passed a resolution calling chiropractic an unscientific cult. To complete the circle, in 1967 the AMA's Judicial Council issued an opinion under Principle 3 holding that it was unethical for a physician to associate professionally with chiropractors.

The AMA's purpose was to prevent medical physicians from referring patients to chiropractors and accepting referrals of patients from chiropractors, to prevent chiropractors from obtaining access to hospital diagnostic services and membership on hospital medical staffs, to prevent medical physicians from teaching at chiropractic colleges or engaging in any joint research, and to prevent any cooperation between the two groups in the delivery of health care services.

Published by order of Susan Getzendanner, US District Judge, Sept 25, 1987.

The AMA believed that the boycott worked—that chiropractic would have achieved greater gains in the absence of the boycott. Since no medical physician would want to be considered unethical by his peers, the success of the boycott is not surprising. However, chiropractic achieved licensing in all 50 states during the existence of the Committee on Quackery.

The Committee on Quackery was disbanded in 1975 and some of the committee's activities became publicly known. . . Several lawsuits were filed by or on behalf of chiropractors and this case was filed in 1976.

Change in AMA's Position on Chiropractic

In 1977, the AMA began to change its position on chiropractic. The AMA's Judicial Council adopted new opinions under which medical physicians could refer patients to chiropractors, but there was still the proviso that the medical physician should be confident that the services to be provided on referral would be performed in accordance with accepted scientific standards. In 1979, the AMA's House of Delegates adopted Report UU which said that not everything that a chiropractor may do is without therapeutic value, but it stopped short of saying that such things were based on scientific standards. It was not until 1980 that the AMA revised its Principles of Medical Ethics to eliminate Principle 3. Until Principle 3 was formally eliminated, there was considerable ambiguity about the AMA's position. The ethics code adopted in 1980 provided that a medical physician "shall be free to choose whom to serve, with whom to associate, and the environment in which to provide medical services."

The AMA settled three chiropractic lawsuits by stipulating and agreeing that under the current opinions of the Judicial Council a physician may, without fear of discipline or sanction by the AMA, refer a patient to a duly licensed chiropractor when he believes that referral may benefit the patient. The AMA confirmed that a physician may also choose to accept or to decline patients sent to him by a duly licensed chiropractor. Finally, the AMA confirmed that a physician may teach at a chiropractic college or seminar. These settlements were entered into in 1978, 1980, and 1986.

The AMA's present position on chiropractic, as stated to the court, is that it is ethical for a medical physician to professionally associate with chiropractors provided the physician believes that such association is in the best interests of his patient. This position has not previously been communicated by the AMA to its members.

Antitrust Laws

Under the Sherman Act, every combination or conspiracy in restraint of trade is illegal. The court has held that the conduct of the AMA and its members constituted a conspiracy in restraint of trade based on the following facts: the purpose of the boycott was to eliminate chiropractic; chiropractors are in competition with some medical physicians; the boycott had substantial anti-competitive effects; there were no pro-competitive effects of the boycott; and the plaintiffs were injured as a result of the conduct. These facts add up to a violation of the Sherman Act.

In this case, however, the court allowed the defendants the opportunity to establish a "patient care defense" which has the following elements:

(1) that they genuinely entertained a concern for what they perceive as scientific method in the care of each person with whom they have entered into a doctor-patient relationship; (2) that this concern is objectively reasonable; (3) that this concern has been the dominant motivating factor in defendants' promulgation of Principle 3 and in the

conduct intended to implement it; and (4) that this concern for scientific method in patient care could not have been adequately satisfied in a manner less restrictive of competition.

The court concluded that the AMA had a genuine concern for scientific methods in patient care, and that this concern was the dominant factor in motivating the AMA's conduct. However, the AMA failed to establish that throughout the entire period of the boycott, from 1966 to 1980, this concern was objectively reasonable. The court reached that conclusion on the basis of extensive testimony from both witnesses for the plaintiffs and the AMA that some forms of chiropractic treatment are effective and the fact that the AMA recognized that chiropractic began to change in the early 1970s. Since the boycott was not formally over until Principle 3 was eliminated in 1980, the court found that the AMA was unable to establish that during the entire period of the conspiracy its position was objectively reasonable. Finally, the court ruled that the AMA's concern for scientific method in patient care could have been adequately satisfied in a manner less restrictive of competition and that a nationwide conspiracy to eliminate a licensed profession was not justified by the concern for scientific method. On the basis of these findings, the court concluded that the AMA had failed to establish the patient care defense.

None of the court's findings constituted a judicial endorsement of chiropractic. All of the parties to the case, including the plaintiffs and the AMA, agreed that chiropractic treatment of diseases such as diabetes, high blood pressure, cancer, heart disease and infectious disease is not proper, and that the historic theory of chiropractic, that there is a single cause and cure of disease is wrong. There was disagreement between the parties as to whether chiropractors should engage in diagnosis. There was evidence that the chiropractic theory of subluxations was unscientific, and evidence that some chiropractors engaged in unscientific practices. The court did not reach the question of whether chiropractic theory was in fact scientific. However, the evidence in the case was that some forms of chiropractic manipulation of the spine and joints was therapeutic. AMA witnesses, including the present Chairman of the Board of Trustees of the AMA, testified that some forms of treatment by chiropractors, including manipulation, can be therapeutic in the treatment of conditions such as back pain syndrome.

Need for Injunctive Relief

Although the conspiracy ended in 1980, there are lingering effects of the illegal boycott and conspiracy which require an injunction. Some medical physicians' individual decisions on whether or not to professionally associate with chiropractors are still affected by the boycott. The injury to chiropractors' reputations which resulted from the boycott has not been repaired. Chiropractors suffer current economic injury as a result of the boycott. The AMA has never affirmatively acknowledged that there are and should be no collective impediments to professional association and cooperation between chiropractors and medical physicians, except as provided by law. Instead, the AMA has consistently argued that its conduct has not violated the antitrust laws.

Most importantly, the court believes that it is important that the AMA members be made aware of the present AMA position that it is ethical for a medical physician to professionally associate with a chiropractor if the physician believes it is in the best interests of his patient, so that the lingering effects of the illegal group boycott against chiropractors finally can be dissipated.

Under the law, every medical physician, institution, and hospital has the right to make an individual decision as to whether or not that physician, institution, or hospital shall associate professionally with chiropractors. Individual choice by a medical physician voluntarily to associate professionally with chiropractors should be governed only by restrictions under state law, if any, and by the individual medical physician's personal judgment as to what is in the best interest of a patient or patients. Professional association includes referrals, consultations, group practice in partnerships, Health Maintenance Organizations, Preferred Provider Organizations, and other alternative health care delivery systems; the provision of treatment privileges and diagnostic services (including radiological and other laboratory facilities) in or through hospital facilities; association and cooperation in educational programs for students in chiropractic colleges; and cooperation in research, health care seminars, and continuing education programs.

An injunction is necessary to assure that the AMA does not interfere with the right of a physician, hospital, or other institution to make an individual decision on the question of professional association.

Form of Injunction

1. The AMA, its officers, agents and employees, and all persons who act in active concert with any of them and who receive actual notice of this order are hereby permanently enjoined from restricting, regulating or impeding, or aiding and abetting others from restricting, regulating or impeding, the freedom of any AMA member or any institution or hospital to make an individual decision as to whether or not that AMA member, institution, or hospital shall professionally associate with chiropractors, chiropractic students, or chiropractic institutions.

2. This Permanent Injunction does not and shall not be construed to restrict or otherwise interfere with the AMA's right to take positions on any issue, including chiropractic, and to express or publicize those positions, either alone or in conjunction with others. Nor does this Permanent Injunction restrict or otherwise interfere with the AMA's right to petition or testify before any public body on any legislative or regulatory measure or to join or cooperate with any other entity in so petitioning or testifying. The AMA's membership in a recognized accrediting association or society shall not constitute a violation of this Permanent Injunction.

3. The AMA is directed to send a copy of this order to each AMA member and employee, first class mail, postage prepaid, within thirty days of the entry of this order. In the alternative, the AMA shall provide the Clerk of the Court with mailing labels so that the court may send this order to AMA members and employees.

4. The AMA shall cause the publication of this order in JAMA and the indexing of the order under "Chiropractic" so that persons desiring to find the order in the future will be able to do so.

5. The AMA shall prepare a statement of the AMA's present position on chiropractic for inclusion in the current reports and opinions of the Judicial Council with an appropriate heading that refers to professional association between medical physicians and chiropractors, and indexed in the same manner that other reports and opinions are indexed. The court imposes no restrictions on the AMA's statement but only requires that it be consistent with the AMA's statements of its present position to the court.

6. The AMA shall file a report with the court evidencing compliance with this order on or before January 10, 1988.

It is so ordered.

Susan Getzendanner
United States District Judge

Naturopathic Medicine

"The work of the naturopathic physician is to elicit healing by helping patients to create or recreate conditions for health to exist within them. Health will occur where the conditions for health exist. Disease is the product of conditions which allow for it."

Jared Zeff, ND[476]

The diagram on this page is derived from the review by Zeff published in 1997 in *Journal of Naturopathic Medicine* entitled "The process of healing: a unifying theory of naturopathic medicine." By my interpretation, the diagram is important for at least three reasons.

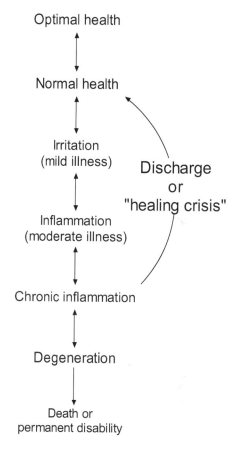

Optimal health

Normal health

Irritation (mild illness)

Inflammation (moderate illness)

Discharge or "healing crisis"

Chronic inflammation

Degeneration

Death or permanent disability

First, whereas the allopathic profession describes the genesis of most diseases as *idiopathic* and therefore [somehow] exclusively serviceable by drugs and surgery, the naturopathic profession describes disease processes as *multifactorial* and *logical* and therefore treatable by the skilled discovery and treatment of the underlying causes. Such underlying causes, which nearly always occur as a plurality, may vary mildly or significantly even within a group of patients with the same diagnosis.

Second, the diagram shows that the development of disease and the restoration of health are both *processes*. The restoration and retention of health requires *intentionality* and *tenacity* in lieu of the simplistic *miracle medicines* and *passive treatments* proffered by the pharmaceutical industry. Generally, disease does not arrive from outside; it is the result of one or more internal imbalances. Chronic illness is generally the result of manifold internal imbalances that culminate in numerous physiologic insults which compromise essential functions to the point that one or more organ systems begin to fail; we as patients and doctors generally label this as some specific "disease" or other, and the general—often erroneous—assumption has been that each *specific disease* (i.e., label, …abstraction, …conceptual entity) requires a *specific treatment* rather than a generalized health-restorative approach. Health is restored through a progressive and stepwise program that addresses as many facets of the illness as possible while vigorously supporting optimal physiologic function.

Third, the fact that Zeff considered the discharge or "healing crisis" so important that it merited inclusion in this diagram shows, indirectly, the naturopathic emphasis on detoxification and the eradication of dysbiosis. Both in the treatment of toxic metal/chemical exposure and in the treatment of chronic infections, patients often go through an acute or subacute phase of feeling ill before experiencing a dramatic alleviation of symptoms; the fact that symptoms may temporarily "get worse before getting better" has been referred to as the "healing crisis." This can occur for at least three reasons. First, in the elimination of chemicals and metals from the body, they must first be released from the tissues; the transition from tissues to blood is similar to a subacute re-exposure which triggers symptoms of toxicity until the toxin is excreted via sweat, urine, bile, or breath. Similarly, improvement in nutritional status—a cornerstone of all naturopathic interventions—expedites/facilitates/restores physiologic processes that have been relatively dormant due to lack of enzymatic cofactors such as vitamins and minerals[477]; optimization of nutritional status provides an opportunity for these pathways (such as detoxification of stored xenobiotics) to function again at which time they must "catch up" on work that has not been performed during the time of nutritional deficiency. The activation of these pathways is an essential step toward health restoration but results in an initial upregulation of hepatic phase-1/oxidative biotransformation which often

---

[476] Zeff JL. The process of healing: a unifying theory of naturopathic medicine. *Journal of Naturopathic Medicine* 1997; 7: 122-5
[477] Ames BN. The metabolic tune-up: metabolic harmony and disease prevention. *J Nutr.* 2003 May;133(5 Suppl 1):1544S-8S

results in the formation of reactive intermediates that temporarily impair physiologic processes and cause an initial exacerbation of symptoms. Third, whether through immunorestoration or the use of botanical/pharmacologic antimicrobial agents, the symptom-exacerbating "die off" reaction—classically called the Jarisch-Herxheimer reaction in the context of treating syphilis—is a result of increased (endo)toxin production/release by bacteria/microbes in response effective antimicrobial processes, whether physiologic or pharmacologic.

Modern naturopathic medicine has grown from deeply rooted European healing traditions reaching back several centuries. Naturopathic physicians have unwaveringly demonstrated respect, love, and appreciation for the healing powers of nature and the process of life itself.[478] Following their coursework in the basic biomedical sciences, naturopathic physicians are trained in urology, oncology, neurology, pediatrics, obstetrics and gynecology, urology, manual physical manipulation (including spinal manipulation), minor surgery, medical procedures, professional ethics, therapeutic diets, clinical and interventional nutrition, botanical medicines, psychological counseling, environmental medicine, and other modalities. Licensed naturopathic physicians commonly practice as generalists and family doctors.[479,480,481,482]

Naturopathic Principles, Concepts, & the *Vis Medicatrix Naturae*

"The healing power of nature is the inherent self-organizing and healing process of living systems… It is the naturopathic physician's role to support, facilitate and augment this process by identifying and removing obstacles to health and recovery, and by supporting the creation of a healthy internal and external environment."[483]

1. **First, Do No Harm *(Primum Non Nocere)*:** Naturopathic physicians use good judgment and compassion to ensure that the treatment does not cause harm to the patient. This contrasts with the effects of allopathic treatment, which collectively kill more than 180,000-220,000 patients per year, at least 493 American patients per day.[484]

2. **Identify and Treat the Causes *(Tolle Causam)*:** *"Illness does not occur without cause."* Naturopathic physicians focus on identifying and addressing the underlying deficiency, toxicity, impairment, or imbalance that is the cause of the health problem or disease.

3. **Treat the Whole Person:** *"The multifactorial nature of health and disease requires a personalized and comprehensive approach to diagnosis and treatment."* On some occasions the illness does take precedence over the person who has it—such in emergency situations like septic arthritis, acute ischemia, and pulmonary edema. In these cases, the situation must be managed appropriately, and these situations are not immediately amenable to long-term lifestyle changes—they require immediate treatment. However, the vast majority of cases in routine outpatient clinical practice will require detailed and bipartite attention to the facets of both **the disease process** and **the person who has the illness**. Our focus as naturopathic physicians on the individual patient is what sets our healing profession apart from others that focus exclusively on the disease and do not consider the manifold intricacies of the individual patient.

4. **The Healing Power of Nature: *Vis Medicatrix Naturae*:** Naturopathic medicine recognizes an inherent self-healing process in the person that is ordered and intelligent. The body has many highly efficient mechanisms for sustaining and regaining health. These mechanisms have their specific and necessary components (e.g., nutrients) and means by which they can be impaired (e.g., xenobiotic

---

[478] Kirchfeld F, Boyle W. Nature Doctors: Pioneers in Naturopathic Medicine. Portland, Oregon; Medicina Biologica (Buckeye Naturopathic Press, East Palestine, Ohio), 1994

[479] Boon HS, Cherkin DC, Erro J, Sherman KJ, Milliman B, Booker J, Cramer EH, Smith MJ, Deyo RA, Eisenberg DM. Practice patterns of naturopathic physicians: results from a random survey of licensed practitioners in two US States. *BMC Complement Altern Med*. 2004;4(1):14

[480] Smith MJ, Logan AC. Naturopathy. *Med Clin North Am*. 2002 Jan;86(1):173-84

[481] Cherkin DC, Deyo RA, Sherman KJ, et al. Characteristics of visits to licensed acupuncturists, chiropractors, massage therapists, and naturopathic physicians. *J Am Board Fam Pract*. 2002 Nov-Dec;15(6):463-72

[482] Cherkin DC, Deyo RA, Sherman KJ, et al. Characteristics of licensed acupuncturists, chiropractors, massage therapists, and naturopathic physicians. *J Am Board Fam Pract*. 2002 Sep-Oct;15(5):378-90

[483] Quoted from the American Association of Naturopathic Physicians website http://aanp.net/Basics/h.naturo.philo.html on February 4, 2001. Other italicized quotes in this section are from the same source. This website has since been replaced by http://naturopathic.org/

[484] "Recent estimates suggest that each year more than 1 million patients are injured while in the hospital and approximately 180,000 die because of these injuries. Furthermore, drug-related morbidity and mortality are common and are estimated to cost more than $136 billion a year." Holland EG, Degruy FV. Drug-induced disorders. *Am Fam Physician*. 1997;56(7):1781-8, 1791-2

immunosuppression). Poor health and disease can result from impairment of these self-healing processes and biologic mechanisms, and thus the body's inherent, natural, self-healing mechanisms—the "healing power of nature"—can be diminished to the state of ineffectiveness or harm (e.g., autoimmunity). Recognizing that the body has this inherent goal of and movement toward self-healing, naturopathic physicians start by identifying and removing "obstacles to cure" rather than ignoring these factors and masking the manifestations of dysfunction with symptom-suppressing drugs.

5. **Prevention**: Healthy lifestyle, proper nutrition, and emotional hygiene go a long way toward preventing (and treating) most conditions. Specific conditions have specific risk factors and causes that have to be considered per patient and condition.

6. **Doctor As Teacher** (*Docere*): Naturopathic physicians explain the situation and the proposed solution to the patient so that the patient is empowered with understanding and with the comfort of knowing what has happened, what is happening, and the proposed course of upcoming events. Naturopathic physicians strive to let their own lives serve as a models for our patients. This does not mean that naturopathic doctors have to feign perfection; the task is to live the best and most conscious life that we can, to be present with our emotions, qualities, and faults and to treat ourselves with respect and acceptance. We can exemplify health (rather than perfection) to our patients by being who we authentically are and by so doing we can facilitate their own acceptance of their current health situation, which is a prerequisite to self-initiated change.

> **"Physician, heal thyself.**
> Thus you help your patient, too.
> Let this be his best medicine that he beholds with his eyes: the doctor who heals himself."
>
> Nietzsche FW. Thus Spoke Zarathustra (1892). [Kaufmann W, translator]. Viking Penguin: 1954, page 77

7. **Re-Establish the Foundation for Health**: An overview of this important naturopathic concept is provided throughout this chapter.

8. **Removing "obstacles to cure"**: *examples*

Obstacle to the optimization of health	Example of possible intervention
o Toxic exposures, medication side-effects	▪ Reduce drug use and dependency
o Toxic relationships, emotional obstacles, past events, unfulfilling occupation,	▪ Improve self-esteem, develop conflict resolution skills, determine life goals and values and a plan for their pursuit
o Social isolation: the typical American has only two friends no-one in whom to confide[485]	▪ Encourage social interaction
o Diet with excess fat, arachidonate, sugar, additives, colorants, and insufficiency of protein, fiber, phytonutrients, and health-promoting fatty acids: ALA, GLA, EPA, DHA, and oleic acid	▪ Diet improvement and nutritional supplementation
o Sedentary lifestyle, lack of exercise	▪ Encourage exercise
o Weight gain/loss as necessary for weight optimization	▪ Encourage self-valuing
o Epidemic exposure to mercury, lead, and xenobiotics	▪ Support detoxification process as a lifestyle

Hierarchy of Therapeutics: This naturopathic concept articulates the importance of addressing *the underlying cause* rather than simply focusing on *the presenting problem*, which is the *symptom of the cause*. Further, interventions are **prioritized**, *for example*:

- Patient-implemented *before* doctor-implemented.

---

[485] McPherson M, Smith-Lovin L, Brashears ME. Social Isolation in America: Changes in Core Discussion Networks over Two Decades. *American Sociological Review* 2006; 71: 353-75 http://www.asanet.org/galleries/default-file/June06ASRFeature.pdf

- Removal of harming agent *before* addition of a therapeutic agent: e.g., stop smoking *before* investing in respiratory therapy; implement healthy diet and exercise before higher-risk and higher-cost drugs for hypertension and hypercholesterolemia.
- Low-force interventions *before* high-force interventions.
- Diet *before* nutritional supplements; nutrients *before* botanicals; botanicals *before* drugs; modulatory drugs *before* suppressive/inhibitory drugs; integrative care *before* surgery.
- *See examples below.*

Hierarchy of Therapeutics (specifically sequential)	Example of possible intervention
1. Reestablishing the foundation for health	• Mental/emotional/spiritual health • Meditation, freeze-frame, "time out" • Relaxation • Positive visualization, positive expectation, affirmation • Counseling, social contact, group work[486] • Family contact and resolution • Dietary intake and nutritional health which addresses the patient's biochemical individuality[487] and correction of deficiencies or excesses • Identification and elimination of food allergies and food sensitivities • Reduce toxin exposure, promote detoxification • Identification and elimination of exposure to gastrointestinal and inhalant xenobiotics • Remove or reduce specific "obstacles to cure"
2. Stimulation of the "healing power of nature" and the "vital force"	• Constitutional hydrotherapy • Homeopathy • Exercise • Acupuncture, Spinal manipulation • Meditation, rest • Tai Chi, Qigong: "energy-cultivation" • Botanical adaptogens
3. Tonification of weakened systems:	• Botanical medicines and other supplements to help restore normal tissue function • Spinal manipulation to address the primary somatovisceral dysfunction and/or secondary musculoskeletal disorders • Hormonal supplementation • Nutritional supplementation • Exercise • Physiotherapy
4. Correction of structural integrity:	• Spinal manipulation, deep tissue massage, visceral manipulation, lymphatic pump to promote immune surveillance[488] • Stretching, balancing, muscle strengthening, and proprioceptive retraining • Surgery, as a last resort

---

[486] See http://www.mkp.org and www.WomanWithin.org for examples.

[487] Williams RJ. Biochemical Individuality: The Basis for the Genetotrophic Concept. Austin and London: University of Texas Press, 1956

[488] "Lymph flow in the thoracic duct increased from 1.57±0.20 mL·min-1 to a peak TDF of 4.80±1.73 mL·min-1 during abdominal pump, and from 1.20±0.41 mL·min-1 to 3.45±1.61 mL·min-1 during thoracic pump." Knott EM, Tune JD, Stoll ST, Downey HF. Increased lymphatic flow in the thoracic duct during manipulative intervention. *J Am Osteopath Assoc.* 2005 Oct;105(10):447-56 http://www.jaoa.org/cgi/content/full/105/10/447

Osteopathic Medicine

Osteopathic medicine and chiropractic are American-born healthcare professions and paradigms that started at nearly the same time in history and from many of the same foundational principles. Both professions were started in the late 1800's and early 1900's and were founded upon the philosophical premise that the body functioned as a whole and that therefore medicine in general and therapeutic interventions in particular needed to be comprehensive in scope and multifaceted in their application. Further, both professions emphasized the importance of structural integrity as a foundational component of health and thus embraced manual manipulative therapy and spinal manipulation.

From their common origins, subtle differences and chance historic events shaped and further separated these professions from each other. Osteopathy was founded by Andrew Taylor Still, a medical doctor who sought to reform what was then called the "Heroic" paradigm of medicine, which embraced bloodletting and the administration of leeches, purgatives, emetics, and poisons such as mercury as means for "rebalancing" what were perceived to be internal causes of disease, namely the "four humours" of the body which were thought to be blood, phlegm, black bile, and yellow bile. In part because of his training within and identification with the medical profession, Still sought to *reform* rather than *directly oppose* the "mainstream medicine" of his day; in contrast, chiropractic's founder Daniel David Palmer was more strongly opposed to the horrific medicine of his time and thus was more *revolutionary* than *evolutionary* in his approach to forging a new paradigm of health and healthcare. Still's willingness to align with the medical profession and the increasingly powerful and influential pharmaceutical industry unquestionably helped his fledgling profession survive the extinction that otherwise would have been swift at the hands of allopathic groups such as **the American Medical Association (AMA), which labeled osteopathic physicians as "cultists" and systematically restricted inclusion of the osteopathic profession into mainstream healthcare by proclamation in 1953 that "...all voluntary associations with osteopaths are unethical." When osteopathic resistance mounted, the AMA and its co-conspirators, who were later found guilty of violating the nation's antitrust laws by illegally suppressing competition and attempting to build a medical monopoly**[489], acquiesced and accepted osteopaths into its ranks—a strategy which the medical profession believed would eventually destroy the osteopathic profession by forcing it to resign its ideals and identity. In his review of osteopathic history, Gevitz[490] writes, **"...the M.D.'s gradually came to believe that the only way to destroy osteopathy was through the absorption of D.O.'s, much as the homeopaths and eclectics [naturopaths] had been swallowed up early in the century."** Even recently, the AMA has listed osteopathic medicine under "alternative medicine"[491] although several osteopathic medical colleges have consistently provided training that is superior to most "conventional" allopathic medical schools.[492] Today, osteopathic physicians practice in most ways similarly to allopaths—i.e., with unlimited scope of practice in all 50 states, full access to the use of drugs and surgery, and with a very pharmacosurgical paradigm of disease and healthcare. Osteopathic medicine is one of the fastest growing healthcare professions in America.

Osteopathic Manipulative Medicine:

Osteopathic manipulative medicine (OMM) is similar to and yet distinct from chiropractic manipulation; the naturopathic profession—true to its eclectic roots—incorporates techniques from all professions. In contrast to chiropractic, OMM terminology and therapeutics focus much more on soft tissues, and the osteopathic lesion—"somatic dysfunction"—is clearly originated from soft tissues in contrast to the chiropractic lesion—the "vertebral subluxation"—which obviously originates from spinal articulations. Whereas the chiropractic intent of correcting or "adjusting" the "subluxation" was historically to improve function of the nervous system, the osteopathic lesion is addressed to more fully improve not only function of the nervous system but also of the vascular, lymphatic, and myofascial systems, too.[493] With regard to the latter, the osteopathic profession has always emphasized the importance of fascia in the genesis of "somatic dysfunction." Indeed, fascia appears to play an

---

[489] Getzendanner S. Permanent injunction order against AMA. *JAMA*. 1988 Jan 1;259(1):81-2

[490] Gevitz N. The D.O.'s: Osteopathic Medicine in America. Johns Hopkins University Press; 1991; pages 100-103

[491] American Medical Association. Report 12 of the Council on Scientific Affairs (A-97) Full Text http://www.ama-assn.org/ama/pub/category/13638.html Accessed November 23, 2006

[492] Special report. America's best graduate schools. Schools of Medicine. The top schools: primary care. *US News World Rep.* 2004 Apr 12;136(12):74

[493] Williams N. Managing back pain in general practice--is osteopathy the new paradigm? *Br J Gen Pract.* 1997 Oct;47(423):653-5
http://www.pubmedcentral.nih.gov/articlerender.fcgi?tool=pubmed&pubmedid=9474832

important and dynamic (not passive) role in neuromusculoskeletal health, particularly as it is a major contributor to proprioception and may also have a more direct effect through the recently described ability of fascia to actively contract in a smooth-muscle-like manner.[494]

From this author's perspective, an unfortunate consequence of the broadness of osteopathic manipulative conceptualizations/techniques (i.e., vertebral, skeletal, vascular, lymphatic, myofascial,...) is the relative lack (compared to chiropractic) of modernization and sophistication and development of its terminology and training textbooks; two of the most widely used osteopathic texts—*Osteopathic Principles in Practice* (1994) by Kuchera and Kuchera[495], and *Outline of Osteopathic Manipulative Procedures* (2006) by Kimberly[496]—both leave very much to be desired with respect to their clarity, terminology, clinical applicability, and referencing to the scientific literature. *Manipulation of the Spine, Thorax and Pelvis: An Osteopathic Perspective* (2006) by Gibbons and Tehan[497] is much more accessible and clinically applicable; however the text focuses exclusively on high-velocity low-amplitude (HVLA) techniques and therefore does not provide sufficient background and training for students in the very techniques that distinguish osteopathic from chiropractic techniques, namely heightened attention to the myofascial dysfunction that (appropriately) underlies the osteopathic lesion.

Ironically, the very growth and "allopathicization" of the profession that has threatened the profession's adherence to its holistic tenets has caused a reflexive re-affirmation of these tenets, and the profession has responded with a well-funded and intentional directive to scientifically investigate the mechanisms and efficacy of osteopathic manipulative medicine.[498,499] Recent findings include improved function and reduced pain in patients treated with a comprehensive manipulative technique for the shoulder[500], as well as the significant efficacy of ankle manipulation for patients with recent ankle injuries.[501] Further, OMM treatment of patients medicated for depression was found to triple the effectiveness of drug monotherapy.[502] Other studies have shown benefit of OMM in the treatment of geriatric pneumonia[503], pediatric asthma[504], pediatric

> ## Osteopathic Interventions need to be Consistent with Osteopathic Philosophy
>
> "In contrast to the description of the osteopathic medical profession by the American Osteopathic Association, namely, "doctors of osteopathic medicine, or D.O.s, apply the philosophy of treating the whole person to the prevention, diagnosis and treatment of illness, disease and injury," [the authors of the article in question] essentially reviewed only pharmacologic treatment.
>
> …
>
> It is hoped that future reviews in this journal can include a more balanced survey of the literature, inclusive of non-pharmacologic and "holistic" interventions that are consistent with osteopathic philosophy."
>
> **Vasquez A.** Interventions need to be Consistent with Osteopathic Philosophy. [Letter] *JAOA: Journal of the American Osteopathic Association* 2006 Sep;106(9):528-9
> http://www.jaoa.org/cgi/content/full/106/9/528

---

[494] "...the existence of an active fascial contractility could have interesting implications for the understanding of musculoskeletal pathologies with an increased or decreased myofascial tonus. It may also offer new insights and a deeper understanding of treatments directed at fascia, such as manual myofascial release therapies or acupuncture." Schleip R, Klingler W, Lehmann-Horn F. Active fascial contractility: Fascia may be able to contract in a smooth muscle-like manner and thereby influence musculoskeletal dynamics. *Med Hypotheses.* 2005;65(2):273-7

[495] Kuchera WA, Kuchera ML. *Osteopathic Principles In Practice, revised second edition.* Kirksville, MO, KCOM Press; 1994

[496] Kimberly PE. *Outline of Osteopathic Manipulative Procedures.The Kimberly Manual 2006.* Kirksville College Osteopathic Medicine. Walsworth Publish. Co., Marceline, Mo

[497] Gibbons P, Tehan P. *Manipulation of the Spine, Thorax and Pelvis: An Osteopathic Perspective. Churchill Livingstone*; 2006. Isbn: 044310039X

[498] Wisnioski SW 3rd. "Circle Turns Round" to "Allopathic Osteopathy." *J Am Osteopath Assoc* 2006; 106: 423-4 http://www.jaoa.org/cgi/content/full/106/7/423

[499] Teitelbaum HS, Bunn WE 2nd, Brown SA, Burchett AW. Osteopathic medical education: renaissance or rhetoric? *J Am Osteopath Assoc.* 2003 Oct;103(10):489-90 http://www.jaoa.org/cgi/reprint/103/10/489

[500] The "seven stages of Spencer" is an organized technique of range-of-motion exercises and post-isometric stretching to improve functionality of the shoulder. This clinical trial showed improved shoulder function in a group of elderly patients treated with this technique. Knebl JA, Shores JH, Gamber RG, Gray WT, Herron KM. Improving functional ability in the elderly via the Spencer technique, an osteopathic manipulative treatment: a randomized, controlled trial. *J Am Osteopath Assoc.* 2002 Jul;102(7):387-96 http://www.jaoa.org/cgi/reprint/102/7/387 See also "CONCLUSION: Manipulative therapy for the shoulder girdle in addition to usual medical care accelerates recovery of shoulder symptoms." Bergman GJ, Winters JC, Groenier KH, Pool JJ, Meyboom-de Jong B, Postema K, van der Heijden GJ. Manipulative therapy in addition to usual medical care for patients with shoulder dysfunction and pain: a randomized, controlled trial. *Ann Intern Med.* 2004 Sep 21;141(6):432-9 http://www.annals.org/cgi/reprint/141/6/432.pdf

[501] This study shows the rapid onset and benefit of manipulative medicine for the treatment of acute ankle sprains: Eisenhart AW, Gaeta TJ, Yens DP. Osteopathic manipulative treatment in the emergency department for patients with acute ankle injuries. *J Am Osteopath Assoc.* 2003 Sep;103(9):417-21 http://www.jaoa.org/cgi/reprint/103/9/417

[502] This study impressively showed that musculoskeletal manipulation improved treatment effectiveness for depression from 33% to 100%. "After 8 weeks, 100% of the OMT treatment group and 33% of the control group tested normal by psychometric evaluation. ... The findings of this pilot study indicate that OMT may be a useful adjunctive treatment for alleviating depression in women." Plotkin BJ, Rodos JJ, Kappler R, Schrage M, Freydl K, Hasegawa S, Hennegan E, Hilchie-Schmidt C, Hines D, Iwata J, Mok C, Raffaelli D. Adjunctive osteopathic manipulative treatment in women with depression: a pilot study. *J Am Osteopath Assoc.* 2001 Sep;101(9):517-23 http://www.jaoa.org/cgi/reprint/101/9/517

[503] This study showed improved clinical outcomes and reduced antibiotic use in elderly patients with pneumonia when treated with manipulative medicine: "The treatment group had a significantly shorter duration of intravenous antibiotic treatment and a shorter hospital stay." Noll DR, Shores JH, Gamber RG, Herron KM, Swift J Jr. Benefits of osteopathic manipulative treatment for hospitalized elderly patients with pneumonia. *J Am Osteopath Assoc.* 2000 Dec;100(12):776-82 http://www.jaoa.org/cgi/reprint/100/12/776

[504] Osteopathic manipulation improved pulmonary function in pediatric patients with asthma: "With a confidence level of 95%, results for the OMT group showed a statistically significant improvement of 7 L per minute to 9 L per minute for peak expiratory flow rates. These results suggest that OMT has a therapeutic effect among this patient population." Guiney PA, Chou R, Vianna A, Lovenheim J. Effects of osteopathic manipulative treatment on pediatric patients with asthma: a randomized controlled trial. *J Am Osteopath Assoc.* 2005 Jan;105(1):7-12 http://www.jaoa.org/cgi/content/full/105/1/7

dysfunctional voiding[505], carpal tunnel syndrome[506], low-back pain[507], and recovery from cardiac bypass surgery.[508] Replication and validation of these studies—many of which are small or of nonrigorous design (e.g., open clinical trials with no control group)—is important to further define and establish the value of osteopathic manipulation in clinical care.

---

[505] "RESULTS: The treatment group exhibited greater improvement in DV symptoms than did the control group (Z=-2.63, p=0.008, Mann-Whitney U-test). Improved or resolution of vesicoureteral reflux and elimination of post-void urine residuals were more prominent in the treatment group." Nemett DR, Fivush BA, Mathews R, Camirand N, Eldridge MA, Finney K, Gerson AC. A randomized controlled trial of the effectiveness of osteopathy-based manual physical therapy in treating pediatric dysfunctional voiding. *J Pediatr Urol.* 2008 Apr;4(2):100-6

[506] Sucher BM, Hinrichs RN, Welcher RL, Quiroz LD, St Laurent BF, Morrison BJ. Manipulative treatment of carpal tunnel syndrome: biomechanical and osteopathic intervention to increase the length of the transverse carpal ligament: part 2. Effect of sex differences and manipulative "priming". *J Am Osteopath Assoc.* 2005 Mar;105(3):135-43. Erratum in: J Am Osteopath Assoc. 2005 May;105(5):238 http://www.jaoa.org/cgi/content/full/105/3/135

[507] "CONCLUSION: OMT significantly reduces low back pain. The level of pain reduction is greater than expected from placebo effects alone and persists for at least three months." Licciardone JC, Brimhall AK, King LN. Osteopathic manipulative treatment for low back pain: a systematic review and meta-analysis of randomized controlled trials. *BMC Musculoskelet Disord.* 2005 Aug 4;6:43 http://www.biomedcentral.com/1471-2474/6/43

[508] This study showed benefit from osteopathic manipulation administered immediately after coronary artery bypass graft surgery: "The observed changes in cardiac function and perfusion indicated that OMT had a beneficial effect on the recovery of patients after CABG surgery. The authors conclude that OMT has immediate, beneficial hemodynamic effects after CABG surgery when administered while the patient is sedated and pharmacologically paralyzed." O-Yurvati AH, Carnes MS, Clearfield MB, Stoll ST, McConathy WJ. Hemodynamic effects of osteopathic manipulative treatment immediately after coronary artery bypass graft surgery. *J Am Osteopath Assoc.* 2005 Oct;105(10):475-81 http://www.jaoa.org/cgi/content/full/105/10/475

Functional Medicine

Note: This section is from the final pre-edited draft which introduces functional medicine in *Vasquez A. Musculoskeletal Pain: Expanded Clinical Strategies* (2008), published by the Institute for Functional Medicine; used here with permission. Slight modifications were made to this section during revisions in 2011.

Introduction: The purpose of this monograph is to provide healthcare professionals with an overview of the "functional medicine" assessment and management strategies that are applicable to painful neuromusculoskeletal disorders. A comprehensive description of functional medicine from the Institute for Functional Medicine (IFM) is provided later in this section, while a more comprehensive explication is provided in *The Textbook of Functional Medicine*.[509] In recognition of the diversity of this document's readership (inclusive of students, recent graduates, experienced professionals, academicians, and policymakers) and the pervasive deficiencies in musculoskeletal knowledge among healthcare providers[510,511,512,513,514,515], this monograph on pain will necessarily review some basic concepts; however, this document alone cannot replace professional training in musculoskeletal medicine nor does it include protocols for

A Functional Medicine Monograph

MUSCULOSKELETAL PAIN:
Expanded Clinical Strategies

Alex Vasquez, DC, ND

THE INSTITUTE FOR FUNCTIONAL MEDICINE

The information in this section on functional medicine is derived from the final pre-edited draft of chapter 1 from Vasquez A. *Musculoskeletal Pain: Expanded Clinical Strategies*, published by the Institute for Functional Medicine in 2008 and available from www.FunctionalMedicine.org

patient management and differential diagnosis for each of the neuromusculoskeletal problems seen in clinical practice. This text should be used in conjunction with the reader's professional training and other reference texts. Clinicians utilizing a functional medicine approach to patient care must be knowledgeable in the details of integrative physiology and nutritional biochemistry and must also posses the clinical acumen necessary to ensure safe and expedient patient care. These traits and skills are of particular necessity when a serious condition is presented. Life-threatening and limb-threatening neuromusculoskeletal problems are notorious for presenting under the guise of an apparently benign complaint such as fatigue, headache, or simple joint pain.

Since approximately 1 of every 7 (14% of total) visits to a primary healthcare provider is for the treatment of musculoskeletal pain or dysfunction[516], every healthcare provider needs to have: 1) knowledge of important concepts related to musculoskeletal medicine, 2) the ability to recognize urgent and emergency conditions, 3) the ability to competently perform orthopedic examination procedures and interpret laboratory assessments, and 4) the knowledge and ability to design and implement effective treatment plans and to coordinate patient management. While this monograph will be thorough in its review of topics discussed, like any other textbook it cannot contain every nuance and examination procedure that clinicians should have in their clinical toolkits. This text should be used in conjunction with the clinician's previous professional training, other textbooks, and best judgment for the delivery of personalized care for each individual patient, including those who present with similar or identical diagnoses. Supportive texts include *Current Medical Diagnosis and Treatment* edited by Tierney

[509] Jones DS (Editor-in-Chief). *Textbook of Functional Medicine*. Institute for Functional Medicine, Gig Harbor, WA 2005
[510] Freedman KB, Bernstein J. The adequacy of medical school education in musculoskeletal medicine. *J Bone Joint Surg Am*. 1998;80(10):1421-7
[511] Freedman KB, Bernstein J. Educational deficiencies in musculoskeletal medicine. *J Bone Joint Surg Am*. 2002;84-A(4):604-8
[512] Joy EA, Hala SV. Musculoskeletal Curricula in Medical Education: Filling In the Missing Pieces. *The Physician and Sportsmedicine*. 2004; 32: 42-45
[513] Matzkin E, Smith ME, Freccero CD, Richardson AB. Adequacy of education in musculoskeletal medicine. *J Bone Joint Surg Am*. 2005 Feb;87-A(2):310-4
[514] Schmale GA. More evidence of educational inadequacies in musculoskeletal medicine. *Clin Orthop Relat Res*. 2005 Aug;(437):251-9
[515] Stockard AR, Allen TW. Competence levels in musculoskeletal medicine: comparison of osteopathic and allopathic medical graduates. *J Am Osteopath Assoc*. 2006 Jun;106(6):350-5
[516] American College of Rheumatology Ad Hoc Committee on Clinical Guidelines. Guidelines for the initial evaluation of the adult patient with acute musculoskeletal symptoms. *Arthritis Rheum*. 1996 Jan;39(1):1-8 See also: **Vasquez A**. Musculoskeletal disorders and iron overload disease: comment on the American College of Rheumatology guidelines. *Arthritis Rheum* 1996;39: 1767-8

et al[517], *Orthopedic Physical Assessment* by Magee[518], and *Integrative Orthopedics* and *Integrative Rheumatology* by Vasquez.[519,520] Further, clinicians can note that this monograph is written primarily for routine outpatient management rather than emergency department management or "playing field" situations.

Musculoskeletal disorders are extremely prevalent and represent a major cause of human suffering, healthcare expenses, and lost productivity. Additionally, many standard medical interventions show high rates of inefficacy and iatrogenesis in addition to their high costs.[521,522,523] The vast majority of painful neuromusculoskeletal disorders can be alleviated and often effectively treated with nutritional interventions, but physicians trained only in standard medicine receive little to no training in nutrition and are therefore generally unable or unwilling to use these science-based interventions to help their patients.[524,525] Further, distain toward nutritional and other nonsurgical and nonpharmacologic interventions is represented in many standard medical textbooks despite proof of efficacy shown in replicable high-quality clinical trials published in top-tier medical journals. For example, despite the more than 800 articles documenting the role of nutritional interventions in the direct or adjunctive treatment of rheumatoid arthritis, the seventeenth edition of *The Merck Manual* published in 1999 wrote that, "Food and diet quackery is common and should be discouraged."[526] Combining these factors with the aforementioned pervasive lack of competence in musculoskeletal knowledge among healthcare providers (exceptions noted[527]), we see that patients with musculoskeletal disorders often face a series of difficult and insurmountable obstacles between their present condition of suffering and the relief that they seek and deserve. Clearly, the field of musculoskeletal medicine is in need of pervasive paradigm shifts in both physician training and patient management to improve patient care.

Background: Historically, prevailing views of disorders of pain and inflammation were conceptually similar to those of most other diseases and premodern accounts of life in general. Our clinical predecessors did the best they could to understand, describe, and treat the health problems with which their patients presented, and the paradigm from which these clinical entities were viewed and addressed was shaped by the social, religious, and scientific views and limitations of their time. Lacking a molecular and physiologic understanding of disease origination, and restrained by metaphysical and simplistic models of "cause and effect", premodern clinicians devised models for the understanding and treatment of disease that generally appear unsatisfactory today in light of the advances in our understanding in disparate yet interrelated fields such as psychoneuroimmunology, molecular biology, nutrigenomics, environmental medicine and toxicology. Despite these advances, we as a human society and as healthcare providers still carry many of these previous conceptualizations and misconceptualizations with us as we move forward toward a future wherein our views and interventions will be much more precise and "objective" in contrast to the generalized and phenomenalistic approaches that typified premodern medicine and which still permeate certain aspects of clinical care today. For example, we still use the term "stroke" to describe acute cerebrovascular insufficiency, although the term originated from the view that affected patients had been "struck" by the gods or fates perhaps as a form of punishment for some ethical or religious transgression. Even today, patients and clinicians commonly interpret disease as some form of punishment or as an extension of spiritual or intrapersonal shortcoming. Advancing science allows us to disassemble complex events that were previously experienced as *phenomena*, that is, as undecipherable and enigmatic events that overwhelmed comprehension. The **Functional Medicine Matrix** provides an extremely useful tool for helping clinicians grasp a multidimensional decipherable view of disease and its corresponding

[517] Tierney ML. McPhee SJ, Papadakis MA (eds). Current Medical Diagnosis and Treatment. New York: Lange Medical Books. Updated annually
[518] Magee DJ. Orthopedic Physical Assessment. Third edition. Philadelphia: WB Saunders, 1997. Newer editions have been published.
[519] Vasquez A. *Integrative Orthopedics: Second Edition*. Fort Worth, Texas; Integrative and Biological Medicine Research and Consulting, 2007 OptimalHealthResearch.com
[520] Vasquez A. *Integrative Rheumatology: Second Edition*. Fort Worth, Texas; Integrative and Biological Medicine Research and Consulting, 2007 OptimalHealthResearch.com
[521] Moseley JB, O'Malley K, Petersen NJ, Menke TJ, Brody BA, Kuykendall DH, Hollingsworth JC, Ashton CM, Wray NP. A controlled trial of arthroscopic surgery for osteoarthritis of the knee. *N Engl J Med* 2002 Jul 11;347(2):81-8
[522] Kolata G. A Knee Surgery for Arthritis Is Called Sham. *The New York Times*, July 11, 2002
[523] Rosner AL. Evidence-based clinical guidelines for the management of acute low-back pain: response to the guidelines prepared for the Australian Medical Health and Research Council. *J Manipulative Physiol Ther*. 2001;24(3):214-20
[524] Lo C. Integrating nutrition as a theme throughout the medical school curriculum. *Am J Clin Nutr*. 2000 Sep;72(3 Suppl):882S-9S
[525] Adams KM, Lindell KC, Kohlmeier M, Zeisel SH. Status of nutrition education in medical schools. *Am J Clin Nutr*. 2006 Apr;83(4):941S-944S
[526] Beers MH, Berkow R (eds). The Merck Manual. Seventeenth Edition. Whitehouse Station; Merck Research Laboratories: 1999, page 419
[527] Humphreys BK, Sulkowski A, McIntyre K, Kasiban M, Patrick AN. An examination of musculoskeletal cognitive competency in chiropractic interns. *J Manipulative Physiol Ther*. 2007;30(1):44-9

treatment which facilitates the achievement of higher clinical efficacy, improved patient outcomes, and more favorable safety and cost-effectiveness profiles.

Whereas the advancement of our scientific knowledge often leads us to discard previous models and interventions, occasionally modern science helps us to understand and revisit previous interventions that may have been prematurely or unduly discarded. For example, Hippocrates' admonition to "Let thy food be thy medicine, and thy medicine be thy food" experienced decades of devaluation when dietary, nutritional, and other natural interventions were misbranded as "quackery." On the contrary to these premature and unsubstantiated condemnations, simple natural interventions such as therapeutic fasting and augmentation of vitamin D3 status (via nutritional supplementation or exposure to ultraviolet-B radiation) have shown remarkable safety and efficacy in the mitigation of chronic hypertension, musculoskeletal pain, and autoimmunity.[528,529,530,531,532,533,534,535,536] Furthermore, the appropriate use of vitamin supplements helps prevent chronic disease by numerous mechanisms including modulation of gene transcription, enhancement of DNA repair and stability, and enhancement of metabolic efficiency.[537,538,539] This document will provide a representative survey of current research in the use of dietary, nutritional, and integrative therapeutics commonly utilized in the clinical management of disorders characterized by pain and inflammation.

State of the Evidence: The bulk of information in this monograph is derived from and referenced to peer-reviewed publications indexed in the database known as Medline/Pubmed provided by the U.S. National Library of Medicine and the National Institutes of Health. For the sake of practicality and publishability, not all statements carry citations, but the most important ones do; citations are always provided when referenced to a particular intervention of importance so that clinicians can access the primary source when refining their clinical decisions. A "blanket statement" to cover all the different assessments and interventions described herein would be necessarily inaccurate and therefore each intervention will be considered on the merits of its own rationale, safety, effectiveness, and cost-effectiveness. Again, however, these considerations must ultimately be viewed within the context of the individual patient's condition and the overall cohesion and comprehensiveness of the treatment plan.

While all clinicians can appreciate the importance of protocols and clinical practice guidelines, we must also perpetually ratify the preeminence of patient individuality and therefore the importance of tailoring treatment to the patient's unique combination of biochemical individuality, comorbid conditions, drug use, personal goals, and willingness to participate in a health-promoting lifestyle. Standardized protocols and practice guidelines are founded on the fallacy of disease homogeneity and the irrelevance of physiologic, psychosocial, and biochemical individuality. As the advancement of biomedical science provides the means for and underscores the importance of customized treatments for each patient, so too has the standard of care begun to shift in the direction of requiring the consideration of these variables before and during the implementation of treatment. Failure to utilize nutritional interventions when such interventions are clinically indicated is inconsistent with the delivery of quality healthcare and may be considered malpractice.[540,541,542,543]

A clinician who is unaware of the political forces that shape healthcare policy and research is analogous to a captain of an oceangoing ship not knowing how to use a compass, sextant, or coastline map. Medical science

[528] Goldhamer A, et al. Medically supervised water-only fasting in the treatment of hypertension. *J Manipulative Physiol Ther* 2001 Jun;24(5):335-9

[529] Goldhamer AC, et al. Medically supervised water-only fasting in the treatment of borderline hypertension. *J Altern Complement Med*. 2002 Oct;8(5):643-50

[530] Goldhamer AC. Initial cost of care results in medically supervised water-only fasting for treating high blood pressure and diabetes. *J Altern Complement Med*. 2002 Dec;8(6):696-7

[531] Krause R, Bühring M, Hopfenmüller W, Holick MF, Sharma AM. Ultraviolet B and blood pressure. *Lancet*. 1998 Aug 29;352(9129):709-10

[532] Pfeifer M, Begerow B, Minne HW, Nachtigall D, Hansen C. Effects of a short-term vitamin D(3) and calcium supplementation on blood pressure and parathyroid hormone levels in elderly women. *J Clin Endocrinol Metab*. 2001 Apr;86(4):1633-7

[533] McCarty MF. A preliminary fast may potentiate response to a subsequent low-salt, low-fat vegan diet in the management of hypertension - fasting as a strategy for breaking metabolic vicious cycles. *Med Hypotheses*. 2003 May;60(5):624-33

[534] Hyppönen E, Läärä E, Reunanen A, Järvelin MR, Virtanen SM. Intake of vitamin D and risk of type 1 diabetes: a birth-cohort study. *Lancet*. 2001 Nov 3;358(9292):1500-3

[535] Fuhrman J, Sarter B, Calabro DJ. Brief case reports of medically supervised, water-only fasting associated with remission of autoimmune disease. *Altern Ther Health Med*. 2002 Jul-Aug;8(4):112, 110-1

[536] Holick MF. Vitamin D deficiency: what a pain it is. *Mayo Clin Proc*. 2003 Dec;78(12):1457-9

[537] Fletcher RH, Fairfield KM. Vitamins for chronic disease prevention in adults: clinical applications. *JAMA*. 2002 Jun 19;287(23):3127-9

[538] Heaney RP. Long-latency deficiency disease: insights from calcium and vitamin D. *Am J Clin Nutr*. 2003 Nov;78(5):912-9

[539] Ames BN. The metabolic tune-up: metabolic harmony and disease prevention. *J Nutr*. 2003 May;133(5 Suppl 1):1544S-8S

[540] Heaney RP. Vitamin D, nutritional deficiency, and the medical paradigm. *J Clin Endocrinol Metab*. 2003 Nov;88(11):5107-8

[541] Fletcher RH, Fairfield KM. Vitamins for chronic disease prevention in adults: clinical applications. *JAMA*. 2002 Jun 19;287(23):3127-9

[542] Berg A. Sliding toward nutrition malpractice: time to reconsider and redeploy. *Am J Clin Nutr*. 1993 Jan;57(1):3-7

[543] Cobb DK, Warner D. Avoiding malpractice: the role of proper nutrition and wound management. *J Am Med Dir Assoc*. 2004 Jul-Aug;5(4 Sup):H11-6

and healthcare policy are influenced by a myriad of powerful private interests which are motivated by their own goals, at times different from the stated goals of medicine, which purports to hold paramount the patient's welfare. Scientific objectivity and the guiding ethical principles of informed consent, beneficence, autonomy, and non-malfeasance are subject to different interpretations depending upon the lens through which a dilemma is viewed. When this "dilemma" is the whole of healthcare, what first appears as order and structure now appears as the disarrayed tug-of-war between factions and private interests, with paradigmatic victory often being awarded to those with the best marketing campaigns and political influence with less importance given to safety, efficacy, and the economic burden to consumers.[544,545,546,547,548,549,550,551,552,553,554,555,556,557,558,559,560,561,562,563,564,565,566,567,568,569,570,571,572,573,574,575] To be ignorant of such considerations is to be blind to the nature of research, policy, and our own biased inclinations for and against particular paradigms, assessments, and interventions. Research articles and sources of authority must be approached with an artist's delicacy, and with a willingness to receive new information as worthy of preeminence over deeply rooted and well ensconced institutionalized fallacies.

Understanding the Multifaceted Nature of Disease Pathogenesis: The Functional Medicine Matrix as Paradigm and Clinical Tool: At its simplest and most practical level, the Functional Medicine Matrix is a teaching tool and clinical method that facilitates consideration of the different contributions of major intrinsic systems and

[544] Editorial. Drug-company influence on medical education in USA. *Lancet*. 2000 Sep 2;356(9232):781

[545] Horton R. Lotronex and the FDA: a fatal erosion of integrity. *Lancet*. 2001 May 19;357(9268):1544-5

[546] Editorial. Politics trumps science at the FDA. *Lancet*. 2005 Nov 26;366(9500):1827

[547] Topol EJ. Failing the public health--rofecoxib, Merck, and the FDA. *N Engl J Med*. 2004 Oct 21;351(17):1707-9

[548] Wolinsky H, Brune T. The Serpent on the Staff: The Unhealthy Politics of the American Medical Association. GP Putnam and Sons, New York, 1994

[549] Wilk CA. Medicine, Monopolies, and Malice: How the Medical Establishment Tried to Destroy Chiropractic. Garden City Park: Avery, 1996

[550] Carter JP. Racketeering in Medicine: The Suppression of Alternatives. Norfolk: Hampton Roads Pub; 1993

[551] National Alliance of Professional Psychology Providers. AMA Seeks To Control and Restrict Psychologist's Scope of Practice. http://www.nappp.org/scope.pdf Accessed November 25, 2006

[552] Daly R, American Psychiatric Association. AMA Forms Coalition to Thwart Non-M.D. Practice Expansion. *Psychiatric News* 2006 March; 41: 17

[553] Angell M. The Truth About the Drug Companies: How They Deceive Us and What to Do About it. Random House; August 2004

[554] Terrett AG. Misuse of the literature by medical authors in discussing spinal manipulative therapy injury. *J Manipulative Physiol Ther*. 1995 May;18(4):203-10

[555] Morley J, Rosner AL, Redwood D. A case study of misrepresentation of the scientific literature: recent reviews of chiropractic. *J Altern Complement Med*. 2001 Feb;7(1):65-78

[556] Wenban AB. Inappropriate use of the title 'chiropractor' and term 'chiropractic manipulation' in the peer-reviewed biomedical literature. *Chiropr Osteopat*. 2006 Aug 22;14:16

[557] Spivak JL. The Medical Trust Unmasked. Louis S. Siegfried Publishers; New York: 1961

[558] Trever W. In the Public Interest. Los Angeles; Scriptures Unlimited; 1972. This is probably the most authoritative documentation of the illegal actions of the AMA up to 1972; contains numerous photocopies of actual AMA documents and minutes of official meetings with overt intentionality of destroying Americans' healthcare options so that the AMA and related organizations would have a monopoly in healthcare.

[559] Getzendanner S. Permanent injunction order against AMA. *JAMA*. 1988 Jan 1;259(1):81-2

[560] "A national study released today reports 20 million American families — or one in seven families — faced hardships paying medical bills last year, which forced many to choose between getting medical attention or paying rent or buying food…" Freeman, Liz. 'Working poor' struggle to afford health care. *Naples Daily News*. Published in Naples, Florida and online at http://www.naplesnews.com/npdn/news/article/0,2071,NPDN_14940_3000546,00.html Accessed July 28, 2004

[561] "The USA's 5.8 million small companies… Health care costs are rising about 15% this year for those with fewer than 200 workers vs. 13.5% for those with 500 or more… But many small employers cite increases of 20% or more. That's made insurance the No. 1 small business problem…" Jim Hopkins. Health care tops taxes as small business cost drain. *USA TODAY*. http://www.usatoday.com/news/health/2003-04-20-small-business-costs_x.htm. Accessed July 28, 2004

[562] "Though the U.S. has slightly fewer doctors per capita than the typical developed nation, we have almost twice as many MRI machines and perform vastly more angioplasties. …at least 31 percent of all the incremental income we'll earn between 1999 and 2010 will go to health care." Pat Regnier, *Money Magazine*. Healthcare myth: We spend too much. October 13, 2003: 11:29 AM EDT http://money.cnn.com/2003/10/08/pf/health_myths_1/ Accessed Monday, July 12, 2004

[563] "Although they spend more on health care than patients in any other industrialized nation, Americans receive the right treatment less than 60 percent of the time, resulting in unnecessary pain, expense and even death…" Ceci Connolly. U.S. Patients Spend More but Don't Get More, Study Finds: Even in Advantaged Areas, Americans Often Receive Inadequate Health Care. *Washington Post*, May 5, 2004; Page A15. On-line at http://www.washingtonpost.com/ac2/wp-dyn/A1875-2004May4 accessed on July 28, 2004

[564] McGlynn EA, Asch SM, Adams J, Keesey J, Hicks J, DeCristofaro A, Kerr EA. The quality of health care delivered to adults in the United States. *N Engl J Med*. 2003 Jun 26;348(26):2635-45

[565] Brennan TA, Leape LL, Laird NM, Hebert L, Localio AR, Lawthers AG, Newhouse JP, Weiler PC, Hiatt HH. Incidence of adverse events and negligence in hospitalized patients: results of the Harvard Medical Practice Study I. 1991. *Qual Saf Health Care*. 2004 Apr;13(2):145-51; discuss 151-2

[566] "Basically, you die earlier and spend more time disabled if you're an American rather than a member of most other advanced countries." Christopher Murray MD PhD, Director of World Health Organization's Global Program on Evidence for Health Policy http://www.who.int/inf-pr-2000/en/pr2000-life.html Accessed July 12, 2004

[567] Shi L. Health care spending, delivery, and outcome in developed countries: a cross-national comparison. *Am J Med Qual* 1997;12(2):83-93

[568] Holland EG, Degruy FV. Drug-induced disorders. *Am Fam Physician*. 1997 Nov 1;56(7):1781-8, 1791-2

[569] Brennan TA, Leape LL, Laird NM, Hebert L, Localio AR, Lawthers AG, Newhouse JP, Weiler PC, Hiatt HH. Incidence of adverse events and negligence in hospitalized patients: results of the Harvard Medical Practice Study I. 1991. *Qual Saf Health Care*. 2004 Apr;13(2):145-51; discuss 151-2

[570] Whitaker R. The case against antipsychotic drugs: a 50-year record of doing more harm than good. *Med Hypotheses*. 2004;62(1):5-13

[571] The relevance of these citations is to show that the misuse of horse estrogens in humans as "hormone replacement therapy" exemplified the application of a strong carcinogen to millions of unsuspecting women: Zhang F, Chen Y, Pisha E, Shen L, Xiong Y, van Breemen RB, Bolton JL. The major metabolite of equilin, 4-hydroxyequilin, autoxidizes to an o-quinone which isomerizes to the potent cytotoxin 4-hydroxyequilenin-o-quinone. *Chem Res Toxicol*. 1999 Feb;12(2):204-13; Pisha E, Lui X, Constantinou AI, Bolton JL. Evidence that a metabolite of equine estrogens, 4-hydroxyequilenin, induces cellular transformation in vitro. *Chem Res Toxicol*. 2001;14(1):82-90; Zhang F, Swanson SM, van Breemen RB, Liu X, Yang Y, Gu C, Bolton JL. Equine estrogen metabolite 4-hydroxyequilenin induces DNA damage in the rat mammary tissues: formation of single-strand breaks, apurinic sites, stable adducts, and oxidized bases. *Chem Res Toxicol*. 2001 Dec;14(12):1654-9

[572] Newman NM, Ling RS. Acetabular bone destruction related to non-steroidal anti-inflammatory drugs. *Lancet*. 1985 Jul 6; 2(8445): 11-4

[573] "In 1983, 2876 people died from medication errors. … By 1993, this number had risen to 7,391 - a 2.57-fold increase." Phillips DP, Christenfeld N, Glynn LM. Increase in US medication-error deaths between 1983 and 1993. *Lancet*. 1998 Feb 28;351(9103):643-4

[574] Smith R. Medical journals are an extension of the marketing arm of pharmaceutical companies. *PLoS Med*. 2005 May;2(5):e138

[575] van der Steen WJ, Ho VK. Drugs versus diets: disillusions with Dutch health care. *Acta Biotheor*. 2001;49(2):125-40

extrinsic influences that are at play in a given disease process or individual patient. When viewed as a diagram, the web of influences can be appreciated to reveal the interconnected nature of influences and body systems and how imbalance or disruption in one area can lead to problems in another. Once homeostatic reserves and compensatory mechanisms are depleted, the patient experiences progressively worsening health (which may be asymptomatic) and the eventual manifestation of clinical disease.

Over the course of many years and discussions and reconsiderations, the faculty at IFM has elucidated eight preeminent systems or loci ("core clinical imbalances") for clinicians to consider when working with any chronic health disorder. These will be listed and described below with particular consideration of the topic of this monograph, which is neuromusculoskeletal pain and inflammation. Interested readers are directed to IFM's monograph series on topics such as "Depression" and "The Role of Gastrointestinal Inflammation in Systemic Disease" to see how this model is applied to disease states in different organ systems.

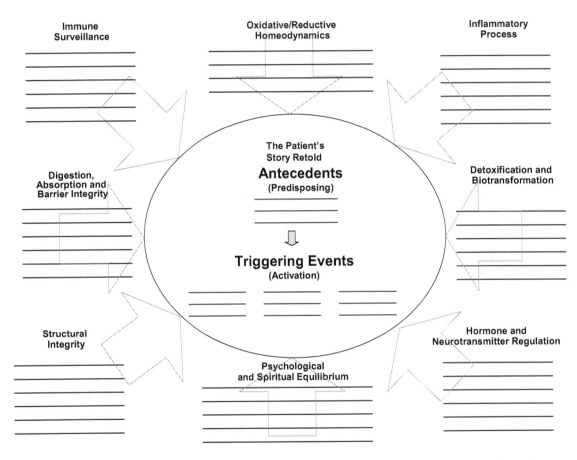

2008 rendering of The Functional Medicine Matrix: A concept, model, and clinical tool for evidence-based clinical care. Copyright Institute for Functional Medicine.

Exploring the Different Aspects of the Functional Medicine Matrix

1. Hormonal and neurotransmitter imbalances: While most clinicians are aware that neurotransmitters can either transmit pain signals or dampen their reception, many clinicians are not aware that neurotransmitter status is somewhat malleable and can be modulated with nutritional supplementation and botanical medicines. The examples that will be considered here are the tryptophan-serotonin-melatonin and the phenylalanine-tyrosine-dopamine-norepinephrine-epinephrine and enkephalin pathways.

   - Tryptophan and 5-hydroxytryptophan (5HTP) are prescription and nonprescription nutritional supplements that are the amino acid precursors for the formation of the neurotransmitter serotonin and, subsequently, the pineal hormone melatonin. Biochemically, these conversions are linear as follows: tryptophan → 5HTP → serotonin → melatonin. Tryptophan depletion and low levels of serotonin are consistently associated with depression, anxiety, exacerbation of eating disorders, and increased sensitivity to acute and chronic pain. Serotonergic pathways are impaired by chronic stress due to increased utilization of serotonin (e.g., serotonin-dependent cortisol release) and increased hepatic degradation of tryptophan by cortisol-stimulated tryptophan pyrrolase.[576] Therapeutically, supplementation with 5HTP augments serotonin and melatonin synthesis and has specific applicability in the alleviation of depression and pain syndromes such as fibromyalgia and headache, including migraine, tension headaches, and juvenile headaches.[577,578] Certainly part of the benefit from 5HTP supplementation is derived from the increased formation of melatonin, as the biological effects of melatonin extend beyond its sleep-promoting role to include powerful antioxidation, anti-infective immunostimulation[579], and preservation of mitochondrial function, a benefit which is of particular relevance to the treatment of fibromyalgia.[580]

- The conditionally essential fatty acids found in fish oil modulate serotonergic and adrenergic activity in the human brain[581], and given the role of serotonin and norepinephrine in the central processing of pain perception[582], a reasonable hypothesis holds that the pain-relieving activity of fish oil supplementation[583] is partly due to central modulation of pain perception and is not wholly due to modulation of eicosanoid production and inflammatory mediator transcription as previously believed.

- Vitamin D3 supplementation may also augment serotonergic activity[584], and this mechanism may partly explain the mood-enhancing and pain-relieving benefits of vitamin D3 supplementation. Attentive readers will note that this brief discussion has already begun to bridge the gaps between nutritional status, neurotransmitter synthesis, pain sensitivity, immune function, and mitochondrial bioenergetics.

- Supplementation with DL-phenylalanine (DLPA; racemic mixture of D- and L-forms of the amino acid phenylalanine derived from synthetic production) has long been used in the treatment of pain and depression.[585] The nutritional L-isomer is converted from phenylalanine to tyrosine to L-dopa to dopamine to norepinephrine and epinephrine. Augmentation of this pathway promotes resistance to fatigue, depression, and pain. The synthetic D-isomer augments pain-relieving enkephalin function by inhibiting enkephalin degradation by the enzyme carboxypeptidase A (enkephalinase); the resultant augmentation of enkephalin levels is generally believed to underlie the analgesic and mood-enhancing benefits of DLPA supplementation.

- Therapeutic massage is yet another means to modulate neurotransmitter synthesis for the alleviation of pain. In a study of patients with chronic back pain, massage increased serotonin and dopamine levels (measured in urine).[586]

Hormonal imbalances are particularly relevant to the discussion of chronic pain caused by inflammation characteristic of autoimmune diseases such as rheumatoid arthritis (RA). Often clinically subtle but nonetheless of extreme importance, these hormonal influences on painful inflammation are worthy of their own detailed discussion and thus will be reviewed later in this monograph in the context of the prototypic inflammatory disease RA. Generally speaking and with a few noted exceptions (such as Sjogren's syndrome), the research literature points to a specific pattern of hormonal imbalances among patients with autoimmunity, and this pattern is consistent with the proinflammatory and

[576] Sandyk R. Tryptophan availability and the susceptibility to stress in multiple sclerosis: a hypothesis. *Int J Neurosci*. 1996 Jul;86(1-2):47-53

[577] Turner EH, Loftis JM, Blackwell AD. Serotonin a la carte: supplementation with the serotonin precursor 5-hydroxytryptophan. *Pharmacol Ther*. 2006 Mar;109(3):325-38

[578] Birdsall TC. 5-Hydroxytryptophan: a clinically-effective serotonin precursor. *Altern Med Rev*. 1998 Aug;3(4):271-80

[579] Gitto E, Karbownik M, Reiter RJ, Tan DX, Cuzzocrea S, Chiurazzi P, Cordaro S, Corona G, Trimarchi G, Barberi I. Effects of melatonin treatment in septic newborns. *Pediatr Res*. 2001 Dec;50(6):756-60

[580] Acuna-Castroviejo D, Escames G, Reiter RJ. Melatonin therapy in fibromyalgia. *J Pineal Res*. 2006 Jan;40(1):98-9

[581] Hibbeln JR, Ferguson TA, Blasbalg TL. Omega-3 fatty acid deficiencies in neurodevelopment, aggression and autonomic dysregulation: opportunities for intervention. *Int Rev Psychiatry*. 2006 Apr;18(2):107-18

[582] Wise TN, Fishbain DA, Holder-Perkins V. Painful physical symptoms in depression: a clinical challenge. *Pain Med*. 2007 Sep;8 Suppl 2:S75-82

[583] Goldberg RJ, Katz J. A meta-analysis of the analgesic effects of omega-3 polyunsaturated fatty acid supplementation for inflammatory joint pain. *Pain*. 2007;129(1-2):210-23

[584] Lansdowne AT, Provost SC. Vitamin D3 enhances mood in healthy subjects during winter. *Psychopharmacology* (Berl). 1998 Feb;135(4):319-23

[585] Russell AL, McCarty MF. DL-phenylalanine markedly potentiates opiate analgesia - an example of nutrient/pharmaceutical up-regulation of the endogenous analgesia system. *Med Hypotheses*. 2000 Oct;55(4):283-8

[586] Hernandez-Reif M, Field T, Krasnegor J, Theakston H. Lower back pain is reduced and range of motion increased after massage therapy. *Int J Neurosci* 2001;106(3-4):131-45

immunodysregulatory effects of estrogens and prolactin and the anti-inflammatory and immunomodulatory effects of cortisol, dehydroepiandrosterone (DHEA), and testosterone. Patients with autoimmune neuromusculoskeletal inflammation generally display a complete or partial pattern of hormonal disturbances typified by elevated estrogen and prolactin and lowered testosterone, DHEA, and cortisol; appropriate therapeutic correction of these imbalances can safely result in disease amelioration. Rectification of endocrinologic imbalances ("orthoendocrinology") will be discussed in the section on RA and has been detailed with broader clinical applicability elsewhere by this author.[587]

2. Oxidation-reduction imbalances and mitochondropathy: Oxidative stress results from the chronic systemic inflammation seen in painful inflammatory disorders such as RA, and oxidative stress contributes to the perpetuation and exacerbation of inflammatory diseases via expedited tissue destruction and alterations in gene transcription and resultant enhancement of inflammatory mediator production.[588] Immune activation increases production of reactive oxygen species (ROS; "free radicals"), and oxidant stress increases activation of pro-inflammatory transcription factors (such as nuclear factor KappaB, NFkB) and also increases spontaneous oxidative modification of endogenous proteins such as cartilage matrix which then undergoes expedited degradation or immunologic attack; thus a vicious cycle of oxidation and inflammation exacerbates and perpetuates various inflammation-associated diseases, resulting in therapeutic recalcitrance and autonomous disease progression.[589,590] A rational clinical approach to breaking this vicious pathogenic cycle can include simultaneous antioxidation and immunomodulation, the former with diet optimization and nutritional supplementation and the latter with allergen avoidance, hormonal correction, xenobiotic detoxification, and specific phytonutritional modulation of pro-inflammatory pathways. Severe and acute inflammation can and often should be suppressed pharmacologically, but sole reliance on pharmacologic immunosuppression leaves the patient vulnerable to iatrogenic immunosuppression and the well-known increased risk for cardiovascular disease, infection, and clinical malignancy while failing to address the underlying biochemical and immunologic imbalances which lie at the bottom of all chronic inflammatory and autoimmune diseases. The contribution of mitochondrial dysfunction to chronic recurrent or persistent pain is most plainly demonstrated in migraine and fibromyalgia (discussed later in this monograph). An important characteristic of migraine is mitochondrial dysfunction, the severity of which correlates positively with the severity of the headache syndrome.[591] In fibromyalgia, numerous abnormalities in cellular bioenergetics are noted, which correlate clinically with the lowered lactate threshold, persistent muscle pain, reduced functional capacity, and the subjective fatigue that characterize the disorder.[592] Nutritional preservation and enhancement of mitochondrial function was termed "mitochondrial resuscitation" by Jeffrey Bland PhD in the 1990s, and clinical implementation of such an approach generally includes, in addition to diet and lifestyle modification, supplementation with coenzyme Q-10, niacin, riboflavin, thiamin, lipoic acid, magnesium, and other nutrients and botanical medicines which enhance production of adenosine triphosphate (ATP).[593]

3. Detoxification and biotransformational imbalances: As our environment becomes increasingly polluted and as researchers and clinicians mature and expand their appreciation and knowledge of the adverse effects of xenobiotics (toxic metals and chemicals), healthcare providers will need to attend to their patients' detoxification capacity and xenobiotic load as a component of the prevention and treatment of disease. By now, senior students and practicing clinicians should be aware of the association of xenobiotics in prototypic diseases such as Parkinson's disease[594,595], adult-onset diabetes mellitus[596,597,598,599],

[587] Vasquez A. _Integrative Rheumatology_. Fort Worth, Texas; Integrative & Biological Medicine Research & Consulting, 2007 OptimalHealthResearch.com
[588] Hitchon CA, El-Gabalawy HS. Oxidation in rheumatoid arthritis. _Arthritis Res Ther_. 2004;6(6):265-78
[589] Tak PP, Zvaifler NJ, Green DR, Firestein GS. Rheumatoid arthritis and p53: how oxidative stress might alter the course of inflammatory diseases. _Immunol Today_. 2000 Feb;21(2):78-82
[590] Kurien BT, Hensley K, Bachmann M, Scofield RH. Oxidatively modified autoantigens in autoimmune diseases. _Free Radic Biol Med_. 2006 Aug 15;41(4):549-56
[591] Lodi R, Kemp GJ, Montagna P, Pierangeli G, Cortelli P, Iotti S, Radda GK, Barbiroli B. Quantitative analysis of skeletal muscle bioenergetics and proton efflux in migraine and cluster headache. _J Neurol Sci_. 1997 Feb 27;146(1):73-80
[592] Park JH, Phothimat P, Oates CT, Hernanz-Schulman M, Olsen NJ. Use of P-31 magnetic resonance spectroscopy to detect metabolic abnormalities in muscles of patients with fibromyalgia. _Arthritis Rheum_. 1998 Mar;41(3):406-13
[593] Pieczenik SR, Neustadt J. Mitochondrial dysfunction and molecular pathways of disease. _Exp Mol Pathol_. 2007 Aug;83(1):84-92
[594] Corrigan FM, Wienburg CL, Shore RF, Daniel SE, Mann D. Organochlorine insecticides in substantia nigra in Parkinson's disease. _J Toxicol Environ Health A_. 2000 Feb 25;59(4):229-34
[595] Fleming L, Mann JB, Bean J, Briggle T, Sanchez-Ramos JR. Parkinson's disease and brain levels of organochlorine pesticides. _Ann Neurol_. 1994 Jul;36(1):100-3

and attention-deficit hyperactivity disorder.[600,601,602] The role of xenobiotic exposure and impaired detoxification in neuromusculoskeletal pain and inflammatory disorders is more subtle and is generally mediated through the resultant immunotoxicity that manifests as autoimmunity. Occasionally, clinicians will encounter patients with musculoskeletal symptomatology that defies standard diagnosis and treatment but which responds remarkably and permanently to empiric clinical detoxification treatment; such a case will be presented in the Case Reports later in this monograph. The numerous roles of xenobiotic exposure in the genesis and perpetuation of chronic health problems and the role of clinical detoxification in the treatment of such problems has been detailed elsewhere by Crinnion[603,604,605,606,607], Rea[608], Bland[609,610], Vasquez[611,612], and others.[613,614]

4. <u>Immune imbalances</u>: Immune imbalances have an obvious role in musculoskeletal inflammation when discussed in the context of autoimmune diseases such as rheumatoid arthritis, ankylosing spondylitis, and systemic lupus erythematosus. While the standard medical approach to this pathophysiology has focused almost exclusively on the pharmacologic suppression of resultant inflammation and tissue destruction, other disciplines such as naturopathic medicine and functional medicine have emphasized the importance of determining and addressing the underlying causes of such immune imbalance. While clinicians of all disciplines must appreciate the important role of pharmacologic immunosuppression in the treatment of inflammatory exacerbations as seen with giant cell arteritis or neuropsychiatric lupus, they should also appreciate that sole reliance on immunosuppression for long-term management of inflammatory disorders is destined to therapeutic failure insofar as it does not correct the underlying cause of the disease and creates dependency upon perpetual immunosuppression with its attendant costs (not uncommonly in the range of $20,000 - 50,000 per year) and adverse effects including infection and increased risk for cancer. Rather than presuming that immune dysfunction and the resultant inflammation and autoimmunity are results of spontaneous generation, astute clinicians seek to identify and correct the causes of these immune imbalances. By identifying and correcting the underlying causes of immune imbalance (when possible), clinicians can lessen or obviate the need for chronic polypharmaceutical treatment with anti-inflammatory and immunosuppressive agents. Vasquez[615] proposed that secondary immune imbalances (distinguished from primary congenital disorders) generally arise from one or more of five main problems: ❶ habitual consumption of a pro-inflammatory diet, ❷ food allergies and intolerances, ❸ microbial dysbiosis, including multifocal polydysbiosis, ❹ hormonal imbalances, and ❺ xenobiotic exposure and accumulation resulting in immunotoxicity via bystander activation and enhanced processing of autoantigens as well as haptenization and neoantigen formation. These influences may act singularly or when combined may be additive and synergistic. While

[596] Fujiyoshi PT, Michalek JE, Matsumura F. Molecular epidemiologic evidence for diabetogenic effects of dioxin exposure in U.S. Air force veterans of the Vietnam war. *Environ Health Perspect*, 2006 Nov;114(11):1677-83

[597] Lee DH, Lee IK, Song K, Steffes M, Toscano W, Baker BA, Jacobs DR Jr. A strong dose-response relation between serum concentrations of persistent organic pollutants and diabetes: results from the National Health and Examination Survey 1999-2002. *Diabetes Care* 2006 Jul;29(7):1638-44

[598] Lee DH, Lee IK, Jin SH, Steffes M, Jacobs DR Jr. Association between serum concentrations of persistent organic pollutants and insulin resistance among nondiabetic adults: results from the National Health and Nutrition Examination Survey 1999-2002. *Diabetes Care*, 2007 Mar;30(3):622-8

[599] Remillard RB, Bunce NJ. Linking dioxins to diabetes: epidemiology and biologic plausibility. *Environ Health Perspect*, 2002 Sep;110(9):853-8

[600] Rauh VA, Garfinkel R, Perera FP, Andrews HF, Hoepner L, Barr DB, Whitehead R, Tang D, Whyatt RW. Impact of prenatal chlorpyrifos exposure on neurodevelopment in the first 3 years of life among inner-city children. *Pediatrics*. 2006 Dec;118(6):e1845-59

[601] Cheuk DK, Wong V. Attention-deficit hyperactivity disorder and blood mercury level: a case-control study in Chinese children. *Neuropediatrics*. 2006 Aug;37(4):234-40

[602] Nigg JT, Knottnerus GM, Martel MM, Nikolas M, Cavanagh K, Karmaus W, Rappley MD. Low blood lead levels associated with clinically diagnosed attention-deficit/hyperactivity disorder and mediated by weak cognitive control. *Biol Psychiatry*. 2008 Feb 1;63(3):325-31

[603] Crinnion W. Results of a Decade of Naturopathic Treatment for Environmental Illnesses: A Review of Clinical Records. *J Naturopathic Medicine* vol. 7; 2, 21-27

[604] Crinnion WJ. Environmental medicine, part 1: the human burden of environmental toxins and their common health effects. *Altern Med Rev*. 2000 Feb;5(1):52-63

[605] Crinnion WJ. Environmental medicine, part 2 - health effects of and protection from ubiquitous airborne solvent exposure. *Altern Med Rev*. 2000 Apr;5(2):133-43

[606] Crinnion WJ. Environmental medicine, part 3: long-term effects of chronic low-dose mercury exposure. *Altern Med Rev*. 2000 Jun;5(3):209-23

[607] Crinnion WJ. Environmental medicine, part 4: pesticides - biologically persistent and ubiquitous toxins. *Altern Med Rev*. 2000 Oct;5(5):432-47

[608] Rea WJ, Pan Y, Johnson AR. Clearing of toxic volatile hydrocarbons from humans. *Bol Asoc Med P R*. 1991 Jul;83(7):321-4

[609] Bland JS, Barrager E, Reedy RG, Bland K. A Medical Food-Supplemented Detoxification Program in the Management of Chronic Health Problems. *Altern Ther Health Med*. 1995 Nov 1;1(5):62-71

[610] Minich DM, Bland JS. Acid-alkaline balance: role in chronic disease and detoxification. *Altern Ther Health Med*. 2007 Jul-Aug;13(4):62-5

[611] Vasquez A. *Integrative Rheumatology: Second Edition*. Fort Worth, Texas; Integrative and Biological Medicine Research and Consulting, 2007 OptimalHealthResearch.com

[612] Vasquez A. Diabetes: Are Toxins to Blame? *Naturopathy Digest* 2007; April

[613] Kilburn KH, Warsaw RH, Shields MG. Neurobehavioral dysfunction in firemen exposed to polycholorinated biphenyls (PCBs): possible improvement after detoxification. *Arch Environ Health*. 1989 Nov-Dec;44(6):345-50

[614] Cecchini M, LoPresti V. Drug residues store in the body following cessation of use: impacts on neuroendocrine balance and behavior--use of the Hubbard sauna regimen to remove toxins and restore health. *Med Hypotheses*. 2007;68(4):868-79

[615] **Vasquez A**. *Integrative Rheumatology: Second Edition*. Fort Worth, Texas; Integrative and Biological Medicine Research and Consulting, 2007 OptimalHealthResearch.com

it is beyond the scope of this monograph to detail each of these here, they will be sufficiently reviewed in later sections dealing with assessment and interventions as well as in the clinical focus subsections, particularly the section on rheumatoid arthritis.

5. <u>Inflammatory imbalances</u>: Inflammatory imbalances may be distinguished from immune imbalances insofar as inflammatory imbalances connote disorders of inflammatory mediator production in the absence of the immunodysfunction that typifies allergy, autoimmunity, or immunosuppression. Here again, long-term consumption of a pro-inflammatory diet[616] is a primary consideration because such a diet typically oversupplies inflammatory precursors such as arachidonate and undersupplies anti-inflammatory phytonutrients such as vitamin D, zinc, selenium, and the numerous phytochemicals that reduce activation of inflammatory pathways.[617,618,619,620] Three of the best examples of correctable inflammatory imbalances are those due to vitamin D deficiency, fatty acid imbalances, and overconsumption of simple sugars and saturated fats. Vitamin D deficiency is a widespread and serious health problem that spans nearly all geographic regions and socioeconomic strata with several important adverse effects. Vitamin D deficiency results in systemic inflammation[621] and chronic musculoskeletal pain[622] which both resolve quickly upon correction of the nutritional deficiency. Similarly and consistent with the Western/American pattern of dietary intake, overconsumption of alpha-linoleic acid and arachidonate along with underconsumption of alpha-linolenic acid (ALA), gamma-linolenic acid (GLA), eicosapentaenoic acid (EPA), docosahexaenoic acid (DHA), and oleic acid subtly yet powerfully shift nutrigenomic tendency and precursor availability in favor of enhanced systemic inflammation. Correction of this imbalance such as with reduced consumption of arachidonate and increased consumption of EPA and DHA has consistently proven to be of significant clinical value in the management of chronic inflammatory disorders.[623,624] Measurable increases in systemic inflammation and oxidative stress follow glucose challenge[625], consumption of saturated fatty acids as found in cream[626], and consumption of a "fast food" breakfast, which triggers the prototypic inflammatory activator NF-kappaB for enhanced production of inflammatory mediators.[627] This triad (vitamin D deficiency, fatty acid imbalance, and overconsumption of sugars and saturated fats) is typical of the Western/American pattern of dietary intake, and the molecular means and clinical consequences of such dietary choices is quite clear, evidenced by burgeoning epidemics of metabolic and inflammatory diseases.

6. <u>Digestive, absorptive, and microbiological imbalances</u>: The grouping of digestive and absorptive considerations suggests that the alimentary tract and its accessory organs of the liver, gall bladder and pancreas will be the focus of these core clinical imbalances, and the addition of microbiological imbalances should remind current clinicians that gastrointestinal dysbiosis is an important and frequent clinical consideration. Impaired digestion begins neither in the stomach nor in the mouth, but it stems rather from any socioeconomic milieu which deprives people of the means to prepare wholesome health-promoting meals and the time to consume those meals in a relaxed parasympathetic-dominant mode, preferably among good company, stimulating conversation, and appropriate ambiance. Poor dentition, xerostomia, hypochlorhydria, cholestasis or cholecystectomy, pancreatic insufficiency, mucosal atrophy,

---

[616] Seaman DR. The diet-induced proinflammatory state: a cause of chronic pain and other degenerative diseases? *J Manipulative Physiol Ther*. 2002 Mar-Apr;25(3):168-79

[617] **Vasquez A**. Reducing Pain and Inflammation Naturally. Part 1: New Insights into Fatty Acid Biochemistry and the Influence of Diet. *Nutritional Perspectives* 2004; October: 5, 7-10, 12, 14

[618] **Vasquez A**. Reducing Pain and Inflammation Naturally. Part 2: New Insights into Fatty Acid Supplementation and Its Effect on Eicosanoid Production and Genetic Expression. *Nutritional Perspectives* 2005; January: 5-16

[619] **Vasquez A**. Reducing pain and inflammation naturally - Part 3: Improving overall health while safely and effectively treating musculoskeletal pain. *Nutritional Perspectives* 2005; 28: 34-38, 40-42

[620] **Vasquez A**. Reducing pain and inflammation naturally - Part 4: Nutritional and Botanical Inhibition of NF-kappaB, the Major Intracellular Amplifier of the Inflammatory Cascade. A Practical Clinical Strategy Exemplifying Anti-Inflammatory Nutrigenomics. *Nutritional Perspectives* 2005;July: 5-12

[621] Timms PM, Mannan N, Hitman GA, Noonan K, Mills PG, Syndercombe-Court D, Aganna E, Price CP, Boucher BJ. Circulating MMP9, vitamin D and variation in the TIMP-1 response with VDR genotype: mechanisms for inflammatory damage in chronic disorders? *QJM*. 2002 Dec;95(12):787-96

[622] Al Faraj S, Al Mutairi K. Vitamin D deficiency and chronic low back pain in Saudi Arabia. *Spine*. 2003 Jan 15;28(2):177-9

[623] James MJ, Gibson RA, Cleland LG. Dietary polyunsaturated fatty acids and inflammatory mediator production. *Am J Clin Nutr*. 2000 Jan;71(1 Suppl):343S-8S

[624] James MJ, Proudman SM, Cleland LG. Dietary n-3 fats as adjunctive therapy in a prototypic inflammatory disease: issues and obstacles for use in rheumatoid arthritis. Prostaglandins *Leukot Essent Fatty Acids*. 2003 Jun;68(6):399-405

[625] Mohanty P, Hamouda W, Garg R, Aljada A, Ghanim H, Dandona P. Glucose challenge stimulates reactive oxygen species (ROS) generation by leucocytes. *J Clin Endocrinol Metab*. 2000 Aug;85(8):2970-3

[626] Mohanty P, Ghanim H, Hamouda W, Aljada A, Garg R, Dandona P. Both lipid and protein intakes stimulate increased generation of reactive oxygen species by polymorphonuclear leukocytes and mononuclear cells. *Am J Clin Nutr*. 2002 Apr;75(4):767-72

[627] Aljada A, Mohanty P, Ghanim H, Abdo T, Tripathy D, Chaudhuri A, Dandona P. Increase in intranuclear nuclear factor kappaB and decrease in inhibitor kappaB in mononuclear cells after a mixed meal: evidence for a proinflammatory effect. *Am J Clin Nutr*. 2004 Apr;79(4):682-90

altered gut motility, and bacterial overgrowth of the small bowel are important and common contributors to impaired digestion and absorption; clinicians should consider these frequently and implement treatment with a low threshold for intervention. The relevance of these problems to pain and the musculoskeletal system is generally that of malnutrition and its macro- and micronutrient consequences. Sunlight-deprived individuals must rely on dietary sources of vitamin D, which are hardly adequate for the prevention of overt deficiency; any impairment in digestion, emulsification, or absorption of this fat-soluble vitamin can readily lead to hypovitaminosis D and its resultant musculoskeletal consequences of osteomalacia and unremitting pain.[628] Consumption of foods to which the individual is sensitized ("food allergies") can trigger migraine and other chronic headaches[629,630] as well as generalized musculoskeletal pain and arthritis.[631,632,633.] Avoidance of the offending foods often results in amelioration or complete remission of the painful syndrome at low cost and high efficacy without reliance on expensive or potentially harmful or addictive pain-reliving drugs. Occasionally, gluten enteropathy (celiac disease) presents with arthritic pain and chronic synovitis; the pain and inflammation remit on a gluten-free diet.[634] Alterations in intestinal microbial balance or an individual's unique response to endogenous bacteria (i.e., dysbiosis) can lead to systemic inflammation, arthritis, vasculitis, and musculoskeletal pain; clinical nuances and molecular mechanisms of gastrointestinal dysbiosis will be surveyed later in this monograph based on a previous review by Vasquez.[635] Clinicians should appreciate that dysbiosis can occur at sites other than the gastrointestinal tract, most importantly the nasopharynx and genitourinary tracts. Eradication of the occult infection or mucosal colonization often results in marked reductions in systemic inflammation and its clinical complications. Interested readers are directed to the excellent review by Noah[636] on the relevance of dysbiosis and its treatment relative to psoriasis; additional citations and clinical applications will be discussed later in this monograph.

7. <u>Structural imbalances from cellular membrane function to the musculoskeletal system</u>: Molecular structural imbalances lie at the heart of the concept of "biochemical individuality" originated by Roger J. Williams[637] in 1956, and this concept was soon thereafter expanded into the theory and practice of "orthomolecular medicine" pioneered by Linus Pauling and colleagues.[638,639] Pauling is considered by many authorities to be the original source of the concept of molecular medicine because he coined the phrase "molecular disease" after his team's discovery in 1949 that sickle cell anemia resulted from a single amino acid substitution that caused physical deformation of the hemoglobin molecule in hypoxic conditions.[640] (One of Pauling's students, Jeffery Bland, continued this legacy with the organization of "functional medicine" which now lives on as the Institute for Functional Medicine.[641]) Single nucleotide polymorphisms (SNP; pronounced "snip") are DNA sequence variations that can result in amino acid substitutions that render the final protein (e.g., structural protein or enzyme) abnormal in structure and therefore function. This aberrancy may or may not cause clinical disease (depending on the severity and importance of the variation), and consequences of the dysfunction may be occult, subtle, or obvious. One of the most powerful and effective means for treating diseases resultant from SNPs that result in enzyme defects is the use of high-dose vitamin supplementation, and this forms the scientific basis for "mega-vitamin therapy" as elegantly and authoritatively reviewed by Bruce Ames, et al.[642] SNP-induced

[628] Basha B, Rao DS, Han ZH, Parfitt AM. Osteomalacia due to vitamin D depletion: a neglected consequence of intestinal malabsorption. *Am J Med*. 2000 Mar;108(4):296-300

[629] Grant EC. Food allergies and migraine. *Lancet*. 1979 May 5;1(8123):966-9

[630] Millichap JG, Yee MM. The diet factor in pediatric and adolescent migraine. *Pediatr Neurol*. 2003 Jan;28(1):9-15

[631] van de Laar MA, Aalbers M, Bruins FG, et al. Food intolerance in rheumatoid arthritis. II. Clinical and histological aspects. *Ann Rheum Dis*. 1992 ;51(3):303-6

[632] Golding DN. Is there an allergic synovitis? *J R Soc Med*. 1990 May;83(5):312-4

[633] Hvatum M, Kanerud L, Hällgren R, Brandtzaeg P. The gut-joint axis: cross reactive food antibodies in rheumatoid arthritis. *Gut*. 2006 Sep;55:1240-7

[634] Bourne JT, Kumar P, Huskisson EC, Mageed R, Unsworth DJ, Wojtulewski JA. Arthritis and coeliac disease. *Ann Rheum Dis*. 1985 Sep;44(9):592-8

[635] **Vasquez A**. Reducing Pain and Inflammation Naturally. Part 6: Nutritional and Botanical Treatments Against "Silent Infections" and Gastrointestinal Dysbiosis, Commonly Overlooked Causes of Neuromusculoskeletal Inflammation and Chronic Health Problems. *Nutr Perspect* 2006; Jan: 5-21

[636] Noah PW. The role of microorganisms in psoriasis. *Semin Dermatol*. 1990 Dec;9(4):269-76

[637] Williams RJ. Biochemical Individuality : The Basis for the Genetotrophic Concept. Austin and London: University of Texas Press, 1956. Page x

[638] Pauling L. On the Orthomolecular Environment of the Mind: Orthomolecular Theory. In: Williams RJ, Kalita DK. A Physician's Handbook on Orthomolecular Medicine. New Cannan; Keats Publishing; 1977. Page 76

[639] Pauling L, Robinson AB, Teranishi R, Cary P. Quantitative analysis of urine vapor and breath by gas-liquid partition chromatography. *Proc Natl Acad Sci U S A*. 1971 Oct;68(10):2374-6

[640] Pauling L, Itano HA, Singer SJ, Wells IC. Sickle cell anemia, a molecular disease. *Science*. 1949 Nov 25;110(2865):543-8

[641] Bland JS. Jeffrey S. Bland, PhD, FACN, CNS: functional medicine pioneer. *Altern Ther Health Med*. 2004 Sep-Oct;10(5):74-81

[642] Ames BN, Elson-Schwab I, Silver EA. High-dose vitamin therapy stimulates variant enzymes with decreased coenzyme binding affinity (increased K(m)): relevance to genetic disease and polymorphisms. *Am J Clin Nutr*. 2002 Apr;75(4):616-58

alterations in enzyme structure reduce affinity for vitamin-derived coenzyme binding; this reduced affinity can be "overpowered" by administration of high doses of the required vitamin cofactor to increase tissue concentrations of the nutrient to promote binding of the enzyme with its ligand for the performance of enzymatic function. Thus, the scientific rationale for nutritional therapy is derived in part from the recognition that altered enzymatic function due to altered enzyme structure can often be corrected by administration of supradietary doses of nutrients. Relatedly, the structure and function of cell membranes is determined by their composition, which is influenced by dietary intake of fatty acids, and which influences production prostaglandins and leukotrienes. This is an important aspect of the scientific rationale for the use of specific fatty acid supplements in the prevention and treatment of painful inflammatory musculoskeletal disease. Cell membrane structure and function can also be altered by systemic oxidative stress; the concomitant alterations in intracellular ions (e.g., calcium) and receptor function along with activation of transcription factors such as NF-kappaB contribute to widespread physiologic impairment which creates a vicious cycle of inflammation, metabolic disturbance, and additional free radical generation.[643,644] Somatic dysfunction, musculoskeletal disorders, and inefficient biomechanics contribute to pain, increased production of inflammatory mediators, and the expedited degeneration of tissues such as collagen and cartilage matrix. Physicians trained in clinical biomechanics and physical medicine appreciate the subtle nuances of musculoskeletal structure-function relationships and address these problems directly with physical and manual means rather than ignoring the physical problem and only treating its biochemical sequelae. While biomechanics, palpatory diagnosis, and manual therapeutics takes years of diligent study for the achievement of proficiency, some of these concepts will be reviewed later in this monograph, particularly in the section on chronic low back pain.

8. Psychological and Spiritual Equilibrium: The connections between physical pain and psychoemotional status and events is worthy of thorough discussion and not merely for the sake of improving upon outdated clinical practices which have typically marginalized these ethereal considerations or considered them only long enough to substantiate psychopharmaceutical intervention. A survey of the literature makes clear the interconnected nature of pain, inflammation, psychoemotional stress, depression, social isolation, and nutritional status; due to space limitations in this monograph, a brief overview must necessarily suffice for the exemplification of representative concepts. Stressful and depressive life events promote the development, persistence, and exacerbation of disorders of pain and inflammation through nutritional, hormonal, immunologic, oxidative, and microbiologic mechanisms. Stated most simply, the perception of stressful events and the resultant neurohormonal cascade results in expedited metabolic utilization and increased urinary excretion of nutrients (e.g., tryptophan , and zinc, magnesium, retinol, respectively) which sum to effect nutritional imbalances and depletion, particularly when the stress response is severe and prolonged.[645,646,647] Specific to the consideration of pain, the depletion of tryptophan (and thus serotonin and melatonin) leaves the patient vulnerable to increased pain from lack of antinociceptive serotonin and to increased inflammation due to impaired endogenous production of anti-inflammatory cortisol, the adrenal release of which requires serotonin-dependent stimulation.[648] Severe stress, inflammation, and drugs used to suppress immune-mediated tissue damage (e.g., cyclosporine) increase urinary excretion of magnesium[649], and the eventual magnesium depletion renders the patient more vulnerable to hyperalgesia, depression, and other central nervous system and psychiatric disorders.[650,651] Furthermore, experimental and clinical data have shown that magnesium deficiency leads to a systemic pro-inflammatory state associated with oxidative stress and increased levels of the

[643] Evans JL, Maddux BA, Goldfine ID. The molecular basis for oxidative stress-induced insulin resistance. *Antioxid Redox Signal.* 2005 Jul-Aug;7(7-8):1040-52

[644] Joseph JA, Denisova N, Fisher D, Shukitt-Hale B, Bickford P, Prior R, Cao G. Membrane and receptor modifications of oxidative stress vulnerability in aging. Nutritional considerations. *Ann N Y Acad Sci.* 1998 Nov 20;854:268-76

[645] Stephensen CB, Alvarez JO, Kohatsu J, Hardmeier R, Kennedy JI Jr, Gammon RB Jr. Vitamin A is excreted in the urine during acute infection. *Am J Clin Nutr.* 1994 Sep;60(3):388-92

[646] Ingenbleek Y, Bernstein L. The stressful condition as a nutritionally dependent adaptive dichotomy. *Nutrition.* 1999 Apr;15(4):305-20

[647] Henrotte JG, Plouin PF, Lévy-Leboyer C, Moser G, Sidoroff-Girault N, Franck G, Santarromana M, Pineau M. Blood and urinary magnesium, zinc, calcium, free fatty acids, and catecholamines in type A and type B subjects. *J Am Coll Nutr.* 1985;4(2):165-72

[648] Sandyk R. Tryptophan availability and the susceptibility to stress in multiple sclerosis: a hypothesis. *Int J Neurosci.* 1996 Jul;86(1-2):47-53

[649] DiPalma JR. Magnesium replacement therapy. *Am Fam Physician.* 1990 Jul;42(1):173-6

[650] Murck H. Magnesium and affective disorders. *Nutr Neurosci.* 2002 Dec;5(6):375-89

[651] Hashizume N, Mori M. An analysis of hypermagnesemia and hypomagnesemia. *Jpn J Med.* 1990 Jul-Aug;29(4):368-72

nociceptive and proinflammatory neurotransmitter substance P.[652] Stress increases secretion of prolactin, a hormone which plays an important pathogenic role in chronic inflammation and autoimmunity.[653,654] An abundance of experimental and clinical research supports the model that chronic psychoemotional stress reduces mucosal immunity, increases intestinal permeability, and allows for increased intestinal colonization by microbes that then stimulate immune responses that cross-react with musculoskeletal tissues and result in the clinical manifestation of autoimmunity and painful rheumatic syndromes which appear clinically as variants of acute and chronic reactive arthritis (formerly Reiter' syndrome[655]) in susceptible patients.[656,657,658,659,660,661,662,663] Very interestingly, certain intestinal bacteria can sense when their human host is stressed, and they take advantage of the situation by becoming more virulent whereas previously these same bacteria may have been incapable of causing disease.[664,665] Psychoemotional stress also reduces mucosal immunity and increases colonization in locations other than the gastrointestinal tract. Microbial colonization of the genitourinary tract ("genitourinary dysbiosis"[666]) appears highly relevant in the genesis and perpetuation of rheumatoid arthritis.[667,668,669,670] Stressful life events also lower testosterone in men and the resultant lack of hormonal immunomodulation can increase the frequency and severity of exacerbations of rheumatoid arthritis[671]; resultant inflammation further suppresses testosterone production and bioavailability[672] leading to a self-perpetuating cycle of hypogonadism and inflammation. Thus, by numerous routes and mechanisms, psychoemotional stress increases the prevalence, persistence, and severity of musculoskeletal inflammation and pain.

Psychiatric codiagnoses are common among patients with painful neuromusculoskeletal disorders, and when the prevailing medical logic cannot solve the musculoskeletal riddle, the disorder is often ascribed to its accompanying mental disorder. The "appropriate" treatment from this perspective is the prescription of psychoactive drugs, generally of the "antidepressant" class. Science-based explanations are needed to expand clinicians' consideration of new possibilities which may someday prevail over commonplace suppositions that leave both clinician and patient trapped within a paradigm of futilely cyclical reasoning and its resultant simplistic symptom-targeting interventions. The following subsections provide alternatives to the "idiopathic pain is caused by its associated depression and both should be treated with antidepressant drugs" hypothesis.

a. <u>Pain, inflammation, and mental depression are final common pathways for nutritional deficiencies and imbalances</u>: As a scientific community we now know that the epidemic problem

---

[652] Weglicki W, Quamme G, Tucker K, Haigney M, Resnick L. Potassium, magnesium, and electrolyte imbalance and complications in disease management. *Clin Exp Hypertens*. 2005 Jan;27(1):95-112

[653] Imrich R. The role of neuroendocrine system in the pathogenesis of rheumatic diseases (minireview). *Endocr Regul*. 2002 Jun;36(2):95-106

[654] Orbach H, Shoenfeld Y. Hyperprolactinemia and autoimmune diseases. Autoimmun Rev. 2007 Sep;6(8):537-42

[655] Panush RS, Wallace DJ, Dorff RE, Engleman EP. Retraction of the suggestion to use the term "Reiter's syndrome" sixty-five years later: the legacy of Reiter, a war criminal, should not be eponymic honor but rather condemnation. *Arthritis Rheum*. 2007 Feb;56(2):693-4

[656] Tlaskalová-Hogenová H, Stepánková R, Hudcovic T, Tucková L, Cukrowska B, Lodinová-Zádníková R, Kozáková H, Rossmann P, Bártová J, Sokol D, Funda DP, Borovská D, Reháková Z, Sinkora J, Hofman J, Drastich P, Kokesová A. Commensal bacteria (normal microflora), mucosal immunity and chronic inflammatory and autoimmune diseases. *Immunol Lett*. 2004 May 15;93(2-3):97-108

[657] Collins SM. Stress and the Gastrointestinal Tract IV. Modulation of intestinal inflammation by stress: basic mechanisms and clinical relevance. *Am J Physiol Gastrointest Liver Physiol*. 2001 Mar;280(3):G315-8

[658] Hart A, Kamm MA. Review article: mechanisms of initiation and perpetuation of gut inflammation by stress. *Aliment Pharmacol Ther*. 2002 Dec;16(12):2017-28

[659] Farhadi A, Fields JZ, Keshavarzian A. Mucosal mast cells are pivotal elements in inflammatory bowel disease that connect the dots: stress, intestinal hyperpermeability and inflammation. *World J Gastroenterol*. 2007 Jun 14;13(22):3027-30

[660] Yang PC, Jury J, Söderholm JD, Sherman PM, McKay DM, Perdue MH. Chronic psychological stress in rats induces intestinal sensitization to luminal antigens. *Am J Pathol*. 2006 Jan;168(1):104-14

[661] Rashid T, Ebringer A. Ankylosing spondylitis is linked to Klebsiella--the evidence. *Clin Rheumatol*. 2007 Jun;26(6):858-64

[662] Vasquez A. *Integrative Rheumatology*. Fort Worth, Texas; Integrative and Biological Medicine Research and Consulting, 2007 OptimalHealthResearch.com

[663] Samarkos M, Vaiopoulos G. The role of infections in the pathogenesis of autoimmune diseases. *Curr Drug Targets Inflamm Allergy*. 2005 Feb;4(1):99-103

[664] Alverdy J, Holbrook C, Rocha F, Seiden L, Wu RL, Musch M, Chang E, Ohman D, Suh S. Gut-derived sepsis occurs when the right pathogen with the right virulence genes meets the right host: evidence for in vivo virulence expression in Pseudomonas aeruginosa. *Ann Surg*. 2000 Oct;232(4):480-9

[665] Wu L, Holbrook C, Zaborina O, Ploplys E, Rocha F, Pelham D, Chang E, Musch M, Alverdy J. Pseudomonas aeruginosa expresses a lethal virulence determinant, the PA-I lectin/adhesin, in the intestinal tract of a stressed host: the role of epithelia cell contact and molecules of the Quorum Sensing Signaling System. *Ann Surg*. 2003;238(5):754-64

[666] **Vasquez A**. *Integrative Rheumatology: Second Edition*. Fort Worth, Texas; Integrative and Biological Medicine Research and Consulting, 2007 OptimalHealthResearch.com

[667] Ebringer A, Rashid T. Rheumatoid arthritis is an autoimmune disease triggered by Proteus urinary tract infection. *Clin Dev Immunol*. 2006 Mar;13(1):41-8

[668] Erlacher L, Wintersberger W, Menschik M, Benke-Studnicka A, Machold K, Stanek G, Söltz-Szöts J, Smolen J, Graninger W. Reactive arthritis: urogenital swab culture is the only useful diagnostic method for the detection of the arthritogenic infection in extra-articularly asymptomatic patients with undifferentiated oligoarthritis. *Br J Rheumatol*. 1995 Sep;34(9):838-42

[669] Rashid T, Ebringer A. Rheumatoid arthritis is linked to Proteus--the evidence. *Clin Rheumatol*. 2007 Jul;26(7):1036-43

[670] Ebringer A, Rashid T, Wilson C. Rheumatoid arthritis: proposal for the use of anti-microbial therapy in early cases. *Scand J Rheumatol*. 2003;32:2-11

[671] James WH. Further evidence that low androgen values are a cause of rheumatoid arthritis: the response of rheumatoid arthritis to seriously stressful life events. *Ann Rheum Dis* 1997;56:566

[672] Karagiannis A, Harsoulis F. Gonadal dysfunction in systemic diseases. *Eur J Endocrinol*. 2005 Apr;152(4):501-13

of vitamin D deficiency leads to both musculoskeletal pain[673] as well as depression[674], and that supplementation with physiologic doses of vitamin D results in an enhanced sense of well-being[675] and high-efficacy alleviation of musculoskeletal pain and depression while providing other major collateral benefits.[676] Since the existence of vitamin D deficiency is more probable than that of antidepressant deficiency, the appropriate intervention for the former is more scientific and rational than that of the latter. Relatedly, research in various fields has shown that Western/American lifestyle and diet patterns diverge radically from human physiologic expectations and human nutritional requirements.[677] With regard to fatty acid intake and the resultant effects on inflammation and neurotransmission, modernized diets are a "set up" for musculoskeletal pain and mental depression, which frequently occur concomitantly and which are both alleviated by corrective fatty acid intervention such as fish oil supplementation as a source of EPA and DHA.[678,679] Correction of fatty acid imbalance is therefore more rational in the comanagement of pain and depression than is sole reliance on antidepressant and anti-inflammatory drugs; the latter have their place in treatment but neither addresses the primary cause of the problem and both drug classes have important adverse effects and significant cost in contrast to the safety, affordability, and collateral benefits derived from fatty acid supplementation. Also relevant to this discussion of chronic pain triggered and perpetuated by nutritional imbalances are the pro-inflammatory nature of the Western/American diet[680] and the pain-sensitizing effects of epidemic magnesium deficiency.[681] Therefore, correction of nutritional deficiencies and optimization of nutritional status might supersede the prescription of drugs in patients with concomitant depression and pain.

b. <u>Pain, inflammation, and depression are final common pathways of physical inactivity</u>: Exercising muscle elaborates cytokines ("myokines") with anti-inflammatory activity; a sedentary lifestyle fails to stimulate this endogenous anti-inflammation and is therefore relatively pro-inflammatory.[682] Further, exercise has antidepressant benefits mediated by positive influences on neurotransmission, growth factor elaboration, endocrinologic function, self-image, and social contact.[683] Patients with musculoskeletal pain should be encouraged to exercise to the extent possible given the individual's capacity and type of injury and/or degree of disability. Thus, a prescription for exercise might supersede the prescription of drugs in patients with concomitant depression and pain. Exercise prescriptions must consider frequency, duration, intensity, variety, safety, enjoyment, accountability and objective measures of compliance and progress, as well as appropriate combinations of components which emphasize aerobic fitness, strengthening, flexibility, muscle balancing, and coordination.

c. <u>Pain and depression are final common pathways of inflammation</u>: Several pro-inflammatory cytokines are psychoactive and cause depression, social withdrawal, impaired cognition, and sickness behavior.[684] As an alternative to the use of antidepressant drugs, correction of the underlying inflammatory disorder by natural, pharmacologic, or integrative means may subsequently promote restoration of normal affect and cognitive function.

---

[673] Plotnikoff GA, Quigley JM. Prevalence of severe hypovitaminosis D in patients with persistent, nonspecific musculoskeletal pain. *Mayo Clin Proc.* 2003 Dec;78(12):1463-70

[674] Wilkins CH, Sheline YI, Roe CM, Birge SJ, Morris JC. Vitamin D deficiency is associated with low mood and worse cognitive performance in older adults. *Am J Geriatr Psychiatry.* 2006 Dec;14(12):1032-40

[675] Vieth R, Kimball S, Hu A, Walfish PG. Randomized comparison of the effects of the vitamin D3 adequate intake versus 100 mcg (4000 IU) per day on biochemical responses and the wellbeing of patients. *Nutr J.* 2004 Jul 19;3:8

[676] **Vasquez A**, Manso G, Cannell J. The clinical importance of vitamin D (cholecalciferol): a paradigm shift with implications for all healthcare providers. *Altern Ther Health Med.* 2004 Sep-Oct;10(5):28-36

[677] O'Keefe JH Jr, Cordain L. Cardiovascular disease resulting from a diet and lifestyle at odds with our Paleolithic genome: how to become a 21st-century hunter-gatherer. *Mayo Clin Proc.* 2004 Jan;79(1):101-8

[678] Kiecolt-Glaser JK, Belury MA, Porter K, Beversdorf DQ, Lemeshow S, Glaser R. Depressive symptoms, omega-6:omega-3 fatty acids, and inflammation in older adults. *Psychosom Med.* 2007 Apr;69(3):217-24

[679] Simopoulos AP. Omega-3 fatty acids in inflammation and autoimmune diseases. *J Am Coll Nutr.* 2002 Dec;21(6):495-505

[680] Aljada A, Mohanty P, Ghanim H, Abdo T, Tripathy D, Chaudhuri A, Dandona P. Increase in intranuclear nuclear factor kappaB and decrease in inhibitor kappaB in mononuclear cells after a mixed meal: evidence for a proinflammatory effect. *Am J Clin Nutr.* 2004 Apr;79(4):682-90

[681] Park JH, Niermann KJ, Olsen N. Evidence for metabolic abnormalities in the muscles of patients with fibromyalgia. *Curr Rheumatol Rep.* 2000 Apr;2(2):131-40

[682] Petersen AM, Pedersen BK. The anti-inflammatory effect of exercise. *J Appl Physiol.* 2005 Apr;98(4):1154-62

[683] Cotman CW, Berchtold NC, Christie LA. Exercise builds brain health: key roles of growth factor cascades and inflammation. *Trends Neurosci.* 2007 Sep;30(9):464-72

[684] Wilson CJ, Finch CE, Cohen HJ. Cytokines and cognition--the case for a head-to-toe inflammatory paradigm. *J Am Geriatr Soc.* 2002 Dec;50(12):2041-56

d. <u>Pain, inflammation, and mental depression are final common pathways for hormonal deficiencies and imbalances</u>: Deficiencies of thyroid hormones, estrogen (insufficiency or excess), testosterone, cortisol, and DHEA can cause depression and impaired neuroemotional status. Hormonal aberrations are common in patients with chronic musculoskeletal pain, particularly of the inflammatory and autoimmune types. Clinical trials have shown that administration of thyroid hormones, testosterone, DHEA, cortisol and suppression prolactin can each provide anti-inflammatory, analgesic, and antidepressant benefits among appropriately selected patients. Thus, identification and correction of hormonal imbalances might supersede the prescription of antidepressant drugs in patients with concomitant depression, inflammation, and pain.

Our cultural and scientific advancements in the knowledge of how the brain and mind function have been paradoxically paralleled by social trends showing increasing depression and social isolation; the typical American has only two friends and no one in whom to confide.[685] In the United States, violent injuries are epidemic, and the level of firearm morbidity and mortality in the US is far higher than anywhere else in the industrialized world.[686] This does to some extent beg the question of the value of "scientific knowledge" of the brain and mind within a social structure that is increasingly violent and fragmented. Further, the mental depression resultant from pandemic social isolation would be better served by physicians' admonition for increased social contact than by the continued overuse of drugs which inhibit neurotransmitter reuptake.

<u>Conclusion</u>: The clinical employment of the functional medicine approach to chronic disease management and health promotion rests upon a foundation of competent patient management and then extends to consider the well documented contributions of the causative *core clinical imbalances* that have allowed the genesis and perpetuation of the problem(s) under consideration. The attainment of wellness, the success of preventive medicine, and the optimization of socioemotional health cannot be attained by pharmacological suppression of the manifestations of dysfunction that result from nutritional and neuroendocrine imbalances, xenobiotic accumulation, sedentary lifestyles, social isolation, and mucosal microbial colonization. Rather, these problems are addressed directly, and these and other causative considerations must remain foremost in the mind of the physician committed to the successful, ethical, and cost-effective long-term prevention and management of chronic health disturbances, particularly those characterized by inflammation and pain.

---

[685] McPherson M, Smith-Lovin L, Brashears ME. Social Isolation in America: Changes in Core Discussion Networks over Two Decades. *American Sociological Review* 2006; 71: 353-75

[686] Preventing firearm violence: a public health imperative. *American College of Physicians. Ann Intern Med.* 1995 Feb 15;122(4):311-3

Functional medicine is a science-based field of health care that is grounded in the following principles:

- **Biochemical individuality** describes the importance of individual variations in metabolic function that derive from genetic and environmental differences among individuals.
- **Patient-centered** medicine emphasizes "patient care" rather than "disease care," following Sir William Osler's admonition that "It is more important to know what patient has the disease than to know what disease the patient has."
- **Dynamic balance** of internal and external factors.
- **Web-like interconnections** of physiological factors – an abundance of research now supports the view that the human body functions as an orchestrated network of interconnected systems, rather than individual systems functioning autonomously and without effect on each other. For example, we now know that immunological dysfunctions can promote cardiovascular disease, that dietary imbalances can cause hormonal disturbances, and that environmental exposures can precipitate neurologic syndromes such as Parkinson's disease.
- **Health as a positive vitality** – not merely the absence of disease.
- **Promotion of organ reserve** as the means to enhance health span.

Functional medicine is anchored by an examination of the core clinical imbalances that underlie various disease conditions. Those imbalances arise as **environmental inputs** such as diet, nutrients (including air and water), exercise, and trauma **are processed** by one's body, mind, and spirit through a unique set of genetic predispositions, attitudes, and beliefs. The **fundamental physiological** processes include communication, both outside and inside the cell; bioenergetics, or the transformation of food into energy; replication, repair, and maintenance of structural integrity, from the cellular to the whole body level; elimination of waste; protection and defense; and transport and circulation. The **core clinical imbalances** that arise from malfunctions within this complex system include:

- **Hormonal and neurotransmitter imbalances**
- **Oxidation-reduction imbalances and mitochondropathy**
- **Detoxification and biotransformational imbalances**
- **Immune imbalances**
- **Inflammatory imbalances**
- **Digestive, absorptive, and microbiological imbalances**
- **Structural imbalances** from cellular membrane function to the musculoskeletal system

Imbalances such as these are the precursors to the signs and symptoms by which we detect and label (diagnose) organ system disease. Improving balance – in the patient's environmental inputs and in the body's fundamental physiological processes – is the precursor to restoring health and it involves much more than treating the symptoms. Functional medicine is dedicated to improving the management of complex, chronic disease by intervening at multiple levels to address these core clinical imbalances and to restore each patient's functionality and health. Functional medicine is not a unique and separate body of knowledge. It is grounded in scientific principles and information widely available in medicine today, combining research from various disciplines into highly detailed yet clinically relevant models of disease pathogenesis and effective clinical management.

      Functional medicine emphasizes a definable and teachable **process** of integrating multiple knowledge bases within a pragmatic intellectual matrix that focuses on functionality at many levels, rather than a single treatment for a single diagnosis. Functional medicine uses the patient's story as a key tool for integrating diagnosis, signs and symptoms, and evidence of clinical imbalances into a comprehensive approach to improve both the patient's environmental inputs and his or her physiological function. It is a clinician's discipline, and it directly addresses the need to transform the practice of primary care.

Chapter 2:
Wellness Promotion
&
Re-Establishing the Foundation for Health

Introduction to Lifestyle Optimization, Wellness Promotion, and Disease Prevention

This section details the lifestyle modifications that support a wellness-promoting whole-health program.

Among the four major primary healthcare professions in the United States—chiropractic, osteopathy, naturopathy, and allopathy—the naturopathic profession stands preeminent in its emphasis upon wellness promotion and lifestyle optimization. This chapter reviews wellness promotion from the current author's perspective and experience—both personal and professional—which is consistent with but not officially representative of the naturopathic profession's concepts "re-establish the foundation of health" and "hierarchy of therapeutics."

This chapter originated many years ago as a handout for patients wherein it explained and described basic concepts that are foundational to health restoration, preservation, and optimization. Over the years that this handout has evolved into a chapter for my books, it has become more detailed and more relevant for clinicians treating patients. In essence, this chapter is a blueprint for the construction of a healthy lifestyle. While it may not cover every consideration, it covers the basics in sufficient detail so as to allow patients to change tracks from the downward descent of the disease-promoting lifestyle to the upward ascent of the health-promoting lifestyle.

Replacing the passive and disempowering drug-surgery paradigm with an active and empowering integrative/functional model of healthcare is one goal of this section.

This section can be thought of as a collection of essays. The review and consideration of a wide range of topics—which might otherwise appear random and nontopical to a reader accustomed to a more limited scope of discussion—is necessary due to the multifaceted nature of human experience and the widely ranging influences on health and disease outcomes.

<u>Topics</u>:

- Re-establishing the Foundation for Health
    - Healthcare, Health, and Wellness
    - **Daily living**
        - Lifestyle habits
        - Motivation: background and clinical applications
        - Exceptional living: the key to exceptional results
        - Recognize and affirm individual uniqueness
        - Individuation & conscious living: alternatives to common paradigms
        - Quality and quantity of sleep: concepts and clinical applications
        - Exercise, obesity, BMI, and proinflammatory activity of adipose tissue
    - **Diet is a powerful tool for the prevention and treatment of disease**
        - Make "whole foods" the foundation of the diet
        - Increase consumption of fruits and vegetables
        - Phytochemicals: food-derived anti-inflammatory nutrients
        - Eat the right amount of protein
        - Reducing consumption of sugars: exceptions for supercompensation
        - Avoiding artificial sweeteners, colors, and other additives, reducing caffeine
        - To the extent possible, eat "organic" foods
        - Recognize the importance of avoiding food allergens
        - Supplement your healthy diet with vitamins, minerals, and fatty acids
        - General guidelines for the safe use of nutritional supplements
    - **Advanced concepts in nutrition**
        - "Biochemical Individuality" and "Orthomolecular Medicine"
        - Nutrigenomics: Nutritional genomics
        - Putting it all together: *the supplemented Paleo-Mediterranean diet*
    - **Emotional, mental, and social health**
        - Stress management and authentic living
        - Stress always has a biochemical/physiologic component
        - The body functions as a whole
        - Healing past experiences
        - Autonomization, intradependence, emotional literacy, corrective experience
    - **Environmental health**
        - Environmental exposures and the importance of detoxification
        - Avoid unnecessary chemical medications and medical procedures
        - Intestinal health, bowel function, and introduction to dysbiosis
- **Natural holistic healthcare contrasted to standard medical treatment**
- **Opposite influences of health promotion vs. disease promotion**
- **Brief Overview of Integrative Primary Healthcare Disciplines**: Chiropractic, Naturopathic Medicine, Osteopathic Medicine, Functional Medicine
- **Previously published essays**
    - Five-Part Nutritional Wellness Protocol That Produces Consistently Positive Results
    - Implementing the Five-Part Nutritional Wellness Protocol for the Treatment of Various Health Problems
    - Common Oversights and Shortcomings in the Study and Implementation of Nutritional Supplementation
    - Revisiting the Five-Part Nutritional Wellness Protocol: The Supplemented Paleo-Mediterranean Diet

Introduction to Wellness Promotion: Re-Establishing the Foundation for Health

"The work of the naturopathic physician is to elicit healing by helping patients to create or recreate conditions for health to exist within them.
Health will occur where the conditions for health exist.
Disease is the product of conditions which allow for it."   *Jared Zeff, N.D.*[1]

One of the most important concepts within the philosophy and practice of naturopathic medicine is that of "re-establishing the foundation for health." This means that instead of first looking to a specific treatment or "magic bullet" to solve a health problem, we first look at the environment in which the problem arose to determine if the patient's environment has initiated or perpetuated the problem. The term *environment* as used here means much more than the patient's immediate surroundings at home and work; it includes all modifiable factors that may have an effect on the patient's health, such as lifestyle, diet, exercise, supplementation, chronic and situational stress, medications with positive and negative effects, exposure to toxicants and microbes, nutritionally-modifiable genetic factors[2], emotions, feelings, and unconscious assumptions[3], and many other considerations. Although the genes that we and our patients have inherited cannot be changed, we can very often modulate the expression of those genes (e.g., via nutrigenomics, described later) by modifying the biochemical, microbial, toxicologic, and neurohormonal milieu that bathes our cells and thus our genes; this concept was expressed in a statement by the US Centers for Disease Control and Prevention in its "Gene-Environment Interaction Fact Sheet" available on-line.[4]

"Optimal health" does not and never will come in a pill or tonic—the human body and the interactions that we each have between our genes, outlooks, environments, and lifestyles are far too complex to ever be addressed wholly and completely by a simplistic paradigm or single treatment. Even a superficial observation of the complexity of human physiology and the complexity of our environments (including noise, toxins such as benzene and mercury, chemicals such as formaldehyde from building materials, work stress and multitasking, radiation exposure, microwaves, etc) shows that **our modern lifestyles subject the human body to many more "stressors" than ever before in the history of human existence.** Each of these stressors depletes our psychic and physiologic reserves, such that daily replenishment and protection are necessary.

Environment—lifestyle, diet, stresses, microbes, toxins—influences genetic expression and the manifestation of health or disease
"Virtually all human diseases result from the interaction of genetic susceptibility factors and modifiable environmental factors, broadly defined to include infectious, chemical, physical, nutritional, and behavioral factors. … "Even so-called single-gene disorders actually develop from the interaction of both genetic and environmental factors. … "We do not inherit a disease state per se. Instead, we inherit a set of a susceptibility factors to certain effects of environmental factors and therefore inherit a higher risk for certain diseases." Gene-Environment Interaction Fact Sheet by the Centers for Disease Control and Prevention, August 2000

Research in nutrition and physiology is revealing the mechanisms by which "simple" lifestyle practices and dietary interventions exert their powerful benefits. For example, whole foods such as fruits and vegetables contain over 8,000 phytochemicals with different physiologic effects[5], and simple practices such as meditation and massage can significantly alter hormone and neurotransmitter levels.[6,7] On the surface, a simple practice such as consumption of fruits and vegetables and a multivitamin/multimineral supplement may seem to be a way to

[1] Zeff JL. The process of healing: a unifying theory of naturopathic medicine. *Journal of Naturopathic Medicine* 1997; 7: 122-5
[2] Kaput J, Rodriguez LR. Nutritional genomics: the next frontier in the postgenomic era. *Physiol Genomics* 16: 166–177 http://physiolgenomics.physiology.org/cgi/content/full/16/2/166
[3] Miller A. The truth will set you free: overcoming emotional blindness and finding your true adult self. New York: Basic Books; 2001
[4] Gene-Environment Interaction Fact Sheet by the Centers for Disease Control and Prevention, August 2000 http://www.ashg.org/pdf/CDC%20Gene-Environment%20Interaction%20Fact%20Sheet.pdf
[5] "We propose that the additive and synergistic effects of phytochemicals in fruit and vegetables are responsible for their potent antioxidant and anticancer activities, and that the benefit of a diet rich in fruit and vegetables is attributed to the complex mixture of phytochemicals present in whole foods." Liu RH. Health benefits of fruit and vegetables are from additive and synergistic combinations of phytochemicals. *Am J Clin Nutr.* 2003 Sep;78(3 Suppl):517S-520S
[6] "The significant decrease of the catecholamine metabolite VMA (vanillic-mandelic acid) in meditators, that is associated with a reciprocal increase of 5-HIAA supports as a feedback necessity the "rest and fulfillment response" versus "fight and flight"." Bujatti M, Riederer P. Serotonin, noradrenaline, dopamine metabolites in transcendental meditation-technique. *J Neural Transm.* 1976;39(3):257-67
[7] "By the end of the study, the massage therapy group, as compared to the relaxation group, reported experiencing less pain, depression, anxiety and improved sleep. They also showed improved trunk and pain flexion performance, and their serotonin and dopamine levels were higher." Hernandez-Reif M, Field T, Krasnegor J, Theakston H. Lower back pain is reduced and range of motion increased after massage therapy. *Int J Neurosci* 2001;106(3-4):131-45

provide merely "good nutrition"; however the clinical effects can include antidepressant[8] and anti-inflammatory benefits[9] by enhancing the efficiency of biochemical reactions[10] and by reducing excess activity of NF-kappaB[11], respectively. The power of interventional nutrition utilizing high-doses and/or synergistic formulations of nutraceuticals and phytonutraceuticals becomes much more clinically apparent when patients first (re)establish a healthy foundation of diet and lifestyle practices upon which these treatments can be added; **I estimate that the effectiveness of treatments for complex illness such as inflammatory diseases and cancer is** *at least* **doubled when patients implement these lifestyle changes in addition to specific treatments rather than relying on specific treatments alone without a healthy supportive lifestyle.** In other words, *"foundation for health* + specific treatments" is much more effective than *"unhealthy lifestyle* + specific treatments." This explains, in part, the discrepancy between the relatively lackluster response seen in *single-intervention* clinical trials* compared to the better results that we attain clinically when using a holistic approach characterized by *multicomponent* treatment plans. The biochemical and "scientific" reasons for this positive/negative synergism will become more clear during the course of this chapter and textbook.

Single-intervention clinical trials (i.e., clinical trials that utilize only one treatment) are the "gold standard" in allopathic drug-based research because in that setting the goal is to quantify and qualify the nature of positive and negative responses to a single intervention, generally a drug. However, this approach loses much of its luster and relevance in clinical settings where neither patients nor their environments and treatment plans can be standardized due to the unique constitution, lifestyle, history, and other nuances of each patient. Single intervention clinical trials have a place in the researching of all treatments, including natural interventions. However, clinicians—especially recent graduates—must pry themselves away from this research tool when it comes to treating individual patients in clinical practice, where **single interventions are the antithesis of holistic treatment**.

Daily Living: Life occurs on a moment-to-moment and daily basis. Choices that we make in relationships, occupations, exercise, and diet have profound and powerful influence over the course of our lives—particularly our health and happiness. Despite the previous and current obfuscation of health information by allopathic groups[12,13,14,15,16] and the pharmaceutical industry[17,18], enough valid information and common sense is available to doctors and the public such that **ignorance is no longer a viable excuse for deferring responsibility for lifestyle-induced disease and misery.**[19] Eating too much sugar and fat while not eating enough fruits and vegetables is making a choice to have an increased probability of developing diabetes, cancer, heart disease, arthritis, and obesity. Exercising regularly, eating a healthy diet, and supplementing the diet with high-quality nutrients and botanicals is making the choice to greatly reduce one's risk of health problems[20,21] and to nurture one's life and one's body so that one can make the most of one's life experience and enjoy life, hobbies, life purpose(s), travel, creativity, community involvement, and time with friends and family.

When we were children, we looked to other people to provide for us and to "take care of us." **As adults, we have to assume responsibility for the course of our own lives, to make decisions based on long-term considerations rather than instant gratification and selective ignorance.** Of course, this does not mean that we

[8] Benton D, Haller J, Fordy J. Vitamin supplementation for 1 year improves mood. *Neuropsychobiology*. 1995;32(2):98-105

[9] Church TS, Earnest CP, Wood KA, Kampert JB. Reduction of C-reactive protein levels through use of a multivitamin. *Am J Med*. 2003;115(9):702-7

[10] Ames BN, Elson-Schwab I, Silver EA. High-dose vitamin therapy stimulates variant enzymes with decreased coenzyme binding affinity (increased K(m)): relevance to genetic disease and polymorphisms. *Am J Clin Nutr*. 2002 Apr;75(4):616-58 http://www.ajcn.org/cgi/content/full/75/4/616

[11] **Vasquez A**. Reducing pain and inflammation naturally - part 4: nutritional and botanical inhibition of NF-kappaB, the major intracellular amplifier of the inflammatory cascade. A practical clinical strategy exemplifying anti-inflammatory nutrigenomics. *Nutritional Perspectives*, July 2005:5-12. www.OptimalHealthResearch.com/part4

[12] Wolinsky H, Brune T. The Serpent on the Staff: The Unhealthy Politics of the American Medical Association. GP Putnam and Sons, New York, 1994

[13] Wilk CA. Medicine, Monopolies, and Malice: How the Medical Establishment Tried to Destroy Chiropractic. Garden City Park: Avery, 1996

[14] Carter JP. Racketeering in Medicine: The Suppression of Alternatives. Norfolk: Hampton Roads Pub; 1993

[15] National Alliance of Professional Psychology Providers. AMA Seeks To Control and Restrict Psychologist's Scope of Practice. http://www.nappp.org/scope.pdf Accessed November 25, 2006

[16] "In an effort to marshal the medical community's resources against the growing threat of expanding scope of practice for allied health professionals, the AMA has formed a national partnership to confront such initiatives nationwide... The committee will use $25,000..." Daly R, American Psychiatric Association. AMA Forms Coalition to Thwart Non-M.D. Practice Expansion. *Psychiatric News* 2006 March; 41: 17 http://pn.psychiatryonline.org/cgi/content/full/41/5/17-a?eaf Accessed November 25, 2006

[17] Angell M. The Truth About the Drug Companies: How They Deceive Us and What to Do About it. Random House; August 2004

[18] "It begins on the first day of medical school... It starts slowly and insidiously, like an addiction, and can end up influencing the very nature of medical decision-making and practice... Attempts to influence the judgment of doctors by commercial interests serving the medical industrial complex are nothing if not thorough." Editorial. Drug-company influence on medical education in USA. *Lancet*. 2000 Sep 2;356(9232):781

[19] "Error is not blindness, error is cowardice. Every acquisition, every step forward in knowledge is the result of courage, of severity towards oneself, of cleanliness with respect to oneself." Nietzsche FW. Ecce Homo: How One Becomes What One Is. [Translator: Hollingdale RJ] Penguin Books:1979,34

[20] Orme-Johnson DW, Herron RE. An innovative approach to reducing medical care utilization and expenditures. *Am J Manag Care*. 1997;3(1):135-44

[21] **Vasquez A**. Five-Part Nutritional Protocol that Produces Consistently Positive Results.*Nutr Wellness* 2005Sept. http://optimalhealthresearch.com/spmd

have to abandon enjoyment; but it does mean that we can make decisions based on priorities, and if health is a priority then we should take steps to attain and maintain it. For people who have chosen to make their health a priority, sugar- and fat-laden food begins to lose its appeal, and exploring new health-building experiences such as healthy cooking, outdoor activities, and community involvement can become an empowering lifestyle that can be transformed into an art—one that is particularly amenable to building relationships and connections with other people. **The improved sense of well-being and improved**

> ### Health living: lifestyle as living art
> "What one should learn from artists: How can we make things beautiful, attractive, and desirable for us when they are not?—and I rather think that in themselves they never are! ... This we should learn from artists, while being wiser than they are in other matters. For with them this subtle power usually comes to an end where art ends and life begins; but we want to be the poets of our lives—first of all in the smallest, most everyday matters."
>
> Nietzsche FW. The Happy Science. 1882. Essay #299.

physical and intellectual performance obtained from consumption of a health-promoting Paleo-Mediterranean diet (described later) supercedes any short-term gratification from the disease-promoting diet commonly referred to as the Standard American Diet (SAD). When people want to be healthy, exercising and spending enjoyable time outdoors becomes more fun than the inactivity and passivity of watching television. When we consider that the average American watches at least 3-4 hours of television per day then we should not be surprised that, with physical inactivity as such a major component of the day, Americans show progressively higher rates of obesity, cancer, heart disease, and diabetes. Such an inactive lifestyle also affects our children: on average, each American child watches more than 23 hours of television per week[22]—a national habit that unquestionably contributes to the high levels of obesity and (social) illiteracy demonstrated by America's youth. Adults who watch average amounts of television are exposed to—some might say "...indoctrinated by...") more than 30 hours of drug advertisements per year—far exceeding their exposure to other, potentially more authentic, health-promoting health information.[23] Not only does television siphon time and energy that could be used more productively, more socially, or more enjoyably, but at a cost of $50-100 per month ($600 to $1,200 per year) **cable television subtracts from the available resources (i.e., time, money, and attention) that could be directed toward health-promoting choices.** Cable television—because of its financial cost and time commitment—is only one of many examples of how everyday lifestyle choices can have an impact on long-term health/disease outcomes. **Clinicians should encourage patients to become mindful of their choices and the impact these choices have on long-term health and vitality.**

<u>Lifestyle habits</u>: Without the conscious decision that **health is a priority** and the realization that **optimal health has to be earned rather than taken for granted**, patients and doctors alike can fall into the belief that healthcare and health maintenance are *burdens* and *inconveniences* rather than opportunities for fulfillment and self-care. Taking an **empowered** and **pro-active** role in one's healthcare may include a coordinated program of diet changes (i.e., eating certain foods, avoiding other foods, modulating total intake), regular exercise, nutritional supplementation, stress reduction, and relationship improvement. Unhealthy habits such as eating junk foods, using tobacco, and watching too much television rob people of the time, energy, motivation, and financial resources that could otherwise be used to improve health and prevent unnecessary illness. As described later in this chapter, the choices that are made on a daily basis from this point forward are the most powerful predictors of future health and are generally more powerful than past habits or genetic inheritance. We can all greatly increase our probability of enjoying a future of high-energy health rather than painful illness by consistently choosing health-promoting options instead of foods, behaviors, and emotional states that promote illness.

---

[22] "American children view over 23 hours of television per week. * Teenagers view an average of 21 to 22 hours of television per week. * By the time today's children reach age 70, they will have spent 7 to 10 years of their lives watching television." American Academy of Pediatrics http://www.aapcal.org/aapcal/tv.html accessed September 30, 2003
[23] "...many ads may be targeted specifically at women and older viewers. Our findings suggest that Americans who watch average amounts of television may be exposed to more than 30 hours of direct-to-consumer drug advertisements each year, far surpassing their exposure to other forms of health communication." Brownfield ED, Bernhardt JM, Phan JL, Williams MV, Parker RM. Direct-to-consumer drug advertisements on network television: an exploration of quantity, frequency, and placement. *J Health Commun.* 2004 Nov-Dec;9(6):491-7

One hour of time per day and/or about $2 - $8 per day:

Active self-care lifestyle	Distraction & inactive lifestyle
1. Meditation 2. Yoga, stretching 3. Walking, jogging, biking, no-cost calisthenics 4. Martial arts, Tai Chi 5. Hot bath 6. Cooking new healthy meals 7. Herbal teas (especially green tea) provide anti-inflammatory, anticancer, and antioxidant benefits 8. Basic nutritional supplementation (less than $2 per day): 1) High-potency multivitamin and multimineral supplement, 2) Complete balanced, fatty acid supplementation, 3) 2,000 – 4,000 IU vitamin D per day for adults, 4) probiotics and/or symbiotic.	1. Cable television 2. 1 pack of cigarettes per day 3. Designer coffee such as Grande Café Latte
Benefits 1. Increased flexibility and joint mobility 2. Reduction in blood pressure 3. Reduced risk of cancer 4. Increased strength 5. Improved cognitive function 6. New and enjoyable meals 7. Relaxation 8. New life skills 9. Improved heart health 10. The opportunity to develop social skills and more friends and a better social support network 11. Reduced risk for Alzheimer's and Parkinson's diseases	**Results** 1. Cable television: Cost $2 - $4 per day = average $1,095 per year) 2. 1 pack of cigarettes per day ($3 per day = $1,095 per year) 3. Grande Café Latte ($4 per day = average $1,460 per year)
Cost: At $2 per day for meditation, stretching, calisthenics, (etc.) and basic supplementation, the total comes to $730 per year.	**Cost:** For cable television, cafe coffee, and cigarettes, the total comes to approximately $3,600 per year.

Motivation: We all have a combination of reasons, feelings, inclinations, and unconscious influences that support and perpetuate our health behaviors.[24,25,26] Getting in touch with those motivations can help us to better understand the healthy/functional (health-promoting) and unhealthy/dysfunctional (illness-promoting) aspects of our psyches. Uncovering and "upgrading" these motivations can help us and our patients to develop more authentic lives and improved health. Self-defeating behaviors, such as 1) a willingness to remain ignorant of factors which influence health, 2) a willingness to frequently consume disease-promoting processed convenience foods, and 3) submission to confinement within the boundaries of one's insurance coverage (which often confines one to drugs and surgery as the only treatment options), reflect—*at best*—the willingness to settle for mediocrity and—*at worst*—an unconscious movement in the direction of illness and early death—masochism and suicide by lifestyle. Conversely, an unencumbered drive toward health will create the greatest opportunity for wellness. Since **actions originate from beliefs and goals**, we can surmise much about undisclosed beliefs and goals in others and ourselves simply by observing outward behavior. Effectively changing actions (such as diet and lifestyle choices) therefore must include not only behavior modification but also careful examination and reconsideration of largely unconscious goals and beliefs that motivate and underlie those behaviors. **When a fully empowered motivation toward health is matched with accurate informational insight, we have the** *potential* **for health-promoting change**—*potential* **which only becomes** *manifest* **after the habitual application of appropriate** *action.* Patients and doctors alike can benefit from considering the factors that incline them *toward* or *away* from behaviors that promote health or disease.

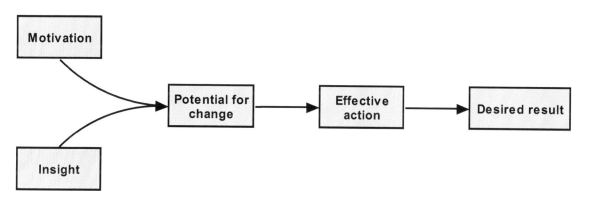

Reasons that I take good care of myself:

_____

_____

_____

_____

_____

Reasons that I don't take good care of myself:

_____

_____

_____

_____

_____

[24] Bradshaw J. Healing the Shame that Binds You [Audio Cassette (April 1990) Health Communications Audio; ISBN: 1558740430]
[25] Miller A. The Drama of the Gifted Child: The Search for the True Self. Basic Books: 1981
[26] Prochaska, JO, Norcross, JC, and DiClemente, CC (1994). Changing for Good: A Revolutionary Six-Stage Program for Overcoming Bad Habits and Moving Your Life Positively Forward. NY, William Morrow and Company; 1994

Motivation: moving from theory to practice: Many recently-graduated doctors start with the erroneous assumption that all patients actually want to become healthier, and furthermore, that all that the doctor has to do is "enlighten" them to the error of their ways and the patient will be dutifully compliant unto the attainment of his or her health-related goals. In reality, many people are surprisingly indifferent about their health. Many people do not care if they are 30 lbs overweight or have hypertension or will die early as a result of their lifestyle; they often have to be encouraged to begin to *consider* making positive changes.

At our 2004 Functional Medicine Symposium, Dr. James Prochaska[27] elucidated the different stages of patient preparedness, and we note that each of these five levels of thought and action produces specific results and requires different types of support from the doctor. I have summarized and modified Dr. Prochaska's lecture in the following table; for additional information and insights, obtain his lecture from the Institute for Functional Medicine (functionalmedicine.org) or obtain his book *Changing for Good*.[28]

Level of preparedness and readiness for change

Stage: representative statement	Doctor's interventions and social support
1. **Pre-contemplation**: "I am not seriously thinking about making a change to be healthier."	▪ Outreach ▪ Retainment
2. **Contemplation**: "I am thinking about making a change, but I am not ready for action."	▪ Resolve resistance ▪ Emphasize benefits ▪ Address ambivalence
3. **Preparation**: "I am getting ready to make a change, but I am not taking effective action yet."	▪ Ensure adequate preparation ▪ Prevent relapse following initial action
4. **Action**: "I am beginning to make changes to become healthier."	▪ Support (group support is best) ▪ Encouragement ▪ Reward system
5. **Maintenance**: "I take action every day and on a consistent basis to reach my goals."	▪ Continued provision for continuation of health changes: facilities, supplements, social support, affirmation

Recognizing the different levels of patient preparedness and addressing individual patients with a customized approach not only for their *disease* but also for their *level of preparedness* for action can help doctors deliver more effective healthcare. Also, patients may have different levels of preparedness for different aspects of their treatment plans. He/she may be ready for **action** with regard to exercise, in **preparation** for dietary change, but in **precontemplation** for the use of supplements and botanicals.

---

[27] Prochaska JO. Changing for good: motivating diabetic patients. The Coming Storm: Reversing the Rising Pandemic of Diabetes and Metabolic Syndrome. The Eleventh International Symposium on Functional Medicine. May 13-15, 2004 in Vancouver, British Columbia, Canada. Pages 173-180. Presented by the Institute for Functional Medicine in Gig Harbor, Washington. www.FunctionalMedicine.org
[28] Prochaska, JO, Norcross, JC, and DiClemente, CC (1994). Changing for Good: A Revolutionary Six-Stage Program for Overcoming Bad Habits and Moving Your Life Positively Forward. NY, William Morrow and Company; 1994

The secret to being exceptionally healthy: *One has to live in an exceptional (unique, personalized) way*. We cannot expect to achieve the goal of being vibrantly healthy or exceptionally happy if we live in the same way as everyone else, particularly when our fellow citizens are likely to be overweight, depressed, socially isolated[29], requiring multiple pharmaceutical medications[30], and experiencing a state of progressively declining health.[31] *Healthy lifestyle* not only includes the basics of adequate sleep, healthy whole-foods diet, supportive relationships, and regular exercise, but it also includes preventive medicine and pro-active healthcare. **Despite the fact that we in the United States (US) spend more on medical treatments than does any other country in the world, Americans have the worst health outcomes of all the major industrialized countries**.[32,33,34] This is largely because *American medicine* is centered on a *disease-oriented model of medicine* which means that instead of having a healthcare system and social structure that proactively promotes health and prevents disease before it happens, our systems are *reactive*—treating disease *after* it occurs rather than emphasizing the prevention of disease *before* it occurs. The dominant allopathic model in the US is also reductionistic: focusing on the small problem (micromanagement) rather than the big picture (macromanagement).

Clearly, the most effective method for avoiding expensive and potentially dangerous medical procedures and drug treatments is for us as a nation and as individuals to shift our thinking from a *disease treatment* model of healthcare to a more logical program of aggressive *disease prevention* and *wellness promotion* via the use of safe natural treatments rather than heroic interventions.[35,36] Of course, this means that our concept and view of health and healthcare will have to change. As noted by Shi[37], **"Redesigning the system of health care delivery in the United States may be the only viable option to improve the quality of health care."** In the meantime, while we work for change on a national level, we are wise to change our personal habits and healthcare choices in favor of natural and preventive healthcare.

> **Americans have poor health outcomes compared to citizens of other industrialized nations**
>
> "Basically, you die earlier and spend more time disabled if you're an American rather than a member of most other advanced countries."
>
> Christopher Murray MD PhD, Director of World Health Organization's Global Program on Evidence for Health Policy. Press release on June 4, 2000. http://www.who.int/inf-pr-2000/en/pr2000-life.html

> **Approximately 493 Americans are killed each day by hospital injuries and drug-prescribing errors**
>
> "Recent estimates suggest that each year more than 1 million patients are injured while in the hospital and approximately 180,000 die because of these injuries. Furthermore, drug-related morbidity and mortality are common and are estimated to cost more than $136 billion a year."
>
> Holland EG, Degruy FV. Drug-induced disorders. *Am Fam Physician*. 1997;56:1781-8, 1791-2

> **Medical drug (in)efficacy**
>
> "The vast majority of drugs —more than 90 percent— only work in 30 or 50 percent of the people."
>
> Allen Roses, M.D., worldwide vice-president of genetics at GlaxoSmithKline. Published Dec 8, 2003 http://commondreams.org/headlines03/1208-02.htm

Healthy lifestyle and biochemical individuality credo: Recognize and affirm that you are a unique individual with unique needs: For each of us, our "personality" extends far beyond and far deeper than our sense of humor and our choice of clothing; we are very unique on a physiologic and biochemical level as well. So-called *normal* and *apparently healthy* individuals vary greatly in their biochemical efficiency and nutritional needs. This is the

---

[29] McPherson M, Smith-Lovin L, Brashears ME. Social Isolation in America: Changes in Core Discussion Networks over Two Decades. *American Sociological Review* 2006; 71: 353-75 http://www.asanet.org/galleries/default-file/June06ASRFeature.pdf

[30] "According to the latest available data, total health care costs reached $1.3 trillion in 2000. This represents a per capita health care expenditure of $4,637. The total prescription drug expenditure in 2000 was $121.8 billion, or approximately $430 per person." Presentation to the U.S. Senate Commerce Committee April 23, 2002 "Drug Pricing & Consumer Costs" Kathleen D. Jaeger, R.Ph., J.D. http://commerce.senate.gov/hearings/042302jaegar.pdf

[31] Zack MM, Moriarty DG, Stroup DF, Ford ES, Mokdad AH. Worsening trends in adult health-related quality of life and self-rated health-United States, 1993-2001. *Public Health Rep*. 2004 Sep-Oct;119(5):493-505 http://www.pubmedcentral.nih.gov/articlerender.fcgi?tool=pubmed&pubmedid=15313113

[32] "[America] also has the fewest hospital days per capita, the highest hospital expenditures per day, and substantially higher physician incomes than the other OECD countries. On the available outcome measures, the United States is generally in the bottom half, and its relative ranking has been declining since 1960." Anderson GF, Poullier JP. Health spending, access, and outcomes: trends in industrialized countries. *Health Aff* (Millwood) 1999 May-Jun;18(3):178-92 http://content.healthaffairs.org/cgi/reprint/18/3/178.pdf

[33] "However, on outcomes indicators such as life expectancy and infant mortality, the United States is frequently in the bottom quartile among the twenty-nine industrialized countries, and its relative ranking has been declining since 1960." Anderson GF. In search of value: an international comparison of cost, access, and outcomes. *Health Aff* 1997 Nov-Dec;16(6):163-71

[34] "Basically, you die earlier and spend more time disabled if you're an American rather than a member of most other advanced countries," says Christopher Murray, MD, PhD, Director of WHO's Global Program on Evidence for Health Policy. http://www.who.int/inf-pr-2000/en/pr2000-life.html

[35] "Systematic access to managed chiropractic care not only may prove to be clinically beneficial but also may reduce overall health care costs." Legorreta A, et al N. Comparative Analysis of Individuals With and Without Chiropractic Coverage. *Archives of Internal Medicine* 2004; 164: 1985-1992

[36] Orme-Johnson DW, Herron RE. An innovative approach to reducing medical care utilization and expenditures. *Am J Manag Care*. 1997;3(1):135-44

[37] Shi L. Health care spending, delivery, and outcome in developed countries: a cross-national comparison. *Am J Med Qual* 1997;12(2):83-93

concept of "biochemical individuality" which was first detailed in 1956 by the renowned scientist Roger J Williams from the University of Texas. In his historic work *Biochemical Individuality: The Basis for the Genetotrophic Concept*, Dr. Williams[38] reviews research that conclusively proves that among *apparently healthy* individuals, we can objectively determine great differences in physiology, organ efficiency, enzyme function, and nutritional needs. For example, variables that promote health include increased enzyme efficiency and efficient digestion and assimilation of nutrients, while internal factors that reduce health can include inadequate digestion, inefficient absorption, increased excretion of nutrients, impaired detoxification, poor enzyme function and "partial genetic blocks"—a term now understood to imply single nucleotide polymorphisms[39] and related enzyme defects, which result in **supradietary requirements for specific vitamins and minerals** for the prevention of disease and maintenance of health.[40] What this means for us as doctors and for our patients in practical terms is that in order for us to become as healthy as possible, we will almost certainly have to give attention to each person's unique biochemical abilities/disabilities in order to maximize the function of the various body systems, enzymes, and to optimize genetic expression.[41] This means that what works for one's neighbor, spouse, or best friend in terms of exercise, diet and nutrition may not work for one's unique physiology. We must all muster the courage to affirm that, in order to attain the goal of stable or progressively better health, we will each have to learn about how our unique bodies work—what conditions of health must be created. We will have to learn to make changes in lifestyle and daily routine which reflect and honor our bodies' ways of working. This may mean modifying work, sleep, and exercise schedules, avoiding some foods and eating others, and customizing nutrient intake to meet the body's needs as they are *in the present*—the health program that appears to have worked last year may not be appropriate at the present time. The process of learning how a person's body works requires time, patience, and the process of trial and error—from patient and doctor—but achieving the goal of improved health and increased energy are well worth the effort.

Individuation and the practice of conscious living: Our visions of reality are influenced by religious institutions, large corporations, advertising networks[42], corporate-owned mass media[43], and what Professors Stevens and Glatstein called "the medical-industrial complex."[44] Some of the paradigms that are advocated are both *unhistorical* (having no historical precedent) and *antihistorical* (contrary to the available historical precedent, which includes sustainability). Some of these companies and organizations offer

> ### The importance of living consciously
> "Consciousness is our basic tool for successful adaptation to reality. The more conscious we are in any situation, the more possibilities we tend to perceive, the more options we have, the more powerful we are — perhaps even the longer we will live.
> Living consciously means seeking to be aware of everything that bears on our actions, purposes, values, and goals — and behaving in accordance with that which we see and know."
>
> Branden N. The Art of Living Consciously. http://nathanielbranden.com Accessed Feb 2011

us a view of reality and vision of our individual potentials that is fashioned in such a way as to promote the financial and political interests of the company or organization. Conversely, the actualization of our true physical, emotional, intellectual, and spiritual potentials may require that we separate from or at least attain a conscious appreciation of the (pseudo)reality that we have been advised to follow.[45,46] Critiques of and reasonable alternatives to our current paradigms of school[47], work[48,49], and money[50] have been discussed elsewhere and are worthy of consideration. Becoming mindful of the paradigms and assumptions under which we live is the first step in true individuation, characterized by choosing (*creating* the best option: freedom) rather than deciding

[38] Williams RJ. Biochemical Individuality : The Basis for the Genetotrophic Concept. Austin and London: University of Texas Press, 1956

[39] Ames BN. Cancer prevention and diet: help from single nucleotide polymorphisms. *Proc Natl Acad Sci U S A*. 1999 Oct 26;96(22):12216-8

[40] Ames BN, Elson-Schwab I, Silver EA. High-dose vitamin therapy stimulates variant enzymes with decreased coenzyme binding affinity (increased K(m)): relevance to genetic disease and polymorphisms. *Am J Clin Nutr*. 2002 Apr;75(4):616-58 http://www.ajcn.org/cgi/content/full/75/4/616

[41] "The combination of biochemical individuality and known functional utilities of allelic variants should converge to create a situation in which nutritional optima can be specified as part of comprehensive lifestyle prescriptions tailored to the needs of each person." Eckhardt RB. Genetic research and nutritional individuality. *J Nutr* 2001;131(2):336S-9S

[42] "Patients' requests for medicines are a powerful driver of prescribing decisions. In most cases physicians prescribed requested medicines but were often ambivalent about the choice of treatment. If physicians prescribe requested drugs despite personal reservations, sales may increase but appropriateness of prescribing may suffer." Mintzes B, Barer ML, Kravitz RL, Kazanjian A, Bassett K, Lexchin J, Evans RG, Pan R, Marion SA. Influence of direct to consumer pharmaceutical advertising and patients' requests on prescribing decisions: two site cross sectional survey. *BMJ*. 2002 Feb 2; 324(7332): 278-9

[43] Manufacturing Consent: Noam Chomsky and the Media. Movie directed by Achbar M and Wintonick P. 1992. See also http://zeitgeistmovie.com/ Stevens CW, Glatstein E. Beware the Medical-Industrial Complex. *Oncologist* 1996;1(4):IV-V http://theoncologist.alphamedpress.org/cgi/reprint/1/4/190-iv.pdf on July 4, 2004

[45] Breton D, Largent C. The Paradigm Conspiracy. Center City; Hazelden: 1996

[46] Pearce JC. Exploring the Crack in the Cosmic Egg: Split Minds and Meta-Realities. New York: Washington Square Press; 1974

[47] Gatto JT. Dumbing us down: the hidden curriculum of compulsory education. Gabriola Island, Canada; New Society Publishers: 2005

[48] "No one should ever work. In order to stop suffering, we have to stop working. That doesn't mean we have to stop doing things. It does mean creating a new way of life based on play..." Black B. The abolition of work and other essays. Port Townsend: Loompanics Unlimited; 1985, pages 17-33

[49] Jarow R. Creating the Work You Love: Courage, Commitment and Career; Inner Traditions Intl Ltd; 1995 [ISBN: 0892815426]

[50] Dominguez JR. Transforming Your Relationship With Money. Sounds True; Book and Cassette edition: 2001 Audio tape.

(*selecting* one of the offered options: the illusion of freedom). Various conscious thoughts and unconscious assumptions create our "working reality" which represents the way that we see things and the paradigm by which we *act in* and *interact with* the larger world. These layers come from our own families, schools, teachers, churches, companies, friends, parents, and ourselves—our previous interpretations and misinterpretations of ourselves and events; in sum, our responses to outer events combined with our internal experiences meld into our perception of ourselves (known as "the genesis of personal identity") and how we as individuals relate to our inner ourselves and [our perception of] the outer world. Becoming conscious of these realities and illusions allows us the opportunity to discard those views that are inaccurate, dysfunctional, and harmful and to accept a truer reality based on what we experience, feel, and know to be real—in the present, as adults. Once we are freed from *unreality*, we can live true to ourselves in a way that is authentically responsible to our own needs *and* the needs of our communities so that we can simultaneously sustain our obligations to society[51,52] while being free to be unique individuals.[53,54]

Examples of commonly accepted paradigms and their reasonable alternatives

Commonly advocated/accepted paradigms ↳ *Implication and effect*	*Alternate paradigm* ↳ *Implication and effect*
It is OK to be irresponsible in daily choices and then blame health problems on bad luck, bad genes, or both. ↳ Many people fail to take responsibility for their lives and thereby become victims of circumstances—negative circumstances that they themselves helped to create.	**Lifestyle, especially diet and nutrition, is the most powerful influence on health outcomes. Therefore, an educated patient is empowered to direct his/her health destiny.** ↳ Optimal health *per individual* is attained when people take responsibility for their lives, seek health information, and then incorporate this information into their daily routine in the form of healthy living: health-promoting lifestyle, eating, exercise, supplementation, relationships, and occupational and social activities, including socio-political involvement to protect the environment and resist the privatization of life and the spoliation of the environment in which we live and upon which our lives and health depend.[55,56]
In general, chemical medications are the answer to nearly all health problems. ↳ The belief in medications as the primary treatment of disease creates a patient population that is apathetic, disempowered, and dependent upon the medical-pharmaceutical industry, which grows richer and more powerful despite so-called 'earnest' attempts at cost containment.[57]	**Many acute and chronic problems can be more effectively managed in terms of prevention, safety, efficacy, and cost-effectiveness when phytonutritional interventions are either used as primary therapy or, when necessary, used in conjunction with medications.** ↳ A reduction in disease prevalence via health-promoting diet and lifestyle along with integrative treatments offers the best opportunity for benefit to patients, doctors, and third-party payers.[58]

---

[51] Bly R. The Sibling Society. Vintage Books USA; Reprint edition (June 1, 1997) ISBN: 0679781285 (Abridged audio edition (May 1, 1996)

[52] Bly R. Where have all the parents gone? A talk on the Sibling Society. New York: Sound Horizons, 1996 Highly recommended.

[53] Bradshaw J. Healing the Shame that Binds You [Audio Cassette (April 1990) Health Communications Audio; ISBN: 1558740430]

[54] Miller A. The truth will set you free: overcoming emotional blindness and finding your true adult self. New York: Basic Books; 2001

[55] "Your lack of interest in the past, your lack of involvement, your unwillingness to develop coherent strategies, your unwillingness to challenge authority - these have created a vacuum in decision-making, that has been filled by professional groups with close relationships with the chemical industries..." Samuel Epstein MD, 1993. Professor of Occupational and Environmental Medicine at the School of Public Health, University of Illinois Medical Center Chicago. http://www.converge.org.nz/pirm/pestican.htm accessed September 11, 2004

[56] Kristin S. Schafer, Margaret Reeves, Skip Spitzer, Susan E. Kegley. Chemical Trespass: Pesticides in Our Bodies and Corporate Accountability. Pesticide Action Network North America. May 2004 Available at http://www.panna.org/campaigns/docsTrespass/chemicalTrespass2004.dv.html on August 1, 2004

[57] "In this paper I offer four hypotheses to help explain why use of pharmaceuticals has continued to grow even as managed care and other cost containment efforts have flourished." Berndt ER. The U.S. pharmaceutical industry: why major growth in times of cost containment? Health Aff (Millwood). 2001 Mar-Apr;20(2):100-14

[58] "Hospital admission rates in the control group were 11.4 times higher than those in the MVAH group for cardiovascular disease, 3.3 times higher for cancer, and 6.7 times higher for mental health and substance abuse. ...MVAH patients older than age 45...had 88% fewer total patients days compared with control patients." Orme-Johnson DW, Herron RE. An innovative approach to reducing medical care utilization and expenditures. Am J Manag Care. 1997 Jan;3(1):135-44

Examples of commonly accepted paradigms and their reasonable alternatives—*continued*

Commonly accepted paradigms ↳ Implication and effect	Alternate paradigm ↳ Implication and effect
Work ethic: a belief that "hard work" has moral value and makes a person "better." ↳ Belief in the principle of "work ethic" encourages people to mindlessly engage in work for the sake of engaging in work without considering the implications of their actions or other alternatives that might produce a more beneficial outcome.[59]	**Work is the means rather than an end unto itself (except when the "work" is enjoyable, in which case it is no longer "work").** ↳ Occupations and professions can be designed for the enhancement of life (health, pleasure, relationships, the environment, care of the poor) rather than as an end to themselves at the expense of the individual, society, and the environment.
It is "normal" for adults to give 10.5-12 hours per day 5 days per week to work. ↳ In most corporate environments, employee's work at least 8.5 hours per day, with 1 additional hour spent in commuting[60] and another hour spent in preparation, transportation, and maintenance of work-related clothing, preparing work-related meals, maintaining the auto that is used for work-related tasks. With 10.5 hours given directly to work, 0.5-1 additional hours are needed for recuperation from work-related stress ("daily decompression"); thus the average amount of time given to work-related activities is much larger than commonly believed.[61] Because of the time and energies devoted to "work" the vast majority of people feel that they do not have sufficient time for themselves, their families and friends, their creativity, learning about the world, political involvement, and other more important aspects of life. "Not enough time" is the most common reason given by patients for not exercising.	**A paradigm of a 4-day workweek is just as valid and perhaps more valid than one that advocates a 5-day workweek. A paradigm of a 6-hour workday is at least as valid as one of an 8-10 hour workday.** ↳ Many people in our culture are chronically overworked, undernourished, tired and suffer from an insufficiency of time to simply be in community, to rest, to be creative. Living with such limitations and pressures should be expected to produce a population that is reactively hedonistic, impulsive, and prone to addiction. Behaviors that are addictive (e.g., drugs, alcohol) and destructive (e.g., over-eating, alcohol, sugar, fat) are simply frustrated and maladaptive coping strategies to combat the stress caused by a damaging, unnatural paradigm from which most people cannot escape.[62] Redesigning our societal structures and expectations in ways that conform to our natural humanity and biologic, nutritional, and emotional needs is more rational than forcing *en masse* all of humanity to contort and conform to an artificial posture and cadence of performance, productivity, "professionalism", and other unnatural expectations. Less time dedicated to work and all that it entails leaves more time for 1) healthy cooking, 2) relaxed, conscious, and enjoyable eating, 3) exercise, 4) creativity and hobbies, 5) keeping informed of and involved with political change, and 6) participation in social relationships.[63]

---

[59] "Conventional wisdom is the habitual, the unexamined life, absorbed into the culture and the fashion of the time, lost in the mad rush of accumulation, lulled to sleep by the easy lies of political hacks and newspaper scribblers, or by priests who wouldn't know a god if they met one." Nisker W. <u>Crazy Wisdom</u>. Berkeley; Ten Speed Press: 1990, page 7

[60] Monday, September 8, 2003 -- The average daily one-way commute to work in the United States takes just over 26 minutes, according to the Bureau of Transportation Statistics' Omnibus Household Survey. Omnibus Household Survey Shows Americans' Average Commuting Time is Just Over 26 Minutes. http://www.bts.gov/press_releases/2003/bts020_03/html/bts020_03.html on August 3, 2004

[61] Dominguez JR. <u>Transforming Your Relationship with Money</u>. Sounds True; Book and Cassette edition: 2001

[62] Breton D, Largent C. <u>The Paradigm Conspiracy: Why Our Social Systems Violate Human Potential-And How We Can Change Them</u>. Hazelden: 1998

Quality and quantity of sleep: A sleep duration of less than 8 hours of deep solid sleep each night is physiologically insufficient for most of people; many people feel best with 9 hours of sleep, yet some people appear to function well on about 6 hours of sleep per night. Not only is it important to get a sufficient *quantity* of sleep, but we need to ensure that the *quality* of the sleep receives appropriate attention, as well. Sleep should be mostly continuous, not "broken" or interrupted. Some experts

> **The Importance of Sleep**
>
> Regulation of sleep-wake cycles and the regular satisfaction of sleep needs are important for preservation of immune function, intellectual performance, emotional stability, and the internal regulation of the body's inflammatory tendency.

believe that people should be able to recall their dreams at night, as this may be a sign of proper neurotransmitter status, especially with regard to serotonin, which is affected by pyridoxine[64] as well as other factors. Going to bed at a regular hour (not later than 10 or 11 at night) helps to synchronize the daily schedule with the body's inherent hormonal rhythms and "physiological clock" which expects one to be in deep sleep by midnight and to be waking at approximately 8 o'clock in the morning. Recent research has shown that **sleep deprivation causes a systemic inflammatory response manifested objectively by increases in high-sensitivity C-reactive protein (hsCRP)**.[65] Correspondingly, sleep apnea, a condition associated with repetitive sleep disturbances, is also associated with an elevation of CRP[66], and effective treatment of sleep apnea results in a normalization of CRP levels.[67] We could therefore conclude that **sleep deprivation creates a proinflammatory condition.** Furthermore, **sleep deprivation has been proven to impair intellectual functioning, emotional state, and immune function**, with abnormalities in immune status already evident the morning after sleep deprivation.[68] Wakefulness and exposure to light at night result in a suppression of melatonin production and may therefore contribute to cancer development since melatonin has anticancer actions that would be abrogated by its reduced endogenous production.[69,70] Limited evidence also suggests that melatonin production is altered in patients with the inflammatory conditions eczema[71] and psoriasis[72] and that this sleep-related hormone has anti-inflammatory/anti-autoimmune benefits that may be relevant for the suppression of diseases such as multiple sclerosis[73] and sarcoidosis.[74]

---

[63] "Take back your time" is a major U.S./Canadian initiative to challenge the epidemic of overwork, over-scheduling and time famine that now threatens our health, our families and relationships, our communities and our environment. http://www.simpleliving.net/timeday/ on August 3, 2004

[64] "...a significant difference in dream-salience scores (this is a composite score containing measures on vividness, bizarreness, emotionality, and color) between the 250-mg condition and placebo over the first three days of each treatment... An hypothesis is presented involving the role of B-6 in the conversion of tryptophan to serotonin." Ebben M, Lequerica A, Spielman A. Effects of pyridoxine on dreaming: a preliminary study. *Percept Mot Skills* 2002 Feb;94(1):135-40

[65] "CONCLUSIONS: Both acute total and short-term partial sleep deprivation resulted in elevated high-sensitivity CRP concentrations... We propose that sleep loss may be one of the ways that inflammatory processes are activated and contribute to the association of sleep complaints, short sleep duration, and cardiovascular morbidity observed in epidemiologic surveys." Meier-Ewert HK, Ridker PM, et al. Effect of sleep loss on C-reactive protein, an inflammatory marker of cardiovascular risk. *J Am Coll Cardiol.* 2004 Feb 18;43(4):678-83

[66] "OSA is associated with elevated levels of CRP, a marker of inflammation and of cardiovascular risk. The severity of OSA is proportional to the CRP level." Shamsuzzaman AS, Winnicki M, Lanfranchi P, Wolk R, Kara T, Accurso V, Somers VK. Elevated C-reactive protein in patients with obstructive sleep apnea. *Circulation.* 2002 May 28;105(21):2462-4

[67] "CONCLUSIONS: Levels of CRP and IL-6 and spontaneous production of IL-6 by monocytes are elevated in patients with OSAS but are decreased by nCPAP." Yokoe T, Minoguchi K, Matsuo H, Oda N, Minoguchi H, Yoshino G, Hirano T, Adachi M. Elevated levels of C-reactive protein and interleukin-6 in patients with obstructive sleep apnea syndrome are decreased by nasal continuous positive airway pressure. *Circulation.* 2003 Mar 4;107(8):1129-34 Available on-line at http://circ.ahajournals.org/cgi/reprint/107/8/1129.pdf on August 2, 2004

[68] "Taken together, SD induced a deterioration of both mood and ability to work, which was most prominent in the evening after SD, while the maximal alterations of the host defence system could be found twelve hours earlier, i.e., already in the morning following SD." Heiser P, Dickhaus B, Opper C, Hemmeter U, Remschmidt H, Wesemann W, Krieg JC, Schreiber W. Alterations of host defense system after sleep deprivation are followed by impaired mood and psychosocial functioning. *World J Biol Psychiatry* 2001 Apr;2(2):89-94

[69] "Observational studies support an association between night work and cancer risk. We hypothesise that the potential primary culprit for this observed association is the lack of melatonin, a cancer-protective agent whose production is severely diminished in people exposed to light at night." Schernhammer ES, Schulmeister K. Melatonin and cancer risk: does light at night compromise physiologic cancer protection by lowering serum melatonin levels? *Br J Cancer.* 2004 Mar 8;90(5):941-3

[70] "This is the first biological evidence for a potential link between constant light exposure and increased human breast oncogenesis involving MLT suppression and stimulation of tumor LA metabolism." Blask DE, Dauchy RT, Sauer LA, Krause JA, Brainard GC. Growth and fatty acid metabolism of human breast cancer (MCF-7) xenografts in nude rats: impact of constant light-induced nocturnal melatonin suppression. *Breast Cancer Res Treat.* 2003 Jun;79(3):313-20

[71] "In 6 patients exhibiting low serum levels of melatonin, the circadian melatonin rhythm was found to be abolished. In 8 patients a diminished nocturnal melatonin increase was observed compared with the controls (n = 40)." Schwarz W, Birau N, Hornstein OP, Heubeck B, Schonberger A, Meyer C, Gottschalk J. Alterations of melatonin secretion in atopic eczema. *Acta Derm Venereol.* 1988;68(3):224-9

[72] "Our results show that psoriatic patients had lost the nocturnal peak and usual circadian rhythm of melatonin secretion." Mozzanica N, Tadini G, Radaelli A, et al. Plasma melatonin levels in psoriasis. *Acta Derm Venereol.* 1988;68(4):312-6

[73] "This hypothesis is supported by the observation that administration of melatonin (3 mg, orally) at 2:00 p.m., when the patient experienced severe blurring of vision, resulted within 15 minutes in a dramatic improvement in visual acuity and in normalization of the visual evoked potential latency after stimulation of the left eye." Sandyk R. Diurnal variations in vision and relations to circadian melatonin secretion in multiple sclerosis. *Int J Neurosci.* 1995 Nov;83(1-2):1-6

[74] Cagnoni ML, Lombardi A, Cerinic MC, Dedola GL, Pignone A. Melatonin for treatment of chronic refractory sarcoidosis. *Lancet.* 1995;346:1229-30

Helping patients improve quality and quantity of sleep

- Schedule sufficient time for sleep; generally this is 9 hours to allow time for "winding down" and "daily decompression" so that a full 8 hours of sleep can ensue.
- Reduce intake of stimulants such as caffeine, tobacco, and aspartame. Some patients will need to reduce intake only in the evening, while others will need to reduce intake even in the morning in order to have improved quality and quantity of sleep later at night.
- Exercise early in the day (morning or early afternoon) to promote restful sleep at night.[75]
- Avoid aggressive or arousing physical activity in the evening to avoid increases in norepinephrine, epinephrine, and cortisol, which can discourage sleep.
- Dim lights at night to promote melatonin production. Beginning one to two hours before bedtime, turn off bright lights and use only dim lighting. Bright lights reduce melatonin secretion and stimulate neocortical activity and thereby inhibit sleep.
- Have an evening ritual/pattern that helps the psyche recognize that the time for sleep has arrived. Such practices can include relaxing warm tea, meditation, prayer, and daily reflection.
- For patients with a pattern of falling asleep and then waking approximately 4-6 hours later with feelings of hunger or anxiety (nocturnal hypoglycemia), they should eat a small meal or snack of complex carbohydrates, protein, and fat before going to bed. For example, the combination of nuts (or nut butter) with whole fruit such as apples provides protein, fat, and complex carbohydrate with a low glycemic index to provide sustenance throughout the night. Protein powders and other sources of "predigested" amino acids should generally be avoided late at night because an excess consumption of high protein foods can reduce tryptophan entry into the brain and thus reduce serotonin and melatonin synthesis. Most amino acid-derived neurotransmitters such as dopamine, glutamate, and norepinephrine are excitatory/stimulatory in nature.
- Vitamin and mineral supplementation is commonly beneficial, particularly with thiamine[76], methylcobalamin (weak evidence[77]), and magnesium (particularly sleep disturbance associated with restless leg syndrome[78]). Vitamins should be taken earlier in the day (with breakfast and lunch; not before bed); however calcium and magnesium can be taken before bed.
- Earplugs, window covers, and a quiet, snore-free environment are generally conducive to better sleep.
- For patients with difficulty falling asleep, consider 5-hydroxytryptophan consumed with simple carbohydrate (50-200 mg for adults, up to 2 mg/kg[79] for children), melatonin (0.5-10 mg), valerian-hops tea or capsules[80] 60-90 minutes before bedtime.

---

[75] "This is the first report to demonstrate that low intensity activity in an elderly population can increase deep sleep and improve memory functioning." Naylor E, Penev PD, Orbeta L, Janssen I, Ortiz R, Colecchia EF, Keng M, Finkel S, Zee PC. Daily social and physical activity increases slow-wave sleep and daytime neuropsychological performance in the elderly. *Sleep*. 2000 Feb 1;23(1):87-95

[76] Wilkinson TJ, Hanger HC, Elmslie J, George PM, Sainsbury R. The response to treatment of subclinical thiamine deficiency in the elderly. *Am J Clin Nutr*. 1997;66(4):925-8

[77] "However, because the percentage of improvement was low and significant improvement was inconsistent, Met-12 might be considered to have a low therapeutic potency and possible use as a booster for other treatment methods of the disorders." Takahashi K, et al. Double-blind test on the efficacy of methylcobalamin on sleep-wake rhythm disorders. *Psychiatry Clin Neurosci*. 1999 Apr;53(2):211-3

[78] "Our study indicates that magnesium treatment may be a useful alternative therapy in patients with mild or moderate RLS-or PLMS-related insomnia." Hornyak M, Voderholzer U, et al. Magnesium therapy for periodic leg movements-related insomnia and restless legs syndrome: an open pilot study. *Sleep*. 1998 Aug 1;21(5):501-5

[79] Bruni O, Ferri R, Miano S, Verrillo E. l-5-Hydroxytryptophan treatment of sleep terrors in children. *Eur J Pediatr*. 2004 May 14

[80] "Sleep improvements with a valerian-hops combination are associated with improved quality of life. Both treatments appear safe and did not produce rebound insomnia upon discontinuation during this study. Overall, these findings indicate that a valerian-hops combination and diphenhydramine might be useful adjuncts in the treatment of mild insomnia." Morin CM, Koetter U, Bastien C, Ware JC, Wooten V. Valerian-hops combination and diphenhydramine for treating insomnia: a randomized placebo-controlled clinical trial. *Sleep*. 2005 Nov 1;28(11):1465-71

Exercise: Human existence has changed radically over the past few millennia, centuries, and decades, and one of the most profound changes has been in our relationship to physical activity. Paleologists and historical scientists agree that physical activity among humans is at its all-time historical low, and that levels of exertion that we now call "vigorous and frequent exercise" would have been *completely normal* in the daily lives of our ancestors, who engaged in at least four times more physical activity than their modern-day progeny.[81] At one time—a time in which vigorous physical activity was a normal part of daily life—probably no word existed for what modern people describe and often resist as "exercise."

Daily exercise is health-promoting and restorative
"The health rewards of exercise extend far beyond its benefits for specific diseases." Exercise reduces blood clotting, lowers blood pressure, lowers cholesterol, improves glucose tolerance and insulin sensitivity, enhances self-image, elevates mood, reduces stress, creates a feeling of well-being, reinforces other positive life-style changes, stimulates creative thinking, increases muscle mass, increases basal metabolic rate, promotes improved sleep, stimulates healthy intestinal function, promotes weight loss, and enhances appearance. "Furthermore, **the ability of exercise to restore function to organs, muscles, joints, and bones is not shared by drugs or surgery.**"   Harold Elrick, MD. Exercise is Medicine. *Physician and Sportsmedicine*. 1996: 24; 2 (February)

Daily exercise is the body's physiological expectation
"Although modern technology has made physical exertion optional, it is still important to exercise as though our survival depended on it, and in a different way it still does. **We are genetically adapted to live an extremely physically active lifestyle.**"   O'Keefe JH Jr, Cordain L. Cardiovascular disease resulting from a diet and lifestyle at odds with our Paleolithic genome: how to become a 21st-century hunter-gatherer. *Mayo Clin Proc.* 2004 Jan;79(1):101-8

Our current mode of compulsory primary and secondary education prioritizes "being still" over physical exertion/expression for the vast majority of students' time. Thus having been separated from their inherent tendency to be physically active and emotionally expressive, many children grow into adults who have to be *retaught to inhabit their bodies* and to engage in physical activity on a daily basis. Basic science has proven that this is true: when animals are restrained, they show less activity when freed and no longer tied down. Conversely, when animals are rigorously exercised, they show higher levels of *spontaneous physical activity* when left to their own discretion. A probable sociological parallel is at work in human cultures where, under the guise of *work* and *entertainment*, people are corralled into lifestyles of physical inactivity in a wide range of apparently divergent activities. Watching television, driving a car, seeing a movie, doing computer/desk work at the office, attending a sports event or educational lecture, seeing the opera—all of these are simply different forms of **sitting**, of physical inactivity. Changing our social structure in a way that prioritizes *life* over *work*, such as moving toward a 4-day work week and/or a 6-hour work day, would allow people more time to live their lives, to pursue healthy diets and relationships, to be creative, and to engage in more physical activity; thus, "escape entertainment" such as fiction books and movies and processed "fast foods"—the latter of which are inherently unhealthy[82]—would become less necessary and less attractive.

Industrialized Westernized societies' disregard for connection with the body
"That I deemed it an imposition to have to make use of my perfectly adequate coordination, or resented—from unexamined principle—the use of time to fill a need, was an arbitrary assignment of values that [this other culture] did not share."   Liedloff J. The Continuum Concept. Cambridge, MA: Da Capo Press; 1977, page 15

---

[81] Eaton SB, Cordain L, Eaton SB. An evolutionary foundation for health promotion. *World Rev Nutr Diet* 2001; 90:5-12
[82] For an additional perspective see movie by Morgan Spurlock (director). Super Size Me. www.supersizeme.com released in 2004

Exploring the spectrum of physical activity from inactivity to athleticism

Inactivity	Minimally active	Active	Healthy	Athletic
• Bed-ridden • Chair-ridden • Minimal activity, such as walking to car or bathroom or to buy groceries • Activity in this category is equivalent to or barely above that which is necessary to sustain life	• Periodic performance of more activity than the minimal needed to sustain life, such as walking around the block after dinner, or taking a brief stroll at a park or at the beach	• Regular performance of low/moderate levels of activity at work or leisure, at least 30-60 minutes of physical activity per day	• 60-120 minutes of vigorous activity such as running, swimming, cycling, or other physical training 4-7 days per week	• More than 2 hours devoted to conditioning, strengthening, and skill-building 4-7 days per week

At least 30-45 minutes of exercise four days per week is the *absolute minimum*. Ideally, patients who have been sedentary and are over age 45 years would have a pre-exercise physical exam that might also include electrocardiography before embarking on a program of vigorous exercise. Patients who have been sedentary for many years can start slowly with their new exercise program, gradually increasing the duration and intensity. With the simple addition of regular exercise to their routine, patients will have significantly reduced risk for problems such as depression, chronic pain, cancer, coronary artery disease, stroke, hypertension, diabetes, arthritis, osteoporosis, dyslipidemia, obesity, chronic obstructive pulmonary disease, constipation, and other problems.[83] Furthermore, successful prevention and treatment of health problems with exercise and lifestyle modifications reduces dependency on pharmaceutical drugs, thereby further saving lives. O'Keefe and Cordain[84] report that **during the hunter-gatherer period, humans averaged 5-10 miles of daily running and walking**. Additionally, **other physical activities such as heavy lifting, digging, and climbing would have been considered "normal" aspects of daily life rather than "exercise"—an achievement for which modern/industrialized people seek recognition.** Thus, when sedentary patients achieve the first-step goal of walking around the block after dinner, we can commend them for making a significant stride forward in ultimately attaining better health, but we cannot stop there nor delude them into believing that this is adequate.

Common physical activities: a buffet of options from which to choose
☑ **"Boot camp"-style aerobics classes**: excellent variety and fast-pace maintains oxygen debt for the entire session (generally 60 minutes) even among reasonably well trained "healthy" people
☑ **Aerobic machines such as elliptical runners and stair-climbing machines**: easy on joints; accessible during inclement weather; easy to integrate with weight-lifting which is commonly available at the same facility
☑ **Baseball**: requires some skill in throwing and batting, but otherwise this is a very inactive sport
☑ **Football**: much of the game is spent in inactivity; most of the fitness comes from preparation for the game, not the game itself; high impact activity wherein injuries are expected
☑ **Hiking**: virtually free of expense; allows for conversation, exploration, and time in nature; mountains required
☑ **Indoor aerobics**: excellent for cardiovascular fitness and weight loss, requires and thus promotes coordination and timing
☑ **Indoor cycling**: excellent for cardiovascular fitness and weight loss, easy on the joints; accessible during inclement weather
☑ **Jogging and running**: easy, accessible, virtually free; allows for conversation and exploration; increases endorphin production and promotes a sense of well-being; detoxification via sweating
☑ **Kayaking and canoeing**: excellent combination of relaxation and exertion; develops upper body strength and balance
☑ **Martial arts**: requires more balance, coordination, timing, strategy, endurance; injuries are to be expected, as is enhanced sense of security and confidence
☑ **Outdoor cycling (mountain and trail)**: same as above; requires more balance and coordination
☑ **Outdoor cycling (road)**: same as above with added bonus of being outdoors; promotes independence from automobiles and petroleum products – thereby reducing pollution and sustaining the environment

---

[83] Harold Elrick, MD. Exercise is Medicine. *The Physician and Sportsmedicine* - Volume 24 - No. 2 - February 1996
[84] O'Keefe JH Jr, Cordain L. Cardiovascular disease resulting from a diet and lifestyle at odds with our Paleolithic genome: how to become a 21st-century hunter-gatherer. *Mayo Clin Proc.* 2004 Jan;79(1):101-8. Available on line at http://www.thepaleodiet.com/articles/Hunter-Gatherer%20Mayo.pdf on May 19, 2004

- ☑ **Rock-climbing (indoor and outdoor)**: requires upper body and grip strength; promotes agility, resourcefulness, courage, and trust; good for building stronger relationships assuming that your partner does not drop the rope or get distracted; carries some inherent risk
- ☑ **Skiing, snowboarding, cross-country skiing**: Require balance and coordination, costly equipment, and appropriate season and climate; risk of traumatic injury due to speed in skiing and snowboarding. Cross-country skiing is generally safe from trauma and provides excellent cardiovascular exertion, in addition to exposure to nature
- ☑ **Soccer**: excellent for lower-body conditioning, teamwork, and coordination, the rapid stops and turns can be hard on joints
- ☑ **Surfing**: paddling requires upper body endurance and strength; some leg strength is required but is not strongly developed during the riding portion of surfing, which is mostly technique and "style"; excellent proprioceptive training
- ☑ **Swimming**: requires access to a pool or suitable body of water; excellent for promoting fitness in a way that is generally easy on joints and muscles and is without impact; requires and thus promotes coordination and timing
- ☑ **Tennis and racket sports**: requires more balance, coordination, timing, strategy, endurance; the rapid stops, starts, and turns can be hard on joints; upper body exertion is asymmetric and can promote muscle imbalance
- ☑ **Volleyball**: good team activity; not highly exertional in terms of either aerobic fitness nor strength acquisition
- ☑ **Walking**: easy, accessible, virtually free; allows for conversation and exploration; allows for time outdoors
- ☑ **Weight lifting, bodybuilding, and powerlifting**: excellent for increasing lean body mass – one of the primary determinants of basal metabolic rate; promotes bone strengthening
- ☑ **Yoga, Calisthenics**: inexpensive, can be done alone or in groups; does not require much/any equipment, therefore costs are low and access is near universal

Obesity: Obesity is a major risk factor for cardiovascular disease, cancer, diabetes mellitus, depression, joint degeneration and pain. Obese people also commonly report difficulties with performing daily activities, and they also report higher rates of depression and social isolation than do people of normal weight. Adipose tissue is biologically active, promoting systemic inflammation and estrogen dominance, thereby promoting the development of inflammatory and malignant diseases such as psoriasis and cancers of the breast, prostate, and colon, respectively.

"Body Mass Index" is a clinically valuable measure of height-weight proportionality and therefore adiposity, since an excess of height-proportionate weight is more commonly due to excess adipose than to excess muscle. To calculate BMI simply chart height and weight in the table below. Numbers greater than 25 correlate with being "overweight" while numbers greater than 30 meet the criteria for "obesity." BMI determinations may not be reflective of disease risk for people who are pregnant, highly muscular, or for young children or the frail elderly.

Body mass index (BMI) interpretation
- ❑ Severely underweight: < 16.5
- ❑ Underweight: 16.5 - 18.4
- ❑ **Normal: 18.5 - 24.9**
- ❑ Overweight: 25 - 29.9
- ❑ Obese Class 1: 30 - 34.9
- ❑ Obese Class 2 (severe obesity): 35 - 39.9
- ❑ Obese Class 3 (morbid obesity): 40 - 47.9
- ❑ Obese Class 4 (supermorbid obesity): ≥ 48

WEIGHT in pounds

HEIGHT	100	110	120	130	140	150	160	170	180	190	200	210	220	230	240	250
5'0"	20	21	23	25	27	29	31	33	35	37	39	41	43	45	47	49
5'1"	19	21	23	25	26	28	30	32	34	36	38	40	42	43	45	47
5'2"	18	20	22	24	26	27	29	31	33	35	37	38	40	42	44	46
5'3"	18	19	21	23	25	27	28	30	32	34	35	37	39	41	43	44
5'4"	17	19	21	22	24	26	27	29	31	33	34	36	38	39	41	43
5'5"	17	18	20	22	23	25	27	28	30	32	33	35	37	38	40	42
5'6"	16	18	19	21	23	24	26	27	29	31	32	34	36	37	39	40
5'7"	16	17	19	20	22	23	25	27	28	30	31	33	34	36	38	39
5'8"	15	17	18	20	21	23	24	26	27	29	30	32	33	35	36	38
5'9"	15	16	18	19	21	22	24	25	27	28	30	31	32	34	35	37
5'10"	14	16	17	19	20	22	23	24	26	27	29	30	32	33	34	36
5'11"	14	15	17	18	20	21	22	24	25	26	27	28	30	32	33	35
6'0"	14	15	16	18	19	20	22	23	24	26	27	28	30	31	33	34
6'1"	13	15	16	17	18	20	21	22	24	25	26	28	29	30	32	33
6'2"	13	14	15	17	18	19	21	22	23	24	26	27	28	30	31	32
6'3"	12	14	15	16	17	19	20	21	22	24	25	26	27	29	30	31
6'4"	12	13	15	16	17	18	19	21	22	23	24	26	27	28	29	30

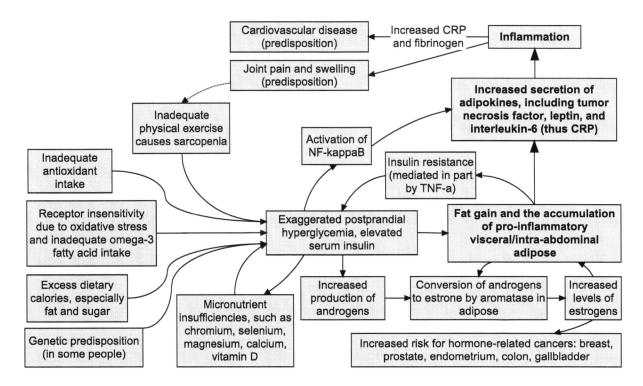

Overview of the proinflammatory and endocrinologic activity of adipose tissue: Adipose tissue is biologically active, promoting systemic inflammation and production of estrogens at the expense of androgens via the enzyme aromatase

The old view that fat (adipose) tissue was merely serving as an inert and inactive depot for lipid/energy storage is now replaced with the view that adipose tissue is biologically-active, influencing overall health via complex mechanisms that are biochemical-inflammatory-endocrinologic and not merely mechanical (i.e., excess weight, excess mass).[85] **Excess fat tissue—especially visceral/abdominal adipose—creates a systemic proinflammatory state** evidenced most readily by the elevations in hsCRP commonly seen in patients with obesity and the metabolic syndrome.[86] Adipokines are cytokines secreted by adipose tissue and include tumor necrosis factor-alpha, interleukin-6, and leptin—a cytokine derived from fat cells that promotes inflammation and immune activation; levels are higher in obese patients and decrease after weight loss. Obese patients also appear to have "leptin resistance" with regard to the suppression of appetite by leptin. **Adipose creates excess estrogens;** concomitant hyperglycemia increases androgen production[87], and these androgens are subsequently converted to estrogens by aromatase in the adipose tissue. For example, the adrenal gland makes androstenedione, which can be converted by aromatase in adipose tissue into estrone.[88] These proinflammatory and hormonal perturbations manifest clinically as an increased risk for breast, prostate, endometrial, colon and gallbladder cancers, and cardiovascular disease. This pattern of inflammation, reduced testosterone, and elevated estrogen is also a predisposition toward the development of autoimmune/inflammatory diseases.

---

[85] "The fat cell is a true endocrine cell that secretes a variety of factors, including metabolites such as lactate, fatty acids, prostaglandin derivatives and a variety of peptides, including cytokines (leptin, tumor necrosis factor, interleukin-1 and -6, adiponectin), angiotensinogen, complement D (adipsin), plasminogen activator inhibitor-1 and undoubtedly many others." Bray GA. The underlying basis for obesity: relationship to cancer. *J Nutr.* 2002 Nov;132(11 Suppl):3451S-3455S

[86] "Our results indicate a strong relationship between adipocytokines and inflammatory markers, and suggest that cytokines secreted by adipose tissue could play a role in increased inflammatory proteins secretion by the liver." Maachi M, Pieroni L, Bruckert E, Jardel C, Fellahi S, Hainque B, Capeau J, Bastard JP. Systemic low-grade inflammation is related to both circulating and adipose tissue TNFalpha, leptin and IL-6 levels in obese women. *Int J Obes Relat Metab Disord.* 2004;28:993-7

[87] Christensen L, Hagen C, Henriksen JE, Haug E. Elevated levels of sex hormones and sex hormone binding globulin in male patients with insulin dependent diabetes mellitus. Effect of improved blood glucose regulation. *Dan Med Bull.* 1997 Nov;44(5):547-50

[88] "The conversion of androstenedione secreted by the adrenal gland into estrone by aromatase in adipose tissue stroma provides an important source of estrogen for the postmenopausal woman. This estrogen may play an important role in the development of endometrial and breast cancer." Bray GA. The underlying basis for obesity: relationship to cancer. *J Nutr.* 2002 Nov;132(11 Suppl):3451S-3455S

The Daily Diet—Powerful Intervention for the Prevention and Treatment of Disease: "Whole foods" should form the foundation and majority of the diet. As doctors and patients, we should emphasize whole fruits, vegetables, nuts, seeds, berries, and lean sources of protein. "Whole foods" are foods that are found in nature, and they should be eaten as closely as possible to their natural state—preferably *unprocessed* and *raw*. Creating a diet based on whole, natural foods by emphasizing the consumption of fruits, vegetables, and lean meats and excluding high-fat factory meats, high-sugar foods like white potatoes, and milled grains like wheat and corn is essential for our efforts of promoting health by matching the human *diet* with the human *genome*.[89] Our genetic make-up was co-created over a period of more than 2.6 million years by interaction with the environment as it exists in its natural state. This environment mandated daily physical activity and a diet that was exclusively composed of 1) fresh fruits, 2) fresh vegetables (mostly uncooked), 3) raw nuts, seeds, berries, roots, and 4) generous portions of lean game meat that was rich in omega-3 fatty acids from free-living animals who were lean because they also ran, fasted, and dealt with limited food supplies. Humans have deviated from this original diet for the sake of ease, conformity, and short-term satisfaction at the expense of health and longevity. Peoples who consume traditional, natural diets have dramatically lower incidences *major* health problems such as cancer, cardiovascular disease, diabetes, obesity and also suffer much less from *milder* problems such as acne, psoriasis, dental cavities, oral malocclusion, and chronic sinus congestion. Societies that are free of these disorders become overwhelmed with them *within only one or two generations* as soon as they adopt the American/Western style of eating. These facts were conclusively documented by Weston Price in his famous 1945 masterpiece *Nutrition and Physical Degeneration*[90] and have been reiterated recently in an excellent review by O'Keefe and Cordain in *Mayo Clinic Proceedings*.[91]

The Supplemented Paleo-Mediterranean Diet

My conclusion after reading several hundred articles on epidemiology, nutritional biochemistry, and dietary intervention studies is that the Paleo-Mediterranean diet—particularly its pesco-vegetarian version—is the single most healthy dietary regimen for the broadest range of patients and for the prevention of the widest range of diseases including cancer, hypertension, diabetes, dermatitis, depression, obesity, arthritis and all inflammatory and autoimmune diseases. By definition, this is a diet that helps patients increase their intake of fruits and vegetables (fiber, antioxidants, phytonutrients), increases their intake of fish (for the anti-inflammatory omega-3 fats EPA and DHA) while reducing intake of the pro-cancer and pro-inflammatory omega-6 fats linoleic acid and arachidonic acid), and it is naturally low in sugars and cholesterol (for alleviating hyperglycemia and dyslipidemia). This dietary pattern helps patients avoid grains, particularly wheat (a common allergen), and it reduces the intake of the high-fermentation carbohydrates in breads, pasta, pastries, potatoes, and sucrose which promote overgrowth of bacteria and yeast in the intestines. Supplementing this pesco-vegetarian diet with vitamins, minerals, fatty acids such as fish oil and GLA (from borage oil), and protein from soy and whey makes this diet effective for both the treatment and prevention of many conditions; I have called this "the Supplemented Paleo-Mediterranean Diet."

1. Vasquez A. A Five-Part Nutritional Protocol that Produces Consistently Positive Results. *Nutritional Wellness* 2005 September
2. Vasquez A. Implementing the Five-Part Nutritional Wellness Protocol for the Treatment of Various Health Problems. *Nutritional Wellness* 2005 November
3. Vasquez A. Revisiting the Five-Part Nutritional Wellness Protocol: The Supplemented Paleo-Mediterranean Diet. *Nutritional Perspectives* 2011 January

The complete texts of these articles are included within this book and on-line at http://optimalhealthresearch.com/spmd.html

Most patients (and doctors) need to increase consumption of fruits and vegetables: Encourage consumption of collard greens, broccoli, kale, spinach, chard, lettuce, onions, red peppers, green beans, carrots, apples, oranges, nuts, blueberries and other fruits and vegetables. Patients can find or make a good low-carbohydrate dressing (such as lemon-garlic tahini[92]) to make these vegetables taste great. Fresh fruits and vegetables are best; but frozen fruits and vegetables are acceptable. Patients can buy a package of (organic) frozen vegetables; then when they are ready for a healthy-and-fast meal, simply thaw the vegetables or warm/steam them on the stovetop. In just a few minutes and with only minimal effort, by regularly eating vegetables, they will have significantly reduced their risk for heart disease, diabetes, cancer, hemorrhoids, constipation, and many other chronic health problems. Using frozen vegetables and eating vegetables only twice per day is not *optimal*—it is *minimal*. For many patients,

[89] O'Keefe JH Jr, Cordain L. Cardiovascular disease resulting from a diet and lifestyle at odds with our Paleolithic genome: how to become a 21st-century hunter-gatherer. *Mayo Clin Proc.* 2004 Jan;79(1):101-8
[90] Price WA. Nutrition and Physical Degeneration. Santa Monica; Price-Pottinger Nutrition Foundation: 1945
[91] O'Keefe JH Jr,Cordain L.Cardiovascular disease resulting from a diet and lifestyle at odds with our Paleolithic genome. *Mayo Clin Proc.*2004;79:101-8
[92] Mollie Katzen. The New Moosewood Cookbook Ten Speed Press; page 103

consuming two servings of vegetables per day is a major lifestyle change. *Ultimately, the goal is for fresh fruits and vegetables to form a major portion of the diet, to be the main course rather than simply a side dish.* A diet based on fruits and vegetables is a powerful nutritional strategy for reducing the risk for cancer, heart disease, and autoimmune and inflammatory disorders.[93]

Phytochemicals—important antioxidant and anti-inflammatory nutrients from fruits, vegetables, nuts, seeds, berries, and many herbs and spices: While we have all commonly thought of the benefits of fruits and vegetables as being derived from the vitamins, minerals, and fiber, we are learning from new research that many if not most of the health-promoting benefits of fruit and vegetable consumption comes from the unique plant-based chemicals—phytochemicals—contained therein. For example, while in the past we might have thought of the benefits of eating apples as being derived from the vitamin C content, we now know that vitamin C only provides 0.4% of the antioxidant action contained within a whole apple—obviously the other components of the apple, namely the phenolic compounds are responsible for most of an apple's antioxidant activity.[94] Recent research has shown that cranberries, apples, red grapes, and strawberries have the most antioxidant power of the fruits[95], while red peppers, broccoli, carrots, and spinach are the best antioxidant vegetables[96]; see the tables that follow. This is a very important concept to appreciate and remember: **the benefits derived from fruits and vegetables are _not_ derived principally from the vitamins and therefore can never be obtained from the use of multivitamin pills as a substitute for whole foods. Multivitamin and multimineral supplements are valuable and worthwhile _supplements_ to a whole-foods diet but should not be used as _substitutes_ for a whole-foods diet. Fruits and vegetables contain more than 8,000 phytochemicals, most of which have anti-inflammatory, anti-proliferative, and anti-cancer benefits[97]—the best and only way to benefit from these chemicals is to change the diet in favor of relying principally on fruits and vegetables as the major component of the diet**, and the easiest way to do this is to eliminate carbohydrate-rich antioxidant-poor foods such as bread, pasta, rice, sweets, crackers, chips and "junk foods."

Phenolic content and antioxidant capacity of common vegetables and fruits[98,99]

Vegetables		Fruits	
Phenolic content	*Antioxidant capacity*	*Phenolic content*	*Antioxidant capacity*
1. Broccoli	1. Red pepper	1. Cranberry	1. Cranberry
2. Spinach	2. Broccoli	2. Apple	2. Apple
3. Yellow onion	3. Carrot	3. Red grape	3. Red grape
4. Red pepper	4. Spinach	4. Strawberry	4. Strawberry
5. Carrot	5. Cabbage	5. Pineapple	5. Peach
6. Cabbage	6. Yellow onion	6. Banana	6. Lemon
7. Potato	7. Celery	7. Peach	7. Pear
8. Lettuce	8. Potato	8. Lemon	8. Banana
9. Celery	9. Lettuce	9. Orange	9. Orange
10. Cucumber	10. Cucumber	10. Pear	10. Grapefruit
		11. Grapefruit	11. Pineapple

[93] "...one of the most consistent research findings is that those who consume higher amounts of fruits and vegetables have lower rates of heart disease and stroke as well as cancer..." Seaman DR. The diet-induced proinflammatory state: a cause of chronic pain and other degenerative diseases? *J Manipulative Physiol Ther.* 2002;25(3):168-79

[94] "We propose that the additive and synergistic effects of phytochemicals in fruit and vegetables are responsible for their potent antioxidant and anticancer activities, and that the benefit of a diet rich in fruit and vegetables is attributed to the complex mixture of phytochemicals present in whole foods." Liu RH. Health benefits of fruit and vegetables are from additive and synergistic combinations of phytochemicals. *Am J Clin Nutr.* 2003 Sep;78(3 Suppl):517S-520S

[95] "Cranberry had the highest total antioxidant activity (177.0 +/- 4.3 micromol of vitamin C equiv/g of fruit), followed by apple, red grape, strawberry, peach, lemon, pear, banana, orange, grapefruit, and pineapple." Sun J, Chu YF, Wu X, Liu RH. Antioxidant and antiproliferative activities of common fruits. *J Agric Food Chem.* 2002 Dec 4;50(25):7449-54

[96] "Red pepper had the highest total antioxidant activity, followed by broccoli, carrot, spinach, cabbage, yellow onion, celery, potato, lettuce, and cucumber." Chu YF, Sun J, Wu X, Liu RH. Antioxidant and antiproliferative activities of common vegetables. *J Agric Food Chem.* 2002 Nov 6;50(23):6910-6

[97] Liu RH. Health benefits of fruit and vegetables are from additive and synergistic combinations of phytochemicals. *Am J Clin Nutr.* 2003 Sep;78(3 Suppl):517S-520S

[98] Chu YF, Sun J, Wu X, Liu RH. Antioxidant and antiproliferative activities of common vegetables. *J Agric Food Chem.* 2002;50:6910-6

[99] Sun J, Chu YF, Wu X, Liu RH. Antioxidant and antiproliferative activities of common fruits. *J Agric Food Chem.* 2002;50:7449-54

Different fruits and vegetables contain different types, quantities, and ratios of vitamins, minerals, and phytochemicals; therefore, *dietary diversity* **will therefore help patients obtain a broad spectrum of and maximum benefit from these different nutrients**. Taking appropriate action with the data that a fruit/vegetable-based diet has powerful health-promoting benefits means that we as doctors and patients have to change our lifestyles with regard to how we plan our meals, what we buy, what we prepare, and what we eat. Behavior modification is a tremendous challenge for people, especially those who lack sufficient motivation or insight. This text is providing the *insight*—the data, references, and concepts. But without *motivation*—from doctors to help their patients attain the highest levels of health, and from patients to change their lifestyles to become as healthy as possible—the research itself does little to promote health.

<u>**Consuming the right amount of protein**</u>: Dietary protein is eaten to provide the body with amino acids, which are the fundamental components that the body uses to create new tissues (such as skin, mucosal surfaces, hair, and nails), heal wounds (e.g., formation of collagen), fight off infections (e.g., formation of immunoglobulin proteins, antibodies), and to create specific hormones (such as insulin and thyroid hormones) and neurotransmitters, such as dopamine, serotonin, norepinephrine, and gamma-aminobutyric acid (GABA). Amino acid profiles in meats, eggs, and milk is similar to that of the human body and such dietary sources have been described as containing relatively more "complete protein" than most plant-based protein sources. For plant-based diets without concomitant use of animal proteins to provide sufficient quantity and quality of protein, foods must be combined with respect to one another's amino acid profiles.

For most people (without kidney or liver problems) the goal for daily protein intake should be 0.50-0.75 grams of protein per pound of lean body weight, depending on activity level and other health needs (see table).

Recommended <u>Grams of Protein</u> Per <u>Pound of Body Weight</u> Per Day[100]	
Infants and children ages 1-6 years[101]	0.68-0.45
RDA for sedentary adult and children ages 6-18 years[102]	0.4
Adult recreational exerciser	**0.5-0.75**
Adult competitive athlete	0.6-0.9
Adult building muscle mass	0.7-0.9
Dieting athlete	0.7-1.0
Growing teenage athlete	0.9-1.0
Pregnant women need additional protein	Add 15-30 grams/day[103]

Sufficient dietary protein is essential for patients with musculoskeletal injuries because tissue healing relies on the constant availability of amino acids and micronutrients[104], which should be supplied by a healthy, balanced, whole-foods diet that may be supplemented with specific vitamins, minerals, and phytonutrients. Low-protein diets suppress immune function, reduce muscle mass, and impair healing[105,106] whereas intakes of higher amounts of protein safely facilitate healing and the maintenance of muscle mass. Increased protein intake does not adversely affect bone health as long as dietary calcium intake is adequate.[107] According to the 1998 review by Lemon[108], "Those involved in strength training might need to consume as much as …1.7 g protein x kg(-1) x day(-

[100] Slightly modified from Nancy Clark, MS, RD. Protein Power. *The Physician and Sportsmedicine* 1996, volume 24, number 4
[101] 1.5-1 g/kg/d (0.68-0.45 grams per pound of body weight. Younger people need proportionately more protein.) Brown ML (ed). <u>Present Knowledge in Nutrition. Sixth Edition.</u> Washington DC: International Life Sciences Institute Nutrition Foundation; 1990 page 68
[102] 0.83 g.kg-1.d-1 (equivalent to 0.37 grams per pound of body weight) Pellet PL. Protein requirements in humans. *Am J Clin Nutr* 1990 May;51:723-37
[103] Weinsier RL, Morgan SL (eds). <u>Fundamentals of Clinical Nutrition</u>. St. Louis: Mosby, 1993 page 50
[104] "Supplementation with protein and vitamins, specifically arginine and vitamins A, B, and C, provides optimum nutrient support of the healing wound." Meyer NA, Muller MJ, Herndon DN. Nutrient support of the healing wound. *New Horiz* 1994 May;2(2):202-14
[105] Castaneda C, Charnley JM, Evans WJ, Crim MC. Elderly women accommodate to a low-protein diet with losses of body cell mass, muscle function, and immune response. *Am J Clin Nutr* 1995 Jul;62(1):30-9 http://www.ajcn.org/cgi/reprint/62/1/30
[106] [No author listed]. Vegetarians and healing. *JAMA* 1995; 273: 910
[107] Heaney RP. Excess dietary protein may not adversely affect bone. *J Nutr* 1998 Jun;128(6):1054-7
[108] Lemon PW. Effects of exercise on dietary protein requirements. *Int J Sport Nutr* 1998 Dec;8(4):426-47

1)...while those undergoing endurance training might need about 1.2 to 1.6 g x kg(-1) x day(-1)... ...**there is no evidence that protein intakes in the range suggested will have adverse effects in healthy individuals.**"

For patients who are completely sedentary, multiply body weight in pounds by 0.4 and this will give the number of grams of protein that should be eaten each day.[109] For patients who are very active (frequent weight lifting, or competitive athlete), multiply body weight in pounds by 0.7-0.9 and this will give the number of grams of protein that should be eaten each day.

Again, compared with sedentary people, *sick people, injured people,* and *athletes* need **more protein** to maintain weight, fight infections, repair injuries, and build and maintain muscle. Not only can insufficient protein intake cause muscle weakness and loss of weight, but recent articles have also suggested that low-protein diets can cause suppression of the immune system[110] and impairment of healing after injury or surgery.[111]

For example, in most instances and according to the data presented in and reviewed for this section, a person weighing 120 pounds should aim for at least 60 grams of protein per day, or 90 grams of protein per day if he/she is more physically active, ill, or injured. A can of tuna has 30 grams of protein; one egg has 6 grams of protein. If she is going to eat eggs as a source of protein for a meal, she might have to eat as many as five eggs to reach a target of 30 grams of protein per meal. When eating meat, visualize the amount of meat in a can of tuna to estimate the amount of protein being eaten—for example, if the portion of meat at a given meal is about the size of a half can of tuna, then we can estimate that the serving contains 15-20 grams of high-quality protein. By knowing the "target intake" for the day, and by estimating the amount of protein eaten with each meal, patients will be able to modify their protein intake to ensure that they reach their protein intake goal.

Protein supplements—most common of which are based on concentrates of or isolated components of egg, soy, or cow's milk— can be used *in conjunction with a healthy diet*. Patients using a protein supplement should eat a healthy diet and then add protein supplements between regular meals. If they substitute a protein supplement for a regular meal, then they may not actually increase protein intake. Whole *real* foods should form the foundation for the diet—patients should not rely too heavily on *protein supplements* when patients can get better results *and improved overall health* with *whole foods*. Whey, casein, and lactalbumin are proteins from milk and dairy products, and may therefore be allergenic in people allergic to cow's milk. Soy protein is safe and a source of high-quality protein for adults[112], and research shows that consumption of soy protein can help reduce the risk of cancer and heart disease[113]; however, I do not recommend the use of large quantities of supplemental soy protein for pregnant women, or for children due to the potential for disrupting endocrine function. Patients may have to experiment with different products until they find one that is suitable in regard to taste, texture, digestibility, hypoallergenicity, nutritional effects, ease of preparation, and affordability.

Recall again that the goal is *improved health*, not simply *adequate protein intake*. If we focus solely on "grams of protein" then we might overlook adverse effects that are associated with certain protein sources. Cow's milk is a high quality protein, but it is commonly allergenic and can exacerbate joint pain in sensitive individuals.[114] Beef, liver, pork and other land animal meats are excellent sources of protein, but they are also generally rich sources of arachidonic acid[115] (if not grass-fed) and iron[116], both of which have been shown to exacerbate joint pain and inflammation. Fish is an excellent source of protein, but fish are often poisoned with mercury and other toxicants, which can be ingested by humans to produce negative health effects.[117,118]

---

[109] Pellet PL. Protein requirements in humans. *Am J Clin Nutr* 1990 May;51(5):723-37
[110] Castaneda C, Charnley JM, Evans WJ, Crim MC. Elderly women accommodate to a low-protein diet with losses of body cell mass, muscle function, and immune response. *Am J Clin Nutr* 1995 Jul;62(1):30-9
[111] Vegetarians and healing. *Journal of the American Medical Association* 1995; 273: 910
[112] "These results indicate that for healthy adults, the isolated soy protein is of high nutritional quality, comparable to that of animal protein sources, and that the methionine content is not limiting for adult protein maintenance." Young VR, Puig M, Queiroz E, Scrimshaw NS, Rand WM. Evaluation of the protein quality of an isolated soy protein in young men: relative nitrogen requirements and effect of methionine supplementation. *Am J Clin Nutr.* 1984 Jan;39(1):16-24
[113] Lissin LW, Cooke JP. Phytoestrogens and cardiovascular health. *J Am Coll Cardiol.* 2000 May;35(6):1403-10
[114] Golding DN. Is there an allergic synovitis? *J R Soc Med* 1990 May;83(5):312-4
[115] Adam O, Beringer C, Kless T, Lemmen C, Adam A, Wiseman M, Adam P, Klimmek R, Forth W. Anti-inflammatory effects of a low arachidonic acid diet and fish oil in patients with rheumatoid arthritis. *Rheumatol Int* 2003 Jan;23(1):27-36
[116] Dabbagh AJ, Trenam CW, Morris CJ, Blake DR. Iron in joint inflammation. *Ann Rheum Dis* 1993; 52:67-73
[117] "These fish often harbor high levels of methylmercury, a potent human neurotoxin." Evans EC. The FDA recommendations on fish intake during pregnancy. *J Obstet Gynecol Neonatal Nurs* 2002 Nov-Dec;31(6):715-20
[118] "Geometric mean mercury levels were almost 4-fold higher among women who ate 3 or more servings of fish in the past 30 days compared with women who ate no fish in that period.." Schober SE, Sinks TH, Jones RL, Bolger PM, McDowell M, Osterloh J, Garrett ES, Canady RA, Dillon CF, Sun Y, Joseph CB, Mahaffey KR. Blood mercury levels in US children and women of childbearing age, 1999-2000. *JAMA* 2003 Apr 2;289(13):1667-74

Eat complex carbohydrates to stabilize blood sugar, mood, and energy: Choose items with a "low glycemic index"[119] to stabilize blood sugar and—for many people—to lower triglycerides and cholesterol levels. Foods with a low Glycemic Index (GI < 55)[120] include yogurt, apple (36), whole orange (43), peach (28), legumes, lentils (28), and soybeans (18), cherries, dried apricots, nuts, most meats, and most vegetables. Healthy foods that have both a low *glycemic index* as well as a low *glycemic load* include: apples, carrots, chick peas, grapes, green peas, kidney beans, oranges, peaches, peanuts, pears, pinto beans, red lentils, and strawberries.[121]

Reduce or eliminate simple sugars from the diet (as necessary): Nearly everyone should minimize intake of table sugar (sucrose), fructose and high-fructose corn syrup, and all artificial sweeteners. Of important and recent note, high-fructose corn syrup has been shown to be contaminated by mercury due to the manufacturing process[122], and fructose has been shown to induce hypertension and the metabolic syndrome in humans.[123] Chronic overconsumption of refined carbohydrates promotes disease by 1) increasing urinary excretion of magnesium and calcium, 2) inducing oxidative stress, 3) promoting fat deposition and obesity, which then generally leads to insulin resistance and hyperinsulinemia with an increase in production of cholesterol, triglycerides, and proinflammatory adipokines[124], and 4) reducing function of leukocytes.[125] Among sweeteners, honey is the best choice since it is the only natural sweetener available with a wide range of health-promoting benefits including anti-inflammatory, antibacterial, antioxidant and anti-allergy effects.[126] Also consider the herb stevia as a non-caloric and nutritive sweetener. Occasional intake of sweets is likely to be of little consequence for people who are generally healthy and who are willing to sustain relatively short-term endothelial dysfunction[127], oxidative stress[128], increased LDL oxidation[129], and activation of NF-kappaB[130] as a result of their self-induced hyperglycemia. Postexertional hyperglycemia can be used to enhance athletic performance by sustaining and inducing glycogen storage following and during exercise (i.e., carbohydrate loading for glycogen "supercompensation"[131,132]). Similarly, consumption of "simple" carbohydrate without protein can be used to

[119] For more information on glycemic index, consult a nutrition book or website such as http://www.stanford.edu/~dep/gilists.htm last accessed August 16, 2003
[120] Janette Brand-Miller, Kaye Foster-Powell. Diets with a low glycemic index: from theory to practice. *Nutrition Today* 1999 March. Accessed on-line at: http://www.findarticles.com/cf_dls/m0841/2_34/54654508/p1/article.jhtml on August 16, 2003.
[121] Mendosa D. Glycemic Values of Common American Foods http://www.mendosa.com/common_foods.htm Accessed on August 4, 2004
[122] "Average daily consumption of high fructose corn syrup is about 50 grams per person in the United States. With respect to total mercury exposure, it may be necessary to account for this source of mercury in the diet of children and sensitive populations." Dufault R, LeBlanc B, Schnoll R, Cornett C, Schweitzer L, Wallinga D, Hightower J, Patrick L, Lukiw WJ. Mercury from chlor-alkali plants: measured concentrations in food product sugar. *Environ Health.* 2009 Jan 26;8:2. See also: "High fructose corn syrup has been shown to contain trace amounts of mercury as a result of some manufacturing processes, and its consumption can also lead to zinc loss." Dufault R, Schnoll R, Lukiw WJ, Leblanc B, Cornett C, Patrick L, Wallinga D, Gilbert SG, Crider R. Mercury exposure, nutritional deficiencies and metabolic disruptions may affect learning in children. *Behav Brain Funct.* 2009 Oct 27;5:44.
[123] News release from American Heart Association's 63rd High Blood Pressure Research Conference. High-sugar diet increases men's blood pressure; gout drug protective. Abstract P127. Sept. 23, 2009. http://americanheart.mediaroom.com/index.php?s=43&item=829 Accessed December 19, 2009
[124] "Because visceral and subcutaneous adipose tissues are the major sources of cytokines (adipokines), increased adipose tissue mass is associated with alteration in adipokine production (eg, overexpression of tumor necrosis factor-a, interleukin-6, plasminogen activator inhibitor-1, and underexpression of adiponectin in adipose tissue)." Aldhahi W, Hamdy O. Adipokines, inflammation, and the endothelium in diabetes. *Curr Diab Rep.* 2003 Aug;3(4):293-8
[125] Sanchez A, Reeser JL, Lau HS, Yahiku PY, Willard RE, McMillan PJ, Cho SY, Magie AR, Register UD. Role of sugars in human neutrophilic phagocytosis. *Am J Clin Nutr.* 1973 Nov;26(11):1180-4
[126] Al-Waili NS. Effects of daily consumption of honey solution on hematological indices and blood levels of minerals and enzymes in normal individuals. *J Med Food.* 2003 Summer;6(2):135-4
[127] "Modest hyperinsulinemia, mimicking fasting hyperinsulinemia of insulin-resistant states, abrogates endothelium-dependent vasodilation in large conduit arteries, probably by increasing oxidant stress. These data may provide a novel pathophysiological basis to the epidemiological link between hyperinsulinemia/insulin-resistance and atherosclerosis in humans." Arcaro G, Cretti A, Balzano S, Lechi A, Muggeo M, Bonora E, Bonadonna RC. Insulin causes endothelial dysfunction in humans: sites and mechanisms. *Circulation.* 2002 Feb 5;105(5):576-82
[128] "Hyperglycemia increased plasma MDA concentrations, but the activities of GSH-Px and SOD were significantly higher after a larger dose of glucose only. Plasma catecholamines were unchanged. These results indicate that the transient increase of plasma catecholamine and insulin concentrations did not induce oxidative damage, while glucose already in the low dose was an important triggering factor for oxidative stress." Koska J, Blazicek P, Marko M, Grna JD, Kvetnansky R, Vigas M. Insulin, catecholamines, glucose and antioxidant enzymes in oxidative damage during different loads in healthy humans. *Physiol Res.* 2000;49 Suppl 1:S95-100
[129] "In conclusion, insulin at physiological doses is associated with increased LDL peroxidation independent of the presence of hyperglycemia." Quinones-Galvan A, Sironi AM, Baldi S, Galetta F, Garbin U, Fratta-Pasini A, Cominacini L, Ferrannini E. Evidence that acute insulin administration enhances LDL cholesterol susceptibility to oxidation in healthy humans. *Arterioscler Thromb Vasc Biol.* 1999 Dec;19(12):2928-32
[130] "These data show that the intake of a mixed meal results in significant inflammatory changes characterized by a decrease in IkappaBalpha and an increase in NF-kappaB binding, plasma CRP, and the expression of IKKalpha, IKKbeta, and p47(phox) subunit." Aljada A, Mohanty P, Ghanim H, Abdo T, Tripathy D, Chaudhuri A, Dandona P. Increase in intranuclear nuclear factor kappaB and decrease in inhibitor kappaB in mononuclear cells after a mixed meal: evidence for a proinflammatory effect. *Am J Clin Nutr.* 2004 Apr;79(4):682-90
[131] "A significant glycogen sparing, as well as supercompensation within 24 h of recovery, was observed after [carbohydrate] supplementation." Brouns F, Saris WH, Beckers E, Adlercreutz H, van der Vusse GJ, Keizer HA, Kuipers H, Menheere P, Wagenmakers AJ, ten Hoor F. Metabolic changes induced by sustained exhaustive cycling and diet manipulation. *Int J Sports Med.* 1989 May;10 Suppl 1:S49-62
[132] "The accepted method of increasing muscle glycogen stores is by "glycogen loading," which classically involves depletion of muscle glycogen, usually by exercise, followed by consumption of a high-CHO diet for several days (e.g., 3, 39). ...increase muscle glycogen concentrations ([glycogen]) to between 150 and 200% of normal resting levels." Robinson TM, Sewell DA, Hultman E, Greenhaff PL. Role of submaximal exercise in promoting creatine and glycogen accumulation in human skeletal muscle. *J Appl Physiol.* 1999 Aug;87(2):598-604

promote entry of tryptophan across the blood-brain barrier and into the brain to promote serotonin synthesis.[133] In summary, *habitual overconsumption* of simple carbohydrates promotes disease by oxidative and proinflammatory mechanisms, while conversely *periodic consumption* of simple carbohydrates can be used to promote athletic performance and to increase intracerebral serotonin synthesis for the promotion of enhanced mood and cognitive performance and for the regulation of food intake.

Avoid artificial sweeteners, colors and other additives: Absolutely never use **aspartame**—this is a synthetic chemical that is easily converted to the toxin formaldehyde.[134] Aspartame causes cancer in animals and is strongly linked to brain tumors in humans.[135,136] **Sodium benzoate** is a food preservative that can cause asthma[137] and skin rashes[138] in sensitive individuals. **Tartrazine (yellow dye #5)** is a food/drug coloring agent that can cause asthma and skin rashes in sensitive individuals.[139] **Carrageenan** is a naturally-occurring carbohydrate extracted from red seaweed. Common sources of carrageenan are certain brands of "rice milk" and "soy milk." In addition to suppressing immune function[140], carrageenan causes intestinal ulcers and inflammatory bowel disease in animals[141] and some research indicates that carrageenan consumption is associated with an increased risk for cancer in humans.[142,143]

Consume sufficient daily water in the form of water and health-promoting teas and juices: Daily "water" intake should be approximately 30 ml/kg; thus, for a 150-lb (70-kg) person, fluid intake should be at least 2.1 liters, and for a person who weighs 220 lbs (100 kg) the daily intake should be approximately 3 liters. More fluids may be used during times of exercise, heat exposure, illness, or detoxification, while fluid restriction can be indicated in patients with heart failure, renal failure, anasarca (generalized edema), and hyponatremia.

Consider reducing or eliminating caffeine: This is especially important for people with reactive hypoglycemia, insomnia, anxiety, hypertension, low-back pain, and for women with fibrocystic breast disease. Caffeine ingestion also leads to the activation of brain noradrenergic receptors, which can cause inhibition of dopaminergic pathways.[144] For people who are in good health, 1-3 servings of caffeine per day are not harmful. Herbal teas and green tea appear to have significant health-promoting effects due to their phytonutrient components and antioxidant, anti-inflammatory, and anticancer properties.

To the extent possible, eat "organic" foods rather than industrially-produced foods: Organic foods (i.e., foods which are *naturally grown* rather than being treated with insect poisons, synthetic fertilizers, and chemicals to enhance shelf-life) tend to cost more than chemically-produced foods; but the increased phytonutrient content justifies the cost. Organic foods contain more nutrients than do chemically-produced foods.[145] More importantly,

---

[133] "Our results suggest that high-carbohydrate meals have an influence on serotonin synthesis. We predict that carbohydrates with a high glycemic index would have a greater serotoninergic effect than carbohydrates with a low glycemic index." Lyons PM, Truswell AS. Serotonin precursor influenced by type of carbohydrate meal in healthy adults. *Am J Clin Nutr*. 1988 Mar;47(3):433-9

[134] Trocho C, Pardo R, Rafecas I, Virgili J, Remesar X, Fernandez-Lopez JA, Alemany M. Formaldehyde derived from dietary aspartame binds to tissue components in vivo. *Life Sci*. 1998;63(5):337-4949

[135] Compared to other environmental factors putatively linked to brain tumors, the artificial sweetener aspartame is a promising candidate to explain the recent increase in incidence and degree of malignancy of brain tumors. ...exceedingly high incidence of brain tumors in aspartame-fed rats compared to no brain tumors in concurrent controls..." Olney JW, Farber NB, Spitznagel E, Robins LN. Increasing brain tumor rates: is there a link to aspartame? *J Neuropathol Exp Neurol* 1996;55(11):1115-23

[136] Russell Blaylock MD. Excitotoxins. Health Press; December 1996 [ISBN: 0929173252] Pages 211-214

[137] "Adverse reactions to benzoate in this patient required avoidance of some drugs, some of those classically prescribed under the form of syrups in asthma." Petrus M, Bonaz S, Causse E, Rhabbour M, Moulie N, Netter JC, Bildstein G. [Asthma and intolerance to benzoates] [Article in French] *Arch Pediatr*. 1996;3(10):984-7

[138] Munoz FJ, et al. Perioral urticaria from sodium benzoate in a toothpaste. *Contact Dermatitis*. 1996 Jul;35(1):51

[139] "Tartrazine sensitivity is most frequently manifested by urticaria and asthma... Vasculitis, purpura and contact dermatitis infrequently occur as manifestations of tartrazine sensitivity." Dipalma JR. Tartrazine sensitivity. *Am Fam Physician*. 1990 Nov;42(5):1347-50

[140] "Impairment of complement activity and humoral responses to T-dependent antigens, depression of cell-mediated immunity, prolongation of graft survival and potentiation of tumour growth by carrageenans have been reported." Thomson AW, Fowler EF. Carrageenan: a review of its effects on the immune system. *Agents Actions*. 1981;11(3):265-73

[141] Watt J, Marcus R. Experimental ulcerative disease of the colon. *Methods Achiev Exp Pathol*. 1975;7:56-71

[142] Tobacman JK. Review of harmful gastrointestinal effects of carrageenan in animal experiments. *Environ Health Perspect*. 2001 Oct;109(10):983-94

[143] "However, the gum carrageenan which is comprised of linked, sulfated galactose residues has potent biological activity and undergoes acid hydrolysis to poligeenan, an acknowledged carcinogen." Tobacman JK, Wallace RB, Zimmerman MB. Consumption of carrageenan and other water-soluble polymers used as food additives and incidence of mammary carcinoma. *Med Hypotheses*. 2001 May;56(5):589-98

[144] "The results suggest that noradrenergic innervation of dopamine cells can directly inhibit the activity of dopamine cells." Paladini CA, Williams JT. Noradrenergic inhibition of midbrain dopamine neurons. *J Neurosci*. 2004 May 12;24(19):4568-75

[145] Smith B. Organic Foods versus Supermarket Foods: element levels. *Journal of Applied Nutrition* 1993; 45(1), p35-9

recent research has also indicated that organic foods are better able to prevent the genetic damage that can lead to cancer than are foods that have been grown in an environment of artificial fertilizers and pesticides.[146]

Recognize the importance of avoiding food allergens: Biomedical research has established that adverse food reactions, regardless of the underlying mechanisms or classification of allergy, intolerance, or sensitivity, can exacerbate a wide range of human illnesses, including thyroid disease[147], mental depression[148,149], asthma, rhinitis,[150] recurrent otitis media[151], migraine[152,153,154], attention deficit and hyperactivity disorders[155], epilepsy[156,157,158], gastrointestinal inflammation[159], hypertension[160], joint pain and inflammation[161,162,163,164,165,166,167,168] and a wide range of other health problems. Any program of health promotion and health maintenance must include consideration of food allergies, food intolerances, and food sensitivities. The elimination-and-challenge technique is the most cost-effective and it also teaches patients how to identify their own food allergies and intolerances, which may change for the better or worse over time; when the patient is empowered with this technique, he/she can take an active and on-going role in his/her own healthcare. Patients may be allergic to foods that are generally considered healthy, including whole organic foods. The more common food allergens—exemplified here by a list of offending foods identified in a study of patients with migraine[169]—are wheat (78%), orange (65%), eggs (45%), tea and coffee (40% each), chocolate and milk (37%) each), beef (35%), and corn, cane sugar, and yeast (33% each).

Supplement the health-promoting whole-foods diet with specific vitamins, minerals, fatty acids, and probiotics: Despite the fact that America is one of the richest nations on earth, and that we produce more than enough food to feed ourselves and many other nations with a healthy diet, Americans tend to have poor dietary habits and inadequate levels of nutritional intake that do not meet the minimal standards, such as the Recommended Daily Allowance (RDA, now Daily Reference Intake (DRI)).[170] Many people are under the misperception that if they appear healthy or are even overweight then they could not possibly have nutritional deficiencies. The truths of this matter are that 1) gross/obvious nutritional deficiencies are common among "apparently healthy" individuals, 2) common situations like stress, poor diets, and use of medications predispose people to nutritional deficiencies, 3) hereditary/genetic disorders affect a large portion of the population and lead

---

[146] "Against BaP, three species of OC vegetables showed 30-57% antimutagenecity, while GC ones did only 5-30%." Ren H, Endo H, Hayashi T. The superiority of organically cultivated vegetables to general ones regarding antimutagenic activities. *Mutat Res*. 2001 Sep 20;496(1-2):83-8

[147] Sategna-Guidetti C, Volta U, Ciacci C, Usai P, Carlino A, De Franceschi L, Camera A, Pelli A, Brossa C. Prevalence of thyroid disorders in untreated adult celiac disease patients and effect of gluten withdrawal: an Italian multicenter study. *Am J Gastroenterol*. 2001 Mar;96(3):751-7

[148] "The detection and treatment of psychological dysfunction related to food intolerance with particular reference to the problem of objective evaluation is discussed... Long-term follow-up revealed maintenance of marked improvements in psychological and physical functioning." Mills N. Depression and food intolerance: a single case study. *Hum Nutr Appl Nutr*. 1986 Apr;40(2):141-5

[149] "OBJECTIVE: To describe a patient with food intolerance probably contributing to depressive symptoms, intolerance to psychotropic medication and treatment resistance... RESULTS: The patient's course improved considerably with an elimination diet." Parker G, Watkins T. Treatment-resistant depression: when antidepressant drug intolerance may indicate food intolerance. *Aust N Z J Psychiatry*. 2002 Apr;36(2):263-5

[150] Speer F. The allergic child. *Am Fam Physician*. 1975 Feb;11(2):88-94

[151] Juntti H, Tikkanen S, Kokkonen J, Alho OP, Niinimaki A. Cow's milk allergy is associated with recurrent otitis media during childhood. *Acta Otolaryngol*. 1999;119(8):867-73

[152] "Foods which provoked migraine in 9 patients with severe migraine refractory to drug therapy were identified... These observations confirm that a food-allergic reaction is the cause of migraine in this group of patients." Monro J, Carini C, Brostoff J. Migraine is a food-allergic disease. *Lancet*. 1984 Sep 29;2(8405):719-21

[153] Egger J, Carter CM, Wilson J, et al. Is migraine food allergy? A double-blind controlled trial of oligoantigenic diet treatment. *Lancet*. 1983 Oct 15;2(8355):865-9

[154] Monro J, Brostoff J, Carini C, Zilkha K. Food allergy in migraine. Study of dietary exclusion and RAST. *Lancet*. 1980 Jul 5;2(8184):1-4

[155] Boris M, Mandel FS. Foods and additives are common causes of the attention deficit hyperactive disorder in children. *Ann Allergy*. 1994 May;72(5):462-8

[156] Egger J, Carter CM, Soothill JF, Wilson J. Oligoantigenic diet treatment of children with epilepsy and migraine. *J Pediatr*. 1989;114(1):51-8

[157] Pelliccia A, Lucarelli S, Frediani T, D'Ambrini G, Cerminara C, Barbato M, Vagnucci B, Cardi E. Partial cryptogenetic epilepsy and food allergy/intolerance. A causal or a chance relationship? Reflections on three clinical cases. *Minerva Pediatr*. 1999 May;51(5):153-7

[158] Frediani T, Lucarelli S, Pelliccia A, Vagnucci B, et al. Allergy and childhood epilepsy: a close relationship? *Acta Neurol Scand*. 2001;104(6):349-52

[159] Marr HY, Chen WC, Lin LH. Food protein induced enterocolitis syndrome: report of one case. *Acta Paediatr Taiwan*. 2001;42(1):49-52

[160] Grant EC. Food allergies and migraine. *Lancet*. 1979 May 5;1(8123):966-9

[161] "Food allergy appeared to be responsible for the joint symptoms in three patients and in one it was possible to precipitate swelling of a knee due to synovitis with effusion by drinking milk a few hours beforehand, the synovial fluid having mildly inflammatory features and a relatively high eosinophil count." Golding DN. Is there an allergic synovitis? *J R Soc Med*. 1990 May;83(5):312-4

[162] Panush RS. Food induced ("allergic") arthritis: clinical and serologic studies. *J Rheumatol*. 1990 Mar;17(3):291-4

[163] Pacor ML, Lunardi C, Di Lorenzo G, Biasi D, Corrocher R. Food allergy and seronegative arthritis: report of two cases. *Clin Rheumatol*. 2001;20(4):279-81

[164] Schrander JJ, Marcelis C, de Vries MP, van Santen-Hoeufft HM. Does food intolerance play a role in juvenile chronic arthritis? *Br J Rheumatol*. 1997 Aug;36(8):905-8

[165] van de Laar MA, van der Korst JK. Food intolerance in rheumatoid arthritis. I. A double blind, controlled trial of the clinical effects of elimination of milk allergens and azo dyes. *Ann Rheum Dis*. 1992 Mar;51(3):298-302

[166] Haugen MA, Kjeldsen-Kragh J, Forre O. A pilot study of the effect of an elemental diet in the management of rheumatoid arthritis. *Clin Exp Rheumatol*. 1994;12(3):275-9

[167] van de Laar MA, Aalbers M, Bruins FG, et al. Food intolerance in rheumatoid arthritis. II. Clinical and histological aspects. *Ann Rheum Dis*. 1992;51(3):303-6

[168] Panush RS, Stroud RM, Webster EM. Food-induced (allergic) arthritis. Inflammatory arthritis exacerbated by milk. *Arthritis Rheum* 1986; 29(2): 220-6

[169] Grant EC. Food allergies and migraine. *Lancet*. 1979 May 5;1(8123):966-9

[170] "Most people do not consume an optimal amount of all vitamins by diet alone. Pending strong evidence of effectiveness from randomized trials, it appears prudent for all adults to take vitamin supplements." Fletcher RH, Fairfield KM. Vitamins for chronic disease prevention in adults: clinical applications. *JAMA* 2002 Jun 19;287(23):3127-9

to an increased need for nutritional intake which can generally only be met with supplementation in addition to a healthy whole-foods diet. Taking a "one-a-day" multivitamin is insufficient for people who truly desire significant benefit from supplementation. These one-a-day preparations generally only provide the minimum daily allowance—this dose is not large enough to provide truly preventive medicine results; also, such one-a-day products tend to contain low-quality nutrients, such as ergocalciferol rather than cholecalciferol[171], cyanocobalamin rather than the hydroxyl-, methyl-, or adenosyl- forms[172], and DL-tocopherol or exclusively L-alpha-tocopherol rather than a mix of tocopherols with a high concentration (generally approximately 40%) of gamma tocopherol.[173]

For people still not convinced of the importance of a multi-vitamin/mineral supplement as part of the basic foundation of the health plan, please consider the following data from the medical research:

- Many people think that eating a "healthy diet" will supply them with the nutrients that they need and that they do not need to take a vitamin supplement. This may have been true 2000 years ago, but today's industrially produced "foods" are generally stripped of much of their nutritional value long before they leave the factory. Industrially-produced fruits and vegetables contain lower quantities of nutrients than does naturally raised "organic" produce. [174]

- The reason that people can be of normal weight or can even be overweight and obese and still have nutrient deficiencies is that the body lowers the metabolic rate when the intake of vitamins and minerals is low. This is referred to as the "physiologic adaptation to marginal malnutrition." Even though people may eat enough calories and protein, they can still suffer from growth retardation and behavioral problems as a result of micronutrient malnutrition, even though they *appear* nourished.[175]

- Most nutrition-oriented doctors will agree that magnesium is one of the most important nutrients, especially for helping prevent heart attack and stroke. **Magnesium deficiency is an epidemic in so-called "developed" nations, with 20-40% of different populations showing objective laboratory evidence of magnesium deficiency.**[176,177,178,179]

- Add to the above that every day we are confronted with more chronic emotional stress and toxic chemicals than has ever before existed on the planet, and it becomes easy to see that basic nutritional support and an organic whole foods diet is just the start of attaining improved health.

General Guidelines for the Safe Use of Nutritional Supplements: Supplementation with vitamins and minerals is generally safe, especially if the following guidelines are followed:

- Vitamins and minerals should generally be taken with food in order to eliminate the possibility of nausea and to increase absorption: Most vitamins and other supplements should be taken with food so that nausea is avoided.

- Iron is potentially harmful: Iron promotes the formation of reactive oxygen species ("free radicals") and is thus implicated in several diseases, such as infections, cancer, liver disease, diabetes, and cardiovascular disease. Iron supplements should not be consumed except by people who have been definitively

---

[171] "Vitamin D(2) potency is less than one third that of vitamin D(3). Physicians resorting to use of vitamin D(2) should be aware of its markedly lower potency and shorter duration of action relative to vitamin D(3)." Armas LA, Hollis BW, Heaney RP. Vitamin D2 is much less effective than vitamin D3 in humans. *J Clin Endocrinol Metab*. 2004 Nov;89(11):5387-91

[172] Freeman AG. Cyanocobalamin--a case for withdrawal: discussion paper. *J R Soc Med*. 1992 Nov;85(11):686–687 http://www.ncbi.nlm.nih.gov/pmc/articles/PMC1293728/pdf/jrsocmed00105-0046.pdf

[173] "gamma-tocopherol is the major form of vitamin E in many plant seeds and in the US diet, but has drawn little attention compared with alpha-tocopherol, the predominant form of vitamin E in tissues and the primary form in supplements. However, recent studies indicate that gamma-tocopherol may be important to human health and that it possesses unique features that distinguish it from alpha-tocopherol." Jiang Q, Christen S, Shigenaga MK, Ames BN. gamma-tocopherol, the major form of vitamin E in the US diet, deserves more attention. *Am J Clin Nutr*. 2001 Dec;74(6):714-22 http://www.ajcn.org/content/74/6/714.full.pdf

[174] Smith B. Organic Foods versus Supermarket Foods: element levels. *Journal of Applied Nutrition* 1993; 45(1), p35-9. I recently found that this article is also available on-line at http://journeytoforever.org/farm_library/bobsmith.html as of June 19, 2004

[175] Allen LH. The nutrition CRSP: what is marginal malnutrition, and does it affect human function? *Nutr Rev* 1993 Sep;51(9):255-67

[176] "The American diet is low in magnesium, and with modern water systems, very little is ingested in the drinking water." Innerarity S. Hypomagnesemia in acute and chronic illness. *Crit Care Nurs Q*. 2000 Aug;23(2):1-19

[177] "Altogether 43% of 113 trauma patients had low magnesium levels compared to 30% of noninjured cohorts." Frankel H, Haskell R, Lee SY, Miller D, Rotondo M, Schwab CW. Hypomagnesemia in trauma patients. *World J Surg*. 1999 Sep;23(9):966-9

[178] "There was a 20% overall prevalence of hypomagnesemia among this predominantly female, African American population." Fox CH, Ramsoomair D, Mahoney MC, Carter C, Young B, Graham R. An investigation of hypomagnesemia among ambulatory urban African Americans. *J Fam Pract*. 1999 Aug;48(8):636-9

[179] "Suboptimal levels were detected in 33.7 per cent of the population under study. These data clearly demonstrate that the Mg supply of the German population needs increased attention." Schimatschek HF, Rempis R. Prevalence of hypomagnesemia in an unselected German population of 16,000 individuals. *Magnes Res*. 2001 Dec;14(4):283-90

diagnosed with iron deficiency by measurement of serum ferritin. Iron supplementation without documentation of iron deficiency by measurement of serum ferritin is inappropriate. [180]

- <u>Vitamin A is one of the only vitamins with the potential for serious toxicity even at low doses</u>: Attention should be given to vitamin A intake so that toxicity is avoided. Total intake of vitamin A must account for all sources—foods, fish oils, and vitamin supplements. Manifestations of vitamin A toxicity include: skin problems (dry skin, flaking skin, chapped or split lips, red skin rash, hair loss), joint pain, bone pain, headaches, anorexia (loss of appetite), edema (water retention, weight gain, swollen ankles, difficulty breathing), fatigue, and/or liver damage. Whenever vitamin A is used in high doses, it must be used for a defined period of time in order to avoid the toxicity that will result from high-dose long-term vitamin A supplementation.

  - <u>Adults</u>: Women who are pregnant or might become pregnant and who are planning to carry the baby to full term delivery should not ingest more than 10,000 IU of vitamin A per day. Vitamin A toxicity is seen with chronic ingestion of therapeutic doses (for example: 25,000 IU per day for 6 years, or 100,000 IU per day for 2.5 years[181]). Most patients should not consume more than 25,000 IU of vitamin A per day for more than 2 months without express supervision by a healthcare provider. Vitamin A is present in some multivitamins, in animal liver and products such as fish liver oil, and in other supplements—read labels to ensure that the total daily intake is not greater than 25,000 IU per day.

  - <u>Infants and Children</u>: Different studies have used either daily or monthly schedules of vitamin A supplementation. In a study with extremely low-birth weight infants, 5,000 IU of vitamin A per day for 28 days was safely used.[182] In another study conducted in sick children, those aged less than 12 months received 100,000 IU on two consecutive days, while children between ages 12-60 months received a larger dose of 200,000 IU on two consecutive days.[183]

- <u>Preexisting kidney problems (such as renal insufficiency) increase the risks associated with nutritional supplementation</u>: Supplementation with vitamins and minerals does not cause kidney damage. However, if a patient already has kidney problems, then nutritional supplementation may become hazardous; this is particularly true with magnesium and potassium and perhaps also with vitamin C. Assessment of renal function with serum or urine tests is encouraged before beginning an aggressive plan of supplementation. Conditions which cause kidney damage include use of specific drugs (e.g., acetaminophen, aspirin, contrast and chemotherapy agents, cocaine), acute or chronic high blood pressure, diabetes mellitus and other diseases such as lupus (SLE), polycystic kidney disease, and scleroderma.

- <u>Pre-existing medical conditions may make supplementation unsafe</u>: A few rare medical conditions may cause nutritional supplementation to be unsafe, including severe liver disease, renal failure, electrolyte imbalances, hyperparathyroidism and other vitamin D hypersensitivity syndromes.

- <u>Several drugs/medications may adversely interact with vitamin/mineral supplements and with botanical medicines</u>: Vitamins/minerals may reduce the effectiveness of some prescription medications. For example, taking certain antibiotics such as ciprofloxacin or tetracycline with calcium reduces absorption of the drugs, therefore rendering the drugs much less effective. Taking botanical medicines with medications may make the drugs dangerously less effective (such as when St. John's Wort is combined with protease inhibitor drugs[184]) or may make the drug dangerously more effective (such when Kava is

---

[180] Hollán S, Johansen KS. Adequate iron stores and the 'Nil nocere' principle.*Haematologia* (Budap). 1993;25(2):69-84

[181] "The smallest continuous daily consumption leading to cirrhosis was 25,000 IU during 6 years, whereas higher daily doses (greater than or equal to 100,000 IU) taken during 2 1/2 years resulted in similar histological lesions. ... The data also indicate that prolonged and continuous consumption of doses in the low "therapeutic" range can result in life-threatening liver damage." Geubel AP, De Galocsy C, Alves N, Rahier J, Dive C. Liver damage caused by therapeutic vitamin A administration: estimate of dose-related toxicity in 41 cases. *Gastroenterology*. 1991 Jun;100(6):1701-9

[182] "Infants with birth weight < 1000 g were randomised at birth to receive oral vitamin A supplementation (5000 IU/day) or placebo for 28 days." Wardle SP, Hughes A, Chen S, Shaw NJ. Randomised controlled trial of oral vitamin A supplementation in preterm infants to prevent chronic lung disease. *Arch Dis Child Fetal Neonatal Ed*. 2001 Jan;84(1):F9-F13 Available on-line at http://adc.bmjjournals.com/cgi/content/full/fetalneonatal%3b84/1/F9

[183] "Children were assigned to oral doses of 200 000 IU vitamin A (half that dose if <12 months) or placebo on the day of admission, a second dose on the following day, and third and fourth doses at 4 and 8 months after discharge from the hospital, respectively." Villamor E, Mbise R, Spiegelman D, Hertzmark E, Fataki M, Peterson KE, Ndossi G, Fawzi WW. Vitamin A supplements ameliorate the adverse effect of HIV-1, malaria, and diarrheal infections on child growth. *Pediatrics*. 2002 Jan;109(1):E6

[184] Piscitelli SC, Burstein AH, Chaitt D, Alfaro RM, Falloon J. Indinavir concentrations and St John's wort. *Lancet*. 2000 Feb 12;355(9203):547-8

combined with the anti-anxiety drug alprazolam[185]). If vitamin D is used in doses greater than 1,000 IU/d in patients taking hydrochlorothiazide or other calcium-retaining drugs, serum calcium should be monitored at least monthly until safety (i.e., lack of hypercalcemia) has been established per patient.[186] Patients should not combine nutritional or botanical medicines with chemical/synthetic drugs without specific advice from a knowledgeable doctor. Do not increase vitamin K consumption from supplements or dietary improvements in patients taking coumadin/warfarin. A reasonable recommendation is that nutritional supplements be taken 2 hours away from pharmaceutical medications to avoid complications such as intraintestinal drug-nutrient binding.

---

[185] Almeida JC, Grimsley EW. Coma from the health food store: interaction between kava and alprazolam. *Ann Intern Med*. 1996 Dec 1;125(11):940-1
[186] **Vasquez A**, Manso G, Cannell J. The clinical importance of vitamin D (cholecalciferol): a paradigm shift with implications for all healthcare providers. *Altern Ther Health Med*. 2004 Sep-Oct;10(5):28-36 http://optimalhealthresearch.com/monograph04.html

Advanced concepts in nutrition—an introduction

Biochemical Individuality and Orthomolecular Medicine:

"Biochemical individuality" was the term coined by biochemist Dr. Roger Williams of the University of Texas[187] to describe the genetic and physiologic variations in human beings that produced different nutritional needs among individuals. Because we all have different genes, each of our bodies therefore creates different protein enzymes, and many of these enzymes—which are essential for proper cellular function—are adversely affected by defects in their construction (i.e., amino acid sequence) that reduce their efficiency. Dr. Linus Pauling[188] noted that single amino acid substitutions could produce dramatic alterations in protein function. Pauling discovered that sickle cell disease was caused by a single amino acid substitution in the hemoglobin molecule, and for this discovery he won the Nobel Prize in Chemistry in 1954.[189] With recognition of the importance of individual molecules in determining health or disease, Pauling coined the phrase "orthomolecular medicine" based on his thesis that many diseases could be effectively prevented and treated if we used the "right molecules" to correct abnormal physiologic function. Pauling contrasted the clinical use of nutrients for the improvement of physiologic function (orthomolecular medicine) with the use of chemical drugs, which generally work by interfering with normal physiology (toximolecular medicine). Since nutrients are the fundamental elements of the human body from which all enzymes, chemicals, and cellular structures are formed, Pauling advocated that the use of customized nutrition and nutritional supplements could promote optimal health by optimizing cellular function and efficiency. More recently, Dr. Bruce Ames has thoroughly documented the science of the orthomolecular precepts[190] and has advocated optimal diets along with nutritional supplementation as a highly efficient and cost-effective method for preventing disease and optimizing health.[191,192] In sum, we see that 1) the foundational diet must be formed from whole foods such as fruits, nuts, seeds, vegetables, and lean

Orthomolecular precepts
• The functions of the body are dependent upon thousands of enzymes. Because of genetic defects that are common in the general population, some of these enzymes are commonly defective – even if only slightly – in large portions of the human population.
• Enzyme defects reduce the function and efficiency of important chemical reactions. Because enzymes are so important for normal function and the prevention of disease, defects in enzyme function can result in disruptions in physiology and the creation of what later manifests as "disease."
• Rather than treating these diseases with synthetic chemical drugs, it is commonly possible to prevent and treat disease with high-doses of vitamins, minerals, and other nutrients to compensate for or bypass metabolic dysfunctions, thus allowing for the promotion of optimal health by promoting optimal physiologic function.
Recent independent review: Ames BN, Elson-Schwab I, Silver EA. High-dose vitamin therapy stimulates variant enzymes with decreased coenzyme binding affinity (increased K(m)): relevance to genetic disease and polymorphisms. *Am J Clin Nutr.* 2002 Apr;75(4):616-58

meats, 2) processed and artificial foods should be avoided, and 3) the use of nutritional supplements is necessary to provide sufficiently high levels of nutrition to overcome defects in enzymatic activity.

---

[187] "Every individual organism that has a distinctive genetic background has distinctive nutritional needs which must be met for optimal well-being. …[N]utrition applied with due concern for individual genetic variations…offers the solution to many baffling health problems." Williams RJ. Biochemical Individuality : The Basis for the Genetotrophic Concept. Austin and London: University of Texas Press, 1956. Page x

[188] "…the concentration of coenzyme [vitamins and minerals] needed to produce the amount of active enzyme required for optimum health may well be somewhat different for different individuals. …many individuals may require a considerably higher concentration of one or more coenzymes than other people do for optimum health…" Pauling L. On the Orthomolecular Environment of the Mind: Orthomolecular Theory. In: Williams RJ, Kalita DK. A Physician's Handbook on Orthomolecular Medicine. New Cannan; Keats Publishing: 1977. Page 76

[189] http://www.nobel.se/chemistry/laureates/1954/pauling-bio.html on April 4, 2004

[190] "About 50 human genetic dis-eases due to defective enzymes can be remedied or ameliorated by the administration of high doses of the vitamin component of the corresponding coenzyme, which at least partially restores enzymatic activity." Ames BN, Elson-Schwab I, Silver EA. High-dose vitamin therapy stimulates variant enzymes with decreased coenzyme binding affinity (increased K(m)): relevance to genetic disease and polymorphisms. *Am J Clin Nutr.* 2002 Apr;75(4):616-58

[191] "An optimum intake of micronutrients and metabolites, which varies with age and genetic constitution, would tune up metabolism and give a marked increase in health, particularly for the poor and elderly, at little cost." Ames BN. The metabolic tune-up: metabolic harmony and disease prevention. *J Nutr.* 2003 May;133(5 Suppl 1):1544S-8S

[192] "Optimizing micronutrient intake [through better diets, fortification of foods, or multivitamin-mineral pills] can have a major impact on public health at low cost." Ames BN. Cancer prevention and diet: help from single nucleotide polymorphisms. *Proc Natl Acad Sci* U S A. 1999 Oct 26;96(22):12216-8

Nutrigenomics—Nutritional Genomics:

"Genome" refers to all of the genetic material in an organism, and "genomics" is the field of study of this information. The field of nutritional genomics—nutrigenomics—refers to the clinical synthesis of 1) research on the human genome (e.g., the Human Genome Project[193]), and 2) the advancing science of clinical nutrition, including research on nutraceuticals (nutritional medicines) and phytomedicinals (botanical medicines). Nutrigenomics represents a major advance in our understanding of the underlying biochemical and physiologic mechanisms of the effects of nutrition.

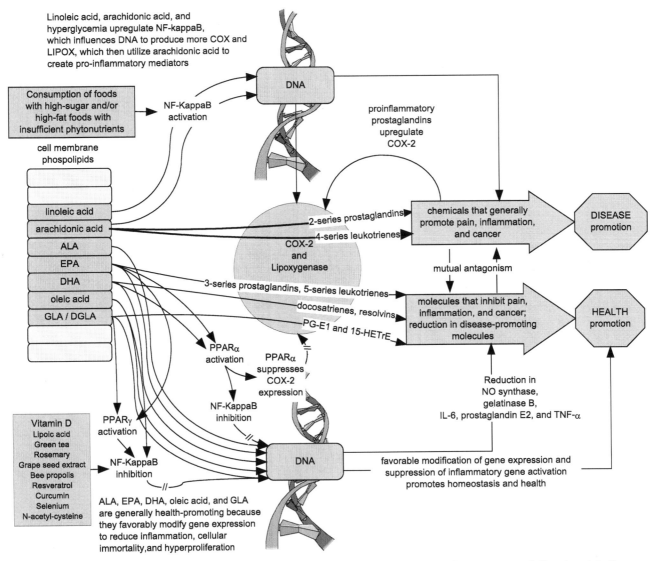

Nutrigenomics—a conceptual diagram: Nutrients influence gene transcription as well as post-translational metabolism.

---

[193] "Begun formally in 1990, the U.S. Human Genome Project is a 13-year effort coordinated by the U.S. Department of Energy and the National Institutes of Health. The project originally was planned to last 15 years, but rapid technological advances have accelerated the expected completion date to 2003. Project goals are to identify all the approximate 30,000 genes in human DNA..." See the official Human Genome website at http://www.ornl.gov/sci/techresources/Human_Genome/home.shtml

Nutrition is far more than "fuel" for our biophysiologic machine; we know now that nutrition—the consumption of specific proteins, amino acids, vitamins, minerals, fatty acids, and phytochemicals—can alter genetic expression and can thus either promote health or disease at the very fundamental level of genetic expression. The commonly employed excuse that many patients use—"I just have bad genes"—now takes on a whole new meaning; it may be that these patients suffer from the expression of "bad genes" *because of the food that they eat*.

The concept and phenomenon of nutrigenomics can be described by saying that each of us has the genes for health, as well as the genes for disease; what largely determines our level of health is how we treat our genes with environmental inputs, especially nutrition. We appear able, to a large extent, to "turn on" disease-promoting genes with poor nutrition and a pro-inflammatory lifestyle[194,195], while, to a lesser extent, we are able to activate or "turn on" health-promoting genes with a healthy diet[196] and with proper nutritional supplementation.[197] For additional details, see the literature cited in this section and the review article by Vasquez available on-line.[198]

Putting it all together with "the supplemented Paleo-Mediterranean diet": The health-promoting diet of choice for the majority of people is a diet based on abundant consumption of fruits, vegetables, seeds, nuts, omega-3 and monounsaturated fatty acids, and lean sources of protein such as lean meats, fatty cold-water fish, soy and whey proteins. This diet prohibits and obviates overconsumption of chemical preservatives, artificial sweeteners, and carbohydrate-dominant foods such as candies, pastries, breads, potatoes, grains, and other foods with a high glycemic load and high glycemic index. This "Paleo-Mediterranean Diet" is a combination of the "Paleolithic" or "Paleo diet" and the well-known "Mediterranean diet", both of which are well described in peer-reviewed journals and the lay press. The Mediterranean diet is characterized by increased proportions of legumes, nuts, seeds, whole grain products, fruits, vegetables (including potatoes), fish and lean meats, and monounsaturated and n-3 fatty acids.[199] Consumption of the Mediterranean diet is associated with improvements in insulin sensitivity and reductions in cardiovascular disease, diabetes, cancer, and all-cause mortality when contrasted to the effects of *ad libitum* eating, particularly in the standard American diet (SAD) eating pattern.[200] The Paleolithic diet detailed by collaborators Eaton[201], O'Keefe[202], and Cordain[203] is similar to the Mediterranean diet except for stronger emphasis on fruits and vegetables (preferably raw or minimally cooked), omega-3-rich lean meats, and reduced consumption of starchy foods such as potatoes and grains, the latter of which were not staples in the human diet until the last few thousand years. Emphasizing the olive oil and red wine of the Mediterranean diet and the absence of grains and potatoes per the Paleo diet appears to be the way to get the best of both dietary worlds; the remaining diet is characterized by fresh whole fruits, vegetables, nuts (especially almonds), seeds, berries, olive oil, lean meats rich in n-3 fatty acids, and red wine in moderation. In sum, this dietary plan along with the inclusion of garlic and dark chocolate (a rich source of cardioprotective, antioxidative, antihypertensive, and anti-inflammatory polyphenolic flavonoids[204,205]) is expected to reduce adverse cardiovascular events by more than 76%.[206] Biochemical justification for this type of diet is ample and is well supported by numerous long-term studies in humans wherein both Mediterranean and Paleolithic diets result in statistically significant and

[194] Rusyn I, Bradham CA, Cohn L, Schoonhoven R, Swenberg JA, Brenner DA, Thurman RG. Corn oil rapidly activates nuclear factor-kappaB in hepatic Kupffer cells by oxidant-dependent mechanisms. *Carcinogenesis*. 1999 Nov;20(11):2095-100 http://carcin.oxfordjournals.org/cgi/content/full/20/11/2095
[195] Aljada A, Mohanty P, Ghanim H, Abdo T, Tripathy D, Chaudhuri A, Dandona P. Increase in intranuclear nuclear factor kappaB and decrease in inhibitor kappaB in mononuclear cells after a mixed meal: evidence for a proinflammatory effect. *Am J Clin Nutr*. 2004 Apr;79(4):682-90
[196] OKeefe JH Jr,Cordain L.Cardiovascular disease resulting from a diet and lifestyle at odds with our Paleolithic genome.*Mayo Clin Proc*.2004;79:101-8
[197] Kaput J, Rodriguez LR. Nutritional genomics: the next frontier in the postgenomic era. *Physiol Genomics* 16: 166–177 http://physiolgenomics.physiology.org/cgi/content/full/16/2/166
[198] Vasquez A.Reducing pain and inflammation naturally - Part 4: Nutritional and Botanical Inhibition of NF-kappaB, the Major Intracellular Amplifier of the Inflammatory Cascade.A Clinical Strategy Exemplifying Anti-Inflammatory Nutrigenomics.*Nutr Perspec* 2005;Jul:5-12 http://optimalhealthresearch.com/part4
[199] Curtis BM, O'Keefe JH Jr. Understanding the Mediterranean diet. Could this be the new "gold standard" for heart disease prevention? *Postgrad Med*. 2002 Aug;112(2):35-8, 41-5 http://www.postgradmed.com/issues/2002/08_02/curtis.htm
[200] Knoops KT, de Groot LC, Kromhout D, Perrin AE, Moreiras-Varela O, Menotti A, van Staveren WA. Mediterranean diet, lifestyle factors, and 10-year mortality in elderly European men and women: the HALE project. *JAMA*. 2004 Sep 22;292(12):1433-9
[201] Eaton SB, Shostak M, Konner M. The Paleolithic Prescription: A program of diet & exercise and a design for living, New York: Harper & Row, 1988
[202] O'Keefe JH Jr, Cordain L. Cardiovascular disease resulting from a diet and lifestyle at odds with our Paleolithic genome: how to become a 21st-century hunter-gatherer. *Mayo Clin Proc*. 2004 Jan;79(1):101-8
[203] Cordain L. The Paleo Diet: Lose Weight and Get Healthy by Eating the Food You Were Designed to Eat. Indianapolis; John Wiley and Sons, 2002
[204] Schramm DD, Wang JF, Holt RR, Ensunsa JL, Gonsalves JL, Lazarus SA, Schmitz HH, German JB, Keen CL. Chocolate procyanidins decrease the leukotriene-prostacyclin ratio in humans and human aortic endothelial cells. *Am J Clin Nutr*. 2001;73(1):36-40
[205] Engler MB, Engler MM, Chen CY, et al. Flavonoid-rich dark chocolate improves endothelial function and increases plasma epicatechin concentrations in healthy adults. *J Am Coll Nutr*. 2004;23(3):197-204
[206] Franco OH, Bonneux L, de Laet C, Peeters A, Steyerberg EW, Mackenbach JP. The Polymeal: a more natural, safer, and probably tastier (than the Polypill) strategy to reduce cardiovascular disease by more than 75%. *BMJ*. 2004;329(7480):1447-50

clinically meaningful reductions in disease-specific and all-cause mortality.[207,208,209,210] Diets rich in fruits and vegetables are sources of more than 8,000 phytochemicals, many of which have antioxidant, anti-inflammatory, and anti-cancer properties.[211] Oleic acid, squalene, and phenolics in olive oil and phenolics and resveratrol in red wine have antioxidant, anti-inflammatory, and anti-cancer properties and also protect against cardiovascular disease.[212] N-3 fatty acids have numerous health benefits via multiple mechanisms as described in the sections that follow. Increased intake of dietary fiber from fruits and vegetable favorably modifies gut flora, promotes xenobiotic elimination (via flora modification, laxation, and overall reductions in enterohepatic recirculation), and is associated with reductions in morbidity and mortality. Such a "Paleolithic diet" can also lead to urinary alkalinization (average urine pH of ≥ 7.5 according to Sebastian et al[213]) which increases renal *retention of minerals* for improved musculoskeletal health[214,215,216] and which increases *urinary elimination of many toxicants and xenobiotics* for a tremendous reduction in serum levels and thus adverse effects from chemical exposure or drug overdose.[217] Furthermore, therapeutic alkalinization was recently shown in an open trial with 82 patients to reduce symptoms and disability associated with low-back pain and to increase intracellular magnesium concentrations by 11%.[218] **Ample intake of amino acids via dietary proteins supports phase-2 detoxification** (amino acid and sulfate conjugation) for proper xenobiotic elimination[219,220], **provides amino acid precursors for neurotransmitter synthesis** and maintenance of mood, memory, and cognitive performance[221,222,223,224], **and prevents the immunosuppression and decrements in musculoskeletal status caused by low-protein diets.**[225] Described originally by the current author[226], the "supplemented Paleo-Mediterranean diet" provides patients the best of current knowledge in nutrition by relying on a foundational diet plan of fresh fruits, vegetables, nuts, seeds, berries, fish, and lean meats which is adorned with olive oil for its squalene, phenolic antioxidant/anti-inflammatory and monounsaturated fatty acid content. Inclusive of medical foods such as red wine, garlic, and dark chocolate which may synergize to effect at least a 76% reduction in cardiovascular disease[227], this diet also reduces the risk for cancer[228] and can be an integral component of a health-promoting lifestyle.[229] Competitive athletes are allowed increased carbohydrate consumption before and after training and competition to promote glycogen storage supercompensation.[230,231,232]

---

[207] de Lorgeril M, Salen P, Martin JL, Monjaud I, Boucher P, Mamelle N. Mediterranean dietary pattern in a randomized trial: prolonged survival and possible reduced cancer rate. *Arch Intern Med.* 1998 Jun 8;158(11):1181-7

[208] Knoops KT, de Groot LC, Kromhout D, Perrin AE, Moreiras-Varela O, Menotti A, van Staveren WA. Mediterranean diet, lifestyle factors, and 10-year mortality in elderly European men and women: the HALE project. *JAMA.* 2004 Sep 22;292(12):1433-9

[209] Lindeberg S, Cordain L, and Eaton SB. Biological and clinical potential of a Paleolithic diet. *J Nutri Environ Med* 2003; 13:149-160

[210] O'Keefe JH Jr, Cordain L, Harris WH, Moe RM, Vogel R. Optimal low-density lipoprotein is 50 to 70 mg/dl: lower is better and physiologically normal. *J Am Coll Cardiol.* 2004 Jun 2;43(11):2142-6

[211] Liu RH. Health benefits of fruit and vegetables are from additive and synergistic combinations of phytochemicals. *Am J Clin Nutr.* 2003;78(3 Sup):517S-520S

[212] Alarcon de la Lastra C, Barranco MD, Motilva V, Herrerias JM. Mediterranean diet and health: biological importance of olive oil. *Curr Pharm Des.* 2001;7:933-50

[213] Sebastian A, Frassetto LA, Sellmeyer DE, Merriam RL, Morris RC Jr. Estimation of the net acid load of the diet of ancestral preagricultural Homo sapiens and their hominid ancestors. *Am J Clin Nutr* 2002;76:1308-16

[214] Sebastian A, Harris ST, Ottaway JH, Todd KM, Morris RC Jr. Improved mineral balance and skeletal metabolism in postmenopausal women treated with potassium bicarbonate. *N Engl J Med.* 1994;330(25):1776-81

[215] Tucker KL, Hannan MT, Chen H, Cupples LA, Wilson PW, Kiel DP. Potassium, magnesium, and fruit and vegetable intakes are associated with greater bone mineral density in elderly men and women. *Am J Clin Nutr.* 1999;69(4):727-36

[216] Whiting SJ, Boyle JL, Thompson A, Mirwald RL, Faulkner RA. Dietary protein, phosphorus and potassium are beneficial to bone mineral density in adult men consuming adequate dietary calcium. *J Am Coll Nutr.* 2002;21(5):402-9

[217] Proudfoot AT, Krenzelok EP, Vale JA. Position Paper on urine alkalinization. *J Toxicol Clin Toxicol.* 2004;42(1):1-26

[218] "The results show that a disturbed acid-base balance may contribute to the symptoms of low back pain. The simple and safe addition of an alkaline multimineral preparate was able to reduce the pain symptoms in these patients with chronic low back pain." Vormann J,Worlitschek M,Goedecke T,Silver B. Supplementation with alkaline minerals reduces symptoms in patients with chronic low back pain. J Trace Elem Med Biol. 2001;15:179-83

[219] Liska DJ. The detoxification enzyme systems. *Altern Med Rev.* 1998;3:187-9

[220] Anderson KE, Kappas A. Dietary regulation of cytochrome P450. *Annu Rev Nutr.* 1991;11:141-67

[221] Rogers RD, Tunbridge EM, Bhagwagar Z, Drevets WC, Sahakian BJ, Carter CS. Tryptophan depletion alters the decision-making of healthy volunteers through altered processing of reward cues. *Neuropsychopharmacology.* 2003;28:153-62 Accessed at http://www.acnp.org/sciweb/journal/Npp062402336/default.htm on November 10, 2004

[222] Arnulf I, Quintin P, Alvarez JC, Vigil L, Touitou Y, Lebre AS, Bellenger A, Varoquaux O, Derenne JP, Alilaire JF, Benkelfat C, Leboyer M. Mid-morning tryptophan depletion delays REM sleep onset in healthy subjects. *Neuropsychopharmacology.* 2002;27(5):843-51 http://www.nature.com/npp/journal/v27/n5/pdf/1395948a.pdf

[223] Thomas JR,Lockwood PA,Singh A, Deuster PA.Tyrosine improves working memory in a multitasking environment.*Pharmacol Biochem Behav.*1999;64:495-500

[224] Markus CR, Olivier B, Panhuysen GE, Van Der Gugten J, Alles MS, Tuiten A, Westenberg HG, Fekkes D, Koppeschaar HF, de Haan EE. The bovine protein alpha-lactalbumin increases the plasma ratio of tryptophan to the other large neutral amino acids, and in vulnerable subjects raises brain serotonin activity, reduces cortisol concentration, and improves mood under stress. *Am J Clin Nutr.* 2000;71:1536-44

[225] Castaneda C, Charnley JM, Evans WJ, Crim MC. Elderly women accommodate to a low-protein diet with losses of body cell mass, muscle function, and immune response. *Am J Clin Nutr.* 1995;62:30-9

[226] **Vasquez A.** Five-Part Nutritional Protocol that Produces Consistently Positive Results. *Nutritional Wellness* 2005 Sept. http://optimalhealthresearch.com/protocol

[227] Franco OH, Bonneux L, de Laet C, Peeters A, Steyerberg EW, Mackenbach JP. The Polymeal: a more natural, safer, and probably tastier (than the Polypill) strategy to reduce cardiovascular disease by more than 75%. *BMJ.* 2004;329(7480):1447-50

[228] "The combination of 4 low risk factors lowered the all-cause mortality rate to 0.35 (95% CI, 0.28-0.44). In total, lack of adherence to this low-risk pattern was associated with a population attributable risk of 60% of all deaths, 64% of deaths from coronary heart disease, 61% from cardiovascular diseases, and 60% from cancer." Knoops KT, de Groot LC, Kromhout D, et al. Mediterranean diet, lifestyle factors, and 10-year mortality in elderly European men and women: the HALE project. *JAMA.* 2004 Sep 22;292(12):1433-9

[229] Orme-Johnson DW, Herron RE. An innovative approach to reducing medical care utilization and expenditures. *Am J Manag Care.* 1997;3(1):135-44

[230] Cordain L, Friel J. The Paleo Diet for Athletes : A Nutritional Formula for Peak Athletic Performance: Rodale Books (September 23, 2005)

Profile of the Supplemented Paleo-Mediterranean Diet[233]

<u>Foods to consume</u>: whole, natural, minimally processed foods include:	<u>Foods to avoid</u>: factory products, high-sugar foods, and chemicals

☺ <u>**Lean sources of protein**</u>
  • Fish (avoiding tuna which is commonly loaded with mercury)
  • Chicken and turkey
  • Lean cuts of free-range grass-fed meats: beef, buffalo, lamb are occasionally acceptable
  • Soy protein[234] and whey protein[235,236]
☺ <u>**Fruits and fruit juices**</u>
☺ <u>**Vegetables and vegetable juices**</u>
☺ <u>**Nuts, seeds, berries**</u>
☺ <u>**Generous use of olive oil**</u>: On sautéed vegetables and fresh salads
☺ <u>**Daily vitamin/mineral supplementation**</u>: With a high-potency broad-spectrum multivitamin and multimineral supplement[237]
☺ <u>**Sun exposure or vitamin D3 supplementation**</u>: To ensure provision of 2,000-5,000 IU of vitamin D3 per day for adults[238]
☺ <u>**Balanced broad-spectrum fatty acid supplementation**</u>: With ALA, GLA, EPA, and DHA[239]
☺ <u>**Water, tea, home-made fruit/vegetable juices**</u>: Commercial vegetable juices are commonly loaded with sodium chloride; choose appropriately. Fruit juices can be loaded with natural and superfluous sugars. Herbal teas can be selected based on the medicinal properties of the plant that is used.
	☒ **Avoid as much as possible fat-laden arachidonate-rich meats like beef, liver, pork, and lamb, as well as high-fat cream and other dairy products with emulsified, readily absorbed saturated fats and arachidonic acid**
	☒ <u>**High-sugar pseudofoods**</u>:
	  • Corn syrup
	  • Cola and soda
	  • Donuts, candy, etc...."junk food"
	☒ <u>**Grains such as wheat, rye, barley**</u>: These have only existed in the human diet for less than 10,000 years and are consistently associated with increased prevalence of degenerative diseases due to the allergic response they invoke and because of their high glycemic load and high glycemic index.
	☒ <u>**Potatoes and rice**</u>: High in sugar, low in phytonutrients
	☒ <u>**Avoid allergens**</u>: Determined per individual
	☒ <u>**Chemicals to avoid**</u>:
	  • <u>Pesticides, Herbicides, Fungicides</u>
	  • <u>Carcinogenic sweeteners</u>: aspartame[240]
	  • <u>Artificial flavors</u>
	  • <u>Artificial colors</u>: tartrazine
	  • <u>Preservatives</u>: benzoate
	  • <u>Flavor enhancers</u>: carrageenan and monosodium glutamate

[231] "A significant glycogen sparing, as well as supercompensation within 24 h of recovery, was observed after [carbohydrate] supplementation." Brouns F, Saris WH, Beckers E, Adlercreutz H, van der Vusse GJ, Keizer HA, Kuipers H, Menheere P, Wagenmakers AJ, ten Hoor F. Metabolic changes induced by sustained exhaustive cycling and diet manipulation. *Int J Sports Med.* 1989 May;10 Suppl 1:S49-62

[232] "The accepted method of increasing muscle glycogen stores is by "glycogen loading," which classically involves depletion of muscle glycogen, usually by exercise, followed by consumption of a high-CHO diet for several days (e.g., 3, 39). ...increase muscle glycogen concentrations ([glycogen]) to between 150 and 200% of normal resting levels." Robinson TM, Sewell DA, Hultman E, Greenhaff PL. Role of submaximal exercise in promoting creatine and glycogen accumulation in human skeletal muscle. *J Appl Physiol.* 1999 Aug;87(2):598-604

[233] **Vasquez A**. Five-Part Nutritional Protocol that Produces Consistently Positive Results. *Nutritional Wellness* 2005 Sept. and Vasquez A. Revisiting the Five-Part Nutritional Wellness Protocol: The Supplemented Paleo-Mediterranean Diet. *Nutritional Perspectives* 2011 January. Both of these articles are included in this textbook and/or on-line at http://optimalhealthresearch.com/spmd.html

[234] "These results indicate that for healthy adults, the isolated soy protein is of high nutritional quality, comparable to that of animal protein sources, and that the methionine content is not limiting for adult protein maintenance." Young VR, Puig M, Queiroz E, Scrimshaw NS, Rand WM. Evaluation of the protein quality of an isolated soy protein in young men: relative nitrogen requirements and effect of methionine supplementation. *Am J Clin Nutr.* 1984 Jan;39(1):16-24

[235] Bounous G. Whey protein concentrate (WPC) and glutathione modulation in cancer treatment. *Anticancer Res.* 2000 Nov-Dec;20(6C):4785-92

[236] Markus CR, Olivier B, Panhuysen GE, Van Der Gugten J, Alles MS, Tuiten A, Westenberg HG, Fekkes D, Koppeschaar HF, de Haan EE. The bovine protein alpha-lactalbumin increases the plasma ratio of tryptophan to the other large neutral amino acids, and in vulnerable subjects raises brain serotonin activity, reduces cortisol concentration, and improves mood under stress. *Am J Clin Nutr.* 2000 Jun;71(6):1536-44 http://www.ajcn.org/cgi/content/full/71/6/1536

[237] "Most people do not consume an optimal amount of all vitamins by diet alone. ...it appears prudent for all adults to take vitamin supplements." Fletcher RH, Fairfield KM. Vitamins for chronic disease prevention in adults: clinical applications. *JAMA.* 2002;287:3127-9

[238] **Vasquez A**, MansoG,CannellJ.The clinical importance of vitamin D (cholecalciferol).*Altern Ther Health Med.*2004Sep10:28-36 www.optimalhealthresearch.com

[239] **Vasquez A**. New Insights into Fatty Acid Supplementation and Its Effect on Eicosanoid Production and Genetic Expression. *Nutr Perspectives* 2005; Jan: 5-16

[240] "In the past two decades brain tumor rates have risen in several industrialized countries, including the United States... Compared to other environmental factors putatively linked to brain tumors, the artificial sweetener aspartame is a promising candidate to explain the recent increase in incidence and degree of malignancy of brain tumors." Olney JW, Farber NB, Spitznagel E, Robins LN. Increasing brain tumor rates: is there a link to aspartame? *J Neuropathol Exp Neurol* 1996 Nov;55(11):1115-23

Emotional, Mental, and Social Health

Stress management and authentic living: Mental, emotional, and physical "stress" describes any unpleasant living condition which can lead to negative effects on health, such as increased blood pressure, depression, apathy, increased muscle tension, and, according to some research, increased risk of serious health problems such as early death from cardiovascular disease and cancer. Many people find that their modern lives are characterized by excess amounts of multitasking, job responsibilities, family responsibilities, commuter traffic, financial pressures in combination with an insufficient amount of relaxation, sleep, community support, exercise, time in nature, healthy nutrition, and time to simply *be* rather than *do*. Stress comes in many different forms and includes malnutrition, trauma, insufficient exercise (epidemic), excess exercise (rare), sleep deprivation, emotional turmoil, and exposure to chemicals and radiation. When most people talk about "stress" they are referring to either chronic anxiety (such as with high-pressure work situations or dysfunctional interpersonal relationships) or the acute stress reaction that is typical of unpredictable rapid-onset events such as an injury, accident, or other physically threatening situation. **These "different types of stress" are not separate from each other; rather, they are interconnected:**

- Emotional stress causes nutritional depletion[241],
- Sleep deprivation alters immune response[242],
- Chemical exposure can disrupt endocrine function.[243]

Therefore, **any type of stress can cause other types of stress**. Avoiding stressful situations is, of course, an effective way to avoid being bothered or harmed by them. If work-related stress is the problem, then finding a new position or occupation is certainly an option worth considering and implementing. High-stress jobs are often high-paying jobs; but if in the process of making money, a person ruins her health and loses years from her life, then no one would ever say, "It was worth it." **Money, success, and freedom only have value for the person alive and healthy to enjoy them.**

Toxic relationships, whether at home or work, are relationships that cause more harm than good by re-injuring old emotional wounds and by creating new emotional injuries. We can all benefit from affirming our right to a happy and healthy life by minimizing/eliminating contact with people who cause emotional harm to us—this requires conscious effort.[244] Engel[245] provides a clear articulation and description of abusive relationships, along with checklists for their recognition and exercises for their remediation. Healthy relationships are difficult to create and maintain these days, and probably a few basic components contribute to this phenomenon. ❶ With the society-wide disintegration of the extended family, most people in our society have never even seen a healthy family unit and therefore have no model and no available mentors to help them recreate a lasting family structure. ❷ Due specifically to the structure of our educational systems and (pseudo)culture of entertainment, most people have very short attention spans and are accustomed to inattention, distraction, and externally derived entertainment and gratification. ❸ Modern schools and fragmented families both fail to teach conflict resolution and relationship skills. ❹ Poor nutritional status—very common in the general population—promotes impulsivity, irritability, depression, and mood instability.

> "**Good relationships make you feel loved, wanted, and cared for**."
>
> Malcolm LL. Health Style. Thorsons: 2001, p 133

---

[241] Ingenbleek Y, Bernstein L. The stressful condition as a nutritionally dependent adaptive dichotomy. *Nutrition* 1999 Apr;15(4):305-20
[242] Heiser P, e. Alterations of host defense system after sleep deprivation are followed by impaired mood and psychosocial functioning. *World J Biol Psychiatry* 2001 Apr;2(2):89-94
[243] "Evidence suggests that environmental exposure to some anthropogenic chemicals may result in disruption of endocrine systems in human and wildlife populations." http://www.epa.gov/endocrine on March 7, 2004
[244] Bryn C. Collins. *How to Recognize Emotional Unavailability and Make Healthier Relationship Choices*. [Mjf Books; ISBN: 1567313442] Recently reprinted as: Emotional Unavailability: Recognizing It, Understanding It, and Avoiding Its Trap [McGraw Hill - NTC (April 1998); ISBN: 0809229145]
[245] Engel B. *The Emotionally Abusive Relationship: How to Stop Being Abused and How to Stop Abusing*. Wiley Publishers: 2003

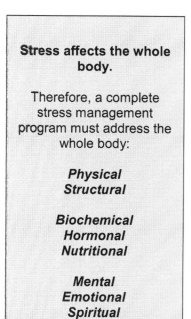

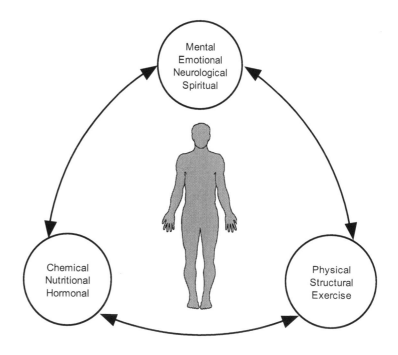

An important concept is that **stress is a "whole body" phenomenon**: affecting the mind, the brain, emotional state, the physical body (including musculoskeletal, immune, and cardiovascular systems), as well as the nutritional status of the individual. The adverse effects of stress can be reduced with an integrated combination of therapeutics that addresses each of the major body systems affected by stress, which are 1) mental/emotional, 2) physical, and 3) nutritional/biochemical.

Approaching stress management from a tripartite perspective

	Mental/emotional	Physical	Nutritional/biochemical
Therapeutic considerations	• Social support • Re-parenting • Conversational style[246] • Meditation, prayer • Healthy boundaries • Books, tapes, groups • Expressive writing[247] • Time to simply rest and relax	• Yoga • Massage • Exercise • Stretching • Swimming • Resting • Biking • Hiking • Affection	• Vitamins, including vitamin C[248] • Fish oil[249] • Hormones, cytokines, neurotransmitters, and eicosanoids • Tryptophan, pyridoxine • Botanical medicines such as *kava*[250], *Ashwaganda,* and *Eleutherococcus*

[246] Rick Brinkman ND and Rick Kirschner ND. *How to Deal With Difficult People* [Audio Cassette. Career Track, 1995]

[247] Smyth JM, Stone AA, Hurewitz A, Kaell A. Effects of writing about stressful experiences on symptom reduction in patients with asthma or rheumatoid arthritis: a randomized trial. *JAMA.* 1999 Apr 14;281(14):1304-9

[248] Brody S, Preut R, Schommer K, Schurmeyer TH. A randomized controlled trial of high dose ascorbic acid for reduction of blood pressure, cortisol, and subjective responses to psychological stress. *Psychopharmacology* (Berl). 2002 Jan;159(3):319-24

[249] Hamazaki T, Itomura M, Sawazaki S, Nagao Y. Anti-stress effects of DHA. *Biofactors.* 2000;13(1-4):41-5

[250] Cagnacci A, et al. Kava-Kava administration reduces anxiety in perimenopausal women. *Maturitas.* 2003 Feb 25;44(2):103-9

Sometimes a stressful situation can be modified into one that is less stressful or dysfunctional, so that the benefits are retained, yet the negative aspects are reduced. Of course, the best example of this is interpersonal relationships, which easily lend themselves to improvement with the application of conscious effort. Many audiotapes, books, and seminars are available for people interested in having improved interpersonal relationships. Selected resources are listed here:

- Men and Women: Talking Together by Deborah Tannen and Robert Bly [Sound Horizons, 1992. ISBN: 1879323095] A lively discussion of the different communication and relationship styles of men and women by two respected experts in their fields.
- How to Deal with Difficult People by Drs. Rick Brinkman and Rick Kirschner. [Audio Cassette. Career Track, 1995] An entertaining format with solutions to common workplace and situational difficulties. Authored and performed by two naturopathic physicians.
- Men are From Mars, Women are From Venus by John Gray. [Audio Cassette and Books]. Phenomenally popular concepts in understanding, accepting, and effectively integrating the differences between men and women.
- The ManKind Project (www.mkp.org). An international organization hosting events for men and women. The men's events, formats, and groups are authentic, clear, and healthy. The ManKind Project has an organization for women called The WomanWithin (www.womanwithin.org). No book or tape can substitute for the dynamics and personal attention that can be experienced by a conscious, empowered, and well-intended group.

When "the problem" cannot be avoided, and the interaction/relationship with the problem cannot be improved, a remaining option is to supplement the internal environment so that it is somewhat "strengthened" to deal with the stress of the bothersome event or situation. For example, when dealing with emotional stress, we can use counseling, support groups, or various relaxation techniques.[251] If we determine that the emotional stress has a biochemical component, then we can use specific botanical and nutritional supplementation to safely and naturally support and restore normal function. Moving deeper into the issue of "stress management" requires that we ask why a person is in a stressful situation to begin with. Of course, with *random acts of chaos* like car accidents, we cannot always ascribe the problem to the person, unless the accident resulted from their own negligence. But **when people are chronically stressed and unhappy about their jobs and/or relationships, then we need to employ more than stress reduction techniques**, and as clinicians we need to offer more than the latest adaptogen. **We have to ask why a person would subject himself/herself to such a situation, and what fears or limitations (self-imposed and/or externally applied) keep him/her from breaking free into a life that works.**[252,253,254,255,256,257]

[251] Martha Davis PhD, Matthew McKay MSW, Elizabeth Robbins Eshelman PhD. The Relaxation & Stress Reduction Workbook 5th edition. New Harbinger Publishers; 2000. [ISBN: 1572242140]

[252] Rick Jarow. Creating the Work You Love: Courage, Commitment and Career; Inner Traditions Intl Ltd; 1995 [ISBN: 0892815426]

[253] Breton D, Largent C. The Paradigm Conspiracy: Why Our Social Systems Violate Human Potential-And How We Can Change Them. Hazelden: 1998

[254] Dominguez JR. Transforming Your Relationship With Money. Sounds True; Book and Cassette edition: 2001 Audio tape.

[255] Miller A. The truth will set you free: overcoming emotional blindness and finding your true adult self. New York: Basic Books; 2001

[256] Bradshaw J. Healing the Shame that Binds You [Audio Cassette (April 1990) Health Communications Audio; ISBN: 1558740430]

[257] Miller A. The Drama of the Gifted Child: The Search for the True Self. Basic Books: 1981

Stress always has a biochemical/physiologic component: Regardless of its origins, stress always takes a toll on the body—*the whole body*. Well-documented effects of stress include:

1. Increased levels of cortisol—higher levels are associated with osteoporosis, memory loss, slow healing, and insulin resistance.
2. Reduced function of thyroid hormones[258] (i.e., induction of peripheral/metabolic hypothyroidism)
3. Reduced levels of testosterone (in men)
4. Increased intestinal permeability and "leaky gut"[259]
5. Increased excretion of minerals in the urine
6. Increased need for vitamins, minerals, and amino acids
7. Suppression of immune function and of natural killer cells that fight viral infections and tumors
8. Decreased production of sIgA—the main defense of the lungs, gastrointestinal tract, and genitourinary tract
9. Increased populations of harmful bacteria in the intestines and an associated increased rate of lung and upper respiratory tract infections
10. Increased incidence of food allergies[260]
11. Sleep disturbance

The body functions as a whole—not as independent, autonomous organ systems: Problems with one aspect of health create problems in other aspects of health. Treatment of disease and promotion of wellness must therefore improve overall health and functioning while simultaneously addressing the disease or presenting complaint.

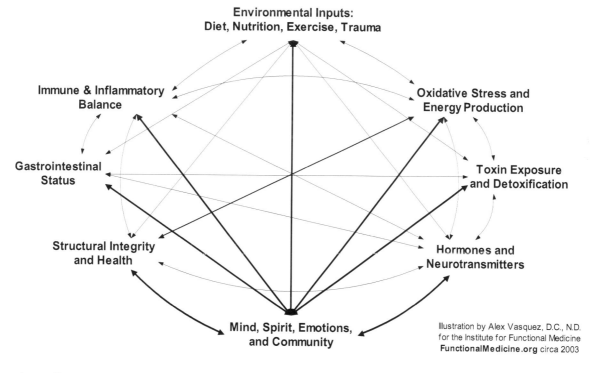

An earlier rendering of the Functional Medicine Matrix, circa 2003: The "Matrix" provides a graphic illustration of the interconnectedness and interdependency of physiologic factors and organ systems; this version was published in *Textbook of Functional Medicine* and published separately as Vasquez A. Web-like Interconnections of Physiological Factors. *Integrative Medicine* 2006, April, 32-37

---

[258] Ingenbleek Y, Bernstein L. The stressful condition as a nutritionally dependent adaptive dichotomy. *Nutrition* 1999 Apr;15(4):305-20
[259] Hart A, Kamm MA. Review article: mechanisms of initiation and perpetuation of gut inflammation by stress. *Aliment Pharmacol Ther* 2002;16(12):2017-28
[260] Anderzen I, Arnetz BB, Soderstrom T, Soderman E. Stress and sensitization in children: a controlled prospective psychophysiological study of children exposed to international relocation. *Journal of Psychosomatic Research* 1997; 43: 259-69

Autonomization, intradependence, emotional literacy, corrective experience:

"None of us are completely developed people when we reach adulthood.
We are each incomplete in our own way." *Merle Fossum*[261]

Consciousness-raising is a keystone gift that holistic physicians can impart to their patients and one which may be necessary for true healing to be manifested and maintained. Healthcare providers are quick to enlighten their patients to the details of diet, exercise, nutrition, medications, surgeries, and other *biomechanical* and *biochemical* aspects of health, but are routinely negligent when it comes to sharing with patients the emotional tools that may be necessary to repair or construct the "self" which is supposed to implement the treatment plan that the doctor has designed. Passivity and ignorance are not hindrances to the success of the *medical paradigm*, which requires that patients are "compliant" rather than self-directed; however, for *authentic, holistic healthcare* to be successful, it must empower the patient sufficiently such that he/she attains/regains appropriate *autonomy*—an "internal locus of control"—sufficient for lifelong internally-driven health maintenance. Health implications of autonomy (or its absence) are obvious and intuitive. Patients with an underdeveloped internal locus of control appear to experience greater degrees of social stress which can lead to hypercortisolemia and hippocampal atrophy.[262] A developed internal locus of control correlates strongly with the success of weight-loss programs, and for nonautonomous patients it is necessary to encourage the development of autonomous self-care behavior in addition to the provision of information about diet and exercise.[263]

> ### Six fundamental components of self-esteem
> 1. Living consciously
> 2. Self-acceptance
> 3. Self-responsibility
> 4. Self-assertiveness
> 5. Living purposefully
> 6. Personal integrity
>
> Branden N. The Six Pillars of Self-Esteem. Bantam: 1995

Completely formed internal identities are the natural result of the *continuum* of positive childhood experiences (inclusive of stability, "unconditional love", healthy parenting, and active, conscious intergenerational social contact) which are ideally merged into adolescent and adulthood experiences of success, acceptance, inclusion, independence, interdependence, and intradependence with the end result being a socially-conscious adult with an internal locus of control. Where the patient has experienced a relative absence of these natural and expected prerequisites, a truncated—wounded, reactive, shame-based, dissatisfied—self is likely to result. The failure to develop self-esteem and an internal locus of control largely explains why so many adult patients feign that they are incapable of action, "can't exercise", and "can't leave" their abusive jobs and relationships, and "can't resist" the dietary habits which daily contribute to their physical and psychoemotional decline. Thus, for more than a few patients, a therapeutic path must be explored which helps to re-create the foundation from which an autonomous adult and authentic self can grow—it is a *process* (not an event) of **emotional recovery**.[264] To this extent, interventional or therapeutic *autonomization* resembles a *recovery program* that can include various forms of conscious action, including goal-setting, positive reinforcement, developing emotional literacy[265] and emotional intelligence[266], and consciousness-raising experiences such as therapy and group work—all of which serve to intentionally (re)create and maintain the necessary climate for authentic selfhood. Therewith, the patient can accept challenges to further develop an *empowered self* by participating in exercises in which the ability to decide, choose, and act responsibly and appropriately are reinforced to eventually become second nature, replacing passivity, inaction, and ineffectiveness.[267]

"Empowerment" can only be authentic if it is built on the foundation of a developed self. While *emotional recovery* and *personal empowerment* are separate spheres of activity and attention, they are not mutually exclusive and indeed are synergistic. However, emotional recovery—that process of recounting one's own history, delving

[261] Fossum M. Catching Fire: Men Coming Alive in Recovery. New York; Harper/Hazelden: 1989, 4-7

[262] "Cumulative exposure to high levels of cortisol over the lifetime is known to be related to hippocampal atrophy... Self-esteem and internal locus of control were significantly correlated with hippocampal volume in both young and elderly subjects." Pruessner JC, Baldwin MW, Dedovic K, Renwick R, Mahani NK, Lord C, Meaney M, Lupien S. Self-esteem, locus of control, hippocampal volume, and cortisol regulation in young and old adulthood. *Neuroimage*. 2005 Dec;28(4):815-26

[263] "Their weight loss was significant and associated with an internal locus of control orientation (P < 0.05)... Participants with an internal orientation could be offered a standard weight reduction programme. Others, with a more external locus of control orientation, could be offered an adapted programme, which also focused on and encouraged the participants' internal orientation." Adolfsson B, Andersson I, Elofsson S, Rossner S, Unden AL. Locus of control and weight reduction. *Patient Educ Couns*. 2005 Jan;56(1):55-61

[264] Bradshaw J. Healing the Shame that Binds You [Audio Cassette (April 1990) Health Communications Audio; ISBN: 1558740430]

[265] Dayton T. Trauma and Addiction: Ending the Cycle of Pain through Emotional Literacy. Deerfield Beach; Health Communications, 2000

[266] Goleman D. Emotional Intelligence. New York; Bantam Books: 1995. Although the book as a whole was considered pioneering for its time, and the book continues to make a valuable contribution, a few of the concepts and author's personal stories are embarrassingly simplistic.

[267] Gatto JT. A Schooling Is Not An Education: interview by Barbara Dunlop. http://www.johntaylorgatto.com/bookstore/index.htm

into the depths of one's own psyche, and integrating what is found into a cohesive, functional and healthy whole—must occur before the program of personal development emphasizes empowerment. *Empowerment* cannot succeed without *recovery* because otherwise the so-called "empowerment" is likely to add to the defense mechanisms that protect against pain and thereby block the development of an authentic self. Stated concisely by Janov[268], **"Anything that builds a stronger defense system deepens the neurosis."**

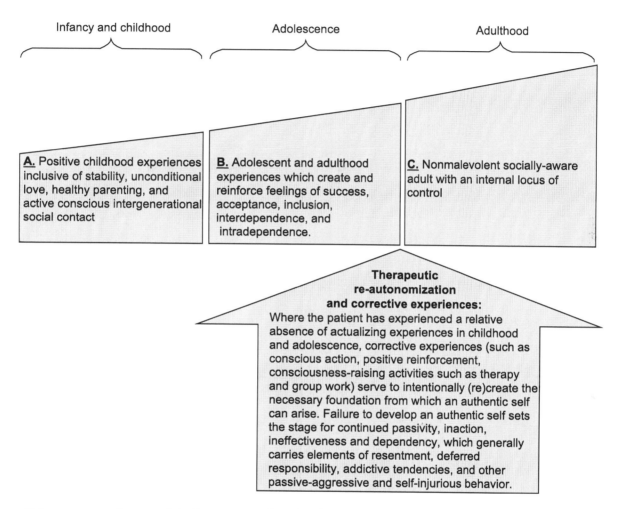

Primary, secondary, and tertiary means for developing an autonomous, authentic self: Ideally, positive childhood experiences (A) merge into adolescent and adult experiences of confidence and maturity (B) for the development of a true adult (C). If A or B is lacking or insufficient, the result is an incomplete self often incapable of *effective* and *appropriate* action. Corrective experiences must then be pursued to re-establish the foundation from which an authentic self can arise.

Patients lacking an internal locus of control are much more likely to succumb to the tantalizing barrage of direct-to-consumer drug advertising[269] which infantilizes patients by 1) oversimplifying diseases, their causes, and treatments, 2) exonerating patients from responsibility and reinforcing the illusion of victimization and helplessness, and 3) encouraging a dependent, passively receptive role by telling patients that they have no proactive role other than to "ask your doctor if a prescription is right for you." Americans consume more prescription and OTC medications per capita than people in any other country.[270,271] With the combined and

[268] Janov A. The Primal Scream. New York; GP Putnam's Sons: 1970, page 20
[269] Aronson E. The Social Animal. San Fransisco; WH Freeman and company: 1972: 21-22, 53
[270] America the medicated. http://www.cbsnews.com/stories/2005/04/21/health/printable689997.shtml and http://www.msnbc.msn.com/id/7503122/ . See also http://usgovinfo.about.com/od/healthcare/a/usmedicated.htm Accessed September 17, 2005.
[271] Kivel P. You Call This a Democracy? Apex Press (August, 2004). ISBN: 1891843265 http://www.paulkivel.com/

synergistic effects of 1) the dissolution of first the extended family and now the nuclear family[272], 2) a society-wide famine of mentors, elders, and community[273,274,275], 3) a dearth of autonomous, genuine exploration from childhood to adulthood, and 4) primary and secondary "educational" institutions designed to squelch independence and autonomy in favor of the more efficient,

predictable, and controllable conformity and "standardization"[276,277], **industrialized societies have raised generations of people who lack completely formed internal identities**. Lacking an internal locus of control and identity from which to think independently and critically, these "adults" are easy prey for slick and flashy drug advertisements that promise the illusion of perfect health in exchange for passivity, abdication, and lifelong medicalization. That the typical American watches four hours of television per day[278] is bad enough, what makes this worse is that "Americans who watch average amounts of television may be exposed to more than 30 hours of direct-to-consumer drug advertisements each year, far surpassing their exposure to other forms of health communication."[279] If we are to wean our suckling culture from undue dependence on the pharmaceutical industry, we have to address our patient population directly and transform them from *passive, nonautonomous, and ignorant about health and disease* to pro-active, autonomous, and well-informed about health and the means required to obtain and sustain it.

Insight into a patient's internal dynamic can provide the clinician with an understanding that explains the phenomena of *non-compliance* and *disease identification*. Rather than seeing non-compliance as "weakness of will", non-compliance as a form of "disobedience" may be a reflection of the patient's unconscious need to wrestle with and resolve parental introjects. For example, if a patient had a rejecting, nonaffirming parent, he/she may need to find another rejecting authority figure in order to continue playing the role of the child; by assuming this role and "setting the stage", the patient is unconsciously attempting to create a situation wherein the primary relationship can be healed.[280] Complicating this is *disease identification*—in which patients use their disease as a source of identity and secondary gain for martyrdom, social support, group participation, acceptance, admiration, purpose, excitement, and drama.

---

[272] Bly R. Iron John. Reading, Mass.: Addison Wesley, 1990

[273] Bly R. The Sibling Society. Vintage Books USA; Reprint edition (June 1, 1997) ISBN: 0679781285 (Abridged audio edition (May 1, 1996), ASIN: 0679451609)

[274] Bly R. Where have all the parents gone? A talk on the Sibling Society. New York: Sound Horizons, 1996 Highly recommended.

[275] Bly R, Hillman J, Meade M. Men and the Life of Desire. Oral Tradition Archives. ISBN: 1880155001. Audio Cassette

[276] Gatto JT. Dumbing Us Down: the Hidden Curriculum of Compulsory Education. Gabriola Island, Canada; New Society Publishers: 2005

[277] Gatto JT. The Paradox of Extended Childhood. [From a presentation in Cambridge, Mass. October 2000] http://www.johntaylorgatto.com/bookstore/index.htm

[278] "American children view over 23 hours of television per week. Teenagers view an average of 21 to 22 hours of television per week. By the time today's children reach age 70, they will have spent 7 to 10 years of their lives watching television." American Academy of Pediatrics http://www.aapca1.org/aapca1/tv.html See also TV-Turnoff Network. Facts and Figures About our TV Habit http://www.tvturnoff.org/factsheets.htm Accessed September 17, 2005

[279] Brownfield ED, et al. Direct-to-consumer drug advertisements on network television. *J Health Commun.* 2004 Nov-Dec;9(6):491-7

[280] Miller A. The Drama of the Gifted Child: The Search for the True Self. Basic Books: 1981, page 88

Helping patients create and maintain authentic selves

An absent or underdeveloped locus of control is the key problem that underlies many anxiety disorders, addictive behavioral traits such as overeating, overworking, codependency, as well as chronic ineffectiveness in the pursuit of one's goals. The solutions to this problem are logical, practical, and accessible to everyone; the major costs associated with each are open-mindedness, attentiveness, discipline and persistence. There is scant mention of this concept and its intervention in the biomedical literature; however, it is well described in the psychological literature, particularly that which focuses on various types of "recovery" such as that from addiction, co-dependence, and low self-esteem, the latter two of which are virtually synonymous with an insufficient internal locus of control.

There is no single path here. There are many paths. The goal is not to choose the right path; rather the goal is to travel several paths to the degree necessary, implement what has been learned, travel other paths, and return to the same path again to retrace one's steps in new ways. The process is similar to that of *ceremonial initiation*, the purpose of which is to formally mark the *beginning* of a process that is *ongoing* and *infinite*.[281] Each path and each process has its gifts, significance, and limitations. However, the ultimate goal of each must be a tangible and positive change in the ways which the patient feels and/or behaves in and interacts with the world on a day-to-day basis.

In no particular order (since the proper sequence will have to be customized to the situation and willingness of the patient), the following are some of the more commonly cited exercises, processes, and sources of additional information:

Apprenticeship and Mentoring: books, tapes, and lectures: Children and non-autonomous adults are pulled into authentic adulthood by mentors, elders, and true adults. The therapeutic encounters thus provided—whether interpersonal or vicarious in the form of lectures, books, or audiotapes— serve as sources of information from which new possibilities can be gleaned, and these therefore serve as infinitely valuable resources for expanding the narrow horizons that characterize an underdeveloped internal locus of control. In essence, books, tapes, and lectures allow the patient to become a student and to choose a vicarious mentor. *Advantages*: Books and tapes allow access to many of the best minds in psychology; books and tapes are inexpensive; allow patients to explore and benefit from many different perspectives; books and tapes are always available and are therefore amenable to various schedules of work and responsibility. *Disadvantages*: Books and tapes do not re-create the interpersonal bridge which is essential for authentic recovery; do not provide a direct and objective means of accountably, thus potentially allowing patients to delude themselves about the effectiveness (or lack thereof) of their recovery process. Examples of better-known books, tapes and recorded lectures on the *process* of emotional recovery:

- *The Six Pillars of Self-Esteem* by Nathaniel Branden PhD. This is a very accessible yet very structured work in which Dr Branden brilliantly elucidates key concepts in psychology relevant to self-efficacy and self-esteem; also available as an audiobook excellently narrated by Dr Branden.
- *Healing the Shame that Binds You* by John Bradshaw [Audio Cassette (April 1990) Health Communications Audio; ISBN: 1558740430] Available as book and cassette with identical titles and different content.
- *A Little Book on the Human Shadow* by Robert Bly. Certainly among the most concise, accessible, and complete books ever written on the processes involved in losing and recovering the self; also available as an audio presentation.
- *The Drama of the Gifted Child* by Alice Miller. This internationally acclaimed book is considered a true classic among therapists and patients alike. Available as book and a brilliantly performed audio cassette.
- *You Can Heal Your Life* by Louise Hay. Another standard for recovery; very "new age."
- *Codependent No More: How to Stop Controlling Others and Start Caring for Yourself* by Melody Beattie. Pioneering for its time.
- *The Artist's Date Book* by Julia Cameron. Each page has a new creative idea for creative expression and "creative recovery."
- *The Psychology of Self-Esteem* by Nathaniel Branden PhD. More advanced and perhaps less widely relevant than his "six pillars" work, this is also an excellent encapsulation of important concepts in personal psychology.

---

[281] Hillman J, Meade M, Some M. Images of initiation. Oral Tradition Archives; 1992

Therapy: *"Therapy is a conversation that matters."* Therapy in this context specifically means face-to-face, active interaction, either one-on-one or in a group setting, with the specific intention to give and/or provide support for personal growth. Whether 12-step groups such as Codependents Anonymous qualify as a form of therapy depends entirely upon the level of engagement of the participant; sitting in a room while *other people* do *their* work provides slow or no benefit for the passive observer. **Recovery is an *active* process, which is why it is antithetical to depression, which is a *passive* state of being.** Patients should go in knowing that this is a *process* and to not expect to be "fixed" after the first hour or even the first month. ***Advantages***: Therapists can provide crucial support and insight while the client wrestles with undecipherable and convoluted emotional and psychic data. Therapists can help the client set goals ("stretches" and "homework") by which the client reaches beyond his/her comfort zone to attain the next expansion in being and experience. Therapists must create a safe space or "container" in which ideas and feelings can be brought forth to intermingle and be consciously appreciated. ***Disadvantages***: Requires a flexible and disciplined schedule; costs money; bad therapists can do more harm than good if they misdirect their clients away from volatile and core issues and authentic expression.[282,283,284,285] Therapy can be disempowering if the patient continues to project his/her locus of control onto the therapist.

Some of the more commonly used tools of the psychotherapeutic trade include:

- **Active listening**
- **Insight, explanation of events**: their origins, reasons, and significance
- **Reminders** of previous conclusions and stories
- **Challenge old ideas and habits**: Therapy that generally or completely lacks confrontation and accountability is ineffective.
- **Encourage exploration and new modes of being and interacting**
- **Creating a safe container wherein the client can review the details, significance, and feelings associated with past events**
- **Modeling the expression of feeling**
- **Defining goals and helping the client focus on what is significant**
- **Correcting distortions of reality**
- **Asking patients to get in touch with and then express their feelings**
- **Support and encourage clients to take calculated risks for the sake of self-expansion**
- **Pointing out errors in logic**
- **Coaching patients in the proper and responsible use of emotional language**
- **Discouraging evasiveness; requiring accountability**[286]

Creativity: All types of self-expression reinforce and validate the patient's sense of self. Creative self-expression, such as writing about thoughts and feelings about significant experiences, can reduce symptomatology in patients with rheumatoid arthritis and asthma.[287]

Experiential: Corrective experiences can be obtained in therapy, with friends and family, in integration groups, and during "experiential" retreats. ***Advantages***: Experiential events orchestrated by therapists and various groups such as ManKind Project (mkp.org) and WomanWithin.org can rapidly facilitate personal growth while also providing an ongoing container and support system that encourages self-development rather than the ego-inflation that accompanies short-term events. ***Disadvantages***: "Adventures" like driving across the nation or climbing a mountain are unconscious and largely impotent attempts at self-initiation; authentic initiation has always been supervised by community elders. However, once a well-founded initiation has taken place, preferably with an on-going community that facilitates continued refinement and self-exploration, then "adventures" can be undertaken consciously to maintain and reinforce the experience of autonomy and competent selfhood. Eventually, transformative and sustentative experiences can be integrated and created in the daily life experience so that dramatic adventures become unnecessary for the continued renewal and "recharging" of the self.

[282] Lee J. Expressing Your Anger Appropriately (Audio Cassette). Sounds True (June 1, 1990); ISBN: 1564550338
[283] Bradshaw J. Healing the Shame that Binds You [Audio Cassette (April 1990) Health Communications Audio; ISBN: 1558740430]
[284] Miller A. The Drama of the Gifted Child: The Search for the True Self. Basic Books: 1981
[285] Miller A. The truth will set you free: overcoming emotional blindness and finding your true adult self. New York: Basic Books; 2001
[286] Kottler JA. The Compleat Therapist. San Francisco; Jossey-Bass publishers; 1991, pages 134-174
[287] Smyth JM, Stone AA, Hurewitz A, Kaell A. Effects of writing about stressful experiences on symptom reduction in patients with asthma or rheumatoid arthritis: a randomized trial. JAMA. 1999 Apr 14;281(14):1304-9

Creating and Re-creating the Self:
An on-going process that involves various types of "therapy" such as healthy formal/informal interpersonal and group relationships, creative expression and exploration, the periodic infusion of new ideas from teachers and mentors, attendance in workshops and seminars (or other forms of on-going consciousness-raising), reflection, and the integration of transformative and sustentative significance into everyday life, in such a way that daily life itself becomes *therapeutic* and *affirmative*.

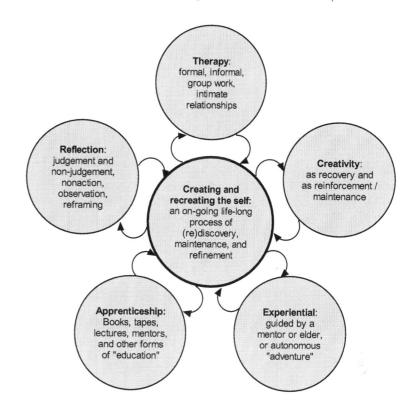

One possible sequence of events for effective, lasting, and authentic autonomization: The caterpillar does not blossom into a butterfly without spending time in its cocoon. The airborne seed descends into the earth for its nourishment before it sprouts and searches for the sun. Similarly, gratification of our ascentionist and impatient ego must be deferred for the sake of allowing the time and descent that provide "grounding" and developing of a solid foundation from which authentic growth can arise. The Western view of "personal development" idealizes a life course of constant ascension that is generally inconsistent with living in a real world fraught with imperfections; two of the major complications arising from such a perfectionistic paradigm are 1) that it causes people to feel anxious and ashamed when confronted with otherwise normal delays and failures, and 2) that it biases people into believing that improvement comes only from advancement rather than also from the return and short-term regression that are characteristic of most historically-proven societal traditions. With modification of the stepwise model proposed by Bradshaw[288], here I propose the following sequence:

1. *Short-term behavior modification*: For people whose behavior is acutely dysfunctional or harmful to themselves or others, they must stop the "acting out" that is the symptom of the underlying emotional injury or schism. Accepting abuse—at work or home—is a form of **acting out** that perpetuates old wounds and saps the strength required for recovery. Enacting addictive behavior is injurious to the psyche because self-injurious behavior reinforces the image of oneself as an object of contempt while also reinforcing the image of psychological dependency and emotional helplessness.

2. *Emotional recovery*: Complete healing is only possible when consciously pursued, and conscious healing can only be pursued after one has become conscious of the wounds, injuries, absences, dynamics, and events that lead to the current state. This process of recovery is referred to mythologically as the "descent" or the time of "eating ashes" that is a recurrent theme in various fairy tales ("Cinderella" literally means "ash girl") and cultural-religious histories (such as Jesus' *descent* into the tomb).[289] The biggest blockades to this process are 1) the ego, which prefers to ascend and to deny intrapersonal "negativity"[290], and 2) the challenge in finding elders and mentors in a society that constantly perpetuates and encourages immaturity, materialism, and superficiality.[291] In the words of famed psychologist Carl Jung, "One does not become enlightened by

---

[288] Bradshaw J. Healing the Shame that Binds You [Audio Cassette (April 1990) Health Communications Audio; ISBN: 1558740430]
[289] Bly R, Hillman J, Meade M. Men and the Life of Desire. Oral Tradition Archives. ISBN: 1880155001
[290] Robert Bly. The Human Shadow. Sound Horizons, New York 1991 [ISBN: 1879323001] and Bly R. A Little Book on the Human Shadow.[ISBN: 0062548476]
[291] Bly R. Where have all the parents gone? A talk on the Sibling Society. New York: Sound Horizons, 1996

imagining figures of light, but by making the darkness *conscious*. The latter procedure, however, is disagreeable, and therefore unpopular." People often have tremendous resistances to the process of self-exploration and internal learning; as Jeffrey Kottler[292] wrote of his own experience in *The Compleat Therapist*, "…like most prospective consumers of therapy, I made up a bunch of excuses for why I could handle this on my own… I was smiling like an idiot…"

3. *Long-term behavior modification and integration*: Insight allows for an illumination of the internal mental-emotional landscape, and effective insight must then be manifested externally by changes/modifications in behavior, habits, and interaction in the world. **Externalized behaviors simultaneously reflect and reinforce thoughts and feelings.** According to Grieneeks[293], patients (and their healthcare providers) can "*think* their way into new ways of *acting*" and "*act* their way into new ways of *thinking*." Eventually, a consciously designed life can be created so that actions, interactions, thoughts, and feelings are melded together in such ways that everyday life itself becomes simultaneously *therapeutic*, *affirmative*, *sustentative*, and *empowering*. In this way, the person and his/her life are unified in such ways as to become self-perpetuating and self-sustaining cycles of ascents and descents, thought-feeling and action, reflection and courage, independence and interdependence—in sum: "a wheel rolling from its own center."[294] At this point the self is established, though it must be maintained and developed with the continuous application of consciousness, reflection, and action.

4. *Metapersonal involvement in community, religion, spirituality, and the world*: Many people are tempted to move from a state of woundedness, relative incompleteness and the feelings of shame and disempowerment to a state of illusory *perfection*, *enlightenment* and *omnipotence* without doing the requisite hard work that makes authentic personal growth possible. People with unhealed emotional wounds often seek to camouflage those deficiencies by becoming pious and projecting an image of completeness and of "having it all figured out" and "having it all together"; religion and the acquisition of power are often misused for this purpose. Many people are successful in wearing this mask for many years; but its crumbling—often manifested as the "midlife crisis"—heralds an opportunity for personal growth if not medicated with anti-depressants, vacations, affairs, gambling, or other distractions.[295] The temptation to bypass Stages 2 [emotional recovery] and 3 [integration] and leapfrog from Stage 1 [woundedness] to Stage 4 [spirituality] should be resisted because the religion or spirituality is then used as a shield *against authenticity* and as a tool for illusory control. Religion can be misused in this way by providing an "identity" and sense of redemption for people with incompletely formed identities and for those with incompletely reconciled shadows and unresolved childhood-parental introjects.[296,297,298] Nietzsche's[299] response to this problem was to encourage self-knowledge and self-reconciliation as prerequisites to religious devotion, hence his admonition, "By all means love your neighbor as yourself – but *first* be such that you love yourself." Historical and recent events remind us of how religion can be misused for misanthropic ends.[300] What is commonly referred to as "spiritual development" — a level of resolution, reconciliation, and autonomy that allows for compassionate interdependence with people, the planet and the larger "world"—is synergistic with and can be supported by religion; but the latter is not a substitute for the former.[301,302] Religion and other forms of metapersonal involvement (e.g., community participation and social generosity) are *important* and *necessary* extensions of self-development. In order for personal development to blossom from the germ of necessary narcissism into its flower of functional completeness, it must eventually manifest in the larger community and the world.

[292] Kottler JA. The Compleat Therapist. San Francisco; Jossey-Bass publishers; 1991, pages 2-3
[293] Keith Grieneeks PhD. "Psychological Assessment" taught in 1998 at Bastyr University.
[294] Friedrich Wilhelm Nietzsche, Walter Kaufmann (Translator). Thus Spoke Zarathustra. Penguin USA; 1978, page 27
[295] Robinson JC. Death of a Hero, Birth of a Soul: Answering the Call of Midlife. Council Oak Books, March 1997 ISBN: 1571780432
[296] Bradshaw J. Healing the Shame that Binds You [Audio Cassette (April 1990) Health Communications Audio; ISBN: 1558740430]
[297] Miller A. The Drama of the Gifted Child: The Search for the True Self. Basic Books: 1981
[298] Miller A. The truth will set you free: overcoming emotional blindness and finding your true adult self. New York: Basic Books; 2001
[299] Nietzsche N. Thus spoke Zarathustra. Read by Jon Cartwright and Alex Jennings and published by Naxos AudioBooks. I think this is among the more brilliant achievements in human history. http://naxosaudiobooks.com/nabusa/pages/432512.htm
[300] Bonhoeffer. (movie documentary by director/writer Martin Doblmeier) http://www.bonhoeffer.com/
[301] Lozoff B. It's a Meaningful Life : It Just Takes Practice. March 1, 2001. ISBN: 0140196242
[302] Bradshaw J. Healing the Shame that Binds You [Audio Cassette (April 1990) Health Communications Audio; ISBN: 1558740430]

5. *Acceptance of mortality and death*: No individual person or any system of thought, whether scientific or religious, can feign completeness without accounting for the end of life and incorporating this account into its overarching paradigm. The event is too significant, and the fear and concerns it provokes are too weighty to not be addressed directly and held in consciousness on a periodic—if not frequent—basis. This topic is of practical importance, too, not only in our own lives and those of our friends and family, but also to the national healthcare system, which currently spends the bulk of its money and resources vainly attempting to preserve life in the last few years and months after which disease or age call unrelentingly for the end of life.

Perhaps if we as individuals and as participants in the healthcare system could accept and deal with our own deaths, then we would not have to panic and participate in such superfluous expenditures of time, energy, emotion, and money when death seeks to arrive, either for our patients, our friends and family, or ourselves. Proximal to the panic and aversion that characterizes the West's relationship to death is the "subclinical" panic and

> "**The event of death is not a tragedy**—to rabbit, fox or man. But the *concept* of death *is* a tragedy, for man, and *indirectly* for poor fox, rabbit, bush, bird, just anything and everything in man's path."
>
> Pearce JC, Exploring the Crack in the Cosmic Egg. Washington Square Press; 1974, page 59

aversion that infiltrate the lives, practices, and policies that we experience every day. Surely, many unconscious events and subconscious influences contribute to the "lives of quiet desperation"[303] and "universal anxiety"[304] that subtly yet powerfully afflict most people; surely, lack of reconciliation with death is a major contributor. Especially in western cultures, death is commonly seen as some type of failure or shortcoming, either on behalf of the patient or his/her doctors, and the most common questions asked on the topic of death are *"how can this be avoided?"* before the event and *"who is to blame?"* after the event. Other cultures accept death as a natural part of life, and indeed, people are seen to have an obligation to die so that the next generations can have their turn in the cycle of life. Alternatives to western hysteria are founded on acceptance of death, and the prerequisites for the acceptance of death are 1) the dedication of sufficient time for its consideration (most people would rather watch a bad movie or attend spectator sports), 2) reframing the event in terms of its being a natural part of our lives, certainly nothing to be ashamed of (discussed below), 3) making necessary logistical preparations (e.g., writing of wills, providing for dependents, and other obvious technicalities), and 4) living as completely, consciously, compassionately, effectively, and authentically as possible so that remorse can be minimized, perhaps completely mitigated. Reframing the event of death begins with its description in general terms so that its enigma, from which its power over the hearts and minds of humanity is derived, can be deciphered and thus deflated. The main characteristics of death which precipitate its fear are 1) the unpredictability of its arrival, 2) the duration of the dying process, and 3) the quality of that process, for example whether it is painful or associated with or precipitated by severe illness or injury. The first characteristic of *timeliness*—the unpredictability of its arrival—stresses people because of their inadequate preparation and the feeling that they have only recently begun to live or have not quite yet begun to live their authentic lives. These concerns are allayed by preparation, both logistical and intrapersonal. Each of us has the responsibility to "become authentically whole" so that we do not inflict our incompleteness onto others, either directly through various forms of transference or deprivation or indirectly though the more subtle means of politics and cultural mores.[305,306] If a person can live with vitality, authenticity, compassion and effectiveness then little is left to want, and fears of death and its

untimely arrival are diminished. The remaining variables are both controllable and uncontrollable; they are uncontrollable to the extent that we are all subject to chaos and accidents, whether in cars, planes, or bathtubs. *Duration* and *quality* are both controllable on an inpatient setting to the extent that palliative care and autonomous decision-making is made available.[307,308]

> "Once accepted, death is an integral component of every event, as the left hand to the right. The cultural death concept could only be instilled in a mind split from its own life flow."
>
> Pearce JC, Exploring the Crack in the Cosmic Egg. Washington Square Press; 1974, page 59

[303] Throeau HD, (Thomas O, ed). Walden and Civil Disobedience. New York: WW Norton and Company; 1966, page 5
[304] Becker E. The Denial of Death. New York: Free Press; 1973, pages 11 and 21
[305] Miller A. The Drama of the Gifted Child: The Search for the True Self. Basic Books: 1981
[306] Robert Bly. The Human Shadow. Sound Horizons, New York 1991 [ISBN: 1879323001] and Bly R. A Little Book on the Human Shadow.[ISBN: 0062548476
[307] Steinbrook R. Medical marijuana, physician-assisted suicide, and the Controlled Substances Act. N Engl J Med. 2004 Sep 30;351(14):1380-3
[308] "Failure to give an effective therapy to seriously ill patients, either adults or children, violates the core principles of both medicine and ethics... Therefore, in the patient's best interest, patients and parents/surrogates, have the right to request medical marijuana under certain circumstances and physicians have the duty to disclose medical marijuana as an

Life can only be authentically and completely experienced after one has created an authentic self and has thereafter accepted life *as it is*. Since death is part of life, the full engagement of life requires *acceptance of* and *reconciliation with* death. Acceptance of death does not necessarily entail that life becomes permeated with nihilistic resignation; on the contrary, it infuses daily events with significance and makes all experiences unique and worthy of appreciation.

Growth, integration, and acceptance: Starting at the top, the progression of personal growth, emotional recovery, integration and daily practice is followed by the more advanced integration of one's chosen purpose, mission, and life work with one's chosen spiritual/religious practice, family and community involvement, and acceptance of and preparation for the end of life and the continuity of society and the environment.

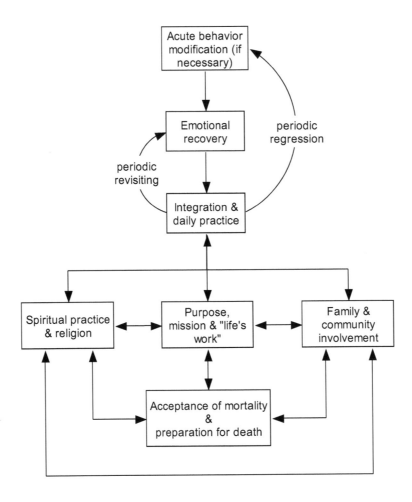

"They say there's no future for us.
They're right,
which is fine with us."   *Rumi*[309]

option and prescribe it when appropriate." Clark PA. Medical marijuana: should minors have the same rights as adults? *Med Sci Monit.*2003;9:ET1-9 www.medscimonit.com/pub/vol_9/no_6/3640.pdf
[309] Rumi in Barks C (translator). The Essential Rumi. HarperSanFransisco: 1995, page 2

Environmental Health, Toxicity, and Detoxification

> "Man's attitude toward nature is today critically important simply because we have now acquired a fateful power to alter and destroy nature. But man is a part of nature, and his war against nature is inevitably a war against himself." *Rachel Carson*[310]

Environmental exposures to chemicals and toxic substances: Studies using blood tests and tissue samples from Americans across the nation have consistently shown that all Americans have toxic chemical accumulation whether or not they work in chemical factories or are obviously exposed at home or work.[311,312] **The recent report from the CDC found toxic chemicals such as pesticides in all Americans, especially minorities, women, and children.**[313] Nearly all of these chemicals are known to contribute to health problems in humans—problems such as cancer, fatigue, poor memory, endocrinopathy, subfertility/infertility, Parkinson's disease, autoimmune diseases like lupus, and many other serious conditions. Therefore, *detoxification programs are a necessity—not a luxury*.

Examples of toxicants commonly found in Americans

Environmental pollutant (population frequency)	*Biologic effects as quoted from HSDB: Hazardous Substances Data Bank. National Library of Medicine, NIH[314] or other reference as noted*
DDE (found in 99% of Americans): DDE is the main metabolite of DDT, a pesticide that was presumably banned in the US in 1972	• DDT is known to be immunosuppressive in animals. • A study published in 2004 showed that increasing levels of DDE in African-American male farmers in North Carolina correlated with a higher prevalence of antinuclear antibodies and up to 50% reductions in serum IgG.[315] • Other studies in humans have suggested an estrogenic or anti-androgenic effect.[316] • Virtually all US women have evidence of DDT/DDE accumulation. Women with higher levels of DDT and/or its metabolites show pregnancy and childbirth complications and have higher rates of infant mortality.[317]

---

[310] Rachel Carson. *Silent Spring*. Boston, Houghton Mifflin Company (2002). ISBN: 0395683297. See also Rachel Carson Dies of Cancer; 'Silent Spring' Author Was 56. New York Times 1956. http://www.rachelcarson.org/ on August 1, 2004

[311] "The average concentration of 2,3,7,8-tetrachlorodibenzo-p-dioxin in the adipose tissue of the US population was 5.38 pg/g, increasing from 1.98 pg/g in children under 14 years of age to 9.40 pg/g in adults over 45." Orban JE, Stanley JS, Schwemberger JG, Remmers JC. Dioxins and dibenzofurans in adipose tissue of the general US population and selected subpopulations. *Am J Public Health* 1994 Mar;84(3):439-45

[312] "Although the use of HCB as a fungicide has virtually been eliminated, detectable levels of HCB are still found in nearly all people in the USA." Robinson PE, Leczynski BA, Kutz FW, Remmers JC. An evaluation of hexachlorobenzene body-burden levels in the general population of the USA. *IARC Sci Publ* 1986;77:183-92

[313] "Many of the pesticides found in the test subjects have been linked to serious short- and long-term health effects including infertility, birth defects and childhood and adult cancers." http://www.panna.org/campaigns/docsTrespass/chemicalTrespass2004.dv.html July 25, 2004

[314] Primary source for this data is the Hazardous Substances Data Bank. National Library of Medicine, National Institutes of Health: http://toxnet.nlm.nih.gov/cgi-bin/sis/htmlgen?HSDB accessed on August 1, 2004

[315] Cooper GS, Martin SA, Longnecker MP, Sandler DP, Germolec DR. Associations between plasma DDE levels and immunologic measures in African-American farmers in North Carolina. *Environ Health Perspect*. 2004 Jul;112(10):1080-4

[316] Dalvie MA, Myers JE, Lou Thompson M, Dyer S, Robins TG, Omar S, Riebow J, Molekwa J, Kruger P, Millar R. The hormonal effects of long-term DDT exposure on malaria vector-control workers in Limpopo Province, South Africa. *Environ Res*. 2004 Sep;96(1):9-19

[317] "The findings strongly suggest that DDT use increases preterm births, which is a major contributor to infant mortality. If this association is causal, it should be included in any assessment of the costs and benefits of vector control with DDT." Longnecker MP, Klebanoff MA, Zhou H, Brock JW. Association between maternal serum concentration of the DDT metabolite DDE and preterm and small-for-gestational-age babies at birth. *Lancet*. 2001 Jul 14;358(9276):110-4

Examples of toxicants commonly found in Americans—*continued*

Environmental pollutant (population frequency)	Biologic effects as quoted from HSDB: Hazardous Substances Data Bank. National Library of Medicine, NIH[318] or other reference
2,5-dichlorophenol (88% nationally and up to 96% in select children populations): Dichlorophenols can occur in tap water as a result of standard chlorination treatment. General population may be exposed to 2,5-dichlorophenol through oral consumption or dermal contact with chlorinated tap water. 2,5-Dichlorophenol was identified in 96% of the urine samples of children residing in Arkansas near an herbicide plant at concentrations of 4-1,200 ppb. The sole manufacturer for herbicide use is Sandoz (Clariant Corporation).	▪ Human Toxicity Excerpts: 1. Burning pain in mouth and throat. White necrotic lesions in mouth, esophagus, and stomach. Abdominal pain, vomiting ... and bloody diarrhea. 2. Pallor, sweating, weakness, headache, dizziness, tinnitus. 3. Shock: Weak irregular pulse, hypotension, shallow respirations, cyanosis, pallor, and a profound fall in body temperature. 4. Possibly fleeting excitement and confusion, followed by unconsciousness. ... 5. Stentorous breathing, mucous rales, rhonchi, frothing at nose and mouth and other signs of pulmonary edema are sometimes seen. Characteristic odor of phenol on the breath. 6. Scanty, dark-colored ... urine ... moderately severe renal insufficiency may appear. 7. Methemoglobinemia, Heinz body hemolytic anemia and hyperbilirubinemia have been reported. ... 8. Death from respiratory, circulatory or cardiac failure. 9. If spilled on skin, pain is followed promptly by numbness. The skin becomes blanched, and a dry opaque eschar forms over the burn. When the eschar sloughs off, a brown stain remains.
Chlorpyrifos (found in 93% of Americans): Insecticide used on corn and cotton and for termite control. Conservative estimates hold that 80% of the chlorpyrifos in the US was produced directly or indirectly by Dow Chemical Corporation.[319] **This pesticide is routinely used in schools and is thus found in blood and tissue samples of nearly all American children.**	▪ Toxic if inhaled, in contact with skin, and if swallowed. ▪ All the organophosphorus insecticides have a cumulative effect by progressive inhibition of cholinesterase. ▪ The symptoms of chronic poisoning due to organophosphorus pesticides include headache, weakness, feeling of heaviness in head, decline of memory, quick onset of **fatigue, disturbed sleep**, loss of appetite, and loss of orientation. Other manifestations of accumulation include **tension, anxiety, restlessness, insomnia, headache, emotional instability, fatigue**... ▪ Chlorpyrifos is a suspected endocrine disruptor.[320] ▪ **Higher chlorpyrifos levels in children correlate with higher incidences attention problems, attention-deficit/hyperactivity disorder, and pervasive developmental disorder.**[321]

[318] Primary source for this data is the Hazardous Substances Data Bank, National Institutes of Health: http://toxnet.nlm.nih.gov/cgi-bin/sis/htmlgen?HSDB accessed on August 1, 2004

[319] Kristin S. Schafer, Margaret Reeves, Skip Spitzer, Susan E. Kegley. Chemical Trespass: Pesticides in Our Bodies and Corporate Accountability. Pesticide Action Network North America. May 2004 Available at http://www.panna.org/campaigns/docsTrespass/chemicalTrespass2004.dv.html on August 1, 2004

[320] http://www.panna.org/resources/documents/factsChlorpyrifos.dv.html accessed August 1, 2004

[321] "Highly exposed children (chlorpyrifos levels of >6.17 pg/g plasma) scored, on average, 6.5 points lower on the Bayley Psychomotor Development Index and 3.3 points lower on the Bayley Mental Development Index at 3 years of age compared with those with lower levels of exposure. Children exposed to higher, compared with lower, chlorpyrifos levels were also significantly more likely to experience Psychomotor Development Index and Mental Development Index delays, attention problems, attention-deficit/hyperactivity disorder problems, and pervasive developmental disorder problems at 3 years of age." Rauh VA, Garfinkel R, Perera FP, Andrews HF, Hoepner L, Barr DB, Whitehead R, Tang D, Whyatt RW. Impact of prenatal chlorpyrifos exposure on neurodevelopment in the first 3 years of life among inner-city children. *Pediatrics*. 2006 Dec;118(6):e1845-59

Examples of toxicants commonly found in Americans—*continued*

Environmental pollutant (population frequency)	Biologic effects as quoted from HSDB: *Hazardous Substances Data Bank. National Library of Medicine, NIH*[322] *or other reference as noted*
Mercury (8% of American women of reproductive age have mercury levels high enough to cause adverse health effects)	▪ Mercury is a well-known neurotoxin, immunotoxin, and nephrotoxin. Mercury toxicity is also a known cause of hypertension in humans. ▪ A recent study published in *JAMA—Journal of the American Medical Association*[323] noted that "Humans are exposed to methylmercury, a well-established neurotoxin, through fish consumption. The fetus is most sensitive to the adverse effects of exposure. … **approximately 8% of women had concentrations higher than the US EPA's recommended reference dose (5.8 microg/L),** below which exposures are considered to be without adverse effects." **The most obvious interpretation of this data published in *JAMA* is that 8% of American women have chronic mercury poisoning—poisoning in this case refers specifically to elevated blood levels of a known toxicant that consistently demonstrates adverse effects on human health.** Logical deduction holds that such a high prevalence of human poisoning should be unacceptable and should lead directly to legislative restrictions on corporate emissions to protect and salvage the health of the public.
2,4-dichlorophenol (found in 87% of Americans): Pesticide	▪ Human Toxicity Excerpts: same as for 2,5-dichlorophenol ▪ In males, significant increases in relative risk ratios for lung cancer, rectal cancer, and soft tissue sarcomas were reported; in females, there were increases in the relative risk of cervical cancer.

"The only thing necessary for the triumph of evil is for good men to do nothing." **Edmond Burke (1729 – 1797)**
"Your lack of interest in the past, your lack of involvement, your unwillingness to develop coherent strategies, your unwillingness to challenge authority - these have created a vacuum in decision-making, that has been filled by professional groups with close relationships with the chemical industries…" Samuel Epstein, M.D.[324]

---

[322] Primary source for this data is the Hazardous Substances Data Bank, National Institutes of Health: http://toxnet.nlm.nih.gov/cgi-bin/sis/htmlgen?HSDB Accessed Aug 1, 2004

[323] Schober SE, Sinks TH, Jones RL, Bolger PM, McDowell M, Osterloh J, Garrett ES, Canady RA, Dillon CF, Sun Y, Joseph CB, Mahaffey KR. Blood mercury levels in US children and women of childbearing age, 1999-2000. *JAMA.* 2003 Apr 2;289(13):1667-74

[324] Samuel Epstein MD, 1993. Professor of Occupational and Environmental Medicine at the School of Public Health, University of Illinois Medical Center Chicago. http://www.converge.org.nz/pirm/pestican.htm accessed September 11, 2004

<u>Toxicity and detoxification—basics</u>: The physiologic processes by which toxins—whether chemicals or metals—are referred to generally as "detoxification." Clinically, doctors can implement treatment interventions to promote and facilitate the removal of chemical and metal toxins; this, too, is generally referred to as detoxification or clinical/therapeutic detoxification programs. Detoxification programs are popular with patients and some doctors and are most often misused and misapplied.

The recent findings that mercury poisoning can result from once-weekly consumption of tuna[325] and that the average American has 13 pesticides in his/her body[326] should be seen as an indication of how dangerously toxic our environment has become, largely due to irresponsible corporate and government policies that value profitability over sustainability.

<u>Detoxification procedures</u>: Though a detailed clinical explanation of detoxification procedures will not be included here (see Chapter 4 of *Integrative Rheumatology*[327]), the general concepts for detoxification are as follows:

1. *Avoidance*: reduced exposure = reduced problem
   a. If there were less chemical pollution, then our environment would be less toxic and therefore we would not have such problems with environmental poisoning.
   b. Limit or eliminate exposure to paint fumes, car exhaust, new carpet, solvents, adhesives, artificial foods, synthetic chemical drugs, copier fumes, pesticides, herbicides, chemical fertilizers, etc.
2. *Depuration*: "The act or process of freeing from foreign or impure matter"[328]
   a. Exercise and sauna
   b. Bowel cleansing, fiber, probiotics, antibiotics, laxatives
   c. Liver and bile stimulators
   d. Cofactors for phase 1 oxidation and phase 2 conjugation
   e. Chelation for heavy metals
   f. Urine alkalinization
3. *Damage control*: managing the consequences of chemical and heavy metal toxicity
   a. Hormone replacement
   b. Antioxidant therapy
   c. Occupational and rehabilitative training
   d. Management of resultant diseases, particularly autoimmune diseases
4. *Political and social action*: Due in large part to corporate influence and government deregulation, environmental contamination with pesticides from American corporations has increased to such an extent over the past few decades that now all Americans show evidence of pesticide accumulation in their bodies. Failure to hold corporations to tight regulatory standards has jeopardized the future of humanity. Voter passivity combined with collusion between multinational corporations and government officials is the underlying problem. Political action is the solution. The past and recent history on this topic is clear and well documented for those who wish to access the facts.[329,330,331,332,333,334,335, 336,337]

---

[325] "The neurobehavioral performance of subjects who consumed tuna fish regularly was significantly worse on color word reaction time, digit symbol reaction time and finger tapping speed (FT)." Carta P, Flore C, Alinovi R, Ibba A, Tocco MG, Aru G, Carta R, Girei E, Mutti A, Lucchini R, Randaccio FS. Sub-clinical neurobehavioral abnormalities associated with low level of mercury exposure through fish consumption. *Neurotoxicology*. 2003 Aug;24(4-5):617-23

[326] "A comprehensive survey of more than 1,300 Americans has found traces of weed- and bug-killers in the bodies of everyone tested, ... The survey, conducted by the U.S. Centers for Disease Control and Prevention, found that the body of the average American contained 13 of these chemicals." Martin Millelstaedt. 13 pesticides in body of average American. *The Globe and Mail*. Friday, May 21, 2004 - Page A17 Available on-line at http://www.theglobeandmail.com/servlet/ArticleNews/TPStory/LAC/20040521/HPEST21/TPEnvironment/ on August 6, 2004

[327] **Vasquez A**. Integrative Rheumatology. IBMRC. http://optimalhealthresearch.com/textbooks/rheumatology.html

[328] Webster's 1913 Dictionary

[329] Robert Van den Bosch. The pesticide conspiracy. Garden City, NY: Doubleday, 1978. ISBN: 0385133847

[330] "Monsanto Corporation is widely known for its production of the herbicide Roundup and genetically engineered Roundup-ready crops... altered to survive a dousing of the toxic herbicide. ...glyphosate, is known to cause eye soreness, headaches, diarrhea, and other flu-like symptoms, and has been linked to non-Hodgkin's lymphoma." Bush Names Former Monsanto Executive as EPA Deputy Administrator. Daily News Archive From March 29, 2001 http://www.beyondpesticides.org/NEWS/daily_news_archive/2001/03_29_01.htm accessed on August 1, 2004

[331] "They pointed to budgets cuts for research and enforcement, to steep declines in the number of cases filed against polluters, to efforts to relax portions of the Clean Air Act, to an acceleration of federal approvals for the spraying of restricted pesticides and more." Patricia Sullivan. Anne Gorsuch Burford, 62, Dies; Reagan EPA Director. *Washington Post*. Thursday, July 22, 2004; Page B06 http://www.washingtonpost.com/wp-dyn/articles/A3418-2004Jul21.html on August 2, 2004

[332] "In fact, amongst the crimes of Reagan and Bush which will go down in history are their emasculation of Federal regulatory apparatus... But in 1988, under the Bush administration, the EPA - illegally, in our view - revoked the Dellaney Law..." Samuel Epstein MD, 1993. Professor of Occupational and Environmental Medicine at the School of Public Health, University of Illinois Medical Center Chicago. http://www.converge.org.nz/pirm/pestican.htm accessed August 1, 2004

[333] "The Environmental Protection Agency will be free to approve pesticides without consulting wildlife agencies to determine if the chemical might harm plants and animals protected by the Endangered Species Act, according to new Bush administration rules.... It also is intended to head off future lawsuits, the officials said." Associated Press. Bush Eases Pesticide Laws http://www.cbsnews.com/stories/2004/07/29/tech/main633009.shtml accessed August 1, 2004

Personal plans for taking responsible action and avoiding political/social passivity that has created the opportunity for regulatory failure and corporate exploitation of the environment that threatens the sustainability of the human species:

_____

_____

_____

_____

_____

_____

_____

_____

_____

_____

_____

_____

_____

_____

_____

_____

_____

_____

_____

_____

_____

_____

_____

_____

_____

_____

_____

_____

_____

_____

_____

_____

_____

_____

_____

_____

_____

_____

_____

_____

_____

_____

_____

[334] "The new policy also could bolster pesticide makers' contention that federal labeling insulates them from suits alleging that their products cause illness or environmental damage, Olson says. 'It . . . could really be disastrous for public health.'" Bush Exempts Pesticide Companies from Lawsuits. Law on Pesticides Reinterpreted: Government Alters Policy in Effort to Protect Manufacturers. Peter Eisler. *USA TODAY*. October 6, 2003 http://www.organicconsumers.org/foodsafety/bushpesticides100703.cfm Accessed Aug 2004

[335] WASHINGTON (AP) — "The Environmental Protection Agency will be free to approve pesticides without consulting wildlife agencies to determine if the chemical might harm plants and animals protected by the Endangered Species Act, according to new Bush administration rules." Bush eases pesticide reviews for endangered species. http://www.usatoday.com/news/washington/2004-07-29-epa-pesticides_x.htm?csp=34 Accessed August 2004

[336] "It is simply intolerable that the EPA, instead of providing an example for open scientific discussion, has continuously violated key environmental legislation, stifling legitimate dissent. The failure of EPA to properly encourage and protect whistleblowing has undermined the ability of the EPA and state environmental agencies to enforce environmental laws." Letter to Carol Browner, Administrator U.S. Environmental Protection Agency from Stephen Kohn, Chair National Whistleblower Center Board of Directors dated March 23, 1999. Availble at http://www.whistleblowers.org/statements.htm on October 10, 2004

[337] "The Bush administration has imposed a gag order on the U.S. Environmental Protection Agency from publicly discussing perchlorate pollution, even as two new studies reveal high levels of the rocket-fuel component may be contaminating the nation's lettuce supply." Peter Waldman. Rocket Fuel Residues Found in Lettuce: Bush administration issues gag order on EPA discussions of possible rocket fuel tainted lettuce. *THE WALL STREET JOURNAL*. See http://www.organicconsumers.org/toxic/lettuce042903.cfm http://www.rhinoed.com/epa's_gag_order.htm http://www.peer.org/press/508.html http://yubanet.com/artman/publish/article_13637.shtml

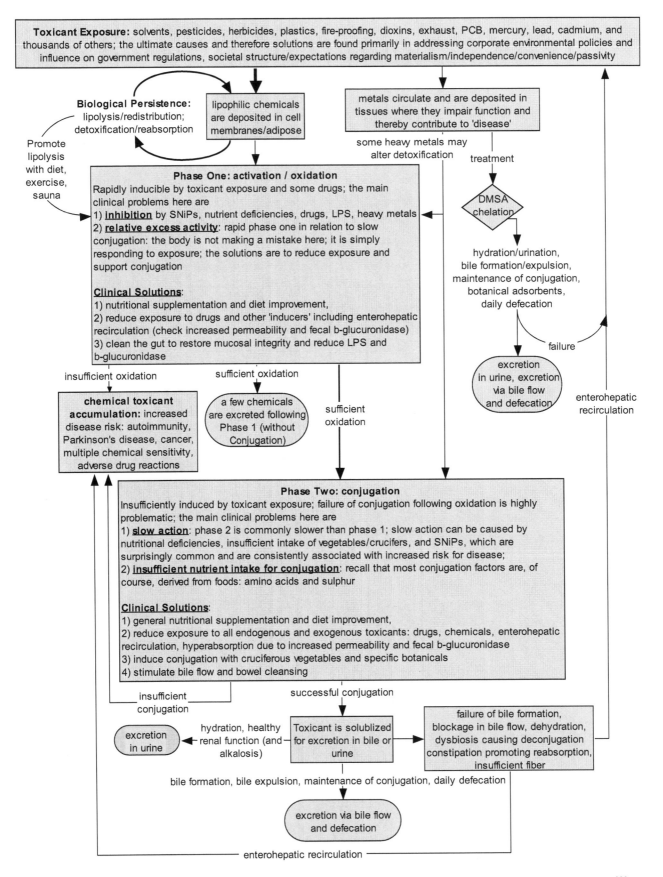

Toxicant Exposure: solvents, pesticides, herbicides, plastics, fire-proofing, dioxins, exhaust, PCB, mercury, lead, cadmium, and thousands of others; the ultimate causes and therefore solutions are found primarily in addressing corporate environmental policies and influence on government regulations, societal structure/expectations regarding materialism/independence/convenience/passivity

Biological Persistence: lipolysis/redistribution; detoxification/reabsorption

lipophilic chemicals are deposited in cell membranes/adipose

metals circulate and are deposited in tissues where they impair function and thereby contribute to 'disease'

Promote lipolysis with diet, exercise, sauna

some heavy metals may alter detoxification

treatment

DMSA chelation

Phase One: activation / oxidation
Rapidly inducible by toxicant exposure and some drugs; the main clinical problems here are
1) **inhibition** by SNiPs, nutrient deficiencies, drugs, LPS, heavy metals
2) **relative excess activity**: rapid phase one in relation to slow conjugation: the body is not making a mistake here; it is simply responding to exposure; the solutions are to reduce exposure and support conjugation

Clinical Solutions:
1) nutritional supplementation and diet improvement,
2) reduce exposure to drugs and other 'inducers' including enterohepatic recirculation (check increased permeability and fecal b-glucuronidase)
3) clean the gut to restore mucosal integrity and reduce LPS and b-glucuronidase

hydration/urination, bile formation/expulsion, maintenance of conjugation, botanical adsorbents, daily defecation

failure

excretion in urine, excretion via bile flow and defecation

enterohepatic recirculation

insufficient oxidation

sufficient oxidation

sufficient oxidation

chemical toxicant accumulation: increased disease risk: autoimmunity, Parkinson's disease, cancer, multiple chemical sensitivity, adverse drug reactions

a few chemicals are excreted following Phase 1 (without Conjugation)

Phase Two: conjugation
Insufficiently induced by toxicant exposure; failure of conjugation following oxidation is highly problematic; the main clinical problems here are
1) **slow action**: phase 2 is commonly slower than phase 1; slow action can be caused by nutritional deficiencies, insufficient intake of vegetables/crucifers, and SNiPs, which are surprisingly common and are consistently associated with increased risk for disease;
2) **insufficient nutrient intake for conjugation**: recall that most conjugation factors are, of course, derived from foods: amino acids and sulphur

Clinical Solutions:
1) general nutritional supplementation and diet improvement,
2) reduce exposure to all endogenous and exogenous toxicants: drugs, chemicals, enterohepatic recirculation, hyperabsorption due to increased permeability and fecal b-glucuronidase
3) induce conjugation with cruciferous vegetables and specific botanicals
4) stimulate bile flow and bowel cleansing

insufficient conjugation

successful conjugation

failure of bile formation, blockage in bile flow, dehydration, dysbiosis causing deconjugation constipation promoting reabsorption, insufficient fiber

excretion in urine

hydration, healthy renal function (and alkalosis)

Toxicant is solublized for excretion in bile or urine

bile formation, bile expulsion, maintenance of conjugation, daily defecation

excretion via bile flow and defecation

enterohepatic recirculation

Overview of toxicant exposure and detoxification/depuration: Details are discussed in *Integrative Rheumatology*.[338]

---

[338] **Vasquez A**. Integrative Rheumatology. IBMRC: 2006, 2009. http://optimalhealthresearch.com/rheumatology.html

Integrative/functional healthcare empowers patients with the ability to understand and effectively participate in the course of their life and health

Drug/surgery-based medicine	Paradigm	Holistic natural healthcare
• Doctor as "savior" and indifferent "objective" observer	Role of the doctor	• Doctor as "teacher" and active caring partner and co-participant in the process
• Helpless victim, disempowered, dependent	Role of the patient	• Active participant, empowered, responsible
• Illness is impossibly complex, and treating this with natural means is generally impossible • Treatment is simple: you have this disease, and you need to take one or more drugs for every problem • Diet and lifestyle modifications are generally viewed as secondary to drugs • The disease is more important than the patient	Nature of illness	• Multifactorial: involving many different aspects of lifestyle, diet, exercise, genetic inheritance, psychology, and environment • Many causes allows for many different treatment approaches and different ways of attaining health • Illness can be modified via selective dietary and lifestyle changes and a custom-tailored treatment plan • The patient is more important than the disease
• Disease-centered, drug-centered	Viewpoint	• Patient-centered, wellness-centered
• Drugs, including chemotherapy • Surgery • Radiation • Electroconvulsive treatment • Vaccinations	Treatment and options	• Diet and lifestyle improvement • Relationship/emotional work • Botanical and nutritional medicines • Physical medicine, chiropractic, exercise • Acupuncture • *Selective* rather than *first-line* use of pharmaceuticals and medical procedures
• Symptom suppression • Drug side-effects are a significant cause of death in the US • Only *treats disease*, does not *promote health*; cannot reach optimal health by only reactively treating established health problems • Enormous expense, often subsidized by private or public "insurance"	Long-term outcome	• Improved health • Potential for successful prevention, treatment or eradication of chronic disease • Potential to become optimally healthy • Proven cost-reduction
• Heightened risk, since drugs are foreign chemicals that have action in the body by interfering with the way that the body normally works • Every drug has side-effects, some of which can be life-threatening • Surgery causes irreparable changes to the body, often for the worse. • Radiation and chemotherapy can cause a secondary cancer to develop	Risks	• Reduced risk, since most of the botanical treatments and all of the nutritional medicines have been a major part of the human diet for centuries/millennia and have proven safety • Delayed onset of action: most treatments are not fast-acting enough to be of value in traumatic or acutely life-threatening situations • Patients must be willing to adopt healthier lifestyles
• Allows a doctor to see many patients within a short amount of time, thus increasing profitability • Since drugs do not cure problems, patients must return for lifelong prescription renewals • Therapeutic passivity: minimal action or effort required by patient and doctor • The doctor holds all the power, and the patient is completely dependent on the doctor for treatment	Benefits	• Improved short-term and long-term health • Empowerment • Understanding of body processes as well as healthcare directions and goals • Options

Health-promoting:

- Frequent exercise and physical activity
- Plenty of sleep
- Maintaining ideal body weight
- Avoiding exposure to chemicals, drugs, pollution, exhaust, tobacco smoke
- Daily consumption of fruits and vegetables
- Ideal protein intake for body size, physical activity, and health status
- Diet high in fiber and complex carbohydrates
- Use of health-promoting beverages such as green tea, fruit/vegetable juices, water, and light consumption of beer or red wine
- Increased intake of ALA, EPA, DHA, GLA, and oleic acid
- Multi-vitamin and multi-mineral supplementation
- Optimal vitamin D and iron status
- Beneficial gastrointestinal flora
- Natural and phytonutraceutical interventions to promote optimal health
- Pro-active healthcare
- Healthy and supportive relationships that foster responsibility, independence, interdependence, health and feelings of being wanted and cared for
- Work environments that promote collaboration and creativity and which appreciate personal time and allow for schedule flexibility

Disease-promoting:

- Physical inactivity and sedentary lifestyle
- Insufficient sleep
- Obesity
- Frequent exposure to chemicals, drugs, pollution, exhaust, tobacco smoke
- Daily consumption of processed and artificial foods
- Insufficient (common) or excessive (rare) protein
- Diet high in simple carbohydrates and sugars
- Use of disease-promoting beverages such as cola, artificially colored/flavored/sweetened drinks, and hard liquor
- Increased intake of linoleic acid (vegetable oils) and arachidonic acid (beef, liver, pork, lamb and most farm-raised land animals)
- Low intake of vitamins and minerals
- Excess iron and insufficient vitamin D
- Dysbiosis: intestinal overgrowth of yeast, parasites, and harmful bacteria
- Use of synthetic chemical drugs to suppress symptoms of poor health
- Reactive healthcare that only responds to problems after they have developed
- Dysfunctional relationships that enable and foster illness, dependency and isolation
- Work environments that promote isolation, pressure, perfectionism and which disapprove of creativity, personal time, and flexibility

Maximize factors that promote health ♦ Minimize factors that promote disease

Opposite influences of health promotion vs. disease promotion: Lifestyle concept: Improved clinical outcomes will be attained when doctors and patients attend to both **prescription of health-promoting activities** and **proscription of disease-promoting activities**. Indeed, attention needs to be given to the **ratio** of these disparate and opposing forces, which ultimately influence genetic expression and physiologic function of many organ systems.

Previously published essays

A Five-Part Nutritional Wellness Protocol That Produces Consistently Positive Results: Brief Review of Scientific Rationale

Alex Vasquez, DC, ND

This article was originally published in *Nutritional Wellness*
http://www.nutritionalwellness.com/archives/2005/sep/09_vasquez.php

When I am lecturing here in the U.S., as well as in Europe, doctors often ask if I will share the details of my protocols with them. Thus, in 2004, I published a 486-page textbook for doctors that includes several protocols and important concepts for the promotion of wellness and treatment of musculoskeletal disorders.[339] In this article, I will share with you what I consider a basic protocol for wellness promotion. I've implemented this protocol as part of the treatment plan for a wide range of clinical problems. In my next column, I will provide several case reports of patients from my office to exemplify the effectiveness of this program and show how it can be the foundation upon which additional treatments can be added as necessary.

Nutrients are required in the proper amounts, forms, and approximate ratios for essential physiologic function; if nutrients are lacking, the body cannot function normally, let alone optimally. Impaired function results in subjective and objective manifestations of what is commonly labeled as "disease." Thus, a powerful and effective alternative to treating diseases with drugs is to re-establish normal/optimal physiologic function by replenishing the body with essential nutrients.

Of course, many diseases are multifactorial and therefore require multicomponent treatment plans, and some diseases actually require the use of drugs. However, while only a relatively small portion of patients actually need drugs for their problems, I am sure we all agree that everyone needs a foundational nutrition plan, as outlined and substantiated below.

1. Health-promoting diet: Following an extensive review of the research literature, I developed what I call the "supplemented Paleo-Mediterranean diet," which I have described in greater detail elsewhere.[340] In essence, this diet plan combines the best of the Mediterranean diet with the best of the Paleolithic diet, the latter of which has been detailed most recently by Dr. Loren Cordain in his book, The Paleo Diet, and his numerous scientific articles.[341] This diet places emphasis on fruits, vegetables, nuts, seeds, and berries that meet the body's needs for fiber, carbohydrates, and most importantly, the 8,000+ phytonutrients that have additive and synergistic health benefits.[342] Preferred protein sources are lean meats such as fish and poultry. In contrast to Cordain's Paleo diet, I also advocate soy and whey for their high-quality protein and anticancer, cardioprotective, and mood-enhancing benefits. Rice and potatoes are discouraged due to their relatively high glycemic indexes and high glycemic loads, and their lack of fiber and phytonutrients (compared to other fruits and vegetables). Generally speaking, grains such as wheat and rye are discouraged due to the high glycemic loads/indexes of most breads and pastries, as well as the allergenicity of gluten, a protein that appears to help trigger disorders such as migraine, celiac disease, psoriasis, epilepsy, and autoimmunity. Sources of simple sugars such as high-fructose corn syrup (e.g., cola, soda) and processed foods (e.g., "TV dinners" and other manufactured snacks and convenience foods) are strictly forbidden. Chemical preservatives, colorants, sweeteners and carrageenan are likewise prohibited. In summary, this diet plan provides plenty of variety, as most dishes comprised of poultry, fish, soy, fruits, vegetables, nuts, berries, and seeds are allowed. The diet also provides plenty of fiber, phytonutrients, carbohydrates, potassium, and protein, while simultaneously being low in fat, sodium, arachidonic acid, and "simple sugars." The diet must be customized with regard to total protein and calorie intake, as determined by the size, status, and activity level of the patient, and individual food allergens should be avoided. Regular consumption of this diet has shown the ability to reduce hypertension, alleviate diabetes, ameliorate migraine headaches, and result in improvement of overall health and a lessening of the severity of many common "diseases." This diet is supplemented with vitamins, minerals, and fatty acids as described below.

2. Multivitamin and multimineral supplementation: Vitamin and mineral supplementation finally received endorsement from "mainstream" medicine when researchers from Harvard Medical School published a review article in Journal of the American Medical Association that concluded, "Most people do not consume an optimal amount of all vitamins by diet alone. ...It appears prudent for all adults to take vitamin supplements."[343] Long-term nutritional insufficiencies experienced by "most people" promote the development of "long-latency deficiency diseases" such as cancer, neuroemotional deterioration, and cardiovascular disease.[344] Impressively, the benefits of multivitamin/multimineral supplementation have been demonstrated in numerous clinical trials. Multivitamin/multimineral supplementation has been shown to improve nutritional status and reduce the risk for chronic diseases[345], improve mood[346], potentiate antidepressant drug treatment[347], alleviate migraine headaches (when used with diet improvement and fatty acids[348]), improve immune

[339] **Vasquez A**. *Integrative Orthopedics: The Art of Creating Wellness While Managing Acute and Chronic Musculoskeletal Disorders*. 2004, 2007
[340] **Vasquez A**. The Importance of Integrative Chiropractic Health Care in Treating Musculoskeletal Pain and Reducing the Nationwide Burden of Medical Expenses and Iatrogenic Injury and Death: A Concise Review of Current Research and Implications for Clinical Practice and Healthcare Policy. *The Original Internist* 2005; 12(4): 159-182
[341] Cordain L. *The Paleo Diet*. (John Wiley and Sons, 2002). Also: Cordain L. Cereal grains: humanity's double edged sword. *World Rev Nutr Diet* 1999;84:19-73 Access to most of Dr Cordain's articles is available at http://thepaleodiet.com/
[342] Liu RH. Health benefits of fruit and vegetables are from additive and synergistic combinations of phytochemicals. *Am J Clin Nutr* 2003;78(3 Suppl):517S-520S
[343] Fletcher RH, Fairfield KM. Vitamins for chronic disease prevention in adults: clinical applications. *JAMA* 2002;287:3127-9
[344] Heaney RP. Long-latency deficiency disease: insights from calcium and vitamin D. *Am J Clin Nutr* 2003;78:912-9
[345] McKay DL, Perrone G, Rasmussen H, Dallal G, Hartman W, Cao G, Prior RL, Roubenoff R, Blumberg JB. The effects of a multivitamin/mineral supplement on micronutrient status, antioxidant capacity and cytokine production in healthy older adults consuming a fortified diet. *J Am Coll Nutr* 2000;19(5):613-21
[346] Benton D, Haller J, Fordy J. Vitamin supplementation for 1 year improves mood. *Neuropsychobiology* 1995;32(2):98-105
[347] Coppen A, Bailey J. Enhancement of the antidepressant action of fluoxetine by folic acid: a randomised, placebo controlled trial. *J Affect Disord* 2000;60:121-30

function and infectious disease outcomes in the elderly[349] (especially diabetics[350]), reduce morbidity and mortality in patients with HIV infection[351,352] alleviate premenstrual syndrome[353,354] and bipolar disorder[355], reduce violence and antisocial behavior in children[356] and incarcerated young adults (when used with essential fatty acids[357]), and improve scores of intelligence in children.[358] Vitamin supplementation has anti-inflammatory benefits, as evidenced by significant reduction in C-reactive protein, (CRP) in a double-blind, placebo-controlled trial.[359] The ability to safely and affordably deliver these benefits makes multimineral-multivitamin supplementation and essential component of any and all health-promoting and disease-prevention strategies. Vitamin A can result in liver damage with chronic consumption of 25,000 IU or more, and intake should generally not exceed 10,000 IU per day in women of childbearing age. Iron should not be supplemented except in patients diagnosed with iron deficiency by a blood test (serum ferritin). Additional vitamin D should be used, as described in the next section.

3. Physiologic doses of vitamin D3: The prevalence of vitamin D deficiency varies from 40 percent (general population) to almost 100 percent (patients with musculoskeletal pain) in the American population. I described the many benefits of vitamin D3 supplementation in the previous issue of Nutritional Wellness and in the major monograph published last year.[360] In summary, vitamin D deficiency causes or contributes to depression, hypertension, seizures, migraine, polycystic ovary syndrome, inflammation, autoimmunity, and musculoskeletal pain such as low-back pain. Clinical trials using vitamin D supplementation have proven the cause-and-effect relationship between vitamin D deficiency and these conditions by showing that each of these could be cured or alleviated with vitamin D supplementation. In our review of the literature, we concluded that daily vitamin D doses should be 1,000 IU for infants, 2,000 IU for children, and 4,000 IU for adults. Cautions and contraindications include the use of thiazide diuretics (e.g., hydrochlorothiazide) or any other medications that can promote hypercalcemia, as well as granulomatous diseases such as sarcoidosis, tuberculosis, and certain types of cancer, especially lymphoma. Effectiveness is monitored by measuring serum 25-OH-vitamin D, and safety is monitored by measuring serum calcium.

4. Balanced and complete fatty acid supplementation: A detailed survey of the literature shows there are at least five health-promoting fatty acids commonly found in the human diet.[361] These are alpha-linolenic acid (ALA; omega-3, from flaxseed oil), eicosapentaenoic acid (EPA; omega-3, from fish oil), docosahexaenoic acid (DHA; omega-3, from fish oil and algae), gamma-linolenic acid (GLA; omega-6, most concentrated in borage oil), and oleic acid (omega-9, from olive oil, also flaxseed and borage oils). Each of these fatty acids has health benefits that cannot be fully attained from supplementing a different fatty acid. The benefits of GLA (borage oil) are not attained by consumption of EPA and DHA (fish oil); in fact, consumption of fish oil can actually promote a deficiency of GLA.[362] Likewise, consumption of GLA alone can reduce EPA levels while increasing levels of proinflammatory arachidonic acid; both of these problems are avoided with co-administration of fish oil any time borage oil is used. Using ALA (flaxseed oil) alone only slightly increases EPA but generally leads to no improvement in DHA status and can lead to a reduction of oleic acid; thus, fish oil, olive oil (and borage oil) should be supplemented when flaxseed oil is used.[363] Obviously, the goal here is a balanced intake of all of the health-promoting fatty acids; using only one or two sources of fatty acids is not balanced and results in suboptimal improvement, at best. In clinical practice, I routinely use combination fatty acid therapy comprised of ALA, EPA, DHA, and GLA for essentially all patients. The product also contains a modest amount of oleic acid, and I encourage use of olive oil for salads and cooking. This approach results in complete and balanced fatty acid intake, and the clinical benefits are impressive.

5. Probiotics /gut flora modification: Proper levels of good bacteria promote intestinal health, proper immune function, and support overall health. Excess bacteria or yeast, or the presence of harmful bacteria, yeast, or "parasites" such as amoebas and protozoas, can cause "leaky gut," systemic inflammation, and a wide range of clinical problems. Intestinal flora can become imbalanced by poor diets, excess stress, immunosuppressive drugs, antibiotics, or exposure to contaminated food or water, all of which are common among American patients. Thus, as a rule, I reinstate the good bacteria by the use of probiotics (good bacteria and yeast), prebiotics (fiber, arabinogalactan, and inulin), and the use of fermented foods such as kefir (in patients not allergic to milk). Harmful yeast, bacteria, and other "parasites" can be eradicated with the combination of dietary change, drugs, and/or herbal extracts. For example, oregano oil in an

[348] Wagner W, Nootbaar-Wagner U. Prophylactic treatment of migraine with gamma-linolenic and alpha-linolenic acids. *Cephalalgia* 1997;17:127-30

[349] Langkamp-Henken B, Bender BS, Gardner EM, Herrlinger-Garcia KA, Kelley MJ, Murasko DM, Schaller JP, Stechmiller JK, Thomas DJ, Wood SM. Nutritional formula enhanced immune function and reduced days of symptoms of upper respiratory tract infection in seniors. *J Am Geriatr Soc* 2004;52:3-12

[350] Barringer TA, Kirk JK, Santaniello AC, Foley KL, Michielutte R. Effect of a multivitamin and mineral supplement on infection and quality of life. A randomized, double-blind, placebo-controlled trial. *Ann Intern Med* 2003;138:365-71

[351] Fawzi WW, Msamanga GI, Spiegelman D, et al. A randomized trial of multivitamin supplements and HIV disease progression and mortality. *N Engl J Med* 2004;351:23-32

[352] Burbano X, Miguez-Burbano MJ, McCollister K, Zhang G, Rodriguez A, Ruiz P, Lecusay R, Shor-Posner G. Impact of a selenium chemoprevention clinical trial on hospital admissions of HIV-infected participants. *HIV Clin Trials* 2002;3:483-91

[353] Abraham GE. Nutritional factors in the etiology of the premenstrual tension syndromes. *J Reprod Med* 1983;28(7):446-64

[354] Stewart A. Clinical and biochemical effects of nutritional supplementation on the premenstrual syndrome. *J Reprod Med* 1987;32:435-41

[355] Kaplan BJ, Simpson JS, Ferre RC, Gorman CP, McMullen DM, Crawford SG. Effective mood stabilization with a chelated mineral supplement: an open-label trial in bipolar disorder. *J Clin Psychiatry* 2001;62:936-44

[356] Kaplan BJ, Crawford SG, Gardner B, Farrelly G. Treatment of mood lability and explosive rage with minerals and vitamins: two case studies in children. *J Child Adolesc Psychopharmacol* 2002;12(3):205-19

[357] Gesch CB, Hammond SM, Hampson SE, Eves A, Crowder MJ. Influence of supplementary vitamins, minerals and essential fatty acids on the antisocial behaviour of young adult prisoners. Randomised, placebo-controlled trial. *Br J Psychiatry* 2002;181:22-8

[358] Benton D. Micro-nutrient supplementation and the intelligence of children. *Neurosci Biobehav Rev* 2001;25:297-309

[359] Church TS, Earnest CP, Wood KA, Kampert JB. Reduction of C-reactive protein levels through use of a multivitamin. *Am J Med* 2003;115:702-7

[360] **Vasquez A**, Manso G, Cannell J. The clinical importance of vitamin D (cholecalciferol): a paradigm shift with implications for all healthcare providers. *Alternative Therapies in Health and Medicine* 2004;10:28-37 http://optimalhealthresearch.com/cholecalciferol.html

[361] **Vasquez A**. Reducing Pain and Inflammation Naturally. Part 2: New Insights into Fatty Acid Supplementation and Its Effect on Eicosanoid Production and Genetic Expression. *Nutritional Perspectives* 2005; January: 5-16 http://optimalhealthresearch.com/part2

[362] Cleland LG, Gibson RA, Neumann M, French JK. The effect of dietary fish oil supplement upon the content of dihomo-gammalinolenic acid in human plasma phospholipids. *Prostaglandins Leukot Essent Fatty Acids* 1990 May;40(1):9-12

[363] Jantti J, Nikkari T, Solakivi T, Vapaatalo H, Isomaki H. Evening primrose oil in rheumatoid arthritis: changes in serum lipids and fatty acids. *Ann Rheum Dis* 1989;48(2):124-7

emulsified, time-released form has proven safe and effective for the elimination of various parasites encountered in clinical practice.[364] Likewise, the herb *Artemisia annua* (sweet wormwood) commonly is used to eradicate specific bacteria and has been used for thousands of years in Asia for the treatment and prevention of infectious diseases, including malaria.[365]

Conclusion:

In this brief review, I have outlined and scientifically substantiated a fundamental protocol that can serve as effective therapy for patients with a wide range of "diseases." Customizing the Paleo-Mediterranean diet to avoid food allergens, using vitamin-mineral supplements along with physiologic doses of vitamin D and broad-spectrum balanced fatty acid supplementation, and ensuring gastrointestinal health with the skillful use of probiotics, prebiotics, and antimicrobial treatments provides an excellent health-promoting and disease-eliminating foundation and lifestyle for many patients. Often, this simple protocol is all that is needed for the effective treatment of a wide range of clinical problems. For other patients with more complex illnesses, of course, additional interventions and laboratory assessments can be used to customize the treatment plan. However, we must always remember that the attainment and preservation of health requires that we meet the body's basic nutritional needs. This five-step protocol begins the process of meeting those needs. In my next article, I'll give you some examples from my clinical practice and additional references to show how safe and effective this protocol can be.

Implementing the Five-Part Nutritional Wellness Protocol for the Treatment of Various Health Problems

Alex Vasquez, DC, ND

This article was originally published in *Nutritional Wellness*
http://www.nutritionalwellness.com/archives/2005/nov/11_vasquez.php

In my last article in *Nutritional Wellness* I described a 5-part nutritional protocol that can be used in the vast majority of patients without adverse effects and with major benefits. For many patients, the basic protocol consisting of 1) the Paleo-Mediterranean diet, 2) multivitamin/multimineral supplementation, 3) additional vitamin D3, 4) combination fatty acid therapy with an optimal balance of ALA, GLA, EPA, DHA, and oleic acid, and 5) probiotics (including the identification and eradication of harmful yeast, bacteria, and other "parasites") is all the treatment that they need. For patients who need additional treatment, this foundational plan still serves as the core of the biochemical aspect of their intervention. Of course, in some cases, we have to use other lifestyle modifications (such as exercise), additional supplements (such as policosanol or antimicrobial herbs), manual treatments (including spinal manipulation) and occasionally select medications (such has hormone modulators) to obtain our goal of maximum improvement.

The following examples show how the 5-part protocol serves to benefit patients with a wide range of conditions. For the sake of saving space, I will use only highly specific citations to the research literature, since I have provided the other references in the previous issue of *Nutritional Wellness* and elsewhere.[366]

- **A Man with High Cholesterol**: This patient is a 41-year-old slightly overweight man with very high cholesterol. His total cholesterol was 290 (normal < 200), LDL cholesterol was 212 (normal <130), and his triglycerides were 148 (optimal <100). I am quite certain that nearly every medical doctor would have put this man on cholesterol-lowering statin drugs for life. **Treatment**: In contrast, I advised a low-carb Paleo-Mediterranean diet because such diets have been shown to reduce cardiovascular mortality more powerfully that "statin" cholesterol-lowing drugs in older patients.[367] Likewise, fatty acid supplementation is more effective than statin drugs for reducing cardiac and all-cause mortality.[368] We added probiotics, because supplementation with *Lactobacillus* and *Bifidobacterium* has been shown to lower cholesterol levels in humans with high cholesterol.[369] Finally, I also prescribed 20 mg of policosanol for its well-known ability to favorably modify cholesterol levels.[370] **Results**: Within **one month** the patient had lost weight, felt better, and his total cholesterol had dropped to normal at 196 (from 290!), LDL was reduced to 141, and triglycerides were reduced to 80. Basically, this treatment plan was "the protocol + policosanol." Drug treatment of this patient would have been more expensive, more risky, and would not have resulted in global health improvements.
- **A Child with Intractable Seizures**: This is a 4-year-old nonverbal boy with 3-5 seizures per day despite being on two anti-seizure medications and having previously had several other "last resort" medical and surgical procedures. He also had a history of food allergies. **Treatment**: Obviously, there was no room for error in this case. We implemented a moderately low-carb hypoallergenic diet since both carbohydrate restriction[371] and allergy avoidance[372] can reduce the frequency and

[364] Force M, Sparks WS, Ronzio RA. Inhibition of enteric parasites by emulsified oil of oregano in vivo. *Phytother Res* 2000;14:213-4

[365] Schuster BG. Demonstrating the validity of natural products as anti-infective drugs. *J Altern Complement Med* 2001;7 Suppl 1:S73-82

[366] **Vasquez A**. Integrative Orthopedics. www.OptimalHealthResearch.com and Chiropractic and Naturopathic Medicine for the Promotion of Optimal Health and Alleviation of Pain and Inflammation. http://optimalhealthresearch.com/monograph05

[367] Knoops KT, et al. Mediterranean diet, lifestyle factors, and 10-year mortality in elderly European men and women: the HALE project. *JAMA*. 2004 Sep 22;292(12):1433-9

[368] Studer M, et al. Effect of different antilipidemic agents and diets on mortality: a systematic review. *Arch Intern Med*. 2005;165:725-30

[369] Xiao JZ, et al. Effects of milk products fermented by Bifidobacterium longum on blood lipids in rats and healthy adult male volunteers.*J Dairy Sci*. 2003;86:2452-61

[370] Cholesterol-lowering action of policosanol compares well to that of pravastatin and lovastatin. *Cardiovasc J S Afr*. 2003;14(3):161

[371] Freeman JM, et al. The efficacy of the ketogenic diet-1998: a prospective evaluation of intervention in 150 children. *Pediatrics*. 1998;102:1358-63

[372] Egger J, Carter CM, Soothill JF, Wilson J. Oligoantigenic diet treatment of children with epilepsy and migraine. *J Pediatr*. 1989;114:51-8

severity of seizures. Since many "anti-seizure" medications actually cause seizures by causing vitamin D deficiency[373], I added 800 IU per day of emulsified vitamin D3 for its antiseizure benefit.[374] We used 1 tsp per day of a combination fatty acid supplement that provides balanced amounts of ALA, GLA, EPA, and DHA, since fatty acids appear to have potential antiseizure benefits.[375] Vitamin B-6 (250 mg of P5P) and magnesium (bowel tolerance) were also added to reduce brain hyperexcitability.[376] Stool testing showed an absence of *Bifidobacteria* and *Lactobacillus*; probiotics were added for their anti-allergy benefits.[377] *Results*: Within about 2 months seizure frequency reduced from 3-5 per day to one seizure every other day: *an 87% reduction in seizure frequency*. Patient was able to discontinue one of the anti-seizure medications. His parents also noted several global improvements: the boy started making eye contact with people, he was learning again, and intellectually he was "making gains every day." His parents considered this an "amazing difference." Going from 30 seizures per week to 4 seizures per week while reducing medication use by 50% is a major achievement. Notice that we simply used the basic wellness protocol with some additional B6 and magnesium. It is highly unlikely that B6 and magnesium alone would have produced such a favorable response.

- **A Young Woman with Full-Body Psoriasis Unresponsive to Drug Treatment**: This is a 17-year-old woman with head-to-toe psoriasis since childhood. She wears long pants and long-sleeved shirts year-round, and the psoriasis is a major interference to her social life. Medications have ceased to help. *Treatment*: The Paleo-Mediterranean diet was implemented with an emphasis on food allergy identification.[1] We used a multivitamin-mineral supplement with 200 mcg selenium to compensate for the nutritional insufficiencies and selenium deficiency that are common in patients with psoriasis; likewise 10 mg of folic acid was added to address the relative vitamin deficiencies and elevated homocysteine that are common in these patients.[378] Combination fatty acid therapy with EPA and DHA from fish oil and GLA from borage oil was used for the anti-inflammatory and skin-healing benefits.[379] Vitamin E (1200 IU of mixed tocopherols) and lipoic acid (1,000 mg per day) were added for their anti-inflammatory benefits and to combat the oxidative stress that is characteristic of psoriasis.[380] Of course, probiotics were used to modify gut flora, which is commonly deranged in patients with psoriasis.[381] *Results*: Within a few weeks, this patient's "lifelong psoriasis" was essentially gone. Food allergy identification and avoidance played a major role in the success of this case. When I saw the patient again 9 months later for her second visit, she had no visible evidence of psoriasis. Her "medically untreatable" condition was essentially cured by the use of my basic protocol, with the addition of a few extra nutrients.

- **A Man with Fatigue and Recurrent Numbness in Hands and Feet**. This 40-year-old man had seen numerous neurologists and had spent tens of thousands of dollars on MRIs, CT scans, lumbar punctures, and other diagnostic procedures. No diagnosis had been found, and no effective treatment had been rendered by medical specialists. *Assessments*: We performed a modest battery of lab tests which revealed elevations of fibrinogen and C-reactive protein (CRP), two markers of acute inflammation. Assessment of intestinal permeability with the lactulose-mannitol assay showed major intestinal damage ("leaky gut"). Follow-up parasite testing on different occasions showed dysbiosis caused by *Proteus, Enterobacter, Klebsiella, Citrobacter*, and *Pseudomonas aeruginosa*—of course, these are gram-negative bacteria that can induce immune dysfunction and autoimmunity, as described elsewhere.[1] Specifically, *Pseudomonas aeruginosa* has been linked to the development of nervous system autoimmunity, such as multiple sclerosis.[382] *Treatment*: We implemented a plan of diet modification, vitamins, minerals, fatty acids, and probiotics. The dysbiosis was further addressed with specific antimicrobial herbs (including caprylic acid and emulsified oregano oil[383]) and drugs (such as tetracycline, Bactrim, and augmentin). The antibiotic drugs proved to be ineffective based on repeat stool testing. *Results*: Within one month we witnessed impressive improvements, both subjectively and objectively. Subjectively, the patient reported that the numbness and tingling almost completely resolved. Fatigue was reduced, and energy was improved. Objectively, the patient's elevated CRP plummeted from abnormally high at 11 down to completely normal at 1. Eighteen months later, the patient's CRP had dropped to less than 1 and fatigue and numbness were no longer problematic. Notice that this treatment plan was basically "the protocol" with additional attention to eradicating the dysbiosis we found with specialized stool testing.

- **A 50-year-old Man with Rheumatoid Arthritis**. This patient presented with a 3-year history of rheumatoid arthritis that had been treated unsuccessfully with drugs (methotrexate and intravenous Remicade). The first time I tested his hsCRP level, it was astronomically high at 124 (normal is <3). Because of the severe inflammation and other risk factors for sudden cardiac death, I referred this patient to an osteopathic internist for immune-suppressing drugs; the patient refused, stating that he was no longer willing to rely on immune-suppressing chemical medications. His treatment was entirely up to me. *Assessments and Treatments*: We implemented the Paleo-Mediterranean diet and a program of vitamins, minerals, optimal combination fatty acid therapy (providing ALA, GLA, EPA, DHA, and oleic acid), and 4000 IU of vitamin D in emulsified form to overcome defects in absorption that are seen in older patients and those with gastrointestinal problems.[384] Hormone testing showed abnormally low DHEA, low testosterone, and slightly elevated estrogen; these problems were corrected with DHEA supplementation and the use of a hormone-modulating drug (Arimidex) that lowers

[373] Ali FE, Al-Bustan MA, Al-Busairi WA, Al-Mulla FA. Loss of seizure control due to anticonvulsant-induced hypocalcemia. *Ann Pharmacother*. 2004;38:1002-5

[374] Christiansen C, Rodbro P, Sjo O."Anticonvulsant action" of vitamin D in epileptic patients? A controlled pilot study. *Br Med J*. 1974 May 4;2(913):258-9

[375] Yuen AW, et al. Omega-3 fatty acid supplementation in patients with chronic epilepsy: A randomized trial. *Epilepsy Behav*. 2005 Sep;7(2):253-8

[376] Mousain-Bosc M, et al. Magnesium VitB6 intake reduces central nervous system hyperexcitability in children. *J Am Coll Nutr*. 2004;23(5):545S-548S

[377] Majamaa H, Isolauri E.Probiotics: a novel approach in the management of food allergy. *J Allergy Clin Immunol*. 1997 Feb;99(2):179-85

[378] Vanizor Kural B, et al. Plasma homocysteine and its relationships with atherothrombotic markers in psoriatic patients. *Clin Chim Acta*. 2003 Jun;332(1-2):23-3

[379] Vasquez A. Reducing Pain and Inflammation Naturally. Part 2: New Insights into Fatty Acid Supplementation and Its Effect on Eicosanoid Production and Genetic Expression. *Nutritional Perspectives* 2005; January: 5-16 www.OptimalHealthResearch.com/part2

[380] Kokcam I, Naziroglu M. Antioxidants and lipid peroxidation status in the blood of patients with psoriasis. *Clin Chim Acta*. 1999 Nov;289(1-2):23-31

[381] Waldman A, et al. Incidence of Candida in psoriasis--a study on the fungal flora of psoriatic patients. *Mycoses*. 2001 May;44(3-4):77-81

[382] Hughes LE, et al. Antibody responses to Acinetobacter spp. and Pseudomonas aeruginosa in multiple sclerosis: prospects for diagnosis using the myelin-acinetobacter-neurofilament antibody index. *Clin Diagn Lab Immunol*. 2001;8(6):1181-8

[383] Force M, Sparks WS, Ronzio RA. Inhibition of enteric parasites by emulsified oil of oregano in vivo. *Phytother Res*. 2000 May;14(3):213-4

[384] **Vasquez A**. Subphysiologic Doses of Vitamin D are Subtherapeutic: Comment on the Study by The Record Trial Group. *TheLancet.com* Accessed June 16, 2005

estrogen and raises testosterone. Specialized stool testing showed absence of *Lactobacillus* and *Bifidobacteria* and intestinal overgrowth of *Citrobacter* and *Enterobacter* which was corrected with probiotics and antimicrobial treatments including undecylenic acid and emulsified oregano oil. Importantly, I also decided to inhibit NF-kappaB (the primary transcription factor that upregulates the pro-inflammatory response[385]) by using a combination botanical formula that contains curcumin, piperine, lipoic acid, green tea extract, propolis, rosemary, resveratrol, ginger, and phytolens (an antioxidant extract from lentils that may inhibit autoimmunity[386])—all of these herbs and nutrients have been shown to inhibit NF-kappaB and to thus downregulate inflammatory responses.[387] ***Results***: Within 6 weeks, this patient had happily lost 10 lbs of excess weight and was able to work without pain for the first time in years. Follow-up testing showed that his previously astronomical hsCRP had dropped from 124 to 7—a drop of 114 points in less than one month: better than had ever been achieved even with the use of intravenous immune-suppressing drugs! This patient continues to make significant progress. Obviously this case was complex, and we needed to do more than the basic protocol. Nonetheless, the basic protocol still served as the foundation for the treatment plan. Note that vitamin D has significant anti-inflammatory benefits and can cause major reductions in inflammation measured by CRP.[388] The correction of the hormonal abnormalities and the dysbiosis, and downregulating NF-kappaB with several botanical extracts were also critical components of this successful treatment plan.[1]

Summary and Conclusions

These examples show how the nutritional wellness protocol that I described in the September issue of *Nutritional Wellness* can be used as the foundational treatment for a wide range of health problems. In many cases, implementation of the basic protocol is all that is needed. In more complex situations, we use the basic protocol and then add more specific treatments to address dysbiosis and hormonal problems, and we can add additional nutrients as needed. However, there will never be a substitute for a healthy diet, sufficiencies of vitamin D and all five of the health-promoting fatty acids (i.e., ALA, GLA, EPA, DHA, and oleic acid), and normalization of gastrointestinal flora. Without these basics, survival and the appearance of health are possible, but true health and recovery from "untreatable" illnesses is not possible. In order to attain optimal health, we have to create the conditions that allow for health to be attained[1,] and we start this process by supplying the body with the nutrients that it needs to function optimally. In the words of naturopathic physician Jared Zeff from the *Journal of Naturopathic Medicine*, "*The work of the naturopathic physician is to elicit healing by helping patients to create or recreate the conditions for health to exist within them. Health will occur where the conditions for health exist. Disease is the product of the conditions which allow for it.*"[389] Although the chiropractic profession has emphasized spinal manipulation as its primary therapeutic tool, the profession has always appreciated holistic, integrative models of therapeutic intervention, health and disease.

Chiropractic was the first healthcare profession in America to specifically claim that the optimization of health requires attention to the spiritual (emotional, psychological), mechanical (physical, structural), and chemical (nutritional, hormonal) aspects of our lives.[1] Chiropractic's founder DD Palmer[390] wrote, "The human body represents the actions of three laws—spiritual, mechanical, and chemical—united as one triune. As long as there is perfect union of these three, there is health." Accordingly, these cornerstones are fundamental to the modern definition of the chiropractic profession recently articulated by the American Chiropractic Association[391]: "*Doctors of Chiropractic are physicians who consider man as an integrated being and give special attention to the physiological and biochemical aspects including structural, spinal, musculoskeletal, neurological, vascular, nutritional, emotional and environmental relationships.*" The cases that I have described in this article demonstrate the importance of attending to the nutritional, hormonal, environmental and gastrointestinal aspects of human physiology for helping our patients attain optimal health.

Common Oversights and Shortcomings in the Study and Implementation of Nutritional Supplementation

Alex Vasquez, D.C., N.D.

This article was originally published in *Naturopathy Digest*
http://www.naturopathydigest.com/archives/2007/jun/vasquez.php

Introduction

An impressive discrepancy often exists between the low efficacy of nutritional interventions reported in the research literature and the higher efficacy achieved in the clinical practices of clinicians trained in the use of interventional nutrition (i.e., chiropractic and naturopathic physicians). This discrepancy is dangerous for at least two reasons. First, it results in an undervaluation of the efficacy of nutritional supplementation, which ultimately leaves otherwise treatable patients untreated. Second, such untreated and undertreated patients are often then forced to use dangerous and expensive pharmaceutical drugs and surgical interventions to treat conditions that could have otherwise been easily and safely treated with nutritional

---

[385] Tak PP, Firestein GS. NF-kappaB: a key role in inflammatory diseases. *J Clin Invest*. 2001 Jan;107(1):7-11

[386] Sandoval M, et al. Peroxynitrite-induced apoptosis in epithelial (T84) and macrophage (RAW 264.7) cell lines: effect of legume-derived polyphenols (phytolens). *Nitric Oxide*. 1997;1(6):476-83

[387] **Vasquez A**. Reducing pain and inflammation naturally - Part 4: Nutritional and Botanical Inhibition of NF-kappaB, the Major Intracellular Amplifier of the Inflammatory Cascade. A Practical Clinical Strategy Exemplifying Anti-Inflammatory Nutrigenomics. *Nutritional Perspectives* 2005;July: 5-12 www.OptimalHealthResearch.com/part4

[388] Timms PM, et al. Circulating MMP9, vitamin D and variation in the TIMP-1 response with VDR genotype. *QJM*. 2002 Dec;95(12):787-96

[389] Zeff JL. The process of healing: a unifying theory of naturopathic medicine. *Journal of Naturopathic Medicine* 1997; 7: 122-5

[390] Palmer DD. *The Science, Art, and Philosophy of Chiropractic*. Portland, OR; Portland Printing House Company, 1910: 107

[391] American Chiropractic Association. What is Chiropractic? http://amerchiro.org/media/whatis/ Accessed January 9, 2005

supplementation and diet modification. Consequently, the burden of suffering, disease, and healthcare expense in the US is higher than it would be if nutritionally-trained clinicians were more fully integrated into the healthcare system.

Obstacles to Efficacy in the Use of Nutritional Supplementation

Below are listed some of the most common causes for the underachievement of nutritional supplementation in practice and in published research. While this list is not all-inclusive, it will serve as a review for clinicians and an introduction for chiropractic/naturopathic students. In both practice and research, the problems listed below often overlap and function synergistically to reduce the efficacy of nutritional supplementation.

1. **Inadequate dosing (quantity)**: Many clinical trials published in major journals and many doctors in clinical practice have used inadequate doses of vitamins (and other natural therapeutics) and have thus failed to achieve the results that would have easily been obtained had they implemented their protocol with the proper physiologic or supraphysiologic dose of intervention. The best example in my experience centers on vitamin D, where so many of the studies are performed with doses of 400-800 IU per day only to conclude that vitamin supplementation is ineffective for the condition being treated. The problem here is that the researchers failed to appreciate that the physiologic requirement for vitamin D3 in adults is approximately 3,000-5,000 IU per day[392] and that therefore their supplemental dose of 400-800 IU is only 10-20% of what is required. Subphysiologic doses are generally subtherapeutic. In this regard, I have had to correct journals such as *The Lancet*[393], *JAMA*[394], and *British Medical Journal*[395] from misleading their readers (many of whom are major policymakers) from concluding that nutritional supplementation is impotent; rather, their researchers and editors were not sufficiently educated in the design and review of studies using nutritional interventions. These journals should hire chiropractic and naturopathic physicians so that they have staff trained in natural treatments and who can thus provide an educated review of studies on these topics.[396]

2. **Inadequate dosing (duration)**: Often the effects of long-term nutritional deficiency are not fully reversible and/or may require a treatment period of months or years to achieve maximal clinical response. For example, full replacement of fatty acids in human brain phospholipids is an ongoing process that occurs over a period of several years; thus studies using fatty acid supplements for a period of weeks or 2-3 months generally underestimate the enhanced effectiveness that can be obtained with administration over many months or several years of treatment. Relatedly, recovery from vitamin D deficiency takes several weeks of high-dose supplementation in order to achieve tissue saturation and subsequent cellular replenishment; studies of short duration are destined to underestimate the results that could have been achieved with supplementation carried out over several months.[397]

3. **Failure to use proper forms of nutrients**: Nutrients are often available in different forms, not the least of which are "active" versus "inactive" and "natural" versus "unnatural." Most vitamin supplements, particularly high-potency B vitamins, are manufactured synthetically and are not from "natural sources" despite the marketing hype promulgated by companies that, for example, mix their synthetic vitamins with a vegetable powder and then call their vitamin supplements "natural." The simple fact is that production of high-potency supplements from purely natural sources would be prohibitively wasteful, inefficient, and expensive. Thus, while it is not necessary for vitamins to be "natural" in order to be useful, it is necessary that the vitamins are useable and preferably not "unnatural." The best example of the use of unnatural supplements is the use of synthetic DL-tocopherol in the so-called "vitamin E" studies; DL-tocopherol is by definition 50% comprised of the L-isomer of tocopherol which is not only unusable by the human body but is actually harmful in that it interferes with normal metabolism and can exacerbate hypertension and cause symptomatic complications (e.g., headaches). Further, tocopherols exist within the body in relationship with the individual forms of the vitamin, such that supplementation with one form (e.g., alpha-tocopherol) can result in a relative deficiency of another form (e.g., gamma-tocopherol). One final example of the failure to use proper forms of nutrients is in the use of pyridoxine HCl as a form of vitamin B6; while this practice itself is not harmful, clinicians need to remember that pyridoxine HCl is ineffective until converted to the more active forms of the vitamin including pyridoxal-5-phosphate. Since this conversion requires co-nutrients such as magnesium and zinc, we can easily see that the reputed failure of B6 supplementation when administered in the form of pyridoxine HCl might actually be due to untreated insufficiencies of required co-nutrients, as discussed in the following section.

4. **Failure to ensure adequacy of co-nutrients**: Vitamins, minerals, amino acids, and fatty acids work together in an intricately choreographed and delicately orchestrated dance that culminates in the successful completion of interconnected physiologic functions. If any of the performers in this event are missing (i.e., nutritional deficiency) or if successive interconversions are impaired due to lack of enzyme function, then the show cannot go on, or—if it does go on—impaired metabolism and defective function will result. So, if we take a patient with "vitamin B6 deficiency" and give him vitamin B6 in the absence of other co-nutrients needed for the proper activation and metabolic utilization of vitamin B6, we cannot honestly expect the "nutritional supplementation" to work in this case; rather, we might see a marginal benefit or perhaps even a negative outcome as an imbalanced system is pushed into a different state of imbalance despite supplementation with the "correct" vitamin. In the case of vitamin B6, necessary co-nutrients include zinc, magnesium, and riboflavin; deficiency of any of these will result in a relative "failure" of B6 supplementation even if a

[392] Heaney RP, Davies KM, Chen TC, Holick MF, Barger-Lux MJ. Human serum 25-hydroxycholecalciferol response to extended oral dosing with cholecalciferol. *Am J Clin Nutr*. 2003 Jan;77(1):204-10 http://www.ajcn.org/cgi/content/full/77/1/204

[393] **Vasquez A**. Subphysiologic Doses of Vitamin D are Subtherapeutic: Comment on the Study by The Record Trial Group. *The Lancet* 2005 Published on-line May 6 http://OptimalHealthResearch.com/lancet

[394] Muanza DN, **Vasquez A**, Cannell J, Grant WB. Isoflavones and Postmenopausal Women. [letter] *JAMA* 2004; 292: 2337

[395] **Vasquez A**, Cannell J. Calcium and vitamin D in preventing fractures: data are not sufficient to show inefficacy. [letter] *BMJ: British Medical Journal* 2005;331:108-9 http://www.optimalhealthresearch.com/reprints/vasquez-cannell-bmj-reprint.pdf

[396] **Vasquez A**. Allopathic Usurpation of Natural Medicine: The Blind Leading the Sighted. *Naturopathy Digest* 2006 February http://www.naturopathydigest.com/archives/2006/feb/vasquez.php

[397] **Vasquez A**, Manso G, Cannell J. The clinical importance of vitamin D (cholecalciferol): a paradigm shift with implications for all healthcare providers. *Altern Ther Health Med*. 2004 Sep-Oct;10(5):28-36 http://optimalhealthresearch.com/monograph04

patient has a B6-responsive condition. Notably, overt magnesium deficiency is alarmingly common among patients and citizens in industrialized nations[398,399,400], and this epidemic of magnesium deficiency is due not only to insufficient intake but also to excessive excretion caused by consumption of high-glycemic foods, caffeine, and a diet that promotes chronic metabolic acidosis with resultant urinary acidification.

5. **Failure to achieve urinary alkalinization**: Western/American-style diets typified by overconsumption of grains, dairy, sugar, and salt result in a state of subclinical chronic metabolic acidosis which results in urinary acidification, relative hypercortisolemia, and consequent hyperexcretion of minerals such as calcium and magnesium.[401 402] Thus, the common conundrum of magnesium replenishment requires not only magnesium supplementation but also dietary interventions to change the internal climate to one that is conducive to bodily retention and cellular uptake of magnesium.[403]

6. **Use of mislabeled supplements**: Even in the professional arena of nutritional supplement manufacturers, some companies habitually underdose their products either in an attempt to spend less in the manufacture of their products or as a consequence of poor quality control. If a product is labeled to contain 1,000 IU of vitamin D but only contains 836 IU of the nutrient, then obviously full clinical efficacy will not be achieved; this was a problem in a recent clinical trial involving vitamin D.[404] The problem for clinicians is in trusting the companies that supply nutritional supplements; some companies do "in house" testing which lacks independent review, while other companies use questionable "independent testing" which is not infrequently performed by a laboratory that is a wholly owned subsidiary of the parent nutritional company. Manufacturing regulations that are sweeping through the industry will cleanse the nutritional supplement world of poorly made products, and these same regulations will sweep some unprepared companies right out the door when they are unable to meet the regulatory requirements.

7. **Assurance of bioavailability and optimal serum/cellular levels**: Clinical trials with nutritional therapies need to monitor serum or cellular levels to ensure absorption, product bioavailability, and the attainment of optimal serum levels. This is particularly relevant in the treatment of chronic disorders such as the autoimmune diseases, wherein so many of these patients have gastrointestinal dysbiosis and often have concomitant nutrient malabsorption.[405] Simply dosing these patients with supplements is not always efficacious; often the gut must be cleared of dysbiosis so that the mucosal lining can be repaired and optimal nutrient absorption can be reestablished.

8. **Coadministration of food with nutritional supplements (sometimes right, sometimes wrong)**: Food can help or hinder the absorption of nutritional supplements. Some supplements, like coenzyme Q10, should be administered with fatty food to enhance absorption. Other supplements, like amino acids, should be administered away from protein-rich foods and are often better administered with simple carbohydrate to enhance cellular uptake; this is especially true with tryptophan.

9. **Correction of gross dietary imbalances enhances supplement effectiveness**: If the diet is grossly imbalanced, then nutritional supplementation is less likely to be effective. The best example of this is in the use of fatty acid supplements, particularly in the treatment of inflammatory disorders. If the diet is laden with dairy, beef, and other sources of arachidonate, then fatty acid supplementation with EPA, DHA, and GLA is much less likely to be effective, or much higher doses of the supplements will need to be used in order to help restore fatty acid balance. Generally speaking, the diet needs to be optimized to enhance the efficacy of nutritional supplementation.

Conclusion

In this brief review, I have listed and discussed some of the most common impediments to the success of nutritional supplementation. I hope that chiropractic and naturopathic students, clinicians, and researchers will find these points helpful in their design of clinical treatment protocols.

---

[398] "Altogether 43% of 113 trauma patients had low magnesium levels compared to 30% of noninjured cohorts." Frankel H, Haskell R, Lee SY, Miller D, Rotondo M, Schwab CW. Hypomagnesemia in trauma patients. *World J Surg*. 1999 Sep;23(9):966-9

[399] "There was a 20% overall prevalence of hypomagnesemia among this predominantly female, African American population." Fox CH, Ramsoomair D, Mahoney MC, Carter C, Young B, Graham R. An investigation of hypomagnesemia among ambulatory urban African Americans. *J Fam Pract*. 1999 Aug;48(8):636-9

[400] "Suboptimal levels were detected in 33.7 per cent of the population under study. These data clearly demonstrate that the Mg supply of the German population needs increased attention." Schimatschek HF, Rempis R. Prevalence of hypomagnesemia in an unselected German population of 16,000 individuals. *Magnes Res*. 2001 Dec;14(4):283-90

[401] Cordain L, Eaton SB, Sebastian A, Mann N, Lindeberg S, Watkins BA, O'Keefe JH, Brand-Miller J. Origins and evolution of the Western diet: health implications for the 21st century. *Am J Clin Nutr*. 2005 Feb;81(2):341-54

[402] Maurer M, Riesen W, Muser J, Hulter HN, Krapf R. Neutralization of Western diet inhibits bone resorption independently of K intake and reduces cortisol secretion in humans. *Am J Physiol Renal Physiol*. 2003 Jan;284(1):F32-40

[403] Vormann J, Worlitschek M, Goedecke T, Silver B. Supplementation with alkaline minerals reduces symptoms in patients with chronic low back pain. *J Trace Elem Med Biol*. 2001;15(2-3):179-83

[404] Heaney RP, Davies KM, Chen TC, Holick MF, Barger-Lux MJ. Human serum 25-hydroxycholecalciferol response to extended oral dosing with cholecalciferol. *Am J Clin Nutr*. 2003 Jan;77(1):204-10 http://www.ajcn.org/cgi/content/full/77/1/204

[405] **Vasquez A**. Reducing Pain and Inflammation Naturally. Part 6: Nutritional and Botanical Treatments Against "Silent Infections" and Gastrointestinal Dysbiosis, Commonly Overlooked Causes of Neuromusculoskeletal Inflammation and Chronic Health Problems. *Nutritional Perspectives* 2006; January http://www.optimalhealthresearch.com/part6

Index

Revisiting the Five-Part Nutritional Wellness Protocol: The Supplemented Paleo-Mediterranean Diet

Alex Vasquez, DC, ND, DO

ABSTRACT: This article reviews the five-part nutritional protocol that incorporates a health-promoting nutrient-dense diet and essential supplementation with vitamins/minerals, specific fatty acids, probiotics, and physiologic doses of vitamin D3. This foundational nutritional protocol has proven benefits for disease treatment, disease prevention, and health maintenance and restoration. Additional treatments such as botanical medicines, additional nutritional supplements, and pharmaceutical drugs can be used atop this foundational protocol to further optimize clinical effectiveness. The rationale for this five-part protocol is presented, and consideration is given to adding iodine-iodide as the sixth component of the protocol.

INTRODUCTION:

In 2004 and 2005 I first published a "five-part nutrition protocol"[1, 2] that provides the foundational treatment plan for a wide range of health disorders. This protocol served and continues to serve as the foundation upon which other treatments are commonly added, and without which those other treatments are likely to fail, or attain suboptimal results at best.[3] Now as then, I will share with you what I consider a basic foundational protocol for wellness promotion and disease treatment. I have used this protocol in my own self-care for many years and have used it in the treatment of a wide range of health-disease conditions in clinical practice.

REVIEW:

This nutritional protocol is validated by biochemistry, physiology, experimental research, peer-reviewed human trials, and the clinical application of common sense. It is the most nutrient-dense diet available, satisfying nutritional needs and thereby optimizing metabolic processes while promoting satiety and weight loss/optimization. Nutrients are required in the proper amounts, forms, and approximate ratios for critical and innumerable physiologic functions; if nutrients are lacking, the body cannot function *normally,* let alone *optimally.* Impaired function results in subjective and objective manifestations of what is eventually labeled as "disease." Thus, a powerful and effective alternative to treating diseases with drugs is to re-establish normal/optimal physiologic function by replenishing the body with essential nutrients, reestablishing hormonal balance ("orthoendocrinology"), promoting detoxification of environmental toxins, and by reestablishing the optimal microbial milieu, especially the eradication of (multifocal) dysbiosis; this multifaceted approach can be applied to several diseases, especially those of the inflammatory and autoimmune varieties.[4]

Of course, most diseases are multifactorial and therefore require multicomponent treatment plans, and some diseases actually require the use of drugs in conjunction with assertive interventional nutrition. However, while only a smaller portion of patients actually need drugs for the long-term management their problems, all clinicians should agree that everyone needs a foundational nutrition plan because nutrients—not drugs—are universally required for life and health. This five-part nutrition protocol is briefly outlined below; a much more detailed substantiation of the underlying science and clinical application of this protocol was recently published in a review of more than 650 pages and approximately 3,500 citations.[5]

1. <u>Health-promoting Paleo-Mediterranean diet</u>: Following an extensive review of the research literature, I developed what I call the "supplemented Paleo-Mediterranean diet." In essence, this diet plan combines the best of the Mediterranean diet with the best of the Paleolithic diet, the latter of which has been best distilled by Dr. Loren Cordain in his book "The Paleo Diet"[6] and his numerous scientific articles.[7, 8, 9] The Paleolithic diet is superior to the Mediterranean diet in nutrient density for promoting satiety, weight loss, and improvements/normalization in overall metabolic function.[10, 11] This diet places emphasis on fruits, vegetables, nuts, seeds, and berries that meet the body's needs for fiber, carbohydrates, and most importantly, the 8,000+ phytonutrients that have additive and synergistic health effects[12]—including immunomodulating, antioxidant, anti-inflammatory, and anti-cancer benefits. High-quality protein sources such as fish, poultry, eggs, and grass-fed meats are emphasized. Slightly modifying Cordain's paleo diet, I also advocate soy and whey protein isolates for their high-quality protein and their anticancer, cardioprotective, and mood-enhancing (due to the high tryptophan content) benefits. Potatoes and other starchy vegetables, wheat and other grains including rice are discouraged due to their high glycemic indexes and high glycemic loads, and their relative insufficiency of fiber and phytonutrients compared to fruits and vegetables. Grains such as wheat, barley, and rye are discouraged due to the high glycemic loads/indexes of most breads, pastries, and other grain-derived products, as well as due to the

immunogenicity of constituents such as gluten, a protein composite (consisting of a prolamin and a glutelin) that can contribute to disorders such as migraine, epilepsy, eczema, arthritis, celiac disease, psoriasis and other types of autoimmunity. Sources of simple sugars and foreign chemicals such as colas/sodas (which contain artificial colors, flavors, and high-fructose corn syrup, which contains mercury[13] and which can cause the hypertensive-diabetic metabolic syndrome[14]) and processed foods (e.g., "TV dinners" and other manufactured snacks and convenience foods) are strictly forbidden. Chemical preservatives, colorants, sweeteners, flavor-enhancers such as monosodium glutamate and carrageenan are likewise avoided. In summary, this diet plan provides plenty of variety, as most dishes comprised of poultry, fish, lean meats, soy, eggs, fruits, vegetables, nuts, berries, and seeds are allowed. The diet provides an abundance of fiber, phytonutrients, carbohydrates, potassium, and protein, while simultaneously being low in fat, sodium, arachidonic acid, and "simple sugars." The diet must be customized with regard to total protein and calorie intake, as determined by the size, status, and activity level of the patient; individual per-patient food allergens should be avoided. Regular consumption of this diet has shown the ability to reduce hypertension, alleviate diabetes, ameliorate migraine headaches, and result in improvement of overall health and a lessening of the severity of many common "diseases", particularly those with an autoimmune or inflammatory component. This Paleo-Mediterranean diet is supplemented with vitamins, minerals, fatty acids, and probiotics—making it the "supplemented Paleo-Mediterranean diet" as described below.

2. Multivitamin and multimineral supplementation: Vitamin and mineral supplementation has been advocated for decades by the chiropractic/naturopathic professions while being scorned by so-called "mainstream medicine." Vitamin and mineral supplementation finally received bipartisan endorsement when researchers from Harvard Medical School published a review article in *Journal of the American Medical Association* that concluded, "Most people do not consume an optimal amount of all vitamins by diet alone. ...it appears prudent for all adults to take vitamin supplements."[15] Long-term nutritional insufficiencies experienced by "most people" promote the development of "long-latency deficiency diseases"[16] such as cancer, neuroemotional deterioration, and cardiovascular disease. Impressively, the benefits of multivita-

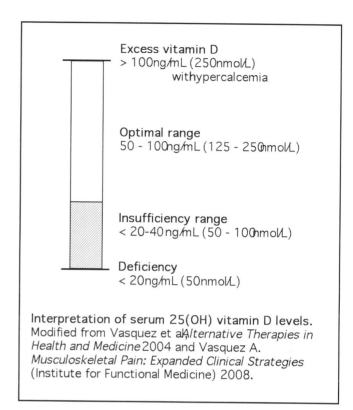

Excess vitamin D
> 100ng/mL (250nmol/L)
with hypercalcemia

Optimal range
50 - 100ng/mL (125 - 250nmol/L)

Insufficiency range
< 20-40ng/mL (50 - 100nmol/L)

Deficiency
< 20ng/mL (50nmol/L)

Interpretation of serum 25(OH) vitamin D levels. Modified from Vasquez et al. *Alternative Therapies in Health and Medicine* 2004 and Vasquez A. *Musculoskeletal Pain: Expanded Clinical Strategies* (Institute for Functional Medicine) 2008.

min/multimineral supplementation have been demonstrated in numerous clinical trials. Multivitamin/multimineral supplementation has been shown to improve nutritional status and reduce the risk for chronic diseases[17], improve mood[18], potentiate antidepressant drug treatment[19], alleviate migraine headaches (when used with diet improvement and fatty acids[20]), improve immune function and infectious disease outcomes in the elderly[21] (especially diabetics[22]), reduce morbidity and mortality in patients with HIV infection[23, 24], alleviate premenstrual syndrome[25, 26] and bipolar disorder[27], reduce violence and antisocial behavior in children[28] and incarcerated young adults (when used with essential fatty acids[29]), and improve scores of intelligence in children.[30] Multivitamin and multimineral supplementation provides anti-inflammatory benefits, as evidenced by significant reduction in C-reactive protein (CRP) in a double-blind, placebo-controlled trial.[31] The ability to safely and affordably deliver these benefits makes multimineral-multivitamin supplementation an essential component of any and all health-promoting and disease-prevention strategies. A few cautions need to be observed; for example, vitamin A can (rarely) result in liver damage with chronic consumption of 25,000 IU or more, and intake should generally not exceed 10,000 IU per day in women of childbearing age. Also, iron should not be supplemented except in patients diagnosed with iron deficiency by a blood test (serum ferritin).

3. <u>Physiologic doses of vitamin D3</u>: The prevalence of vitamin D deficiency varies from 40-80 percent (general population) to almost 100 percent (patients with musculoskeletal pain) among Americans and Europeans. Vasquez, Manso, and Cannell described the many benefits of vitamin D3 supplementation in an assertive review published in 2004.[32] Our publication showed that vitamin D deficiency causes or contributes to depression, hypertension, seizures, migraine, polycystic ovary syndrome, inflammation, autoimmunity, and musculoskeletal pain, particularly low-back pain. Clinical trials using vitamin D supplementation have proven the cause-and-effect relationship between vitamin D deficiency and most of these conditions by showing that each could be cured or alleviated with vitamin D supplementation. In our review of the literature, we concluded that daily vitamin D doses should be 1,000 IU for infants, 2,000 IU for children, and 4,000 IU for adults, although some adults respond better to higher doses of 10,000 IU per day. Cautions and contraindications include the use of thiazide diuretics (e.g., hydrochlorothiazide) or any other medications that promote hypercalcemia, as well as granulomatous diseases such as sarcoidosis, tuberculosis, and certain types of cancer, especially lymphoma. Effectiveness is monitored by measuring serum 25-OH-vitamin D, and safety is monitored by measuring serum calcium. Dosing should be tailored for the attainment of optimal serum levels of 25-hydroxy-vitamin D3, generally 50-100 ng/ml (125-250 nmol/l) as illustrated.

4. <u>Balanced and complete fatty acid supplementation</u>: A detailed survey of the literature shows that five fatty acids have major health-promoting disease-preventing benefits and should therefore be incorporated into the daily diet and/or regularly consumed as dietary supplements.[33] These are alpha-linolenic acid (ALA; omega-3, from flaxseed oil), eicosapentaenoic acid (EPA; omega-3, from fish oil), docosahexaenoic acid (DHA; omega-3, from fish oil and algae), gamma-linolenic acid (GLA; omega-6, most concentrated in borage oil but also present in evening primrose oil, hemp seed oil, black currant seed oil), and oleic acid (omega-9, most concentrated in olive oil, which contains in addition to oleic acid many anti-inflammatory, antioxidant, and anticancer phytonutrients). Supplementing with one fatty acid can exacerbate an insufficiency of other fatty acids; hence the impor-

tance of balanced combination supplementation. Each of these fatty acids has health benefits that cannot be fully attained from supplementing a different fatty acid; hence, again, the importance of balanced combination supplementation. The benefits of GLA are not attained by consumption of EPA and DHA; in fact, consumption of fish oil can actually promote a deficiency of GLA.[34] Likewise, consumption of GLA alone can reduce EPA levels while increasing levels of proinflammatory arachidonic acid; both of these problems are avoided with co-administration of EPA any time GLA is used because EPA inhibits delta-5-desaturase, which converts dihomo-GLA into arachidonic acid. Using ALA alone only slightly increases EPA but generally leads to no improvement in DHA status and can lead to a reduction of oleic acid; thus, DHA and oleic acid should be supplemented when flaxseed oil is used.[35] Obviously, the goal here is physiologically-optimal (i.e., "balanced") intake of all of the health-promoting fatty acids; using only one or two sources of fatty acids is not balanced and results in suboptimal improvement. In clinical practice, I routinely use combination fatty acid therapy comprised of ALA, EPA, DHA, and GLA for essentially all patients; when one appreciates that the average daily Paleolithic intake of n-3 fatty acids was 7 grams per day contrasted to the average daily American intake of 1 gram per day, we can see that—by using combination fatty acid therapy emphasizing n-3 fatty acids—we are simply meeting physiologic expectations via supplementation, rather than performing an act of recklessness or heroism. The product I use also contains a modest amount of oleic acid that occurs naturally in flax and borage seed oils, and I encourage use of olive oil for salads and cooking. This approach results in complete and balanced fatty acid intake, and the clinical benefits are impressive. Benefits are to be expected in the treatment of premenstrual syndrome, diabetic neuropathy, respiratory distress syndrome, Crohn's disease, lupus, rheumatoid arthritis, cardiovascular disease, hypertension, psoriasis, eczema, migraine headaches, bipolar disorder, borderline personality disorder, mental depression, schizophrenia, osteoporosis, polycystic ovary syndrome, multiple sclerosis, and musculoskeletal pain. The discovery in September 2010 that the G protein-coupled receptor 120 (GPR120) functions as an n-3 fatty acid receptor that, when stimulated with EPA or DHA, exerts broad anti-inflammatory effects (in cell experiments) and enhances systemic insulin sensitivity (in animal study) confirms a new mechanism of action of fatty acid supplementation and shows that we as clinician-researchers are still learning the details of the beneficial effects of commonly used treatments.[36]

5. Probiotics /gut flora modification: Proper levels of good bacteria promote intestinal health, support proper immune function, and encourage overall health. Excess bacteria or yeast, or the presence of harmful bacteria, yeast, or "parasites" such as amoebas and protozoas, can cause "leaky gut," systemic inflammation, and a wide range of clinical problems, especially autoimmunity. Intestinal flora can become imbalanced by poor diets, excess stress, immunosuppressive drugs, and antibiotics, and all of these factors are common among American patients. Thus, as a rule, I reinstate the good bacteria by the use of probiotics (good bacteria and yeast), prebiotics (fiber, arabinogalactan, and inulin), and the use of fermented foods such as kefir and yogurt for patients not allergic to milk. Harmful yeast, bacteria, and other "parasites" can be eradicated with the combination of dietary change, antimicrobial drugs, and/or herbal extracts. For example, oregano oil in an emulsified, time-released form has proven safe and effective for the elimination of various parasites encountered in clinical practice.[37] Likewise, the herb Artemisia annua (sweet wormwood) commonly is used to eradicate specific bacteria and has been used for thousands of years in Asia for the treatment and prevention of infectious diseases, including drug-resistant malaria.[38] Restoring microbial balance by providing probiotics, restoring immune function (immunorestoration) and eliminating sources of dysbiosis, especially in the gastrointestinal tract, genitourinary tract, and oropharynx, is a very important component in the treatment plan of autoimmunity and systemic inflammation.[39]

Should combinations of iodine and iodide be the Sixth Component of the Protocol?: Both iodine and iodide have biological activity in humans. An increasing number of clinicians are using combination iodine-iodide products to provide approximately 12 mg/d; this is consistent with the average daily intake of iodine-iodide in countries such as Japan with a high intake of seafood, including fish, shellfish, and seaweed. Collectively, iodine and iodide provide antioxidant, antimicrobial, mucolytic, immunosupportive, antiestrogen, and anticancer benefits that extend far beyond the mere incorporation of iodine into thyroid hormones.[5] Benefits of iodine/iodide in the treatment of asthma[40,41] and systemic fungal infections[42,43] have been documented, and many clinicians use combination iodine/iodide supplementation for the treatment of estrogen-driven conditions such as fibrocystic breast disease.[44] While additional research is needed and already underway to further establish the role of iodine-iodide as a routine component of clinical care, clinicians should begin incorporating this nutrient into their protocols based on the above-mentioned physiologic roles and clinical benefits.

SUMMARY AND CONCLUSIONS:

In this brief review, I have described and substantiated a fundamental protocol that can serve as effective therapy for patients with a wide range of diseases and health disorders. Customizing the Paleo-Mediterranean diet to avoid patient-specific food allergens, using vitamin-mineral supplements along with physiologic doses of vitamin D and broad-spectrum balanced fatty acid supplementation, and ensuring "immunomicrobial" health with the skillful use of probiotics, prebiotics, immunorestoration, and antimicrobial treatments provides an excellent health-promoting and disease-eliminating foundation and lifestyle for many patients. Often, this simple protocol is all that is needed for the effective treatment of a wide range of clinical problems, even those that have been "medical failures" for many years. For other patients with more complex illnesses, of course, additional interventions and laboratory assessments can be used to optimize and further customize the treatment plan. Clinicians should avoid seeking "silver bullet" treatments that ignore overall metabolism, immune function, and inflammatory balance, and we must always remember that the attainment and preservation of health requires that we first meet the body's basic nutritional and physiologic needs. This five-step protocol begins the process of meeting those needs. With it, health can be restored and the need for disease-specific treatment is obviated or reduced; without it, fundamental physiologic needs are not met, and health cannot be obtained and maintained. Addressing core physiologic needs empowers doctors to deliver the most effective healthcare possible, and it allows patients to benefit from such treatment.

Dr Alex Vasquez is a Director of the Medical Board of Advisors for Biotics Research Corporation and is the author of many articles and books for doctors. His professional degrees include Doctor of Chiropractic, (University of Western States, March 1996), Doctor of Naturopathic Medicine (Bastyr University, September 1999), and Doctor of Osteopathic Medicine (University of North Texas Health Science Center, May 2010).

REFERENCES

1. Vasquez A. Integrative Orthopedics: The Art of Creating Wellness While Managing Acute and Chronic Musculoskeletal Disorders. 2004, 2007
2. Vasquez A. A Five-Part Nutritional Protocol that Produces Consistently Positive Results. Nutritional Wellness 2005 September Available in the printed version and on-line at http://www.nutritionalwellness.com/archives/2005/sep/09_vasquez.php
3. Vasquez A. Common Oversights and Shortcomings in the Study and Imple-

mentation of Nutritional Supplementation. Naturopathy Digest 2007 June. http://www.naturopathydigest.com/archives/2007/jun/vasquez.php

4. Vasquez A. Integrative Rheumatology. IBMRC: 2006, 2009. http://optimal-healthresearch.com/rheumatology.html
5. Vasquez A. Chiropractic and Naturopathic Mastery of Common Clinical Disorders. IBMRC: 2009. http://optimalhealthresearch.com/clinical_mastery.html
6. Cordain L. The Paleo Diet. John Wiley and Sons, 2002
7. O'Keefe JH Jr, Cordain L. Cardiovascular disease resulting from a diet and lifestyle at odds with our Paleolithic genome: how to become a 21st-century hunter-gatherer. Mayo Clin Proc. 2004 Jan;79(1):101-8
8. Cordain L. Cereal grains: humanity's double edged sword. World Rev Nutr Diet 1999;84:19-73
9. Cordain L, Eaton SB, Sebastian A, Mann N, Lindeberg S, Watkins BA, O'Keefe JH, Brand-Miller J. Origins and evolution of the Western diet: health implications for the 21st century. Am J Clin Nutr. 2005 Feb;81(2):341-54
10. "A high micronutrient density diet mitigates the unpleasant aspects of the experience of hunger even though it is lower in calories. Hunger is one of the major impediments to successful weight loss. Our findings suggest that it is not simply the caloric content, but more importantly, the micronutrient density of a diet that influences the experience of hunger. It appears that a high nutrient density diet, after an initial phase of adjustment during which a person experiences "toxic hunger" due to withdrawal from pro-inflammatory foods, can result in a sustainable eating pattern that leads to weight loss and improved health." Fuhrman J, Sarter B, Glaser D, Acocella S. Changing perceptions of hunger on a high nutrient density diet. Nutr J. 2010 Nov 7;9:51 http://www.nutritionj.com/content/9/1/51
11. "The Paleolithic group were as satiated as the Mediterranean group but consumed less energy per day (5.8 MJ/day vs. 7.6 MJ/day, Paleolithic vs. Mediterranean, p=0.04). Consequently, the quotients of mean change in satiety during meal and mean consumed energy from food and drink were higher in the Paleolithic group (p=0.03). Also, there was a strong trend for greater Satiety Quotient for energy in the Paleolithic group (p=0.057). Leptin decreased by 31% in the Paleolithic group and by 18% in the Mediterranean group with a trend for greater relative decrease of leptin in the Paleolithic group." Jonsson T, Granfeldt Y, Erlanson-Albertsson C, Ahren B, Lindeberg S. A Paleolithic diet is more satiating per calorie than a Mediterranean-like diet in individuals with ischemic heart disease. Nutr Metab (Lond). 2010 Nov 30;7(1):85.
12. Liu RH. Health benefits of fruit and vegetables are from additive and synergistic combinations of phytochemicals. Am J Clin Nutr 2003;78(3 Suppl):517S-520S
13. "With daily per capita consumption of HFCS in the US averaging about 50 grams and daily mercury intakes from HFCS ranging up to 28 µg, this potential source of mercury may exceed other major sources of mercury especially in high-end consumers of beverages sweetened with HFCS." Dufault R, LeBlanc B, Schnoll R, Cornett C, Schweitzer L, Wallinga D, Hightower J, Patrick L, Lukiw WJ. Mercury from chlor-alkali plants: measured concentrations in food product sugar. Environ Health. 2009 Jan 26;8:2 http://www.ehjournal.net/content/8/1/2
14. Vasquez A. Integrative Medicine and Functional Medicine for Chronic Hypertension: An Evidence-based Patient-Centered Monograph for Advanced Clinicians. IBMRC: 2011. http://optimalhealthresearch.com/hypertension_functional_integrative_medicine.html See also: Reungjui S, Roncal CA, Mu W, Srinivas TR, Sirivongs D, Johnson RJ, Nakagawa T. Thiazide diuretics exacerbate fructose-induced metabolic syndrome. J Am Soc Nephrol. 2007 Oct;18(10):2724-31 http://jasn.asnjournals.org/content/18/10/2724.full.pdf
15. Fletcher RH, Fairfield KM. Vitamins for chronic disease prevention in adults: clinical applications. JAMA 2002;287:3127-9
16. Heaney RP. Long-latency deficiency disease: insights from calcium and vitamin D. Am J Clin Nutr 2003;78:912-9
17. McKay DL, Perrone G, Rasmussen H, Dallal G, Hartman W, Cao G, Prior RL, Roubenoff R, Blumberg JB. The effects of a multivitamin/mineral supplement on micronutrient status, antioxidant capacity and cytokine production in healthy older adults consuming a fortified diet. J Am Coll Nutr 2000;19(5):613-21
18. Benton D, Haller J, Fordy J. Vitamin supplementation for 1 year improves mood. Neuropsychobiology 1995;32(2):98-105
19. Coppen A, Bailey J. Enhancement of the antidepressant action of fluoxetine by folic acid: a randomised, placebo controlled trial. J Affect Disord 2000;60:121-30
20. Wagner W, Nootbaar-Wagner U. Prophylactic treatment of migraine with gamma-linolenic and alpha-linolenic acids. Cephalalgia 1997;17:127-30
21. Langkamp-Henken B, Bender BS, Gardner EM, Herrlinger-Garcia KA, Kelley MJ, Murasko DM, Schaller JP, Stechmiller JK, Thomas DJ, Wood SM. Nutritional formula enhanced immune function and reduced days of symptoms of upper respiratory tract infection in seniors. J Am Geriatr Soc 2004;52:3-12
22. Barringer TA, Kirk JK, Santaniello AC, Foley KL, Michielutte R. Effect of a multivitamin and mineral supplement on infection and quality of life. A randomized, double-blind, placebo-controlled trial. Ann Intern Med 2003;138:365-71
23. Fawzi WW, Msamanga GI, Spiegelman D, et al. A randomized trial of multivitamin supplements and HIV disease progression and mortality. N Engl J Med 2004;351:23-32
24. Burbano X, Miguez-Burbano MJ, McCollister K, Zhang G, Rodriguez A, Ruiz P, Lecusay R, Shor-Posner G. Impact of a selenium chemoprevention clinical trial on hospital admissions of HIV-infected participants. HIV Clin Trials 2002;3:483-91
25. Abraham GE. Nutritional factors in the etiology of the premenstrual tension syndromes. J Reprod Med 1983;28(7):446-64
26. Stewart A. Clinical and biochemical effects of nutritional supplementation on the premenstrual syndrome. J Reprod Med 1987;32:435-41
27. Kaplan BJ, Simpson JS, Ferre RC, Gorman CP, McMullen DM, Crawford SG. Effective mood stabilization with a chelated mineral supplement: an open-label trial in bipolar disorder. J Clin Psychiatry 2001;62:936-44
28. Kaplan BJ, Crawford SG, Gardner B, Farrelly G. Treatment of mood lability and explosive rage with minerals and vitamins: two case studies in children. J Child Adolesc Psychopharmacol 2002;12(3):205-19
29. Gesch CB, Hammond SM, Hampson SE, Eves A, Crowder MJ. Influence of supplementary vitamins, minerals and essential fatty acids on the antisocial behaviour of young adult prisoners. Randomised, placebo-controlled trial. Br J Psychiatry 2002;181:22-8
30. Benton D. Micro-nutrient supplementation and the intelligence of children. Neurosci Biobehav Rev 2001;25:297-309
31. Church TS, Earnest CP, Wood KA, Kampert JB. Reduction of C-reactive protein levels through use of a multivitamin. Am J Med 2003;115:702-7
32. Vasquez A, Manso G, Cannell J. The clinical importance of vitamin D (cholecalciferol): a paradigm shift with implications for all healthcare providers. Alternative Therapies in Health and Medicine 2004;10:28-37 http://optimalhealthresearch.com/cholecalciferol.html
33. Vasquez A. Reducing Pain and Inflammation Naturally - Part 1: New Insights into Fatty Acid Biochemistry and the Influence of Diet. Nutritional Perspectives 2004; October: 5, 7-10, 12, 14 http://optimalhealthresearch.com/reprints/series/
34. Cleland LG, Gibson RA, Neumann M, French JK. The effect of dietary fish oil supplement upon the content of dihomo-gammalinolenic acid in human plasma phospholipids. Prostaglandins Leukot Essent Fatty Acids 1990 May;40(1):9-12
35. Jantti J, Nikkari T, Solakivi T, Vapaatalo H, Isomaki H. Evening primrose oil in rheumatoid arthritis: changes in serum lipids and fatty acids. Ann Rheum Dis 1989;48(2):124-7
36. Oh da Y, Talukdar S, Bae EJ, Imamura T, Morinaga H, Fan W, Li P, Lu WJ, Watkins SM, Olefsky JM. GPR120 is an omega-3 fatty acid receptor mediating potent anti-inflammatory and insulin-sensitizing effects. Cell. 2010 Sep 3;142(5):687-98 http://www.cell.com/abstract/S0092-8674%2810%2900888-3?switch=standard
37. Force M, Sparks WS, Ronzio RA. Inhibition of enteric parasites by emulsified oil of oregano in vivo. Phytother Res 2000;14:213-4
38. Schuster BG. Demonstrating the validity of natural products as anti-infective drugs. J Altern Complement Med 2001;7 Suppl 1:S73-82
39. Vasquez A. Integrative Rheumatology. IBMRC: 2006, 2009. http://optimalhealthresearch.com/rheumatology.html
40. Tuft L. Iodides in bronchial asthma. J Allergy Clin Immunol. 1981 Jun;67(6):497
41. Falliers CJ, McCann WP, Chai H, Ellis EF, Yazdi N. Controlled study of iodotherapy for childhood asthma. J Allergy. 1966 Sep;38(3):183-92
42. Tripathy S, Vijayashree J, Mishra M, Jena DK, Behera B, Mohapatra A. Rhinofacial zygomycosis successfully treated with oral saturated solution of potassium iodide: a case report. J Eur Acad Dermatol Venereol. 2007 Jan;21(1):117-9
43. Bonifaz A, Saúl A, Paredes-Solis V, Fierro L, Rosales A, Palacios C, Araiza J. Sporotrichosis in childhood: clinical and therapeutic experience in 25 patients. Pediatr Dermatol. 2007 Jul-Aug;24(4):369-72
44. Ghent WR, Eskin BA, Low DA, Hill LP. Iodine replacement in fibrocystic disease of the breast. Can J Surg. 1993 Oct;36(5):453-60

This CME article has been brought to you by an educational grant from Biotics Research Corporation.

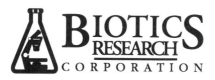

6801 Biotics Research Drive
Rosenberg, TX 77471
Toll Free: 1-800-231-5777
www.bioticsresearch.com

CME
CONTINUING MEDICAL EDUCATION

THE CLINICAL IMPORTANCE OF VITAMIN D (CHOLECALCIFEROL): A PARADIGM SHIFT WITH IMPLICATIONS FOR ALL HEALTHCARE PROVIDERS

Alex Vasquez, DC, ND, Gilbert Manso, MD, John Cannell, MD

Alex Vasquez, DC, ND is a licensed naturopathic physician in Washington and Oregon, and licensed chiropractic doctor in Texas, where he maintains a private practice and is a member of the Research Team at Biotics Research Corporation. He is a former Adjunct Professor of Orthopedics and Rheumatology for the Naturopathic Medicine Program at Bastyr University. **Gilbert Manso**, MD, is a medical doctor practicing integrative medicine in Houston, Texas. In practice for more than 35 years, he is Board Certified in Family Practice and is Associate Professor of Family Medicine at University of Texas Medical School in Houston. **John Cannell**, MD, is a medical physician practicing in Atascadero, California, and is president of the Vitamin D Council (Cholecalciferol-Council.com), a non-profit, tax-exempt organization working to promote awareness of the manifold adverse effects of vitamin D deficiency.

InnoVision Communications is accredited by the Accreditation Council for Continuing Medical Education to provide continuing medical education for physicians. The learner should study the article and its figures or tables, if any, then complete the self-evaluation at the end of the activity. The activity and self-evaluation are expected to take a maximum of 2 hours.

OBJECTIVES
Upon completion of this article, participants should be able to do the following:

1. Appreciate and identify the manifold clinical presentations and consequences of vitamin D deficiency
2. Identify patient groups that are predisposed to vitamin D hypersensitivity
3. Know how to implement vitamin D supplementation in proper doses and with appropriate laboratory monitoring

Reprint requests: InnoVision Communications, 169 Saxony Rd, Suite 103, Encinitas, CA 92024; phone, (760) 633-3910 or (866) 828-2962; fax, (760) 633-3918; e-mail, alternative.therapies@ innerdoorway.com. Or visit our online CME Web site by going to http://www.alternative -therapies.com and selecting the Continuing Education option.

While we are all familiar with the important role of vitamin D in calcium absorption and bone metabolism, many doctors and patients are not aware of the recent research on vitamin D and the widening range of therapeutic applications available for cholecalciferol, which can be classified as both a vitamin and a pro-hormone. Additionally, we also now realize that the Food and Nutrition Board's previously defined Upper Limit (UL) for safe intake at 2,000 IU/day was set far too low and that the physiologic requirement for vitamin D in adults may be as high as 5,000 IU/day, which is less than half of the >10,000 IU that can be produced endogenously with full-body sun exposure.[1,2] With the discovery of vitamin D receptors in tissues other than the gut and bone—especially the brain, breast, prostate, and lymphocytes—and the recent research suggesting that higher vitamin D levels provide protection from diabetes mellitus, osteoporosis, osteoarthritis, hypertension, cardiovascular disease, metabolic syndrome, depression, several autoimmune diseases, and cancers of the breast, prostate, and colon, we can now utilize vitamin D for a wider range of preventive and therapeutic applications to maintain and improve our patients' health.[3] Based on the research reviewed in this article, the current authors believe that assessment of vitamin D status and treatment of vitamin D deficiency with oral vitamin D supplements should become a routine component of clinical practice and preventive medicine. Vitamin D supplementation with doses of 4,000 IU/day for adults is clinically safe and physiologically reasonable since such doses are consistent with physiologic requirements.[2] Higher doses up to 10,000 IU/day appear safe and produce blood levels of vitamin D that are common in sun-exposed equatorial populations.[1,2] Periodic assessment of serum 25-OH-vitamin D [25(OH)D] and serum calcium will help to ensure that vitamin D levels are sufficient and safe for health maintenance and disease prevention. Clinical research supporting the use of vitamin D in the management of type 2 diabetes, osteoporosis, osteoarthritis, hypertension, cardiovascular disease, metabolic syndrome, multiple sclerosis, polycystic ovary syndrome, musculoskeletal pain, depression, epilepsy, and the prevention of cancer and type 1 diabetes is presented along with our proposals for the interpretation of serum 25(OH)D laboratory values, for the design of future research studies, and for supplementation in infants, children, adults, and during pregnancy and lactation.

BASIC PHYSIOLOGY OF VITAMIN D

Vitamin D is obtained naturally from two sources: sunlight and dietary consumption. Vitamin D3 (cholecalciferol) is the form of vitamin D produced in the skin and consumed in the diet. Vitamin D2 (ergocalciferol), which is produced by irradiating fungi, is much less efficient as a precursor to the biologically active 1,25-dihydroxyvitamin D (calcitriol). Additionally, since ergocalciferol shows altered pharmacokinetics compared with D3 and may become contaminated during its microbial production, it is potentially less effective and more toxic than cholecalciferol.[4] Although ergocalciferol is occasionally used clinically and in research studies, cholecalciferol is the preferred form of supplementation and will be implied in this article when supplementation is discussed.

Vitamin D can be described as having two pathways for metabolism: one being "endocrine" and the other "autocrine" (within the cell) and perhaps "paracrine" (around the cell). This elucidation, recently reviewed by Heany,[5] is vitally important in expanding our previously limited conception of vitamin D from only a "bone nutrient with importance only for the prevention of rickets and osteomalacia" to an extraordinary molecule with far-reaching effects in a variety of cells and tissues. Furthermore, Heany's distinction of "short-latency deficiency diseases" such as rickets from "long-latency deficiency diseases" such as cancer provides a conceptual handle that helps us grasp an understanding of the differences between the acute manifestations of severe nutritional deficiencies and the delayed manifestations of chronic subclinical nutritional deficiencies.[5]

In its endocrine metabolism, vitamin D (cholecalciferol) is formed in the skin following exposure to sunlight and then travels in the blood to the liver where it is converted to 25-hydroxyvitamin D (calcidiol, 25(OH)D) by the enzyme vitamin D-25-hydroxylase. 25(OH)D then circulates to the kidney for its final transformation to 1,25-dihydroxyvitamin D (calcitriol) by 25-hydroxyvitamin D3-1alpha-hydroxylase (1-OHase).[6] Calcitriol is the most biologically active form of vitamin D and increases calcium and phosphorus absorption in the intestine, induces osteoclast maturation for bone remodeling, and promotes calcium deposition in bone and a reduction in parathyroid hormone (PTH). While increased calcium absorption is obviously important for nutritional reasons, suppression of PTH by vitamin D is also clinically important since relatively lower levels of PTH appear to promote and protect health, and higher levels of PTH correlate with increased risk for myocardial infarction, stroke, and hypertension.[7,8] Relatedly, Fujita[9] proposed the "calcium paradox" wherein vitamin D or calcium deficiency leads to elevations of PTH which increases intracellular calcium and may thereby promote a cascade of cellular dysfunction that can contribute to the development of diabetes mellitus, neurologic diseases, malignancy, and degenerative joint disease.

In its autocrine metabolism, circulating 25(OH)D is taken up by a wide variety of cells that contain both 1-OHase as well as nuclear vitamin D receptors (VDR). Therefore, these cells are able to make their own calcitriol rather than necessarily relying upon hematogenous supply. Cells and tissues that are known to contain 1-OHase, and which therefore make their own calcitriol, include the breast, prostate, lung, skin, lymph nodes, colon, pancreas, adrenal medulla, and brain (cerebellum and cerebral cortex).[3,10] Cells and tissues with nuclear, cytosolic, or membrane-bound VDR include islet cells of the pancreas, monocytes, transformed B-cells, activated T-cells, neurons, prostate cells, ovarian cells, pituitary cells, and aortic endothelial cells.[11] Indeed, given the wide range of cells and tissues that metabolize vitamin D in an autocrine manner, we see that there is biological potential for vitamin D to influence function and pathophysiology in a wide range of metabolic processes and disease states.

Since many cells and tissues of the body have the ability to metabolize vitamin D, we should not be surprised that vitamin D plays a role in the function of these cells. Calcitriol is known to modulate transcription of several genes, notably those affecting differentiation and proliferation such as c-myc, c-fos, and c-sis,[6] and this may partially explain the inverse relationship between sun exposure (eg, vitamin D) and cancer mortality.[12,13] Vitamin D appears to modulate neurotransmitter/neurologic function as shown by its antidepressant[14] and anticonvulsant[15] benefits. Vitamin D is obviously immunoregulatory as manifested by its ability to reduce inflammation,[16,17] suppress and/or prevent certain autoimmune diseases,[18-20] reduce the risk for cancer,[12] and possibly reduce the severity and frequency of infectious diseases, such as acute pneumonia in children.[21]

CLINICAL APPLICATIONS AND THERAPEUTIC BENEFITS OF VITAMIN D

Support for a broad range of clinical applications for vitamin D supplementation comes from laboratory experiments, clinical trials, and epidemiologic surveys. Despite the imperfections of current data, we can still see significant benefits from vitamin D supplementation in a variety of human diseases, as briefly reviewed below.

Cardiovascular Disease

Deaths from cardiovascular disease are more common in the winter, more common at higher latitudes and more common at lower altitudes, observations that are consistent with vitamin D insufficiency.[22] The risk of heart attack is twice as high for those with 25(OH)D levels less than 34 ng/ml (85 nmol/L) than for those with vitamin D status above this level.[23] Patients with congestive heart failure were recently found to have markedly lower levels of vitamin D than controls,[24] and vitamin D deficiency as a cause of heart failure has been documented in numerous case reports.[25-29]

Hypertension

It has long been known that blood pressure is higher in the winter than the summer, increases at greater distances from the equator and is affected by skin pigmentation—all observations consistent with a role for vitamin D in regulating blood pressure.[30] When patients with hypertension were treated with ultraviolet light three times a week for six weeks their vitamin D levels increased by 162%, and their blood pressure fell significantly.[31] Even small amounts of oral cholecalciferol (800 IU) for eight weeks lowered both blood pressure and heart rate.[32]

Type 2 Diabetes

Hypovitaminosis D is associated with insulin resistance and beta-cell dysfunction in diabetics and young adults who are apparently healthy. Healthy adults with higher serum 25(OH)D levels had significantly lower 60 min, 90 min and 129 min postprandial glucose levels and significantly better insulin sensitivity than those who were vitamin D deficient.[33] The authors noted that, compared with metformin, which improves insulin sensitivity by 13%, higher vitamin D status correlated with a 60% improvement in insulin sensitivity. In a recent clinical trial using 1,332 IU/day for only 30 days in 10 women with type 2 diabetes, vitamin D supplementation was shown to improve insulin sensitivity by 21%.[34]

Osteoarthritis

Many practitioners know that vitamin D helps prevent and treat osteoporosis, but few know that the progression of osteoarthritis, the most common arthritis, is lessened by adequate blood levels of vitamin D. Framingham data showed osteoarthritis of the knee progressed more rapidly in those with 25(OH)D levels lower than 36 ng/ml (90 nmol/L).[35] Another study found that osteoarthritis of the hip progressed more rapidly in those with 25(OH)D levels lower than 30 ng/ml (75 nmol/L).[36]

Multiple Sclerosis

The autoimmune/inflammatory disease multiple sclerosis (MS) is notably rare in sunny equatorial regions and becomes increasingly prevalent among people who live farther from the equator and/or who lack adequate sun exposure. In a clinical trial with 10 MS patients, Goldberg, Fleming, and Picard[19] pre-scribed daily supplementation with approximately 1,000 mg calcium, 600 mg magnesium, and 5,000 IU vitamin D (from 20 g cod liver oil) for up to two years and found a reduction in the number of exacerbations and an absence of adverse effects. This is one of very few studies in humans that employed sufficient daily doses of vitamin D (5,000 IU) and had sufficient duration (2 years). More recently, Mahon et al[37] gave 800 mg calcium and 1,000 IU vitamin D per day for six months to 39 patients with MS and noted a modest anti-inflammatory effect.

Prevention of Type 1 Diabetes

Type 1 diabetes is generally caused by autoimmune/inflammatory destruction of the pancreatic beta-cells. Vitamin D supplementation shows significant preventive and ameliorative benefits in animal models of type 1 diabetes. In a study with more than 10,000 participants, Hypponen et al[18] showed that supplementation in infants (less than one year of age) and children with 2,000 IU of vitamin D per day reduced the incidence of type 1 diabetes by approximately 80%. Relatedly, several studies using cod liver oil as a rich source of vitamin D have also documented significant reductions in the incidence of type 1 diabetes.

Depression

Seasonal affective disorder (SAD) is a particular subtype of depression characterized by the onset or exacerbation of melancholia during winter months when bright light, sun exposure, and serum 25(OH)D levels are reduced. Recently, a dose of 100,000 IU of vitamin D was found superior to light therapy in the treatment of SAD after one month.[38] Similarly, in a study involving 44 subjects, supplementation with 400 or 800 IU per day was found to significantly improve mood within five days of supplementation.[14]

Epilepsy

Seizures can be the presenting manifestation of vitamin D deficiency.[39] Hypovitaminosis D decreases the threshold for and increases the incidence of seizures, and several "anticonvulsant" drugs interfere with the formation of calcitriol in the kidney and further reduce calcitriol levels via induction of hepatic clearance. Therefore, antiepileptic drugs may lead to iatrogenic seizures by causing iatrogenic hypovitaminosis D.[40] Conversely, supplementation with 4,000-16,000 IU per day of vitamin D2 was shown to significantly reduce seizure frequency in a placebo controlled pilot study by Christiansen et al.[15]

Migraine Headaches

Calcium clearly plays a role in the maintenance of vascular tone and coagulation, both of which are altered in patients with migraine. Thys-Jacobs[41] reported two cases showing a reduction in frequency, duration, and severity of menstrual migraine attacks following daily supplementation with 1,200 mg of calcium and 1,200–1,600 IU of vitamin D in women with vitamin D deficiency.

Polycystic Ovary Syndrome

Polycystic ovary syndrome (PCOS) is a disease seen only in humans and is classically characterized by polycystic ovaries, amenorrhea, hirsuitism, insulin resistance, and obesity. Animal studies have shown that calcium is essential for oocyte activation and maturation. Vitamin D deficiency was highly prevalent among 13 women with PCOS, and supplementation with 1,500 mg of calcium per day and 50,000 IU of vitamin D2 on a weekly basis normalized menstruation and/or fertility in nine of nine women with PCOS-related menstrual irregularities within three months of treatment.[42]

Musculoskeletal Pain

Patients with non-traumatic, persistent musculoskeletal pain show an impressively high prevalence of overt vitamin D deficiency. Plotnikoff and Quigley[43] recently showed that 93% of their 150 patients with persistent, nonspecific musculoskeletal pain were overtly deficient in vitamin D. Masood et al[44] found a high prevalence of vitamin D deficiency in children with limb pain, and vitamin D supplementation ameliorated pain within three months. Al Faraj and Al Mutairi[45] found vitamin D deficiency in 83% of their 299 patients with low-back pain, and supplementation with 5,000–10,000 IU of vitamin D per day lead to pain reduction in nearly 100% of patients after three months.

Critical Illness and Autoimmune/Inflammatory Conditions

Deficiency of vitamin D is common among patients with inflammatory and autoimmune disorders and those with prolonged critical illness. In addition to the previously mentioned epidemic of vitamin D insufficiency in patients with MS, we also see evidence of vitamin D insufficiency in a large percentage of patients with Grave's disease,[46] ankylosing spondylitis,[47] systemic lupus erythematosus,[48] and rheumatoid arthritis.[20] Clinical trials with proper dosing and duration need to be performed in these patient groups. C-reactive protein was reduced by 23% and matrix metalloproteinase-9 was reduced by 68% in healthy adults following bolus injections of vitamin D that resulted in an average dose of 547 IU per day for 2.5 years.[17] A recent trial of vitamin D supplementation in patients with prolonged critical illness showed a significant and dose-dependent "anti-inflammatory effect" evidenced by reductions in IL-6 and CRP.[16] However, the insufficient dose of only 400 IU per day (administered intravenously) for only ten days precluded more meaningful and beneficial results, and we present guidelines for future studies later in this paper.

Cancer Prevention and Treatment

The inverse relationship between sunlight exposure and cancer mortality was documented by Apperly in 1941.[13] Vitamin D has anti-cancer effects mediated by anti-proliferative and proapoptotic mechanisms[3] which are augmented by modulation of nuclear receptor function and enzyme action,[49] and limited research shows that synthetic vitamin D analogs may have a role in the treatment of human cancers.[50] Grant[12] has shown that inadequate exposure to sunlight, and hence hypovitaminosis D, is associated with an increased risk of cancer mortality for several malignancies, namely those of the breast, colon, ovary, prostate, bladder, esophagus, kidney, lung, pancreas, rectum, stomach, uterus, and non-Hodgkin lymphoma. He proposes that adequate exposure to ultraviolet light and/or supplementation with vitamin D could save more than 23,000 American lives per year from a reduction in cancer mortality alone.

The aforementioned clinical trials using vitamin D in a wide range of health conditions have helped to expand our concept of vitamin D and to appreciate its manifold benefits. However, in light of new research showing that the physiologic requirement is 3,000–5,000 IU/day for adults and that serum levels plateau only after 3-4 months of daily supplementation,[2] we must conclude that studies using lower doses and/or shorter durations have underestimated the clinical efficacy of vitamin D. Guidelines for the critique and design of clinical trials are proposed later in this article to aid clinicians and researchers in evaluating and designing clinical studies for the determination of the therapeutic efficacy of vitamin D.

ASSESSMENT OF VITAMIN D STATUS WITH MEASUREMENT OF SERUM 25-OH-VITAMIN D

Current laboratory reference ranges for 25(OH)D were erroneously based on average serum levels for the "apparently healthy" nonrachitic, nonosteomalacic American population, a large proportion of which is vitamin D deficient. Currently, laboratories do not report optimal levels so they will mislead the practitioner unless he or she is aware of current research. For the majority of labs, the bottom of the reference range is set too low due to the previous underappreciation of the clinical benefits of and physiologic requirement for higher vitamin D levels, and the top of the range is too low due to previous misinterpretations of the research resulting in an overestimation of vitamin D toxicity.[1,2,51,52] Therefore, new reference ranges need to be determined based on the current research, and we present our proposals in Figure 1 and in the following outline:

• **Vitamin D Deficiency: less than 20 ng/mL (50 nmol/L).**
Serum 25(OH)D levels below 20 ng/mL (50 nmol/L) are clearly indicative of vitamin D deficiency. However, several authorities note that this level appears to be too low; Heaney[5] and Holick[51] both state that 25(OH)D levels should always be greater than 30 ng/mL (75 nmol/L).

• **Vitamin D Insufficiency: less than 40 ng/mL (100 nmol/L).**
According to Zittermann,[11] hypovitaminosis D, wherein tissue levels are depleted and PTH is slightly elevated, correlates with serum levels of 30–40 ng/mL (75–100 nmol/L). Independently, Dawson-Hughes et al[53] showed that serum levels of PTH begin to elevate when 25(OH)D levels fall below 45 ng/mL (110 nmol/L) in elderly men and women, and these findings were supported by Kinyamu et al[54] who found that optimal PTH status deteriorates when 25(OH)D levels fall below 49

ng/mL (122 nmol/L) in elderly women. Therefore, in order to maintain physiologic suppression of PTH, serum levels of 25(OH)D need to be greater than 40 ng/mL (100 nmol/L).

• Optimal Vitamin D Status: 40–65 ng/mL (100–160 nmol/L)

Based on our review of the literature, we propose that the optimal—"sufficient and safe"—range for 25(OH)D correlates with serum levels of 40–65 ng/mL (100–160 nmol/L).[55] This proposed optimal range is compatible with other published recommendations: Zittermann[11] states that serum levels of 40–80 ng/mL (100–200 nmol/L) are "adequate," and Mahon et al[37] recently advocated an optimal range of 40–100 ng/mL (100–250 nmol/L) for patients with multiple sclerosis. The lower end of our proposed range is consistent with suggestions by Mercola[56,57] who advocates an optimal range of 45–50 ng/mL (115–128 nmol/L) and by Holick[51] who states that levels should be 30–50 ng/mL (75–125 nmol/L). The upper end of our proposed optimal range is modified from the previously mentioned ranges offered by Zittermann[11] (up to 80 ng/mL [200 nmol/L]) and Mahon et al[37] (up to 100 ng/mL [250 nmol/L]). According to the authoritative monograph by Vieth,[1] there is no consistent, credible evidence of vitamin D toxicity associated with levels below 80–88 ng/mL (200 –220 nmol/L). Vieth[1] states, "Although not strictly within the 'normal' range for a clothed, sun-avoiding population, serum 25(OH)D concentrations of 220 nmol/L (88 ng/mL) are consistent with certain environments, are not unusual in the absence of vitamin D supplements, and should be regarded as being within the physiologic range for humans." Similarly, in his very thorough review of the literature, Zittermann[11] concludes that serum 25(OH)D concentrations up to 100 ng/mL (250 nmol/L) are subtoxic. Additional support for the safety of this upper limit comes from documentation that sun exposure alone can raise levels of 25(OH)D to more than 80 ng/mL (200 nmol/L)[1] and that oral supplementation with 10,000 IU/day (mimicking endogenous production from sun exposure) in healthy men resulted in serum levels greater than 80 ng/mL (200 nmol/L) with no evidence of toxicity.[2] Until more data becomes available, we have chosen 65 ng/mL (160 nmol/L) rather than 80 ng/mL (200 nmol/L) as the upper end of the optimal range to provide a safety zone between the optimal level and the level which may possibly be associated with toxicity, and to allow for other factors which may promote hypercalcemia, as discussed below. Long-term prospective interventional studies with large groups and clinical trials involving patients with vitamin D-associated illnesses (listed above) will be needed in order to accurately define the optimal range—the serum level of vitamin D that affords protection from illness but which does not cause iatrogenic complications. In reviewing much of the current literature, we found no evidence of adverse effects associated with a 25(OH)D level of 65 ng/mL (160 nmol/L), and we found that this level is considered normal by some medical laboratories[6] and that it can be approximated and safely exceeded with frequent full-body exposure to ultraviolet light[1] or oral administration of physiologic doses of 5,000–10,000 IU cholecalciferol per day for 20 weeks.[2] Prospective studies and interventional clinical trials comparing different serum levels of 25(OH)D with clinical outcomes are necessary to elucidate the exact optimal range in various clinical conditions. While no acute or subacute risks are associated with the 25(OH)D levels suggested here, research shows clear evidence of long-term danger associated with vitamin D levels that are insufficient.

• Vitamin D Excess: Serum Levels Greater than 80 ng/mL (200 nmol/L) with Accompanying Hypercalcemia

Serum levels of 25(OH)D can exceed 80 ng/mL (200 nmol/L) with ultraviolet light exposure in the absence of oral vitamin D supplementation[1,6] and with oral supplementation with 10,000 IU per day as previously mentioned[2]—in neither scenario is toxicity observed. 25(OH)D greater than 80 ng/mL (200 nmol/L) are not indicative of toxicity unless accompanied by clinical manifestations and hypercalcemia. Vieth[1] notes that hypercalcemia due to hypervitaminosis D is always associated with serum 25(OH)D concentrations greater than 88 ng/mL (220 nmol/L), and Holick[6] previously stated, "Vitamin D intoxication does not occur until the circulating levels of 25(OH)D are over 125 ng/mL [312 nmol/L]." Assessment for hypervitaminosis D is performed by measurement of serum 25(OH)D and serum calcium.

MONITORING FOR VITAMIN D TOXICITY WITH 25(OH)D AND SERUM CALCIUM

Hypercalcemia can occur with vitamin D supplementation by either directly causing direct toxicity (rare) or by being associated with a vitamin D hypersensitivity syndrome (more common). If serum calcium becomes abnormally high, then vitamin D supplementation must be discontinued until the cause of the hypercalcemia is identified; however, direct vitamin D toxicity will rarely be the sole cause of the hypercalcemia.

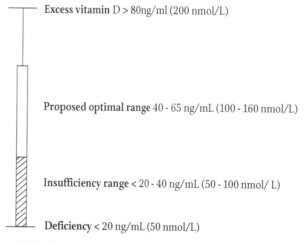

Excess vitamin D > 80ng/ml (200 nmol/L)

Proposed optimal range 40 - 65 ng/mL (100 - 160 nmol/L)

Insufficiency range < 20 - 40 ng/mL (50 - 100 nmol/ L)

Deficiency < 20 ng/mL (50 nmol/L)

* Modified from: Vasquez A. *Integrative Orthopedics: Concepts, Algorithms, and Therapeutics.* Houston; Natural Health Consulting Corporation. 2004: 417-419 with permission.

FIGURE 1. Proposed normal and optimal ranges for serum 25(OH)D levels based on current research*

The most important indicator of direct vitamin D toxicity is elevated serum calcium associated with a 25(OH)D level greater than 90 ng/ml (225 nmol/L). Elevated 1,25(OH)D levels are commonly—though not always—seen with vitamin D toxicity. Severe vitamin D intoxication is rare and usually seen only with industrial accidents, such as overdosing the fortification of milk, or with long-term administration of more than 40,000 IU of vitamin D per day. Severe hypercalcemia may require urinary acidification and corticosteroids to expedite the reduction in serum calcium.[58]

Induction of vitamin D toxicity generally requires 1–4 months of 40,000 IU per day in infants.[58] In adults, toxicity generally requires several months of supplementation of at least 100,000 IU per day. Hypercalcemia appears to be the mechanism of vitamin D toxicity (rather than a direct toxic effect of the vitamin), and 25-OH-vitamin D levels may be normal in patients who are vitamin D toxic and hypercalcemic, particularly with vitamin D hypersensitivity syndrome. It has therefore been suggested that serum calcium be measured on a weekly and then monthly basis in patients receiving high-dose vitamin D. Manifestations attributable to hypervitaminosis D and hypercalcemia include anorexia, nausea, and vomiting followed by weakness, nervousness, pruritus, polyuria, polydipsia, renal impairment, and soft-tissue calcifications.

As a cause of hypercalcemia, vitamin D hypersensitivity syndromes are more common than vitamin D toxicity, and they generally arise when aberrant tissue uncontrollably produces the most active form of the vitamin—calcitriol. Primary hyperparathyroidism, granulomatous disease (such as sarcoidosis, Crohn's disease, and tuberculosis) and various forms of cancer may cause the syndrome. 25(OH)D levels are normal or even low in vitamin D hypersensitivity while serum calcium and 1,25(OH)D levels are elevated. Additional causes include adrenal insufficiency, hyperthyroidism, hypothyroidism, and adverse drug effects, particularly with thiazide diuretics. Whatever the cause, patients with persistent hypercalcemia should discontinue vitamin D supplementation and receive a thorough diagnostic evaluation to determine the cause of the problem.

Interventional Strategies to Treat Vitamin D Deficiency by Increasing Serum Vitamin D Levels

Human physiology adapted to and was shaped by a natural environment with ample exposure to sunlight.[5, 61] Full-body exposure to ultraviolet light on clear days in equatorial latitudes can easily provide the equivalent of 4,000–20,000 IU of vitamin D.[1,61] Slightly longer durations of full-body sun exposure of approximately 30 minutes (3x the minimal erythemal dose) will produce 50,000 IU of vitamin D in lightly pigmented persons, while 5x longer durations are required for more darkly pigmented people to attain the same vitamin D production.[61] The oral dose of vitamin D required to obtain adequate blood levels depends on latitude, sun exposure, body weight, skin pigmentation, dietary sources, efficiency of absorption, presence of intestinal disease (eg, intestinal resection or malabsorption), and medication use, for example with the vitamin D-depleting actions of common anticonvulsant drugs.[40]

Past and Future Vitamin D Studies: Critique and Design

Nearly all published clinical trials have suffered from flawed design, including inadequate dosing, inadequate duration, wrong type of vitamin D (ie, ergocalciferol, D2), failure to test serum vitamin D levels, and/or failure to ensure that serum vitamin D levels entered into the optimal range. The following guidelines are provided for clinicians and researchers using vitamin D in clinical practice and research to improve the quality of research and patient care.

1. Dosages of vitamin D must reflect physiologic requirements and natural endogenous production and should therefore be in the range of 3,000–10,000 IU per day

The physiologic requirement for vitamin D appears to be 3,000–5,000 IU per day in adult males.[2] Full-body exposure to ultraviolet light (eg, sunshine) can produce the equivalent of 10,000–25,000 IU of vitamin D3 per day.[1] Therefore, intervention trials with supplemental vitamin D should use between 4,000 IU/day, which is presumably sufficient to meet physiologic demands, and 10,000 IU/day, which is the physiologic dose attained naturally via full-body sun exposure. Based on these physiologic criteria, we see that the majority of intervention studies in adults have used inadequate, subphysiologic doses of vitamin D. Therefore, studies that failed to identify therapeutic benefits from vitamin D supplementation were flawed due to insufficient therapeutic intervention—the dose of vitamin D was too low.

2. Vitamin D supplementation must be continued for at least 5-9 months for maximum benefit

Since serum 25(OH)D levels do not plateau until after 3-4 months of supplementation,[2] and we would expect clinical and biochemical changes to become optimally apparent some time after the attainment of peak serum levels, any intervention study of less than 5-9 months is of insufficient duration to determine either maximum benefit or that vitamin D supplementation is ineffective for the condition being investigated. Conversely, since vitamin D supplementation can alter intracellular metabolism within minutes of administration,[11] benefits seen in short-term studies should not be inaccurately attributed to statistical error or placebo effect.

3. Supplementation should be performed with D3 rather than D2

Although cholecalciferol (vitamin D3) and ergocalciferol (vitamin D2) are both used as sources of vitamin D, D3 is the human nutrient and is much more efficient in raising and sustaining serum 25[OH]D levels. Vitamin D2 is a fungal metabolite and has been associated with adverse effects due to contamination and altered pharmacokinetics.[4] The type of vitamin D must always be clearly stated in published research reports.

4. Supplements should be tested for potency

Some products do not contain their claimed amount. This problem was illustrated in the study by Heaney et al[2] who found that the vitamin D supplement they used in their study, although produced by a well-known company, contained only 83% of its stated value. To ensure accuracy and consistency of clinical trials, actual dosages must be known.

5. Effectiveness of supplementation must include evaluation of serum vitamin D levels

Supplementation does not maximize therapeutic efficacy unless it raises serum 25(OH)D levels into the optimal range. To assess absorption, compliance, and safety, serum 25(OH)D levels must be monitored in clinical trials involving vitamin D supplementation. Assessment of serum levels is important also to determine the relative dose-effectiveness of different preparations of vitamin D, as some evidence suggests that micro-emulsification facilitates absorption of fat-soluble nutrients.[56,59,60] Measurement of 1,25-dihydroxyvitamin (calcitriol) is potentially misleading and is not recommended for the evaluation of vitamin D status.

6. Serum vitamin D levels must enter the optimal range

The majority of clinical intervention studies using vitamin D have failed to use supplementation of sufficient dosage and duration to attain optimal serum levels of vitamin D. Our proposed optimal range for 25(OH)D is 40–65 ng/mL (100–160 nmol/L) and is presented in Figure 1.

The above-mentioned criteria will aid future researchers in designing interventional studies that can accurately evaluate the relationship between vitamin D status and human illness. Clinicians, who are not conducting research but rather are interested in attaining clinical improvement in their patients, should follow these guidelines as well when using vitamin D supplementation in patients, while remembering to monitor for toxicity with the triad of clinical assessments, serum 25(OH)D, and serum calcium. Clinicians and researchers need to remember, however, that optimal clinical effectiveness often depends on synergism of diet, lifestyle, exercise, emotional health, and other factors. Single intervention studies are a reasonable research tool only for evaluating cause-and-effect relationships based on the presumption of a simplistic, linear model that is generally inconsistent with the complexity and multiplicity of synergistic and interconnected factors that determine health and disease. Thus, single intervention studies with vitamin D supplementation will be useful from an intellectual standpoint insofar as they will help us to further define the role of vitamin D in human physiology and pathophysiology. However, optimal clinical results with individual patients are more easily attained with the use of multicomponent treatment plans that address many facets of the patient's health.[55]

Vitamin D Supplementation in Adults

When 28 men and women were administered 4,000 IU per day for up to five months, in the absence of UVB from the sun, serum 25(OH)D levels reached approximately 40 ng/mL (100 nmol/L), and no toxicity was observed.[4] When 67 men were administered 5,000 and 10,000 IU of cholecalciferol per day for twenty weeks, again in the absence of UVB from the sun, serum levels of 25(OH)D increased to approximately 60 ng/mL (150 nmol/L) and 90 ng/mL (225 nmol/L), respectively, and no toxicity was observed.[2] Therefore, given that endogenous vitamin D production following full-body sun exposure at lower latitudes can produce >10,000 IU[1] and that 4,000 IU per day is a safe level of supplementation[4] that meets physiologic needs in adults,[2] we recommend at least 4,000 IU per day for adults, with efficacy and safety ensured by periodic measurement of 25(OH)D and serum calcium.

Vitamin D Supplementation in Pregnant Women

In 1966, two case reports and a brief review of the literature showed no adverse effects of 100,000 IU per day of vitamin D in hypoparathyroid pregnant women.[62] In 1971, a study of 15 hypoparathyroid pregnant women was reported wherein the women received more than 100,000 IU per day of vitamin D with no adverse effects to the mother or child, leading the authors to conclude that there was "no risk from vitamin D in pregnancy."[63] Doses of vitamin D for pregnant women were extensively reviewed by Hollis and Wagner[61] immediately prior to the completion of this article, and the authors concluded that doses of 100,000 IU per day were safe for pregnant women. The authors write, "Thus, there is no evidence in humans that even a 100,000 IU/day dose of vitamin D for extended periods during pregnancy results in any harmful effects." Data from several placebo-controlled clinical trials with pregnant women show that vitamin D supplementation results in superior health status for the mother and infant. The current daily reference intake (DRI) for vitamin D of 200–400 IU per day is therefore "grossly inadequate," and administration of less than 1,000 IU vitamin D per day to pregnant women is scientifically unjustifiable and ethically questionable. Hollis and Wagner[61] conclude that up to 4,000 IU per day is necessary for pregnant women, and this conclusion is consistent with previously cited research on physiologic requirements[2] and endogenous vitamin D production.[1] In order to ensure safety and efficacy in individual patients, we encourage periodic measurement of serum calcium and 25(OH)D levels.

Vitamin D Supplementation in Infants and Children

In Finland from the mid-1950s until 1964, the recommended daily intake of vitamin D for infants was 4,000–5,000 IU, a dose that was proven safe and was associated with significant protection from type 1 diabetes.[61] More recently, in a study involving more than 10,000 infants and children, daily administration of 2,000 IU per day was safe and effective for reducing the incidence of type 1 diabetes by 80%.[18] Thus, for infants and children, doses of 1,000 IU per day are certainly safe, and higher doses should be monitored by serum calcium and 25(OH)D levels.

Options for Raising Vitamin D Blood Levels

We have two practical options for increasing vitamin D levels in the body: oral supplementation and/or exposure to ultraviolet radiation. Sunlight is commonly unavailable on rainy or cloudy days, during the winter months, and in particular geographic locations. Topical sunscreens block vitamin D production by 97%-100%. Furthermore, since many people work indoors where sunshine is inaccessible, or they are partially or fully clothed when outside, reliance on sunshine to provide optimal levels of vitamin D is generally destined to provide unsatisfactory and inconsistent biochemical and clinical results. The use of UVB tanning beds can increase vitamin D levels; but this option is more expensive and time-consuming than oral supplementation, and excess ultraviolet radiation exposure expedites skin aging and encourages the development of skin cancer. Given the impracticalities and disadvantages associated with relying on sun exposure to provide optimal levels of vitamin D year-round, for the majority of patients, oral vitamin D supplementation is the better option for ensuring that biochemical needs are consistently met.

Vitamin D is either absent or present in non-therapeutic amounts in dietary sources. One of the only major dietary sources of vitamin D is cod-liver oil, but the amount required to obtain a target dose of 4,000 IU per day would require patients to consume at least three tablespoons of cod-liver oil, or the amount contained in >18 capsules of most commercial preparations.[55] Clearly this would be unpalatable and prohibitively expensive for most patients, and it would result in very low compliance. Additionally, such a high dose of cod-liver oil may produce adverse effects with long-term use, particularly with regard to excess vitamin A, and perhaps an increased tendency for bleeding and reduced biological activity of gamma-linolenic acid due to the high content of eicosapentaenoic acid.[55,64] Oral supplementation with "pure" vitamin D supplements allows the dose to be tailored to the individual needs of the patient.

DISCUSSION AND CONCLUSIONS

Vitamin D is not a drug, nor should it be restricted to prescription availability. Vitamin D is not a new or unproven "treatment." Vitamin D is an endogenous, naturally occurring, photochemically-produced steroidal molecule with essential functions in systemic homeostasis and physiology, including modulation of calcium metabolism, cell proliferation, cardiovascular dynamics, immune/inflammatory balance, neurologic function, and genetic expression. Insufficient endogenous production due to lack of sufficient sun exposure necessitates oral supplementation to meet physiologic needs. Failure to meet physiologic needs creates insufficiency/deficiency and results in subtle yet widespread disturbances in cellular function which appear to promote the manifestation of subacute long-latency deficiency diseases such as osteoporosis, cardiovascular disease, hypertension, cancer, depression, epilepsy, type 1 diabetes, insulin resistance, autoimmune disease, migraine, polycystic ovary syndrome, and musculoskeletal pain. In case reports, clinical trials, animal studies, and/or epidemiologic surveys, the provision of vitamin D via sunlight or supplementation has been shown to safely help prevent or alleviate all of the aforementioned conditions.

Vitamin D deficiency/insufficiency is an epidemic in the developed world that has heretofore received insufficient attention from clinicians despite documentation of its prevalence, consequences, and the imperative for daily supplementation at levels above the current inadequate recommendations of 200–600 IU.[65] For example, at least 57% of 290 medical inpatients in Massachusetts, USA were found to be vitamin D deficient,[66] and overt vitamin D deficiency was recently found in 93% of 150 patients with chronic musculoskeletal pain in Minnesota, USA.[43] Other studies in Americans have shown vitamin D deficiency in 48% of patients with multiple sclerosis,[37] 50% of patients with fibromyalgia and systemic lupus erythematosus,[48] 42% of healthy adolescents[67] and African American women,[68] and at least 62% of the morbidly obese.[69] International studies are consistent with the worldwide prevalence of vitamin D deficiency in various patient groups, showing vitamin D deficiency in 83% of 360 patients with chronic low-back pain in Saudi Arabia,[45] 73% of Austrian patients with ankylosing spondylitis,[47] up to 58% of Japanese women with Grave's disease,[46] more than 40% of Chinese adolescent girls,[70] and 40%-70% of Finnish medical patients.[71] As a medically valid diagnosis (ICD-9 code: 268.9 Unspecified vitamin D deficiency) with a high prevalence and clinically significant morbidity, vitamin D deficiency deserves equal attention and status with other diagnoses encountered in clinical practice. Given the depth and breadth of the peer-reviewed research documenting the frequency and consequences of hypovitaminosis D, failure to diagnose and treat this disorder is ethically questionable (particularly in pregnant women[61]) and is inconsistent with the delivery of quality, science-based healthcare. Failure to act prudently based on the research now available in favor of vitamin D supplementation appears likely to invite repetition analogous to the previous failure to act on the research supporting the use of folic acid to prevent cardiovascular disease and neural tube defects—a blunder that appears to have resulted in hundreds of thousands of unnecessary cardiovascular deaths[72] and which has contributed to incalculable human suffering related to otherwise unnecessary neural tube defects, cervical dysplasia, cancer, osteoporosis, and mental depression. Currently, Grant[12] estimates that at least 23,000 and perhaps as many as 47,000 cancer deaths[73] might be prevented each year in America if we employed simple interventions (ie, sunshine or supplementation) to raise vitamin D levels. Of course, additional lives may be saved and suffering reduced by alleviating the morbidity and mortality associated with hypertension, autoimmune disease, depression, epilepsy, migraine, diabetes, polycystic ovary syndrome, musculoskeletal pain, osteoporosis, and cardiovascular disease. Until proven otherwise, the balance of the research clearly indicates that oral supplementation in the range of 1,000 IU/day for infants, 2,000 IU/day for children, and 4,000 IU/day for adults is safe and reasonable to meet physiologic requirements, to promote optimal health, and to reduce the risk of several serious diseases. Safety and effectiveness of supplementation are assured by periodic monitoring of serum 25(OH)D and serum calcium.

References

1. Vieth R. Vitamin D supplementation, 25-hydroxyvitamin D concentrations, and safety. *Am J Clin Nutr.* 1999;69(5):842-56.
2. Heaney RP, Davies KM, Chen TC, Holick MF, Barger-Lux MJ. Human serum 25-hydroxycholecalciferol response to extended oral dosing with cholecalciferol. *Am J Clin Nutr.* 2003;77(1):204-10.
3. Holick MF. Vitamin D: importance in the prevention of cancers, type 1 diabetes, heart disease, and osteoporosis. *Am J Clin Nutr.* 2004;79(3):362-71.
4. Vieth R, Chan PC, MacFarlane GD. Efficacy and safety of vitamin D3 intake exceeding the lowest observed adverse effect level. *Am J Clin Nutr.* 2001;73(2):288-94.
5. Heaney RP. Long-latency deficiency disease: insights from calcium and vitamin D. *Am J Clin Nutr.* 2003;78(5):912-9.
6. Holick MF. Calcium and Vitamin D. Diagnostics and Therapeutics. *Clin Lab Med.* 2000;20(3):569-90.
7. Kamycheva E, Sundsfjord J, Jorde R. Serum parathyroid hormone levels predict coronary heart disease: the Tromso Study. *Eur J Cardiovasc Prev Rehabil.* 2004;11(1):69-74.
8. Sato Y, Kaji M, Metoki N, Satoh K, Iwamoto J. Does compensatory hyperparathyroidism predispose to ischemic stroke? *Neurology.* 2003;60(4):626-9.
9. Fujita T. Calcium paradox: consequences of calcium deficiency manifested by a wide variety of diseases. *J Bone Miner Metab.* 2000;18(4):234-6.
10. Zehnder D, Bland R, Williams MC, McNinch RW, Howie AJ, Stewart PM, Hewison M. Extrarenal expression of 25-hydroxyvitamin d(3)-1 alpha-hydroxylase. *J Clin Endocrinol Metab.* 2001;86(2):888-94.
11. Zittermann A. Vitamin D in preventive medicine: are we ignoring the evidence? *Br J Nutr.* 2003;89(5):552-72.
12. Grant WB. An estimate of premature cancer mortality in the U.S. due to inadequate doses of solar ultraviolet-B radiation. *Cancer.* 2002;94(6):1867-75.
13. Apperly FL. The relation of solar radiation to cancer mortality in North America. *Cancer Res.* 1941;1:191-5.
14. Lansdowne AT, Provost SC. Vitamin D3 enhances mood in healthy subjects during winter. *Psychopharmacology* (Berl). 1998;135(4):319-23.
15. Christiansen C, Rodbro P, Sjo O. "Anticonvulsant action" of vitamin D in epileptic patients? A controlled pilot study. *Br Med J.* 1974;2(913):258-9.
16. Van den Berghe G, Van Roosbroeck D, Vanhove P, Wouters PJ, De Pourcq L, Bouillon R. Bone turnover in prolonged critical illness: effect of vitamin D. *J Clin Endocrinol Metab.* 2003;88(10):4623-32.
17. Timms PM, Mannan N, Hitman GA, Noonan K, Mills PG, Syndercombe-Court D, Aganna E, Price CP, Boucher BJ. Circulating MMP9, vitamin D and variation in the TIMP-1 response with VDR genotype: mechanisms for inflammatory damage in chronic disorders? *QJM.* 2002;95:787-96.
18. Hypponen E, Laara E, Reunanen A, Jarvelin MR, Virtanen SM. Intake of vitamin D and risk of type 1 diabetes: a birth-cohort study. *Lancet.* 2001;358(9292):1500-3.
19. Goldberg P, Fleming MC, Picard EH. Multiple sclerosis: decreased relapse rate through dietary supplementation with calcium, magnesium and vitamin D. *Med Hypotheses.* 1986 Oct;21(2):193-200.
20. Cantorna MT. Vitamin D and autoimmunity: is vitamin D status an environmental factor affecting autoimmune disease prevalence? *Proc Soc Exp Biol Med.* 2000;223(3):230-3
21. Wayse V, Yousafzai A, Mogale K, Filteau S. Association of subclinical vitamin D deficiency with severe acute lower respiratory infection in Indian children under 5 y. *Eur J Clin Nutr.* 2004;58(4):563-7.
22. Scragg R. Seasonality of cardiovascular disease mortality and the possible protective effect of ultra-violet radiation. *Int J Epidemiol.* 1981;10(4):337-41
23. Scragg R, Jackson R, Holdaway IM, Lim T, Beaglehole R. Myocardial infarction is inversely associated with plasma 25-hydroxyvitamin D3 levels: a community-based study. *Int J Epidemiol.* 1990;19(3):559-63.
24. Zittermann A, Schleithoff SS, Tenderich G, Berthold HK, Korfer R, Stehle P. Low vitamin D status: a contributing factor in the pathogenesis of congestive heart failure? *J Am Coll Cardiol.* 2003;41:105-12.
25. Gulati S, Bajpai A, Juneja R, Kabra M, Bagga A, Kalra V. Hypocalcemic heart failure masquerading as dilated cardiomyopathy. *Indian J Pediatr.* 2001;68(3):287-90.
26. Brunvand L, Haga P, Tangsrud SE, Haug E. Congestive heart failure caused by vitamin D deficiency? *Acta Paediatr.* 1995;84(1):106-8.
27. Kini SM, Pednekar SJ, Nabar ST, Varthakavi P. A reversible form of cardiomyopathy. *J Postgrad Med.* 2003;49(1):85-7.
28. Olgun H, Ceviz N, Ozkan B. A case of dilated cardiomyopathy due to nutritional vitamin D deficiency rickets. *Turk J Pediatr.* 2003;45(2):152-4.
29. Price DI, Stanford LC Jr, Braden DS, Ebeid MR, Smith JC. Hypocalcemic rickets: an unusual cause of dilated cardiomyopathy. *Pediatr Cardiol.* 2003;24(5):510-2.
30. Rostand SG. Ultraviolet light may contribute to geographic and racial blood pressure differences. *Hypertension.* 1997;30(2 Pt 1):150-6.
31. Krause R, Buhring M, Hopfenmuller W, Holick MF, Sharma AM. Ultraviolet B and blood pressure. *Lancet.* 1998;352(9129):709-10.
32. Pfeifer M, Begerow B, Minne HW, Nachtigall D, Hansen C. Effects of a short-term vitamin D(3) and calcium supplementation on blood pressure and parathyroid hormone levels in elderly women. *J Clin Endocrinol Metab.* 2001;86(4):1633-7.
33. Chiu KC, Chu A, Vay LWG, Saad MF. Hypovitaminosis D is associated with insulin resistance and beta cell dysfunction. *Am J Clin Nutr.* 2004; 79:820-5.
34. Borissova AM, Tankova T, Kirilov G, Dakovska L, Kovacheva R. The effect of vitamin D3 on insulin secretion and peripheral insulin sensitivity in type 2 diabetic patients. *Int J Clin Pract.* 2003;57(4):258-61.
35. McAlindon TE, Felson DT, Zhang Y, Hannan MT, Aliabadi P, Weissman B, Rush D, Wilson PW, Jacques P. Relation of dietary intake and serum levels of vitamin D to progression of osteoarthritis of the knee among participants in the Framingham Study. *Ann Intern Med.* 1996;125(5):353-9.
36. Lane NE, Gore LR, Cummings SR, Hochberg MC, Scott JC, Williams EN, Nevitt MC. Serum vitamin D levels and incident changes of radiographic hip osteoarthritis: a longitudinal study. Study of Osteoporotic Fractures Research Group. *Arthritis Rheum.* 1999;42(5):854-60.
37. Mahon BD, Gordon SA, Cruz J, Cosman F, Cantorna MT. Cytokine profile in patients with multiple sclerosis following vitamin D supplementation. *J Neuroimmunol.* 2003;134(1-2):128-32.
38. Gloth FM 3rd, Alam W, Hollis B. Vitamin D vs broad spectrum phototherapy in the treatment of seasonal affective disorder. *J Nutr Health Aging.* 1999;3(1):5-7
39. Johnson GH, Willis F. Seizures as the presenting feature of rickets in an infant. *Med J Aust.* 2003;178(9):467; discussion 467-8.
40. Ali FE, Al-Bustan MA, Al-Busairi WA, Al-Mulla FA. Loss of seizure control due to anticonvulsant-induced hypocalcemia. *Ann Pharmacother.* 2004;38(6):1002-5
41. Thys-Jacobs S. Vitamin D and calcium in menstrual migraine. *Headache.* 1994 Oct;34(9):544-6.
42. Thys-Jacobs S, Donovan D, Papadopoulos A, Sarrel P, Bilezikian JP. Vitamin D and calcium dysregulation in the polycystic ovarian syndrome. *Steroids.* 1999;64(6):430-5.
43. Plotnikoff GA, Quigley JM. Prevalence of severe hypovitaminosis D in patients with persistent, nonspecific musculoskeletal pain. *Mayo Clin Proc.* 2003;78(12):1463-70
44. Masood H, Narang AP, Bhat IA, Shah GN. Persistent limb pain and raised serum alkaline phosphatase the earliest markers of subclinical hypovitaminosis D in Kashmir. *Indian J Physiol Pharmacol.* 1989;33(4):259-61.
45. Al Faraj S, Al Mutairi K. Vitamin D deficiency and chronic low back pain in Saudi Arabia. *Spine.* 2003;28(2):177-9.
46. Yamashita H, Noguchi S, Takatsu K, Koike E, Murakami T, Watanabe S, Uchino S, Yamashita H, Kawamoto H. High prevalence of vitamin D deficiency in Japanese female patients with Graves' disease. *Endocr J.* 2001;48(1):63-9.
47. Falkenbach A, Tripathi R, Sedlmeyer A, Staudinger M, Herold M. Serum 25-hydroxyvitamin D and parathyroid hormone in patients with ankylosing spondylitis before and after a three-week rehabilitation treatment at high altitude during winter and spring. *Wien Klin Wochenschr.* 2001;113(9):328-32.
48. Huisman AM, White KP, Algra A, Harth M, Vieth R, Jacobs JW, Bijlsma JW, Bell DA. Vitamin D levels in women with systemic lupus erythematosus and fibromyalgia. *J Rheumatol.* 2001;28(11):2535-9.
49. Banerjee P, Chatterjee M. Antiproliferative role of vitamin D and its analogs--a brief overview. *Mol Cell Biochem.* 2003;253(1-2):247-54.
50. Trouillas P, Honnorat J, Bret P, Jouvet A, Gerard JP. Redifferentiation therapy in brain tumors: long-lasting complete regression of glioblastomas and an anaplastic astrocytoma under long term 1-alpha-hydroxycholecalciferol. *J Neurooncol.* 2001;51(1):57-66
51. Holick MF. Vitamin D deficiency: what a pain it is. *Mayo Clin Proc.* 2003;78(12):1457-9
52. Wright JV. Vitamin D: Its Role in Autoimmune Disease and Hypertension. *Townsend Letter for Doctors and Patients.* 2004; May #250: 75-78.
53. Dawson-Hughes B, Harris SS, Dallal GE. Plasma calcidiol, season, and serum parathyroid hormone concentrations in healthy elderly men and women. *Am J Clin Nutr.* 1997;65(1):67-71.
54. Kinyamu HK, Gallagher JC, Rafferty KA, Balhorn KE. Dietary calcium and vitamin D intake in elderly women: effect on serum parathyroid hormone and vitamin D metabolites. *Am J Clin Nutr.* 1998;67(2):342-8.
55. Vasquez A. *Integrative Orthopedics: Concepts, Algorithms, and Therapeutics.* Houston; Natural Health Consulting Corporation (www.OptimalHealthResearch.com): 2004. Pages 417-419 and website updates.
56. Mercola J. Available at: http://www.mercola.com/forms/vitamind.htm. Accessed July 23, 2004.
57. Mercola J. Test Values and Treatment for Vitamin D Deficiency. Available at: http://www.mercola.com/2002/feb/23/vitamin_d_deficiency.htm. Accessed July 23, 2004.
58. Berkow R, Fletcher AJ. *The Merck Manual of Diagnosis and Therapy.* Fifteenth Edition. Rathway; Merck Sharp and Dohme Research Laboratories. 1987: 928, 974-5.
59. Bucci LR, Pillors M, Medlin R, Henderson R, Stiles JC, Robol HJ, Sparks WS. Enhanced uptake in humans of coenzyme Q10 from an emulsified form. Third International Congress of Biomedical Gerontology; Acapulco, Mexico: June 1989.
60. Bucci LR, Pillors M, Medlin R, Klenda B, Robol H, Stiles JC, Sparks WS. *Enhanced blood levels of coenzyme Q-10 from an emulsified oral form.* In Faruqui SR and Ansari MS (editors). Second Symposium on Nutrition and Chiropractic Proceedings. April 15-16, 1989 in Davenport, Iowa
61. Hollis BW, Wagner CL. Assessment of dietary vitamin D requirements during pregnancy and lactation. *Am J Clin Nutr.* 2004;79(5):717-26.
62. O'Leary JA, Klainer LM, Neuwirth RS. The management of hypoparathyroidism in pregnancy. *Am J Obstet Gynecol.* 1966;94(8):1103-7.
63. Goodenday LS, Gordon GS. No risk from vitamin D in pregnancy. *Ann Intern Med.* 1971;75(5):807-8.
64. Horrobin DF. Interactions between n-3 and n-6 essential fatty acids (EFAs) in the regulation of cardiovascular disorders and inflammation. *Prostaglandins Leukot Essent Fatty Acids.* 1991;44(2):127-31.
65. Utiger RD. The need for more vitamin D. *N Engl J Med.* 1998;338:828-9
66. Thomas MK, Lloyd-Jones DM, Thadhani RI, Shaw AC, Deraska DJ, Kitch BT, Vamvakas EC, Dick IM, Prince RL, Finkelstein JS. Hypovitaminosis D in medical inpatients. *N Engl J Med.* 1998;338(12):777-83.
67. Gordon CM, DePeter KC, Feldman HA, Grace E, Emans SJ. Prevalence of vitamin D deficiency among healthy adolescents. *Arch Pediatr Adolesc Med.* 2004;158(6):531-7.
68. Nesby-O'Dell S, Scanlon KS, Cogswell ME, Gillespie C, Hollis BW, Looker AC, Allen C, Doughertly C, Gunter EW, Bowman BA. Hypovitaminosis D prevalence and determinants among African American and white women of reproductive age: third National Health and Nutrition Examination Survey, 1988-1994. *Am J Clin Nutr.* 2002;76:187-92.
69. Buffington C, Walker B, Cowan GS Jr, Scruggs D. Vitamin D Deficiency in the Morbidly Obese. *Obes Surg.* 1993;3:421-424.
70. Fraser DR. Vitamin D-deficiency in Asia. *J Steroid Biochem Mol Biol.* 2004;89-90:491-5
71. Kauppinen-Makelin R, Tahtela R, Loyttyniemi E, Karkkainen J, Valimaki MJ. A high prevalence of hypovitaminosis D in Finnish medical in- and outpatients. *J Intern Med.* 2001;249(6):559-63.
72. Ellis A. Inertia on folic acid has caused thousands of unnecessary deaths. *BMJ.* 2003;326(7398):1054.
73. Grant WB. Personal communication by email, "My current estimate is 47,000 premature cancer deaths/year." June 3, 2004.

CME
CONTINUING MEDICAL EDUCATION

CME TEST INSTRUCTIONS

To receive 2.0 hours of CME credit for this article, visit www.cecmeonline.com, log in, purchase the CME course for $10 and take the online test. This test is valid for 1 year from the date of publication. Within 3 to 4 weeks of InnoVision Communications receiving your completed online test, you will receive a CME certificate.

InnoVision Communications is accredited by the Accreditation Council for Continuing Medical Education to provide continuing medical education for physicians. InnoVision Communications designates these educational activities on an hour-for-hour basis toward category 1 credit of the AMA Physician's Recognition Award. Each physician should claim only those hours of credit that he/she actually spent in the educational activity.

CME TEST QUESTIONS*

THE CLINICAL IMPORTANCE OF VITAMIN D (CHOLECALCIFEROL): A PARADIGM SHIFT WITH IMPLICATIONS FOR ALL HEALTHCARE PROVIDERS

In the following questions, only one answer is correct.

1. In clinical trials, augmentation of vitamin D levels with ultraviolet light exposure or oral supplementation has been shown to benefit which of the following conditions:
   A. Osteoporosis; Hypertension
   B. Depression; Multiple sclerosis
   C. Back pain; Insulin resistance
   D. All of the above

2. In the absence of vitamin D supplementation, ultraviolet light exposure (ie, sunshine) can produce 25(OH)D levels that exceed current laboratory reference ranges:
   A. True
   B. False

3. Which of the following can cause hypercalcemia?
   A. Sarcoidosis and Crohn's disease
   B. Adrenal insufficiency and hypothyroidism
   C. Coadministration of vitamin D and thiazide diuretics
   D. All of the above

4. According to the current research literature reviewed in this article, which of the following may be considered long-latency deficiency diseases associated with insufficiency of vitamin D?
   A. Metabolic syndrome
   B. Autoimmune disease such as multiple sclerosis and type 1 diabetes
   C. Depression and cancer
   D. All of the above

5. If a patient has hypovitaminosis D and a vitamin D-responsive condition such as depression, hypertension, insulin resistance, or multiple sclerosis, which of the following is appropriate first-line treatment?
   A. Drugs only
   B. Vitamin D only
   C. Correction of the vitamin D deficiency, and co-administration of medications if necessary
   D. Use of synthetic vitamin D analogs

6. Since vitamin D is highly effective for the prevention and alleviation of several health problems, and because it has a wide range of safety, physiologic doses should be regulated as a prescription drug and prohibited from public access:
   A. True
   B. False

7. Given the prevalence and consequences of vitamin D deficiency, failure to test for and treat vitamin D insufficiency is ethical:
   A. True
   B. False

8. Since vitamin D has a wide margin of safety, patients should be administered vitamin D routinely and receive which of the following types of monitoring:
   A. Periodic measurement of serum 1,25-dihydroxyvitamin D (calcitriol) and urinary creatinine
   B. Periodic measurement of serum 25-hydroxyvitamin D (calcidiol) and serum calcium
   C. Clinical assessments only
   D. Liver function tests and electrocardiography

See page 94 for Self-Assessment answers

Reducing Pain and Inflammation Naturally
Part I: New Insights into Fatty Acid Biochemistry and the Influence of Diet

Alex Vasquez, DC, ND

PAIN AND INFLAMMATION ARE NEUROCHEMICAL MANIFESTATIONS of physiologic imbalances which originate biochemically, structurally, and/or neurologically. Beyond the obvious relevance to the treatment of conditions associated with pain and inflammation, the implications of the data presented will provide therapeutic insight for doctors treating a wide range of complex chronic illnesses. Given the strength and momentum of this research, combined with the public's increasing interest in alternatives to dangerous, expensive, and often ineffective pharmaceutical treatments, the time has come for the chiropractic profession to assume a more empowered leadership position in the provision of healthcare and the prevention and treatment of most chronic health problems.

INTRODUCTION:

Since its inception, the chiropractic profession has recognized and affirmed the importance and benefits of whole-patient healthcare.[1,2] In contrast to the medical model of disease, which generally seeks to use synthetic drugs to target isolated biochemical pathways, the holistic model of health and disease appreciates that a multifaceted approach including physical (structural, biomechanical, anatomical), biochemical (nutritional, hormonal, neurochemical), and psychoemotional assessments and interventions is commonly safer, more effective, and less expensive in the long-term for the restoration and preservation of optimal health.[3] Extensive documentation in support of these concepts and their clinical applications has recently been compiled by the current author in a 486-page manuscript.[4]

While the benefits, safety, and cost-effectiveness of physical medicine and spinal manipulation have been well established in journal articles and commissioned reports,[5,6] it is only within the past few years that we have seen a literal explosion of high-quality research supporting the concept that skillful phytonutritional interventions can have a powerful and beneficial influence on patient outcomes for a wide range of health concerns. Thus, as the only nationally-licensed healthcare providers with training in nutrition, chiropractic physicians should claim their proper position of leadership in the management of chronic health disorders.

The research increasingly points to inflammation as a common determinant of many diseases, including cancer, cardiovascular disease, neurologic conditions, diabetes, arthritis, and the so-called autoimmune diseases such as rheumatoid arthritis, lupus, and multiple sclerosis. Additionally, new research is also documenting the powerful influence of nutrition on optimal cell membrane dynamics, neurotransmitter/hormone receptor function, and modification of gene expression. The most powerful, cost-effective, and fundamental means for effectively addressing all of these processes—1) inflammation, 2) cell membrane dynamics, 3) neurotransmitter/hormone receptor function, and 4) gene expression—is with skillful nutritional intervention: dietary improvement and phytonutritional supplementation. In particular, modulation of fatty acid metabolism by supplementation with nutritional oils is the most efficient means to achieve all four of the above-mentioned goals.

FOOD AND INFLAMMATION:

The adage "One man's food is another man's poison" finds particular relevance when we are dealing with patients experiencing pain and inflammation. Although dietary recommendations must always be customized for each individual patient, we can confidently make certain general recommendations to help these patients overcome their health problems and to feel and function better. Conceptually, we can organize our ideas about foods into the following categories: 1) foods to avoid, 2) foods to consume, 3) customized recommendations with regard to allergies, sensitivities, and intolerances.

Foods to Avoid: Many doctors and patients are unaware of the pro-inflammatory nature of many commonly eaten foods.[7] As long as patients continue to consume pro-inflammatory chemicals in their foods on a daily basis, then they will continue to fight an uphill battle against pain and inflammation. Generally speaking, eating is itself a pro-inflammatory event, with sugars and fats inducing more inflammation than protein-containing foods.[8] Therefore, simple sugars and high-fat foods should be avoided. Two fatty acids in particular, linoleic acid (LA) and arachidonic acid (ARA) from the n-6 family should be reduced or eliminated from the diet to the extent possible. LA increases inflammation by several mechanisms, one of which is activation of NF-kappaB.[9] (Phytonutritional modulation of NF-kappaB[10] will be reviewed in upcoming articles in this series.) Therefore, rich sources of LA should be avoided as much as possible. LA is abundant in most nut, seed, and vegetable oils such as canola oil (21%), safflower oil (76%), sunflower oil (71%), corn oil (57%), soybean oil (54%), and cottonseed oil (54%). Similarly, ARA is the direct precursor to the isoprostanes—chemicals that are formed from the non-enzymatic oxidation of ARA and which exacerbate pain and inflammation. ARA is the precursor for and increases the production of inflammatory and noxious chemicals, particularly the prostaglandins and leukotrienes. Additionally, laboratory research has found that ARA also promotes activation of NF-kappaB and can cause a 400% increase in superoxide production in Kupffer cells.[9] The most obvious method for *reducing production of chemicals derived from ARA* is to *reduce dietary intake of ARA;* this means avoiding the richest sources of ARA such as whole milk, beef, liver, pork, lamb, and to a lesser extent turkey and chicken. Additionally, many of these problematic foods, especially beef, liver, pork, and lamb, are also major sources of dietary iron, which promotes joint inflammation independently from its contribution to iron overload and hemochromatoic arthropathy. Indeed, as I have discussed in this journal[11] and elsewhere[12], all patients with polyarthropathy should be tested for iron overload. In summary, patients with inflammatory conditions should avoid foods that are high in fat, simple carbohydrates, linoleic acid, arachidonic acid, and iron. Artificial and processed foods should also be avoided since they are commonly rich in *trans*-fatty acids and are depleted of antioxidants.

Foods to Consume: Fruits and vegetables are rich sources of health-promoting nutrients such as vitamins, minerals, fiber, fatty acids such as squalene, and—perhaps most important—a wide range of phytochemicals including limonoids, carotenoids, terpinoids, isothiocyanates, flavonoids, proanthocyanidins and other polyphenols. Dietary antioxidants have important anti-inflammatory benefits that extend beyond their abilities to quench free radicals. Additionally, components of whole foods, such as the sterols and sterolins found in vegetables, have significant immune-modulating effects and have shown benefit in alleviating the inflammation of rheumatoid arthritis. Fruits and vegetables contain over 5,000 different phytochemicals that act additively and synergistically to maximize antioxidant protection and to protect health.[13] Vegetarian, vegan, and plant-based whole-foods diets are naturally low in fat, linoleic acid, arachidonic acid, iron, and trans-fatty acids. Extra virgin olive oil contains oleic acid, squalene, and phenolic compounds which work synergistically to reduce inflammation, pain, and cardiovascular disease. Whey, soy, and cold-water fatty fish provide health benefits in addition to the provision of high-quality protein. Green tea shows anti-inflammatory, antioxidant, and anti-cancer actions. Diets with a strong foundation of whole fruits and vegetables help patients increase their intake of antioxidant and anti-inflammatory vitamins, minerals, fiber, and phytonutrients while helping to reduce intake of pro-inflammatory iron and fatty acids. Lastly, a significant portion of the health benefits and anti-inflammatory effects of increased consumption of fruits and vegetables is due to favorable alterations in gastrointestinal microflora[14] rather than the direct nutritive values of foods.

Customized Recommendations and Food Allergies: We are all aware that, in certain patients, specific foods and combinations of foods may exacerbate joint pain and inflammation.[15,16] Therefore the diet must be customized for each patient with regard to food allergies, food sensitivities, and food intolerances. Not only must problematic foods be avoided, but patients' gastrointestinal and immune status must be evaluated and improved.[4] Although many doctors are aware of the elimination-and-challenge technique, most doctors do not direct sufficient attention to improving gastrointestinal status and immune function so that the immune system is no longer hyper-responsive to benign food constituents.[4]

AN INTRODUCTION TO FATTY ACID METABOLISM

We can think of the major biologically active fatty acids as originating from three major categories or "families" based on their molecular configuration and thus their physiologic properties. We can then ascribe general properties to these families and the individual members within each group. The most clinically important fatty acids are "unsaturated", meaning they have one or more carbon-to-carbon double bonds rather than carbon-to-carbon single bonds, the latter being "saturated" with the full number of hydrogen molecules. Double bonds strongly influence the biochemical and clinical effects of fatty acids, making these fatty acids more reactive and biologically active than their saturated counterparts, as well as more prone to oxidation, rancidification, and hydrogenation.

Within each family, fatty acids progress from predecessors to progeny by a series of enzymatic steps catalyzed by desaturase and elongase enzymes. The desaturase enzymes are very slow in their conversions compared to the elongase enzymes, and the clinical relevance of this difference will become apparent as this article and series of articles progresses. We also note that fatty acids never change from one family to another: e.g., an omega-3 fatty acid will always remain in the omega-3 family and will never become a member of the omega-6 or omega-9 family. This is because the defining characteristic on a molecular level is never altered: omega-3 fatty acids have their first carbon-to-carbon double bond starting at the third carbon from the methyl group; omega-6 fatty acids have their first carbon-to-carbon double bond starting at the sixth carbon from the methyl group; omega-9 fatty acids have their first carbon-to-carbon double bond starting at the ninth carbon from the methyl group. For the sake of efficiency and accordance with nomenclature conventions, we will hereafter abbreviate "omega" as "n" for the n-3, n-6, and n-9 fatty acids, respectively.

N-3 fatty acids: The n-3 family of fatty acids begins with alpha-linolenic acid, commonly referred to as one of the two "essential fatty acids" because it cannot be produced within the human body and must therefore be provided by the diet. Manifestations of n-3 fatty acid deficiencies are generally subtle when contrasted to those of the n-6 family and include behavioral and visual impairment, endocrinologic alterations, and a tendency toward the development and progression of several chronic degenerative diseases.[17]

Abundant in flax oil (~57%), alpha-linolenic acid (ALA) is converted to stearidonic acid by delta-6-desaturase. Stearidonic acid (SDA) is elongated to n-3 eicosatetraenoic acid, which is then converted to eicosapentaenoic acid (EPA) by delta-5-desaturase. EPA is elongated to n-3 docosapentaenoic acid (n-3 DPA), which is then converted to docosahexaenoic acid (DHA) by delta-4-desaturase. These substrates and conversions are illustrated in Figure 1 (modified with permission from Integrative Orthopedics[4]).

N-6 fatty acids: The n-6 family of fatty acids begins

with linoleic acid (LA), also referred to as an "essential fatty acid" because it cannot be synthesized *de novo* within the human body. LA is abundant in most nut, seed, and vegetable oils such as canola oil (21%), safflower oil (76%), sunflower oil (71%), corn oil (57%), soybean oil (54%), and cottonseed oil (54%).[18] LA is converted by delta-6-desaturase to gamma-linolenic acid (GLA), which is quickly elongated to dihomo-gamma-linolenic acid (DGLA). DGLA is slowly converted by delta-5-desaturase to arachidonic acid (ARA), which is elongated to adrenic acid, which is finally converted to n-6 docosapentaenoic acid by delta-4-desaturase. These substrates and conversions are illustrated in Figure 2 (modified with permission

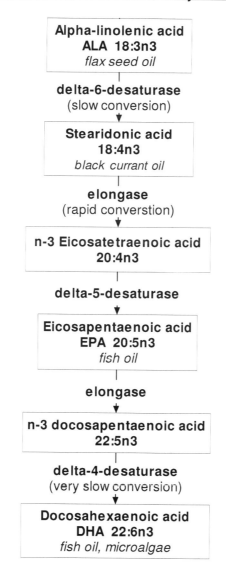

Figure 1. Metabolism of n-3 fatty acids

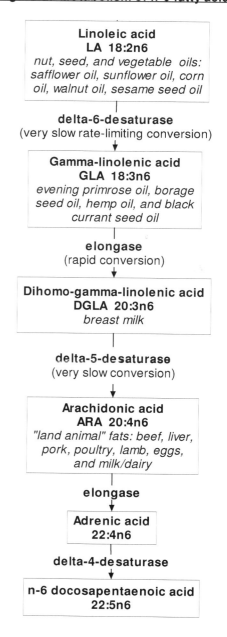

Figure 2. Metabolism of n-6 fatty acids

from Integrative Orthopedics[4]).

Note that the term "eicosatetraenoic acid" can apply to both 20:4n6 (arachidonic acid) of the omega-6 fatty acid family[19] and to 20:4n3 of the omega-3 fatty acid family.[20] Therefore, to avoid the confusion that would result from the use of the term "eicosatetraenoic acid" by itself, "n-6 eicosatetraenoic acid" should be used when referring to 20:4n6 (arachidonic acid) and "n-3 eicosatetraenoic acid" should be used when referring to 20:4n3. Similarly, 22:5n3 of the omega-3 fatty acid family[21,22] and 22:5n6 of the omega-6 fatty acid family[23,24,25] are both referred to as "docosapentaenoic acid." Therefore using the term "docosapentaenoic acid" will be ambiguous unless the appropriate n-3 or n-6 designation is stated. "N-3 docosapentaenoic acid" should be used to refer to 22:5n3 and "n-6 docosapentaenoic acid" should be used for 22:5n6.

N-9 fatty acids: The primary n-9 fatty acid in the human diet is oleic acid, the predominant monounsaturated fatty acid in olive oil. While oleic acid is certainly biologically active and therefore clinically important, due to the complexity of olive oil as the primary source of oleic acid, we are not yet able to clearly determine from epidemiological studies how much of the benefit of olive oil consumption is due to the oleic acid compared to the benefits derived from the powerful antioxidant and anti-inflammatory actions of the phenolics, the relatively high content of squalene, or other confounding variables in diet and lifestyle.[26,27]

ENZYMATIC CONVERSION: CHEMICAL FLOWCHARTS VERSUS THE REALITY OF CLINICAL EFFECTIVENESS

If conversion of one fatty acid to the next proceeded as efficiently as depicted in biochemical flow charts, then n-3 ALA and n-6 LA could be supplemented to provide all of the downstream fatty acids and their metabolites, presumably in the proper ratios. However, clearly this is not the case due to intrinsic as well as genotypic (inherited) and phenotypic (manifested) defects in enzyme effectiveness. Clinicians need to understand the individual characteristics of these enzymes in order to successfully employ therapies which modulate fatty acid metabolism. Since the conversions catalyzed by elongase are quite efficient and are almost never discussed as cause for concern in the medical and nutritional literature, we will focus on the desaturase enzymes, which are noted to have significant variances in phenotypic expression and which can be adversely affected by common vitamin and mineral deficiencies.

Delta-6-desaturase: The first step in the n-3 and n-6 pathways is the action of delta-6-desaturase (D6D) in converting ALA to SDA and LA to GLA, respectively. Enzymatic conversions by D6D are rate-limiting due to 1)

its strong need for several vitamin and mineral co-factors, 2) its genotypic impairment, such as in patients with eczema,[28] 3) its phenotypic impairment in patients with diabetes,[29] and its impairment by trans-fatty acids,[30] stress neurotransmitters,[31] and other environmental and nutritional influences.[4] The slow conversions by D6D explain why, as Horrobin noted, "…it is impossible to produce any significant elevation of DGLA levels in humans by increasing linoleic acid intake."[32] Similarly, conversion of ALA to the downstream and clinically desirable fatty acids EPA and DHA is unreliable, with most studies showing only a modest increase in EPA and no increase in DHA following supplementation with ALA. Cofactors required for efficient action of D6D include iron, zinc, magnesium, pyridoxine, riboflavin, and niacin; when these vitamins and minerals are deficient, D6D function will be impaired and defects in fatty acid metabolism will result.[33]

Delta-5-desaturase: Delta-5-desaturase (D5D) slowly converts n-3 eicosatetraenoic acid to EPA, and in the n-6 pathway, DGLA to ARA. Supplementation with GLA has been shown to result in a slight to modest increase in ARA that may or may not be clinically significant. Impairment of D5D is seen in patients with the blinding eye disease retinitis pigmentosa, resulting in marked reduction in retinal DHA levels.[34]

Delta-4-desaturase: Delta-4-desaturase (D4D), like the other desaturase enzymes, is also very slow-acting. While impaired conversion of adrenic acid to n-6 docosapentaenoic acid appears to be of little or no consequence, reduced bioavailability of DHA due to its slow conversion from n-3 docosapentaenoic acid has tremendous implications in the etiology of schizophrenia, a disease associated with impaired D4D activity.[35]

By understanding the biochemical efficiency of these enzymes, doctors are better able to understand how to implement clinical strategies for modulating fatty acid balance in their patients. In the n-3 family, supplementation with ALA increases (in order of decreasing efficiency) ALA, SDA, and EPA but does not consistently elevate DHA. Therefore, although consumption of flax oil has many important benefits and may be used to modestly increase EPA levels, it cannot be relied upon to increase DHA levels.[36] Supplementation with SDA increases EPA levels, but DHA is not significantly increased due to the slow conversion by D4D.[37] Supplementation with EPA proportionately increases EPA but does not consistently increase DHA.[38] DHA supplementation is the most effective and reliable means for increasing DHA levels.[39]

In the n-6 family, supplementation with LA does not lead to clinically significant increases in GLA or DGLA.[32] Supplementation with GLA greatly increases DGLA and leads to a modest increase in ARA.[40] Diets high in ARA lead to increased tissue levels of ARA. Consumption of EPA lowers levels of GLA/DGLA[29] and oleic acid[41]; likewise, consumption of GLA lowers levels of EPA.[40] **Overall, the implications are that when a particular fatty acid is desired for its physiologic effect and clinical benefits, it should be supplied directly from the diet or supplements.**

CONCLUSION:

In this brief article, we have introduced and reviewed the foundational terminology and concepts which will facilitate the introduction of more advanced concepts as presented in the upcoming articles in this series. Dietary improvement and custom-tailored prescription of individual fatty acids is consistently providing patients and doctors with greater health and superior clinical results. Alleviation, prevention, and effective treatment of many diseases previously considered to be "untreatable" is now possible with fatty acid supplementation, diet modification, and the use of other vitamins, minerals, and botanical medicines. The skillful use of these interventions by the chiropractic profession, whether as adjunctive treatment to spinal manipulation or as primary therapy, is in accord with our holistic philosophy and promises to advance the prominence of our profession in the healthcare arena. Since the pharmaceutical-surgical paradigm delivers many unnecessary risks and unsatisfactory outcomes in the management of chronic disease[42-49], now is the time for chiropractic physicians to step forward and deliver the safest, most effective and cost-effective therapies ever before seen in American healthcare for the management of chronic health problems.

REFERENCES:

1. "Doctors of Chiropractic are physicians who consider man as an integrated being and give special attention to the physiological and biochemical aspects including structural, spinal, musculoskeletal, neurological, vascular, nutritional, emotional and environmental relationships." Available at http://www.amerchiro.org/media/whatis/ on March 11, 2004

2. Beckman JF, Fernandez CE, Coulter ID. A systems model of health care: a proposal. J Manipulative Physiol Ther. 1996 Mar-Apr;19(3):208-15

3. Orme-Johnson DW, Herron RE. An innovative approach to reducing medical care utilization and expenditures. Am J Manag Care 1997 Jan;3(1):135-44

4. Vasquez A. Integrative Orthopedics: Concepts, Algorithms, and Therapeutics. Houston; Natural Health Consulting Corporation (www.OptimalHealthResearch.com): 2004

5. Manga, Pran; Angus, Doug; Papadopoulos, Costa; Swan, William. The Effectiveness and Cost-Effectiveness of Chiropractic Management of Low-Back Pain. Richmond Hill, Ontario: Kenilworth Publishing, 1993

6. American Chiropractic Association. See http://www.amerchiro.org/media/research/ and http://www.amerchiro.org/media/research/more_research.shtml for citations; available on March 3, 2004

7. Seaman DR. The diet-induced proinflammatory state: a cause of chronic pain and other degenerative diseases? J Manipulative Physiol Ther. 2002 Mar-Apr;25(3):168-79

8. Aljada A, Mohanty P, Ghanim H, Abdo T, Tripathy D, Chaudhuri A, Dandona P. Increase in intranuclear nuclear factor kappaB and decrease in inhibitor kappaB in mononuclear cells after a mixed meal: evidence for a proinflammatory effect. Am J Clin Nutr. 2004 Apr;79(4):682-90

9. Rusyn I, Bradham CA, Cohn L, Schoonhoven R, Swenberg JA, Brenner DA, Thurman RG. Corn oil rapidly activates nuclear factor-kappaB in hepatic Kupffer cells by oxidant-dependent mechanisms. Carcinogenesis. 1999 Nov;20(11):2095-100

10. Tak PP, Firestein GS. NF-kappaB: a key role in inflammatory diseases. J Clin Invest. 2001 Jan;107(1):7-11

11. Vasquez A. High body iron stores: causes, effects, diagnosis, and treatment. Nutritional Perspectives 1994; 17: 13, 15-7, 19, 21, 28

12. Vasquez A. Musculoskeletal disorders and iron overload disease: comment on the American College of Rheumatology guidelines for the initial evaluation of the adult patient with acute musculoskeletal symptoms. Arthritis & Rheumatism: Official Journal of the American College of Rheumatology 1996; 39:1767-8

13. Liu RH. Health benefits of fruit and vegetables are from additive and synergistic combinations of phytochemicals. Am J Clin Nutr. 2003 Sep;78(3 Suppl):517S-520S

14. Nenonen MT, Helve TA, Rauma AL, Hanninen OO. Uncooked, lactobacilli-rich, vegan food and rheumatoid arthritis. Br J Rheumatol. 1998 Mar;37(3):274-81

15. Panush RS. Food induced ("allergic") arthritis: clinical and serologic studies. J Rheumatol. 1990 Mar;17(3):291-4

16. Pacor ML, Lunardi C, Di Lorenzo G, Biasi D, Corrocher R. Food allergy and seronegative arthritis: report of two cases. Clin Rheumatol. 2001;20(4):279-81

17. Tapiero H, Ba GN, Couvreur P, Tew KD. Polyunsaturated fatty acids (PUFA) and eicosanoids in human health and pathologies. Biomed Pharmacother. 2002 Jul;56(5):215-22

18. Morris DH. Canola and the good news about dietary

fat. Published by the Canola Council at http://www.canola-council.org/pubs/GNs.pdf available as of March 3, 2004

19. Mimouni V, Christiansen EN, Blond JP, Ulmann L, Poisson JP, Bezard J. Elongation and desaturation of arachidonic and eicosapentaenoic acids in rat liver. Effect of clofibrate feeding. Biochim Biophys Acta. 1991 Nov 27;1086(3):349-53

20. Erasmus U. Fats that heal, fats that kill. British Columbia Canada: Alive Books, 1993 Page 276

21. Williard DE, Harmon SD, Kaduce TL, Preuss M, Moore SA, Robbins ME, Spector AA. Docosahexaenoic acid synthesis from n-3 polyunsaturated fatty acids in differentiated rat brain astrocytes. J Lipid Res. 2001 Sep;42(9):1368-76

22. Takahashi R, Nassar BA, Huang YS, Begin ME, Horrobin DF. Effect of different ratios of dietary N-6 and N-3 fatty acids on fatty acid composition, prostaglandin formation and platelet aggregation in the rat. Thromb Res. 1987 Jul 15;47(2):135-46

23. Retterstol K, Haugen TB, Christophersen BO. The pathway from arachidonic to docosapentaenoic acid (20:4n-6 to 22:5n-6) and from eicosapentaenoic to docosahexaenoic acid (20:5n-3 to 22:6n-3) studied in testicular cells from immature rats. Biochim Biophys Acta. 2000 Jan 3;1483(1):119-31

24. Ahmad A, Murthy M, Greiner RS, Moriguchi T, Salem N Jr. A decrease in cell size accompanies a loss of docosahexaenoate in the rat hippocampus. Nutr Neurosci. 2002 Apr;5(2):103-13

25. Mimouni V, Narce M, Huang YS, Horrobin DF, Poisson JP. Adrenic acid delta 4 desaturation and fatty acid composition in liver microsomes of spontaneously diabetic Wistar BB rats. Prostaglandins Leukot Essent Fatty Acids. 1994 Jan;50(1):43-7

26. Stark AH, Madar Z. Olive oil as a functional food: epidemiology and nutritional approaches. Nutr Rev. 2002 Jun;60(6):170-6

27. Newmark HL. Is oleic acid or squalene the important preventive agent? Am J Clin Nutr. 2000 Aug;72(2):502

28. Manku MS, Horrobin DF, Morse N, Kyte V, Jenkins K, Wright S, Burton JL. Reduced levels of prostaglandin precursors in the blood of atopic patients: defective delta-6-desaturase function as a biochemical basis for atopy. Prostaglandins Leukot Med. 1982 Dec;9(6):615-28

29. Horrobin DF. Fatty acid metabolism in health and disease: the role of delta-6-desaturase. Am J Clin Nutr. 1993 May;57(5 Suppl):732S-736S

30. Simopoulos AP. Essential fatty acids in health and chronic disease. Am J Clin Nutr. 1999 Sep;70(3 Suppl):560S-569S

31. Mamalakis G, Kafatos A, Tornaritis M, Alevizos B. Anxiety and adipose essential fatty acid precursors for prostaglandin E1 and E2. J Am Coll Nutr. 1998 Jun;17(3):239-43

32. Horrobin DF. Interactions between n-3 and n-6 essential fatty acids (EFAs) in the regulation of cardiovascular disorders and inflammation. Prostaglandins Leukot Essent Fatty Acids. 1991 Oct;44(2):127-31

33. Serfontein WJ, de Villiers LS, Ubbink J, Rapley C. Delta-6-desaturase enzyme co-factors and atherosclerosis. S Afr Med J. 1985 Jul 20;68(2):67-8

34. Hoffman DR, DeMar JC, Heird WC, Birch DG, Anderson RE. Impaired synthesis of DHA in patients with X-linked retinitis pigmentosa. J Lipid Res. 2001 Sep;42(9):1395-401

35. Mahadik SP, Shendarkar NS, Scheffer RE, Mukherjee S, Correnti EE. Utilization of precursor essential fatty acids in culture by skin fibroblasts from schizophrenic patients and normal controls. Prostaglandins Leukot Essent Fatty Acids. 1996 Aug;55(1-2):65-70

36. Francois CA, Connor SL, Bolewicz LC, Connor WE. Supplementing lactating women with flaxseed oil does not increase docosahexaenoic acid in their milk. Am J Clin Nutr. 2003 Jan;77(1):226-33

37. James MJ, Ursin VM, Cleland LG. Metabolism of stearidonic acid in human subjects: comparison with the metabolism of other n-3 fatty acids. Am J Clin Nutr. 2003 May;77(5):1140-5

38. Park Y, Harris W. EPA, but not DHA, decreases mean platelet volume in normal subjects. Lipids. 2002 Oct;37(10):941-6

39. Mori TA, Burke V, Puddey IB, Watts GF, O'Neal DN, Best JD, Beilin LJ. Purified eicosapentaenoic and docosahexaenoic acids have differential effects on serum lipids and lipoproteins, LDL particle size, glucose, and insulin in mildly hyperlipidemic men. Am J Clin Nutr. 2000 May;71(5):1085-94

40. Jantti J, Nikkari T, Solakivi T, Vapaatalo H, Isomaki H. Evening primrose oil in rheumatoid arthritis: changes in serum lipids and fatty acids. Ann Rheum Dis. 1989 Feb;48(2):124-7

41. Haban P, Zidekova E, Klvanova J. Supplementation with long-chain n-3 fatty acids in non-insulin-dependent diabetes mellitus (NIDDM) patients leads to the lowering of oleic acid content in serum phospholipids. Eur J Nutr. 2000 Oct;39(5):201-6

42. "Basically, you die earlier and spend more time disabled if you're an American rather than a member of most other advanced countries." Christopher Murray MD PhD, Director of World Health Organization's Global Program on Evidence for Health Policy Press Release: Washington, D.C. and Geneva, Switzerland on 4 June 2000. Available at http://www.who.int/inf-

pr-2000/en/pr2000-life.html on March 2, 2004

43. "In this controlled trial involving patients with osteoarthritis of the knee, the outcomes after arthroscopic lavage or arthroscopic debridement were no better than those after a placebo procedure." Moseley JB, O'Malley K, Petersen NJ, Menke TJ, Brody BA, Kuykendall DH, Hollingsworth JC, Ashton CM, Wray NP. A controlled trial of arthroscopic surgery for osteoarthritis of the knee. N Engl J Med 2002 Jul 11;347(2):81-8

44. "In 1983, 2876 people died from medication errors. ... By 1993, this number had risen to 7,391 - a 2.57-fold increase." Phillips DP, Christenfeld N, Glynn LM. Increase in US medication-error deaths between 1983 and 1993. Lancet. 1998 Feb 28;351(9103):643-4

45. "A senior executive with Britain's biggest drugs company has admitted that most prescription medicines do not work on most people who take them. Allen Roses, worldwide vice-president of genetics at GlaxoSmithKline, said fewer than half of the patients prescribed some of the most expensive drugs actually derived any benefit from them." Connor S. Glaxo Chief: Our Drugs Do Not Work on Most Patients. Published on Monday, December 8, 2003 by the Independent/UK. Available on-line at http://www.commondreams.org/headlines03/1208-02.htm on February 28, 2004

46. "Recent estimates suggest that each year more than 1 million patients are injured while in the hospital and approximately 180,000 die because of these injuries. Furthermore, drug-related morbidity and mortality are common and are estimated to cost more than $136 billion a year." Holland EG, Degruy FV. Drug-induced disorders. Am Fam Physician. 1997 Nov 1;56(7):1781-8, 1791-2. Available on-line at http://aafp.org/afp/971101ap/holland.html

47. "...lush advertisements from companies with obvious vested interests, and authoritative testimonials from biased investigators who presumably believe in their own work to the point of straining credulity and denying common sense... (translate: economic improvement, not biological superiority)." Stevens CW, Glatstein E. Beware the Medical-Industrial Complex. Oncologist 1996;1(4):IV-V

48. "Conservative calculations estimate that approximately 107,000 patients are hospitalized annually for nonsteroidal anti-inflammatory drug (NSAID)-related gastrointestinal (GI) complications and at least 16,500 NSAID-related deaths occur each year among arthritis patients alone. The figures for all NSAID users would be overwhelming, yet the scope of this problem is generally under-appreciated." Singh G. Recent considerations in nonsteroidal anti-inflammatory drug gastropathy. Am J Med. 1998 Jul 27; 105(1B): 31S-38S

49. "Although the standard of care in developed countries is to maintain schizophrenia patients on neuroleptics, this practice is not supported by the 50-year research record for the drugs. A critical review reveals that this paradigm of care worsens long-term outcomes..." Whitaker R. The case against antipsychotic drugs: a 50-year record of doing more harm than good. Med Hypotheses. 2004;62(1):5-13 available

ABOUT THE AUTHOR:

Dr. Alex Vasquez is a licensed naturopathic physician in Washington and Oregon, and licensed chiropractor in Texas, where he maintains a private practice and is a member of the research team at Biotics Research Corporation. As former Adjunct Professor of Orthopedics and Rheumatology for the Naturopathic Medicine Program at Bastyr University, he is the author of more than 18 published articles and a recently published 486-page textbook for the chiropractic and naturopathic professions, "Integrative Orthopedics: The Art of Creating Wellness While Managing Acute and Chronic Musculoskeletal Disorders" available from OptimalHealthResearch.com.

ACKNOWLEDGEMENTS:

Pepper Grimm BA and Mike Owen DC of Biotics Research Corporation reviewed this manuscript before submission.

Reducing Pain and Inflammation Naturally.
Part II: New Insights into Fatty Acid Supplementation and Its Effect on Eicosanoid Production and Genetic Expression

Alex Vasquez, D.C., N.D.

Abstract: Doctors and patients can achieve significant success in the treatment of pain and inflammation by using dietary modification along with nutritional, botanical, and fatty acid supplementation. The first article in this series reviewed recent diet research and the basic biochemistry of fatty acid metabolism, and this second article will provide doctors with a profound understanding of the importance of optimal fatty acid supplementation and will review the clinical benefits of this essential therapy. This review contains the most concise, detailed, up-to-date, and clinically relevant description of fatty acid metabolism that has ever been published in a single article.

INTRODUCTION

Chiropractic and naturopathic physicians are the only doctorate-level healthcare providers with graduate-level training in therapeutic nutrition and are emerging as the leaders in the treatment and prevention of long-term health disorders, including nearly all of the chronic diseases seen in clinical practice such as obesity, hypertension, adult-onset diabetes, hypercholesterolemia, allergies, asthma, arthritis, depression and a long list of other musculoskeletal and non-musculoskeletal conditions.[1,2] With the increasing substantiation of the effectiveness and cost-effectiveness of the nutritional management of these problems, and the documentation of the excessive cost and adverse effects generally associated with pharmaceutical medications, we are approaching a paradigm shift in healthcare which will eventually (re)position the practitioners of holistic natural healthcare in their proper place—at the forefront of patient management.

Healthcare providers of all disciplines are obligated to act responsibly to protect the health of the public. Current research published in peer-reviewed medical journals suggests that over-utilization of allopathic medical care endangers patients' health by exposing patients to prescribing errors[3], hospital injuries, and what is described as "substandard care."[4] A recent article in the *New England Journal of Medicine*[5] concluded that deficits in allopathic medical care pose "serious threats to the health of the American public." A 1997 review published by the American Academy of Family Physicians[6] stated, "Recent estimates suggest that each year more than 1 million patients are injured while in the hospital and approximately 180,000 die because of these injuries. Furthermore, drug-related morbidity and mortality are common and are estimated to cost more than $136 billion a year." New research also shows that several popular "antidepressant" drugs actually increase the risk for suicide in children[7] and adults[8,9,] and, similarly, "antipsychotic" drugs may worsen clinical outcomes in a large percentage of patients with mental illness.[10] Chiropractic diet therapy—not drugs—is the most effective treatment for chronic hypertension.[11, 12] Many anti-inflammatory drugs for the treatment of joint pain actually promote joint destruction[13, 14, 15] and the newer selective cyclooxygenase inhibitors carry an unjustifiable cost[16, 17] and fail to deliver improved efficacy[18] despite significantly increasing the risk for kidney damage, hypertension, myocardial infarction, stroke, and sudden death.[19, 20, 21] On the other hand, natural treatments such as dietary improvements and fatty acid supplementation have been shown to safely reduce the need for medical treatments, to improve health, to alleviate many common diseases, and to prolong life at lower cost, negligible risk, and with improved overall outcomes.[22, 23] **In order to reduce costs, promote health, and reduce iatrogenic disease, our healthcare paradigm must change from "disease treatment with drugs and surgery" to "health promotion with therapeutic nutrition and lifestyle improvements."** It is safe and reasonable to predict that in the near future, customized dietary improvement, therapeutic nutrition, lifestyle modification, and fatty acid supplementation will be viewed as integral components of patient care for all patients with all diseases. Doctors must therefore be informed of new research on how to use these interventions skillfully.

The combination of dietary improvement and skillful nutritional intervention as reviewed by the current author in the first article in this series[24] and in greater detail elsewhere[25] is the single most powerful approach for the effective treatment of a wide range of conditions. Following closely behind general dietary modification, fatty acid supplementation offers clinicians the opportunity to improve the health of their patients in ways that no other single treatment can.

FATTY ACID SUPPLEMENTATION: UNDERSTANDING IS THE KEY TO MASTERY

An accurate and detailed understanding of fatty acid metabolism is important for the complete and effective management of many clinical conditions including mental depression, coronary artery disease, hypertension, diabetes, other inflammatory/autoimmune disorders, and many of the musculoskeletal conditions encountered in clinical practice. The practical application of this information is relatively straightforward, and with a detailed understanding of precursors and modulators of fatty acid, prostaglandin, and leukotriene metabolism, clinicians can facilitate or restrict the production of bioactive chemicals to promote the desired clinical result. The basics of fatty acid metabolism were reviewed previously; here we focus on clinical applications. We will focus on the fatty acids with the greatest promise for clinical benefit: alpha-linolenic acid, gamma-linolenic acid, eicosapentaenoic acid, docosahexaenoic acid, and oleic acid. Biochemical pathways and clinical implications of fatty acid metabolism are detailed in Figures 1 and 2.

Figure 1. Metabolism of omega-3 fatty acids and related eicosanoids

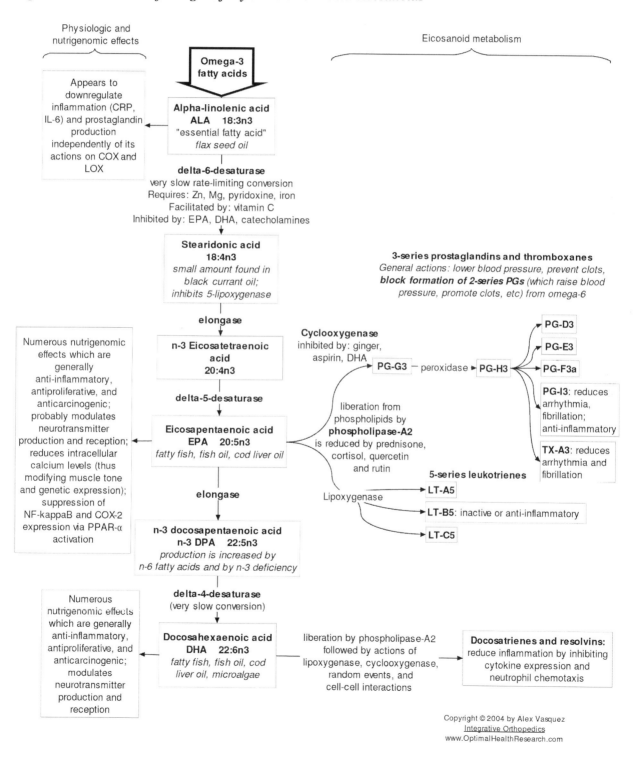

Figure 2. *Metabolism of omega-6 fatty acids and related eicosanoids*

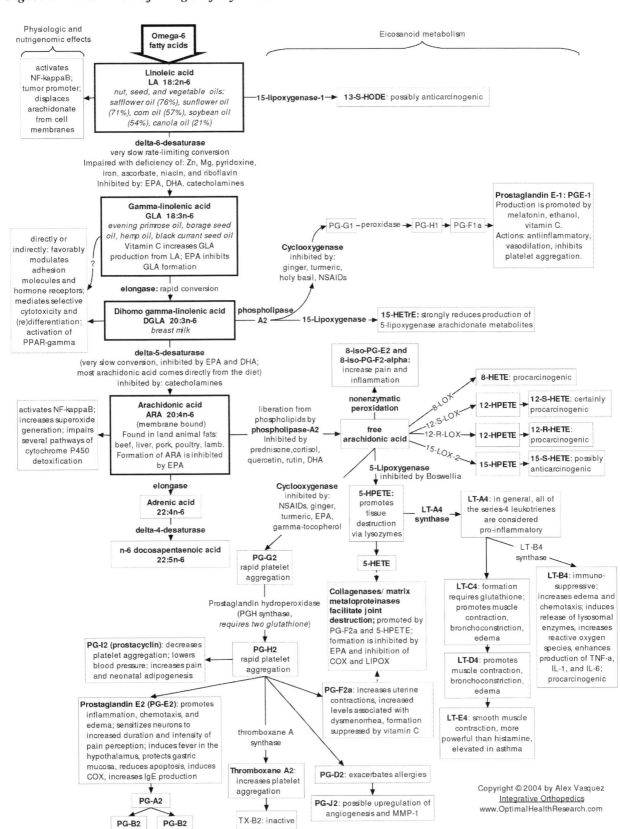

THE HEALTH-PROMOTING FATTY ACIDS: ALA, EPA, DHA, GLA, AND OLEIC ACID

- *Alpha-linolenic acid: ALA, α-LNA, ALNA, 18:3n3:* ALA is an essential fatty acid as it is the "first in line" in the family of omega-3 polyunsaturated fatty acids (PUFA). Sources include flax seed oil (57% ALA), canola oil (9% ALA), soy oil, breast milk, English/black walnuts, soybeans, pine nuts, green vegetables, and beans. Conversion of ALA to the more biologically active EPA and DHA does not reliably or efficiently occur in humans.[26] No increase in DHA has been consistently observed in humans after supplementation of ALA[27]; in fact, supplementation with flax seed oil has actually been shown to reduce DHA levels in humans.[28] Although ALA can reduce blood pressure and cardiovascular mortality[26], it does not reduce serum lipids as do EPA and DHA. In a study of men with metabolic syndrome, ALA was shown to have anti-inflammatory benefits independent of its conversion to EPA or DHA.[29] The mechanism of action appears to be downregulation of NF-KappaB (the main "amplifier" for the expression of proinflammatory gene products[30]) rather than the direct modulation of eicosanoid biosynthesis. One study using flax oil as a source of ALA to treat rheumatoid arthritis found no clinical or biochemical benefit (i.e., no change in Hgb, CRP, ESR)[31]; however, the poor results of this study may have been due to the inferior quality of the flax oil product that was used which only supplied 32% ALA compared with the much higher concentration of 57% found in most products. Moderate intakes of ALA from flax oil profoundly reduce production of proinflammatory prostaglandins (e.g., PG-E2, measured by urinary excretion) by 52% to 85% in humans[32] which is superior to the 42% reduction induced by rofecoxib (the drug "Vioxx").[33] In summary, increased intake of ALA appears to provide cardioprotective[34] and anti-inflammatory benefits[29,32], and ALA can help reduce the frequency and severity of migraine headaches when used as part of a comprehensive natural treatment plan that includes diet change and nutritional supplementation.[35]

- *Eicosapentaenoic acid: EPA, 20:5n3:* EPA is essentially absent in vegan diets since the major dietary source is fish oil. Dietary EPA is incorporated into cell membranes where it modulates neurotransmitter and hormone receptor function and where it is stored before liberation by phospholipase for eicosanoid production. EPA-derived eicosanoids have anti-inflammatory properties, including a reduction in the production of proinflammatory eicosanoids such as LT-B4, PAFs, and cytokines such as TNF-alpha and IL-1, and a large reduction in PG-E2 and TX-B2.[36] Unfortunately, EPA can decrease production of DGLA, the metabolite of GLA that has health-promoting properties.[37] EPA doses of at least 4 grams per day are needed to increase bleeding time.[38] EPA supplementation reduces urinary excretion of calcium in patients with hypercalciuria and may therefore help prevent the development of calcium urolithiasis.[39] Due to its anti-inflammatory, membrane-enhancing, and other nutrigenomic benefits, EPA supplementation has proven beneficial for patients with lupus[40], cancer[41], borderline personality disorder[42], mental depression[43,44,45], schizophrenia[46], and osteoporosis (when used with GLA).[47]

- *Docosahexaenoic acid: DHA, 20:6n-3:* DHA is found only in plants of the sea, phytoplankton/microalgae, and consumers of microalgae (such as fish). Like EPA, DHA is an important component of cell membranes and generally appears to improve cell membrane function via improving receptor function and signal transduction. In late 2003, bioactive metabolites of DHA—the docosatrienes and resolvins—were discovered to mediate potent anti-inflammatory benefits.[48] Animal studies have shown that induction of DHA deficiency causes memory deficits and a reduction in hippocampal cell size[49], and DHA deficiency in humans is consistently associated with mental depression, learning disorders (e.g., ADD/ADHD), and other neuropsychiatric disorders such as schizophrenia. DHA levels are reduced by ethanol consumption.[50] DHA appears essential for optimal cognitive function in infants and adults, and DHA also provides protection against thrombosis, arrhythmia, cardiovascular death, Alzheimer's disease[51], otitis media (when used with nutritional supplementation[52]), and coronary restenosis following angioplasty.[53] Supplementation with DHA (often in the form of fish oil, which includes EPA) has been shown to benefit patients with bipolar disorder[54], Crohn's disease[55], rheumatoid arthritis[56,57,58], lupus[59], cardiovascular disease[60], psoriasis[61], and cancer.[62] DHA appears to have an "anti-stress" benefit manifested by 30% reductions in norepinephrine and improved resilience to psychoemotional stress.[63,64] Supplementation with EPA+DHA is extremely safe and reduces all-cause mortality.[60]

- *Gamma (γ)-linolenic acid: GLA, 18:3n6:* The

most powerful health-promoting n-6 fatty acid, GLA is found in varying concentrations in evening primrose oil, borage seed oil, hemp seed oil, and black currant seed oil. Most if not all of the actions of GLA are mediated following its elongation to the biologically active DGLA, from which eicosanoids that have cardioprotective and anti-inflammatory benefits are derived. Low levels of DGLA are associated with increased risk for stroke and myocardial infarction.[37] DGLA metabolites reduce the formation of the arachidonate-derived 2-series prostaglandins, 4-series leukotrienes and platelet-activating factor.[65] GLA supplementation results in the formation of two biologically active metabolites from DGLA formed by cyclooxygenase and lipoxygenase. Prostaglandin E-1 (PG-E1) is the main metabolite formed from DGLA by cyclooxygenase and its production is increased by vitamin C.[66] PG-E1 decreases platelet aggregation[37], inhibits vascular smooth muscle cell proliferation *in vitro*[67], causes vasodilation[36], and thus helps lower blood pressure.[37] PG-E1 has anti-inflammatory benefits and is probably the most potent prostaglandin with respect to bronchodilation.[66] Additionally, PG-E1 may have a mood elevating effect insofar as levels are elevated in patients with mania, reduced in patients with depression, and are elevated by ethanol intake.[68] Production of PG-E1 is increased by n-3 fatty acids.[69] 15-HETrE is the second main metabolite from GLA/DGLA and is formed from DGLA via 15-lipoxygenase. 15-HETrE has potent anti-inflammatory action by inhibiting the conversion of arachidonic acid to leukotrienes via inhibition of 5-lipoxygenase and 12-lipoxygenase.[37, 70] Clinically, this is very important because several common and serious health problems including allergy, asthma, cardiovascular disease, and cancer are at least partially dependent upon the function of lipoxygenase for the production of leukotrienes. Notably, prostate cancer cells can be rapidly killed *in vitro* by lipoxygenase inhibition.[71] Clinical benefit associated with GLA supplementation is seen in patients with, eczema[72], breast cancer (when used with tamoxifen[73]), premenstrual syndrome[74], rheumatoid arthritis[75, 76], diabetic neuropathy[77], migraine headaches (when used with ALA[35]), and respiratory distress syndrome (when used with EPA).[78]

- *Oleic acid:* N-9 oleic acid appears to have health-promoting benefits, namely cardioprotection and anti-inflammation which are both partially mediated via suppression of NF-kappaB.[79] Most studies that have used oleic acid have used olive oil, which

is a complex mixture of oleic acid, squalene, and phenolic antioxidants/anti-inflammatories; therefore, determination of the benefits of oleic acid alone (i.e., without squalene and phenolics) is difficult. Other sources of oleic acid include flax seed oil and borage oil. Olive oil should be consumed in the diet to attain sufficient quantity of oleic acid along with the health-promoting, anti-inflammatory, anti-cancer, and cardioprotective squalene and phenolic antioxidants. Dietary consumption of olive oil is consistently associated with reductions in cancer and cardiovascular disease, particularly when used as a component of a health-promoting diet.[80, 81]

NUTRIGENOMICS: MODULATION OF GENETIC EXPRESSION VIA INTERVENTIONAL NUTRITION

The study of how dietary components and nutritional supplements influence genetic expression is referred to as "nutrigenomics" or "nutritional genomics" and has been described as "the next frontier in the postgenomic era."[82] Various nutrients have been shown to modulate genetic expression and thus alter phenotypic manifestations of disease by upregulating or downregulating specific genes, interacting with nuclear receptors, altering hormone receptors, and modifying the influence of transcription factors, such as proinflammatory NF-kappaB. Indeed, the previous view that nutrients only interact with human physiology at the metabolic/post-transcriptional level must be updated in light of current research showing that nutrients can, in fact, modify human physiology and phenotype at the genetic/pre-transcriptional level. Whereas pharmaceutical modulation of genetic expression will require billions of dollars and decades of research before clinical implementation, the power of health-promoting nutritional interventions is available to us immediately at comparatively negligible cost.

Fatty acids and their end-products modulate genetic expression in several ways, as these examples will illustrate. In general, n-3 fatty acids decrease inflammation and promote health while n-6 fatty acids (except for GLA, which is generally health-promoting) increase inflammation, oxidative stress, and the manifestation of disease. Corn oil, probably as a result of its high n-6 LA (linoleic acid) content, rapidly activates NF-kappaB and thus promotes tumor development, atherosclerosis, and elaboration of pro-inflammatory mediators such as TNFa.[83, 84, 85] Similarly n-6 arachidonic acid increased production of the free radical superoxide approximately 4-fold when added to isolated Kupffer cells *in vitro*. Prostaglandin-E2 is produced from arachidonic acid by cyclooxygenase and increases genetic expression of cyclooxygenase and IL-6; thus, inflammation manifested by an increase in PG-E2 leads to additive expression of cyclooxygenase, which further increases inflammation and elevates C-reactive protein.[86] The unique health-promoting effects of GLA are nutrigenomically mediated via activation of PPAR-gamma, inhibition of NF-kappaB, and impairment of estrogen receptor function.[87, 88] Supplementation with ALA leads to a dramatic reduction of prostaglandin formation in humans[32], and this effect is probably mediated by down-regulation of proinflammatory transcription, as evidenced by reductions in CRP, IL-6, and SAA.[29] EPA appears to exert much of its anti-inflammatory benefit by suppressing NF-kappaB activation via activation of PPAR-alpha[89] and

thus reducing elaboration of proinflammatory mediators.[90] EPA also indirectly modifies gene expression and cell growth by reducing intracellular calcium levels and thus activating protein kinase R which impairs eukaryotic initiation factor-2alpha and inhibits protein synthesis at the level of translation initiation, thereby mediating an anti-cancer benefit.[91] DHA is the precursor to docosatrienes and resolvins which downregulate gene expression for proinflammatory IL-1, inhibit TNFa, and reduce neutrophil entry to sites of inflammation.[48] Therefore, we see that fatty acids directly affect gene expression by complex and multiple mechanisms. These effects are summarized in Figure 3.

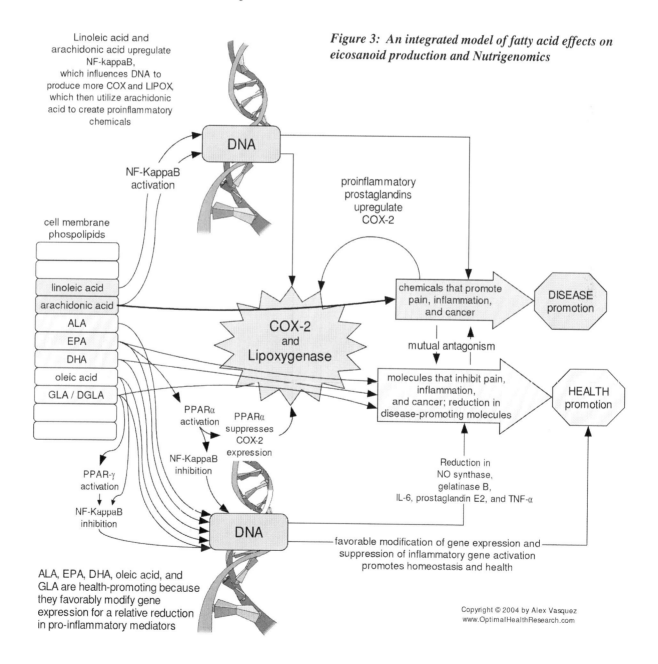

Figure 3: An integrated model of fatty acid effects on eicosanoid production and Nutrigenomics

BIOCHEMICAL AND CLINICAL SUPERIORITY OF USING FATTY ACIDS IN BALANCED COMBINATION

For the majority of clinical situations, the use of fatty acids in isolation is inferior to using fatty acids in balanced combination for several reasons. First, fatty acid defects/deficiencies generally occur *in combination* rather than in isolation, and therefore more than one fatty acid is generally needed when fatty acid supplementation is required. Second, since fatty acids compete for space in cell membranes, supplementation with a single fatty acid can exacerbate depletion of other fatty acids. Supplementation with EPA and DHA (ie, fish oil) leads to a reduction in DGLA and deprives patients of the benefits of PG-E1 and 15-HETrE[92]; therefore GLA should be supplemented when EPA and DHA are used. ALA supplementation[32] and fish oil supplementation[93] both reduce tissue levels of oleic acid and this is believed to have negative effects; therefore ALA and fish oil supplementation should include additional oleic acid. GLA supplementation causes a harmful reduction in EPA and a harmful increase in arachidonic acid unless EPA and DHA are supplemented along with the GLA.[94] Because of these adverse effects noted with the use of single sources of fatty acids, **the current trend in the research literature and in clinical practice is to use fatty acids *in combination*.** In other words, clinical benefits are generally improved significantly when doctors and patients use a fatty acid supplement that contains the health-promoting omega-3, -6, and -9 fatty acids *in combination* and *in their proper ratios*.

Clinical studies using mixed fatty acid preparations have shown clinically powerful benefits. The combination of ALA and GLA was shown to dramatically reduce the severity, frequency, and duration of migraine headaches when used with vitamin supplementation and a reduction in dietary arachidonate.[35] Combination therapy with EPA, DHA, GLA, and arachidonate was found beneficial for children with symptoms of ADD/ADHD.[95] Combination therapy with EPA and GLA improved biochemical and clinical indexes in adult patients with acute respiratory distress syndrome.[78] Supplementation with GLA, EPA, and calcium is superior to calcium alone in the treatment and prevention of osteoporosis.[47] In a recent placebo-controlled trial with pregnant women, the combination of EPA, DHA, and GLA appeared to protect women from eclampsia and edema.[96] Similarly, in patients with asthma, the combination of EPA and GLA was well tolerated and reduced leukotriene-B4 production.[97] Recently, the combination of EPA+DHA in a 2:1 ratio with GLA was estimated to reduce the risk for myocardial infarction in women by 43%.[98] Thus, using combinations of health-promoting fatty acids from the n-3 family (i.e., ALA, EPA, DHA) and

n-6 family (i.e., GLA) along with n-9 oleic acid to prevent the decrease in oleic acid that occurs with ALA, EPA, and DHA supplementation will most certainly prove clinically beneficial for the treatment and prevention of an impressively wide range of health disorders; the research is already showing a clear trend in this direction.

CONCLUSIONS AND CLINICAL IMPLEMENTATION

Fatty acid imbalances and deficiencies are common in industrialized societies such as America that consume nutritionally deficient diets with a lack of vitamins, minerals, and n-3 fatty acids and a superabundance of artificial foods and over-reliance upon grains.[99, 100] The consistent theme in the research is that supplementation with ALA, EPA, DHA, GLA, and oleic acid provides clinically significant health-promoting benefits in a wide range of patient groups with various health disorders. In the treatment of inflammatory, cardiovascular, and malignant diseases, concomitant reduction in dietary arachidonic acid accentuates the benefits of ALA, EPA, DHA, and GLA supplementation.[101] Paradoxically, preservation of or an increase in tissue levels of arachidonic acid can be uniquely beneficial in patients with neuropsychiatric illness such as depression, attention deficit / hyperactivity disorder, and schizophrenia when treated with fatty acid supplementation.[95, 102, 103]

The safety of fatty acid supplementation is high and has been well established in numerous clinical studies. Drug interactions are extremely rare with fatty acids. The low frequency of drug interactions and adverse effects is to be expected from these fatty acids which are synthesized within the body and/or available from common foods, though in insufficient amounts to be clinically therapeutic. Very high doses of n-3 fatty acids may have a clinically significant anticoagulant effect and should be used cautiously in patients with bleeding tendencies and those taking anticoagulant medications such as coumadin/warfarin, aspirin, or plavix/clopidogrel.

Supplementation with *all* of the health-promoting fatty acids—ALA, EPA, DHA, GLA, and oleic acid—is expected to provide doctors and patients with benefits superior to those attained with the use of single fatty acids in isolation. Doses are tailored to patient size/weight and health status and are kept within the safe boundaries established in published research. Oleic acid is safe at high doses as its is consumed *ad libitum* in Mediterranean diets. The highest daily dose of ALA reported in the literatures is 10,700 mg used in a 4-week study of lactating women.[27] Two studies have used 13,000 mg EPA+DHA per day without adverse effects in hypertensive patients[104] and cancer patients.[105] Four grams per day of GLA has been safely used in adults, and proof of safety was established in a study of infants with eczema given doses of 3 grams per day.[72] Clinical effectiveness of fatty acid supplementation for most conditions (e.g., cancer and all inflammatory/autoimmune diseases) will be increased by implementing a diet low in linoleic and arachidonic acids, which is achieved via avoidance of vegetable oils, nut oils, milk/dairy, and most grain-fed beef, liver, pork, lamb, and, to a lesser extent, turkey and chicken. Food allergens are avoided and the underlying immune dysfunction is addressed with orthomolecular immunomodulation.[25] Balanced, complete fatty acid supplementation along with a health-promoting diet[24,25], multivitamin supplementation[106], and assurance of optimal vitamin D status[25,107] forms the foundational treatment plan for nearly all patients with all diseases. For many patients, regardless of their official "diagnosis", this simple, safe, cost-effective approach of overall health improvement is all the treatment they require. Doctors who use this approach will have achieved a significant clinical advantage in the treatment of patients with premenstrual syndrome, diabetic neuropathy, respiratory distress syndrome, Crohn's disease, lupus, rheumatoid arthritis, cardiovascular disease, hypertension, psoriasis, eczema, migraine headaches[108], bipolar disorder[109], borderline personality disorder, mental depression[110] schizophrenia, osteoporosis[111], polycystic ovary syndrome[112], multiple sclerosis[113], and musculoskeletal pain.[25,114,115] Patients with highly complex illnesses and multiple health disorders may require additional treatment, as will be described in future articles in this journal following a comprehensive synthesis of current research for chiropractic and naturopathic physicians.[25]

ABOUT THE AUTHOR:

Dr. Alex Vasquez is a licensed naturopathic physician in Washington and Oregon, and licensed chiropractor in Texas, where he maintains a private practice and is a member of the Research Team at Biotics Research Corporation. As former Adjunct Professor of Orthopedics and Rheumatology for the Naturopathic Medicine Program at Bastyr University, he is the author of more than 20 published articles and a recently published 486-page textbook for the chiropractic and naturopathic professions, *"Integrative Orthopedics: The Art of Creating Wellness While Managing Acute and Chronic Musculoskeletal Disorders"* available from OptimalHealthResearch.com.

ACKNOWLEDGEMENTS:

Pepper Grimm BA and Mike Owen DC of Biotics Research Corporation reviewed this manuscript before submission.

REFERENCES:

1. Kessler RC, Davis RB, Foster DF, Van Rompay MI, Walters EE, Wilkey SA, Kaptchuk TJ, Eisenberg DM. Long-term trends in the use of complementary and alternative medical therapies in the United States. Ann Intern Med 2001;135:262-268

2. Eisenberg DM, Davis RB, Ettner SL, Appel S, Wilkey S, Van Rompay M, Kessler RC. Trends in alternative medicine use in the United States, 1990-1997: results of a follow-up national survey. JAMA 1998 Nov 11;280(18):1569-75

3. Phillips DP, Christenfeld N, Glynn LM. Increase in US medication-error deaths between 1983 and 1993. Lancet. 1998 Feb 28;351(9103):643-4

4. "CONCLUSIONS: There is a substantial amount of injury to patients from medical management, and many injuries are the result of substandard care." Brennan TA, Leape LL, Laird NM, Hebert L, Localio AR, Lawthers AG, Newhouse JP, Weiler PC, Hiatt HH. Incidence of adverse events and negligence in hospitalized patients: results of the Harvard Medical Practice Study I. 1991. Qual Saf Health Care. 2004 Apr;13(2):145-51

5. "Participants received 54.9 percent (95 percent confidence interval, 54.3 to 55.5) of recommended care." McGlynn EA, Asch SM, Adams J, Keesey J, Hicks J, DeCristofaro A, Kerr EA. The quality of health care delivered to adults in the United States. N Engl J Med. 2003 Jun 26;348(26):2635-45

6. Holland EG, Degruy FV. Drug-induced disorders. Am Fam Physician. 1997 Nov 1;56(7):1781-8, 1791-2 Available at http://aafp.org/afp/971101ap/holland.html on September 8, 2004

7. "...failed to show paroxetine to be more efficacious than placebo. In addition, the pooled results showed that suicidal thoughts, suicide attempts and episodes of self-harm were more frequent among the paroxetine users (5.3% of 378 children) than among those in the placebo group (2.8% of 285 children)." Wooltorton E. Paroxetine (Paxil, Seroxat): increased risk of suicide in pediatric patients. CMAJ. 2003 Sep 2;169(5):446

8. "The risk of suicidal behavior is increased in the first month after starting antidepressants, especially during the first 1 to 9 days." Jick H, Kaye JA, Jick SS. Antidepressants and the risk of suicidal behaviors. JAMA. 2004 Jul 21;292(3):338-43

9. Jick SS, Dean AD, Jick H. Antidepressants and suicide. BMJ. 1995 Jan 28;310(6974):215-8

10. "The evidence consistently reveals that maintaining all schizophrenia patients on antipsychotics produces poor long-term outcomes..." Whitaker R. The case against antipsychotic drugs: a 50-year record of doing more harm than good. Med Hypotheses. 2004;62(1):5-13

11. Goldhamer A, et al. Medically supervised water-only fasting in the treatment of hypertension. J Manipulative Physiol Ther 2001 Jun;24(5):335-9

12. Goldhamer AC, et al. Medically supervised water-only fasting in the treatment of borderline hypertension. J Altern Complement Med. 2002 Oct;8(5):643-50

13. "At...concentrations comparable to those... in the synovial fluid of patients treated with the drug, several NSAIDs suppress proteoglycan synthesis... These NSAID-related effects on chondrocyte metabolism ... are much more profound in osteoarthritic cartilage than in normal cartilage, due to enhanced uptake of NSAIDs by the osteoarthritic cartilage." Brandt KD. Effects of nonsteroidal anti-inflammatory drugs on chondrocyte metabolism in vitro and in vivo. Am J Med. 1987 Nov 20; 83(5A): 29-34

14. "This highly significant association between NSAID use and acetabular destruction gives cause for concern, not least because of the difficulty in achieving satisfactory hip replacements in patients with severely damaged acetabula." Newman NM, Ling RS. Acetabular bone destruction related to non-steroidal anti-inflammatory drugs. Lancet. 1985 Jul 6; 2(8415): 11 4

15. Brandt KD. Effects of nonsteroidal anti-inflammatory drugs on chondrocyte metabolism in vitro and in vivo. Am J Med. 1987 Nov 20; 83(5A): 29-34

16. Nelson R. Coxibs not cost-effective for arthritis in most patients. Lancet 2003; May 24: 1796

17. Spiegel BM, Targownik L, Dulai GS, Gralnek IM. The cost-effectiveness of cyclooxygenase-2 selective inhibitors in the management of chronic arthritis. Ann Intern Med. 2003 May 20;138(10):795-806

18. "In these trials rofecoxib 12.5-25 mg/day was no more effective than the comparators (ibuprofen or diclofenac) used at maximal recommended doses." Rofecoxib: new preparation. A disappointing NSAID analgesic. Prescrire Int 2000 Dec;9(50):166-7, 169

19. "The results from VIGOR showed that the relative risk of developing a confirmed adjudicated thrombotic cardiovascular event (myocardial infarction, unstable angina, cardiac thrombus, resuscitated cardiac arrest, sudden or unexplained death, ischemic stroke, and transient ischemic attacks) with rofecoxib treatment compared with naproxen was 2.38." Mukherjee D, Nissen SE, Topol EJ. Risk of cardiovascular events associated with selective COX-2 inhibitors. JAMA 2001; 286(8):954-9

20. "Systolic blood pressure increased significantly in 17% of rofecoxib- compared with 11% of celecoxib-treated patients (P = 0.032) at any study time point." Whelton A, Fort JG, Puma JA, Normandin D, Bello AE, Verburg KM; SUCCESS VI Study Group.Cyclooxygenase-2—specific inhibitors and cardiorenal function: a randomized, controlled trial of celecoxib and rofecoxib in older hypertensive osteoarthritis patients. Am J Ther 2001 Mar-Apr;8(2):85-95

21. Topol EJ, Falk GW. A coxib a day won't keep the doctor away. Lancet. 2004 Aug 21;364(9435):639-40

22. Orme-Johnson DW, Herron RE. An innovative approach to reducing medical care utilization and expenditures. Am J Manag Care. 1997 Jan;3(1):135-44

23. Ornish D, et al. Intensive lifestyle changes for reversal of coronary heart disease. JAMA. 1998 Dec 16;280(23):2001-7

24. Vasquez A. Reducing Pain and Inflammation Naturally. Part 1: New Insights into Fatty Acid Biochemistry and the Influence of Diet. Nutritional Perspectives 2004; October pages 3-14

25. Vasquez A. Integrative Orthopedics: The Art of Creating Wellness While Managing Acute and Chronic Musculoskeletal Disorders. Houston; Natural Health Consulting Corporation. (www.OptimalHealthResearch.com): 2004

26. "Indu and Ghafoorunissa showed that while keeping the amount of dietary LA constant, 3.7 g ALA appears to have biological effects similar to those of 0.3 g long-chain n-3 PUFA with conversion of 11 g ALA to 1 g long-chain n-3 PUFA." Simopoulos AP. Essential fatty acids in health and chronic disease. Am J Clin Nutr. 1999 Sep;70(3 Suppl):560S-569S

27. Francois CA, Connor SL, Bolewicz LC, Connor WE. Supplementing lactating women with flaxseed oil does not increase docosahexaenoic acid in their milk. Am J Clin Nutr. 2003 Jan;77(1):226-33

28. "Linear relationships were found between dietary alpha-LA and EPA in plasma fractions and in cellular phospholipids. … There was an inverse relationship between dietary alpha-LA and docosahexaenoic acid concentrations in the phospholipids of plasma, neutrophils, mononuclear cells, and platelets." Mantzioris E, James MJ, Gibson RA, Cleland LG. Differences exist in the relationships between dietary linoleic and alpha-linolenic acids and their respective long-chain metabolites. Am J Clin Nutr. 1995 Feb;61(2):320-4

29. "CONCLUSIONS: Dietary supplementation with ALA for 3 months decreases significantly CRP, SAA and IL-6 levels in dyslipidaemic patients. This anti-inflammatory effect may provide a possible additional mechanism for the beneficial effect of plant n-3 polyunsaturated fatty acids in primary and secondary prevention of coronary artery disease." Rallidis LS, Paschos G, Liakos GK, Velissaridou AH, Anastasiadis G, Zampelas A. Dietary alpha-linolenic acid decreases C-reactive protein, serum amyloid A and interleukin-6 in dyslipidaemic patients. Atherosclerosis. 2003 Apr;167(2):237-42

30. Tak PP, Firestein GS. NF-kappaB: a key role in inflammatory diseases. J Clin Invest. 2001 Jan;107(1):7-11

31. "Thus, 3-month's supplementation with alpha-LNA did not prove to be beneficial in rheumatoid arthritis." Nordstrom DC, Honkanen VE, Nasu Y, Antila E, Friman C, Konttinen YT. Alpha-linolenic acid in the treatment of rheumatoid arthritis. A double-blind, placebo-controlled and randomized study: flaxseed vs. safflower seed. Rheumatol Int. 1995;14(6):231-4

32. Adam O, Wolfram G, Zollner N. Effect of alpha-linolenic acid in the human diet on linoleic acid metabolism and prostaglandin biosynthesis. J Lipid Res. 1986 Apr;27(4):421-6

33. Van Hecken A, Schwartz JI, Depre M, De Lepeleire I, Dallob A, Tanaka W, Wynants K, Buntinx A, Arnout J, Wong PH, Ebel DL, Gertz BJ, De Schepper PJ. Comparative inhibitory activity of rofecoxib, meloxicam, diclofenac, ibuprofen, and naproxen on COX-2 versus COX-1 in healthy volunteers. J Clin Pharmacol. 2000 Oct;40(10):1109-20

34. Hu FB, Stampfer MJ, Manson JE, Rimm EB, Wolk A, Colditz GA, Hennekens CH, Willett WC. Dietary intake of alpha-linolenic acid and risk of fatal ischemic heart disease among women. Am J Clin Nutr. 1999 May;69(5):890-7

35. Wagner W, Nootbaar-Wagner U. Prophylactic treatment of migraine with gamma-linolenic and alpha-linolenic acids. Cephalalgia. 1997 Apr;17(2):127-30

36. Tapiero H, et al. Polyunsaturated fatty acids (PUFA) and eicosanoids in human health and pathologies. Biomed Pharmacother. 2002 Jul;56(5):215-22

37. Horrobin DF. Interactions between n-3 and n-6 essential fatty acids (EFAs) in the regulation of cardiovascular disorders and inflammation. Prostaglandins Leukot Essent Fatty Acids. 1991 Oct;44(2):127-31

38. "A dose of 1.8 g EPA/d did not result in any prolongation in bleeding time, but 4 g/d increased bleeding time and decreased platelet count with no adverse effects. In human studies, there has never been a case of clinical bleeding…" Simopoulos AP. Essential fatty acids in health and chronic disease. Am J Clin Nutr. 1999 Sep;70(3 Suppl):560S-569S

39. Yasui T, Tanaka H, Fujita K, Iguchi M, Kohri K. Effects of eicosapentaenoic acid on urinary calcium excretion in calcium stone formers. Eur Urol. 2001 May;39(5):580-5

40. Duffy EM, Meenagh GK, McMillan SA, Strain JJ, Hannigan BM, Bell AL. The clinical effect of dietary supplementation with omega-3 fish oils and/or copper in systemic lupus erythematosus. J Rheumatol. 2004 Aug;31(8):1551-6

41. Wigmore SJ, Barber MD, Ross JA, Tisdale MJ, Fearon KC. Effect of oral eicosapentaenoic acid on weight loss in patients with pancreatic cancer. Nutr Cancer. 2000;36(2):177-84

42. Zanarini MC, Frankenburg FR. omega-3 Fatty acid treatment of women with borderline personality disorder: a double-blind, placebo-controlled pilot study. Am J Psychiatry. 2003 Jan;160(1):167-9

43. Nemets B, Stahl Z, Belmaker RH. Addition of omega-3 fatty acid to maintenance medication treatment for recurrent unipolar depressive disorder. Am J Psychiatry. 2002 Mar;159(3):477-9

44. Puri BK, Counsell SJ, Hamilton G, Richardson AJ, Horrobin DF. Eicosapentaenoic acid in treatment-resistant depression associated with symptom remission, structural brain changes and reduced neuronal phospholipid turnover. Int J Clin Pract. 2001 Oct;55(8):560-3

45. Peet M, Horrobin DF. A dose-ranging study of the effects of ethyl-eicosapentaenoate in patients with ongoing depression despite apparently adequate treatment with standard drugs. Arch Gen Psychiatry. 2002 Oct;59(10):913-9

46. Emsley R, Myburgh C, Oosthuizen P, van Rensburg SJ. Randomized, placebo-controlled study of ethyl-eicosapentaenoic acid as supplemental treatment in schizophrenia. Am J Psychiatry. 2002 Sep;159(9):1596-8

47. Kruger MC, Coetzer H, de Winter R, Gericke G, van Papendorp DH. Calcium, gamma-linolenic acid and eicosapentaenoic acid supplementation in senile osteoporosis. Aging (Milano). 1998 Oct;10(5):385-94

48. Hong S, Gronert K, Devchand PR, Moussignac RL, Serhan CN. Novel docosatrienes and 17S-resolvins generated from docosahexaenoic acid in murine brain, human blood, and glial cells. Autacoids in anti-inflammation. J Biol Chem. 2003 Apr 25;278(17):14677-87

49. Ahmad A, Murthy M, Greiner RS, Moriguchi T, Salem N Jr. A decrease in cell size accompanies a loss of docosahexaenoate in the rat hippocampus. Nutr Neurosci. 2002 Apr;5(2):103-13

50. Pawlosky RJ, Bacher J, Salem N Jr. Ethanol consumption alters electroretinograms and depletes neural tissues of docosahexaenoic acid in rhesus monkeys: nutritional consequences of a low n-3 fatty acid diet. Alcohol Clin Exp Res. 2001 Dec;25(12):1758-65

51. Horrocks LA, Yeo YK. Health benefits of docosahexaenoic acid (DHA). Pharmacol Res. 1999 Sep;40(3):211-25

52. Linday LA, Dolitsky JN, Shindledecker RD, Pippenger CE. Lemon-flavored cod liver oil and a multivitamin-mineral supplement for the secondary prevention of otitis media in young children: pilot research. Ann Otol Rhinol Laryngol. 2002 Jul;111(7 Pt 1):642-52

53. Bairati I, Roy L, Meyer F. Double-blind, randomized, controlled trial of fish oil supplements in prevention of recurrence of stenosis after coronary angioplasty. Circulation. 1992 Mar;85(3):950-6

54. Stoll AL, Severus WE, Freeman MP, Rueter S, Zboyan HA, Diamond E, Cress KK, Marangell LB. Omega 3 fatty acids in bipolar disorder: a preliminary double-blind, placebo-controlled trial. Arch Gen Psychiatry. 1999 May;56(5):407-12

55. Belluzzi A, Brignola C, Campieri M, Pera A, Boschi S, Miglioli M. Effect of an enteric-coated fish-oil preparation on relapses in Crohn's disease. N Engl J Med. 1996 Jun 13;334(24):1557-60

56. Adam O, Beringer C, Kless T, Lemmen C, Adam A, Wiseman M, Adam P, Klimmek R, Forth W. Anti-inflammatory effects of a low arachidonic acid diet and fish oil in patients with rheumatoid arthritis. Rheumatol Int. 2003 Jan;23(1):27-36

57. Lau CS, Morley KD, Belch JJ. Effects of fish oil supplementation on non-steroidal anti-inflammatory drug requirement in patients with mild rheumatoid arthritis—a double-blind placebo controlled study. Br J Rheumatol. 1993 Nov;32(11):982-9

58. Kremer JM, Jubiz W, Michalek A, Rynes RI, Bartholomew LE, Bigaouette J, Timchalk M, Beeler D, Lininger L. Fish-oil fatty acid supplementation in active rheumatoid arthritis. A double-blinded, controlled, crossover study. Ann Intern Med. 1987 Apr;106(4):497-503

59. Walton AJ, Snaith ML, Locniskar M, Cumberland AG, Morrow WJ, Isenberg DA. Dietary fish oil and the severity of symptoms in patients with systemic lupus erythematosus. Ann Rheum Dis. 1991 Jul;50(7):463-6

60. "The recent GISSI (Gruppo Italiano per lo Studio della Sopravvivenza nell'Infarto miocardico)-Prevention study of 11,324 patients showed a 45% decrease in risk of sudden cardiac death and a 20% reduction in all-cause mortality in the group taking 850 mg/d of omega-3 fatty acids." O'Keefe JH Jr, Harris WS. From Inuit to implementation: omega-3 fatty acids come of age. Mayo Clin Proc. 2000 Jun;75(6):607-14

61. Bittiner SB, Tucker WF, Cartwright I, Bleehen SS. A double-blind, randomised, placebo-controlled trial of fish oil in psoriasis. Lancet. 1988 Feb 20;1(8582):378-80

62. Gogos CA, Ginopoulos P, Salsa B, Apostolidou E, Zoumbos NC, Kalfarentzos F. Dietary omega-3 polyunsaturated fatty acids plus vitamin E restore immunodeficiency and prolong survival for severely ill patients with generalized malignancy: a randomized control trial. Cancer. 1998 Jan 15;82(2):395-402

63. Hamazaki T, Itomura M, Sawazaki S, Nagao Y. Anti-stress effects of DHA. Biofactors. 2000;13(1-4):41-5

64. Sawazaki S, Hamazaki T, Yazawa K, Kobayashi M. The effect of docosahexaenoic acid on plasma catecholamine concentrations and glucose tolerance during long-lasting psychological stress: a double-blind placebo-controlled study. J Nutr Sci Vitaminol (Tokyo). 1999 Oct;45(5):655-65

65. Fan YY, Chapkin RS. Importance of dietary gamma-linolenic acid in human health and nutrition. J Nutr. 1998 Sep;128(9):1411-4

66. Horrobin DF. Ascorbic acid and prostaglandin synthesis. Subcell Biochem. 1996;25:109-15

67. Fan YY, Chapkin RS. Importance of dietary gamma-linolenic acid in human health and nutrition. J Nutr. 1998 Sep;128(9):1411-4

68. Horrobin DF, Manku MS. Possible role of prostaglandin E1 in the affective

disorders and in alcoholism. Br Med J. 1980 Jun 7;280(6228):1363-6

69. Rubin D, Laposata M. Cellular interactions between n-6 and n-3 fatty acids: a mass analysis of fatty acid elongation/desaturation, distribution among complex lipids, and conversion to eicosanoids. J Lipid Res. 1992 Oct;33(10):1431-40

70. .Fan YY, Chapkin RS. Importance of dietary gamma-linolenic acid in human health and nutrition. J Nutr. 1998 Sep;128(9):1411-4

71. Ghosh J, Myers CE. Inhibition of arachidonate 5-lipoxygenase triggers massive apoptosis in human prostate cancer cells. Proc Natl Acad Sci U S A. 1998 Oct 27;95(22):13182-7

72. Fiocchi A, Sala M, Signoroni P, Banderali G, Agostoni C, Riva E. The efficacy and safety of gamma-linolenic acid in the treatment of infantile atopic dermatitis. J Int Med Res. 1994 Jan-Feb;22(1):24-32

73. Kenny FS, Pinder SE, Ellis IO, Gee JM, Nicholson RI, Bryce RP, Robertson JF. Gamma linolenic acid with tamoxifen as primary therapy in breast cancer. Int J Cancer. 2000 Mar 1;85(5):643-8

74. Puolakka J, Makarainen L, Viinikka L, Ylikorkala O. Biochemical and clinical effects of treating the premenstrual syndrome with prostaglandin synthesis precursors. J Reprod Med. 1985 Mar;30(3):149-53

75. Brzeski M, Madhok R, Capell HA. Evening primrose oil in patients with rheumatoid arthritis and side-effects of non-steroidal anti-inflammatory drugs. Br J Rheumatol. 1991 Oct;30(5):370-2

76. Rothman D, DeLuca P, Zurier RB. Botanical lipids: effects on inflammation, immune responses, and rheumatoid arthritis. Semin Arthritis Rheum. 1995 Oct;25(2):87-96

77. Jamal GA, Carmichael H. The effect of gamma-linolenic acid on human diabetic peripheral neuropathy: a double-blind placebo-controlled trial. Diabet Med. 1990 May;7(4):319-23

78. Pacht ER, DeMichele SJ, Nelson JL, Hart J, Wennberg AK, Gadek JE. Enteral nutrition with eicosapentaenoic acid, gamma-linolenic acid, and antioxidants reduces alveolar inflammatory mediators and protein influx in patients with acute respiratory distress syndrome. Crit Care Med. 2003 Feb;31(2):491-500

79. Massaro M, Carluccio MA, De Caterina R. Direct vascular antiatherogenic effects of oleic acid: a clue to the cardioprotective effects of the Mediterranean diet. Cardiologia. 1999 Jun;44(6):507-13

80. de Lorgeril M, Salen P, Martin JL, Monjaud I, Boucher P, Mamelle N. Mediterranean dietary pattern in a randomized trial: prolonged survival and possible reduced cancer rate. Arch Intern Med. 1998 Jun 8;158(11):1181-7

81. Alarcon de la Lastra C, Barranco MD, Motilva V, Herrerias JM. Mediterranean diet and health: biological importance of olive oil. Curr Pharm Des. 2001 Jul;7(10):933-50

82. Kaput J, Rodriguez RL. Nutritional genomics: the next frontier in the postgenomic era. Physiol Genomics. 2004 Jan 15;16(2):166-77

83. Rusyn I, Bradham CA, Cohn L, Schoonhoven R, Swenberg JA, Brenner DA, Thurman RG. Corn oil rapidly activates nuclear factor-kappaB in hepatic Kupffer cells by oxidant-dependent mechanisms. Carcinogenesis. 1999 Nov;20(11):2095-100

84. Rose DP, Hatala MA, Connolly JM, Rayburn J. Effect of diets containing different levels of linoleic acid on human breast cancer growth and lung metastasis in nude mice. Cancer Res. 1993 Oct 1;53(19):4686-90

85. Dichtl W, Ares MP, Jonson AN, Jovinge S, Pachinger O, Giachelli CM, Hamsten A, Eriksson P, Nilsson J. Linoleic acid-stimulated vascular adhesion molecule-1 expression in endothelial cells depends on nuclear factor-kappaB activation. Metabolism. 2002 Mar;51(3):327-33

86. Bagga D, Wang L, Farias-Eisner R, Glaspy JA, Reddy ST. Differential effects of prostaglandin derived from omega-6 and omega-3 polyunsaturated fatty acids on COX-2 expression and IL-6 secretion. Proc Natl Acad Sci U S A. 2003 Feb 18;100(4):1751-6. Available at http://www.pnas.org/cgi/reprint/100/4/1751.pdf

87. Menendez JA, Colomer R, Lupu R. Omega-6 polyunsaturated fatty acid gamma-linolenic acid (18:3n-6) is a selective estrogen-response modulator in human breast cancer cells: gamma-linolenic acid antagonizes estrogen receptor-dependent transcriptional activity, transcriptionally represses estrogen receptor expression and synergistically enhances tamoxifen and ICI 182,780 (Faslodex) efficacy in human breast cancer cells. Int J Cancer. 2004 May 10;109(6):949-54

88. Jiang WG, Redfern A, Bryce RP, Mansel RE. Peroxisome proliferator activated receptor-gamma (PPAR-gamma) mediates the action of gamma linolenic acid in breast cancer cells. Prostaglandins Leukot Essent Fatty Acids. 2000 Feb;62(2):119-27

89. Mishra A, Chaudhary A, Sethi S. Oxidized omega-3 fatty acids inhibit NF-kappaB activation via a PPARalpha-dependent pathway. Arterioscler Thromb Vasc Biol. 2004 Sep;24(9):1621-7

90. Zhao Y, Joshi-Barve S, Barve S, Chen LH. Eicosapentaenoic acid prevents LPS-induced TNF-alpha expression by preventing NF-kappaB activation. J Am Coll Nutr. 2004 Feb;23(1):71-8

91. Palakurthi SS, Fluckiger R, Aktas H, Changolkar AK, Shahsafaei A, Harneit S, Kilic E, Halperin JA. Inhibition of translation initiation mediates the anticancer effect of the n-3 polyunsaturated fatty acid eicosapentaenoic acid. Cancer Res. 2000 Jun 1;60(11):2919-25

92. "...intake of fish oil caused a significant depression in the content of DGLA... Since DGLA is the precursor of PGE1, which has been shown to

be anti-inflammatory, our findings suggest that the anti-inflammatory effects of fish oil consumption could be mitigated by an associated reduction in DGLA." Cleland LG, Gibson RA, Neumann M, French JK. The effect of dietary fish oil supplement upon the content of dihomo-gammalinolenic acid in human plasma phospholipids. Prostaglandins Leukot Essent Fatty Acids. 1990 May;40(1):9-12

93. "Supplementation with long-chain n-3 FAs in NIDDM patients leads to the lowering of oleic acid SPL content." Haban P, Zidekova E, Klvanova J. Supplementation with long-chain n-3 fatty acids in non-insulin-dependent diabetes mellitus (NIDDM) patients leads to the lowering of oleic acid content in serum phospholipids. Eur J Nutr. 2000 Oct;39(5):201-6

94. "The decrease in serum eicosapentaenoic acid and the increase in arachidonic acid concentrations induced by evening primrose oil may not be favourable effects in patients with rheumatoid arthritis in the light of the roles of these fatty acids as precursors of eicosanoids." Jantti J, Nikkari T, Solakivi T, Vapaatalo H, Isomaki H. Evening primrose oil in rheumatoid arthritis: changes in serum lipids and fatty acids. Ann Rheum Dis. 1989 Feb;48(2):124-7

95. Stevens L, Zhang W, Peck L, Kuczek T, Grevstad N, Mahon A, Zentall SS, Arnold LE, Burgess JR. EFA supplementation in children with inattention, hyperactivity, and other disruptive behaviors. Lipids. 2003 Oct;38(10):1007-21

96. D'Almeida A, Carter JP, Anatol A, Prost C. Effects of a combination of evening primrose oil (gamma linolenic acid) and fish oil (eicosapentaenoic + docahexaenoic acid) versus magnesium, and versus placebo in preventing pre-eclampsia. Women Health. 1992;19(2-3):117-31

97. Surette ME, Koumenis IL, Edens MB, Tramposch KM, Clayton B, Bowton D, Chilton FH. Inhibition of leukotriene biosynthesis by a novel dietary fatty acid formulation in patients with atopic asthma: a randomized, placebo-controlled, parallel-group, prospective trial. Clin Ther. 2003 Mar;25(3):972-9

98. Laidlaw M, Holub BJ. Effects of supplementation with fish oil-derived n-3 fatty acids and gamma-linolenic acid on circulating plasma lipids and fatty acid profiles in women. Am J Clin Nutr. 2003 Jan;77(1):37-42

99. Simopoulos AP. Essential fatty acids in health and chronic disease. Am J Clin Nutr. 1999 Sep;70(3 Suppl):560S-569S

100. O'Keefe JH Jr, Cordain L. Cardiovascular disease resulting from a diet and lifestyle at odds with our Paleolithic genome: how to become a 21st-century hunter-gatherer. Mayo Clin Proc 2004 Jan;79(1):101-8

101. Adam O, Beringer C, Kless T, Lemmen C, Adam A, Wiseman M, Adam P, Klimmek R, Forth W. Anti-inflammatory effects of a low arachidonic acid diet and fish oil in patients with rheumatoid arthritis. Rheumatol Int. 2003 Jan;23(1):27-36

102. Horrobin DF, Jenkins K, Bennett CN, Christie WW. Eicosapentaenoic acid and arachidonic acid: collaboration and not antagonism is the key to biological understanding. Prostaglandins Leukot Essent Fatty Acids. 2002 Jan;66(1):83-90

103. Peet M, Horrobin DF; E-E Multicentre Study Group. A dose-ranging exploratory study of the effects of ethyl-eicosapentaenoate in patients with persistent schizophrenic symptoms. J Psychiatr Res. 2002 Jan-Feb;36(1):7-18

104. Du Plooy WJ, Venter CP, Muntingh GM, Venter HL, Glatthaar II, Smith KA. The cumulative dose response effect of eicosapentaenoic and docosahexaenoic acid on blood pressure, plasma lipid profile and diet pattern in mild to moderate essential hypertensive black patients. Prostaglandins Leukot Essent Fatty Acids 1992 Aug;46(4):315-21

105. Burns CP, Halabi S, Clamon GH, Hars V, Wagner BA, Hohl RJ, Lester E, Kirshner JJ, Vinciguerra V, Paskett E. Phase I clinical study of fish oil fatty acid capsules for patients with cancer cachexia: cancer and leukemia group B study 9473. Clin Cancer Res. 1999 Dec;5(12):3942-7

106. Fletcher RH, Fairfield KM. Vitamins for chronic disease prevention in adults: clinical applications. JAMA. 2002 Jun 19;287(23):3127-9

107. Vasquez A, Manso M, Cannell J. The Clinical Importance of Vitamin D (Cholecalciferol): A Paradigm Shift with Implications for All Healthcare Providers. Alternative Therapies in Health and Medicine 2004; 10: 28-37

108. Grant EC. Food allergy and migraine. Lancet. 1979 Aug 18;2(8138):358-9

109. Kaplan BJ, Simpson JS, Ferre RC, Gorman CP, McMullen DM, Crawford SG. Effective mood stabilization with a chelated mineral supplement: an open-label trial in bipolar disorder. J Clin Psychiatry. 2001 Dec;62(12):936-44

110. Lansdowne AT, Provost SC. Vitamin D3 enhances mood in healthy subjects during winter. Psychopharmacology (Berl). 1998;135(4):319-23

111. Holick MF. Vitamin D: importance in the prevention of cancers, type 1 diabetes, heart disease, and osteoporosis. Am J Clin Nutr. 2004;79(3):362-71

112. Thys-Jacobs S, Donovan D, Papadopoulos A, Sarrel P, Bilezikian JP. Vitamin D and calcium dysregulation in the polycystic ovarian syndrome. Steroids. 1999;64(6):430-5

113. Goldberg P, Fleming MC, Picard EH. Multiple sclerosis: decreased relapse rate through dietary supplementation with calcium, magnesium and vitamin D. Med Hypotheses. 1986 Oct;21(2):193-200

114. Al Faraj S, Al Mutairi K. Vitamin D deficiency and chronic low back pain in Saudi Arabia. Spine. 2003;28(2):177-9

115. Vasquez A. Integrative Orthopedics and Vitamin D: Testing, Administration, and New Relevance in the Treatment of Musculoskeletal Pain. Townsend Letter for Doctors and Patients 2004; October, 75-77

Reducing Pain and Inflammation Naturally – Part 3: Improving Over-all Health While Safely and Effectively Treating Musculoskeletal Pain

Alex Vasquez, D.C., N.D.

Abstract: Following the optimization of diet and fatty acid balance, the next therapeutic steps in the treatment of pain and inflammation can include the use of vitamin D, chondroitin sulfate, niacinamide, and botanical medicines such as Boswellia. In direct contrast to so-called "anti-inflammatory drugs" which always have significant toxicity, each of these natural treatments has been proven in controlled clinical trials to significantly reduce pain and inflammation without major adverse effects. Chondroitin sulfate has actually been shown to reduce cardiovascular mortality in humans while it safely and effectively ameliorates the pain and inflammation of osteoarthritis. Similarly, vitamin D supplementation has been proven effective in the treatment of hypertension, depression, migraine headaches, polycystic ovary syndrome and in the prevention of type-1 diabetes. By failing to fully cover chiropractic and naturopathic healthcare services, insurance companies which comprise and contribute to the American healthcare system are losing profitability and forcing patients to use drug and surgical treatments that are commonly less effective, more dangerous, and more expensive than the natural treatments described in this paper. Services provided by chiropractic and naturopathic physicians are supported by peer-reviewed research and deserve equitable coverage and status in America's healthcare system.

INTRODUCTION

As primary care providers with specialized training in musculoskeletal medicine, chiropractic physicians typically play a dual role in clinical practice on a daily basis, generally striving to simultaneously accomplish two related goals in each patient: 1) promoting overall wellness and professionally-supervised patient-implemented preventive healthcare, and 2) alleviating acute and chronic musculoskeletal pain. Both of these goals are important given the tremendous financial and social impact of musculoskeletal pain and the progressive deterioration of Americans' health. At any given time, nearly thirty percent of the American population suffers from musculoskeletal pain, joint swelling, or limitation of movement, and approximately 1 of every 7 (14% of total) visits to a primary healthcare provider is for the treatment of musculoskeletal pain or dysfunction. Resulting in more than $100 billion in US healthcare costs each year, back pain is the most prevalent medical problem in the US, is the leading cause of long-term disability, and is the second leading cause of restricted activity and the use of prescription and non-prescription drugs.[1] The preventive healthcare and wellness promotion advocated and implemented by chiropractic and naturopathic physicians is now more important than ever since the health of the American population is consistently and progressively declining: obesity and diabetes are "ever-growing" epidemics among children and adults,[2] infant mortality has recently increased for the first time in 40 years,[3] and self-reported health status and health-related quality of life among adults are declining.[4] In the 25 years between 1975 and 2000, the incidence of cancer increased significantly, and the number of people diagnosed with cancer is expected to double in the next several decades.[5] Despite these negative health trends, America spends more on healthcare than does any other nation—an unprecedented $1.55 trillion, which is roughly 15% of the US gross domestic product.[6] From the perspective of cost-effectiveness, the medically-dominated American healthcare system delivers a very poor return on investment, and it appears that assertive wellness promotion and increased utilization of chiropractic and naturopathic healthcare may provide improved outcomes and decreased overall healthcare costs.[7,8]

Numerous adverse effects are produced as a direct result of medical/pharmaceutical management of benign musculoskeletal pain. According to a 1998 review by Singh,[9] "Conservative calculations estimate that approximately 107,000 patients are hospitalized annually for nonsteroidal anti-inflammatory drug (NSAID)-related gastrointestinal (GI) complications and at least 16,500 NSAID-related deaths occur each year among arthritis patients alone. The figures for all NSAID users would be overwhelming, yet the scope of this problem is generally under-appreciated." More recently following the withdrawal of the arthritis drug rofecoxib (Vioxx) in late September 2004, Topol[10] extrapolated that as many as 160,000 adverse cardiovascular events (including stroke, myocardial infarction, and death) may have resulted from the collusion of Merck's intentional failure to withdraw what was known for years to be a dangerous drug, the FDA's failure to enforce regulatory standards to protect the public, and the overutilization of Vioxx by the medical profession, which was well informed of the lethality of Vioxx for several years[11] before Merck's confessionary and belated withdrawal of the drug. Soon thereafter, several other so-called "anti-inflammatory drugs" such as valdecoxib (Bextra),[12] celecoxib (Celebrex),[13] and naproxen (Aleve)[14] were likewise associated with excess cardiovascular injury and death. Although the advertising-induced feeding frenzy on Celebrex made it the most successful drug launch in US history with more than 7.4 million prescriptions written within its first 6 months,[15] within 2 years of its release, evidence linking the drug to increased cardiovascular events (including death) was accumulating,[11] and the drug has since been linked to a wide range of adverse effects such as membranous glomerulopathy and acute interstitial nephritis,[16] acute cholestatic hepatitis,[17] and toxic epidermal necrolysis.[18] When compared with placebo in cardiac surgery patients, Bextra/valdecoxib is associated with a 3-fold to 4-fold increased risk of heart attack, stroke, and death,[19] and currently 7 million arthritis patients, many of whom are already at high risk for cardiovascular disease, are being treated with this drug.[12]

Increasingly aware of the negative effects of pharmaceutical management of musculoskeletal pain, patients and healthcare providers alike are looking to natural treatments and chiropractic healthcare[20,21] with the hopes of avoiding the risks of iatrogenic disease, such as drug-induced renal failure,[22] hepatotoxicity,[23] gastrointestinal ulceration and hemorrhage,[24] osteonecrosis,[25,26] joint degeneration,[27,28] hypertension,[28] myocardial infarction,[11] and premature death[11,12] that are associated with the non-steroidal anti-inflammatory drugs ("NSAIDs"), non-NSAID analgesics such as acetaminophen, and the relatively new selective cyclooxygenase-2 inhibitors (cox-2 inhibitors, or "coxibs"). It is tragically paradoxical that many of the pharmaceutical drugs used for the suppression of arthritis symptoms and advertised as "arthritis relief" actually exacerbate joint destruction and chronic inflammation by interfering with the biosynthesis of the glycosaminoglycans that are essential components of joint cartilage while also promoting destruction of subchondral bone.[25,26,27,28] This places chiropractic physicians in an ethical dilemma when helping patients who have been prescribed potentially dangerous medications by their medical doctors. On the one hand, chiropractic physicians are aware of the research showing that, for example, coxibs provide little clinical benefit while promoting increased cardiovascular mortality and other potentially lethal adverse effects. On the other hand, if a chiropractic physician advises discontinuation of the medication, he or she may be reprimanded for "practicing medicine." It appears that chiropractic physicians will need to obtain limited prescription rights for the sake of helping protect their patients from iatrogenic and drug-induced disease. Given that chiropractic physicians are already duly trained in basic and clinical sciences sufficient for primary care, post-graduate certification courses in pharmacology would be sufficient if additional training is deemed necessary to obtain these prescription rights.

The first two articles in this series reviewed the importance of diet and fatty acids in the alleviation of pain and inflammation. This article reviews the most commonly used and well-researched nutritional and botanical interventions for the treatment of pain and inflammation,

namely vitamin D, glucosamine and chondroitin sulfate, niacinamide, vitamin D, proteolytic enzymes, Devil's Claw (*Harpagophytum procumbens*), Willow bark (*Salix* spp), and Boswellia (*Boswellia serrata*). This review will provide chiropractic and naturopathic physicians with clinically useful information to help their patients attain improved health and well-being. Osteoarthritis and chronic low-back pain, the two most prevalent musculoskeletal afflictions, will serve as prototypes for this discussion.

SELECTED NUTRITIONAL AND BOTANICAL THERAPEUTICS FOR THE ALLEVIATION OF JOINT PAIN AND INFLAMMATION

Subsequent to the overall health improvement and anti-inflammatory benefits provided by the supplemented Paleo-Mediterranean diet described previously, many patients who require additional anti-inflammatory interventions can be safely and effectively treated with the following phytonutraceuticals, each of which is supported by experimental and clinical data in humans. Mechanism(s) of action, indications, contraindications, dosage, and common drug interactions (if any) are listed for each.

Glucosamine and chondroitin sulfate: Glucosamine and chondroitin are the "building blocks" from which cartilage is built and oral supplementation is intended to enhance cartilage anabolism and to thus counteract the enhanced cartilage catabolism seen in destructive arthritic processes. Clinical trials with glucosamine and chondroitin sulfates have shown consistently positive results in clinical trials involving patients with osteoarthritis of the hands, hips, knees, temporomandibular joint, and low-back.[29,30,31,32,33,34] For example, glucosamine sulfate was superior to placebo for pain reduction and preservation of joint space in a 3-year clinical trial in patients with knee osteoarthritis.[36] Arguments against the use of glucosamine due to inflated concern about inefficacy or exacerbation of diabetes[37] are without scientific merit[38,39] as evidenced by a 90-day trial[40] of diabetic patients consuming 1500 mg of glucosamine hydrochloride with 1200 mg of chondroitin sulfate which showed no significant alterations in serum glucose or hemoglobin A1c and by the previously cited 3-year study which found significant clinical benefit and no adverse effects on glucose homeostasis. The adult dose of glucosamine sulfate is generally 1500-2000 mg per day in divided doses, and the dose of chondroitin sulfate is approximately 1000 mg daily. Both treatments are safe for multiyear use, and rare adverse effects include allergy and nonpathologic gastrointestinal upset. Clinical benefit is generally significant following 4-6 weeks of treatment and is maintained for the duration of treatment. In contrast to coxib and other mislabeled "anti-inflammatory" drugs that consistently elevate the incidence of cardiovascular disease, death, and other adverse effects, supplementation with chondroitin sulfate appears to safely reduce the pain and disability associated with osteoarthritis while simultaneously reducing incidence of cardiovascular morbidity and mortality.[41,42] In a study with animals that spontaneously develop atherosclerosis,[43] administration of chondroitin sulfate appears to have induced regression of existing atherosclerosis. In a six-year study with 120 patients with established cardiovascular disease, 60 chondroitin-treated patients suffered 6 coronary events and 4 deaths compared to 42 events and 14 deaths in a comparable group of 60 patients receiving "conventional" therapy; chondroitin-treated patients reported enhancement of well-being while no adverse clinical or laboratory effects were noted during the 6 years of treatment.[44]

Vitamin D (cholecalciferol): Vitamin D insufficiency is epidemic in the United States and is extremely prevalent (>90%) among patients with chronic musculoskeletal pain[45] limb pain,[46] and low-back pain.[47] The mechanism by which this pain is produced has been clearly elucidated: 1) vitamin D deficiency causes a reduction in calcium absorption, 2) production of parathyroid hormone (PTH) is increased to maintain blood calcium levels, 3) PTH results in increased urinary excretion of phosphorus, which leads to hypophosphatemia, 4) insufficient calcium phosphate results in deposition of unmineralized collagen matrix on the endosteal (inside) and periosteal (outside) of bones, 5) when the collagen matrix hydrates and swells, it causes pressure on the sensory-innervated periosteum resulting in pain.[48] In patients with vitamin D deficiency, oral supplementation with vitamin D clearly produces anti-inflammatory benefits,[49,50] and treatment with vitamin D can safely lead to dramatic reductions in musculoskeletal pain in a large percentage of patients.[46,47] Routine annual measurement of vitamin D status should be the standard of care[51] since failure to diagnose vitamin D deficiency and to provide adequate replacement doses are both ethically questionable and scientifically unjustifiable in light of the low cost, manifold benefits, rare adverse effects, and high prevalence of vitamin D deficiency.[52,53] Physiologic requirements are approximately 4,000 IU per day in men[54] and can only be achieved with high-dose oral supplementation or full-body sun exposure on a frequent or preferably daily basis. As reviewed in the recent monograph by Vasquez et al,[55] relative contraindications include the use of thiazide diuretics or presence of a vitamin D hypersensitivity syndrome such as primary hyperparathyroidism, adrenal insufficiency, hyperthyroidism, hypothyroidism, or granulomatous disease such as sarcoidosis, Crohn's disease, or tuberculosis). Serum calcium is periodically monitored in patients receiving moderate doses of vitamin D (adult range 4,000 – 10,000 IU per day), since hypercalcemia is the best laboratory indicator of vitamin D excess.

High doses of vitamin D (up to 100,000 IU per day) have been safely used during pregnancy[56,57] periodic testing of serum calcium is required to monitor and for hypercalcemia. Vitamin D supplementation has been proven effective in the treatment of hypertension, depression, migraine headaches, polycystic ovary syndrome and in the prevention of cancer and type-1 diabetes. [55]

Figure 2. Normal and optimal ranges for serum 25(OH) vitamin D levels based on current research. Used with permission from Vasquez A. Integrative Orthopedics. (OptimalHealthResearch.com): 2004

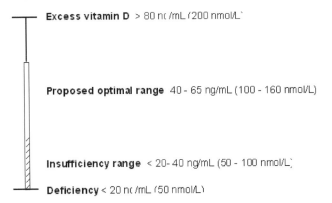

Proteolytic enzymes: Oral administration of proteolytic enzymes (such as pancreatin, bromelain, papain, trypsin and alpha-chymotrypsin) for therapeutic purposes is well established on physiologic, biochemical, and clinical grounds, and a brief review of their historical use is warranted. One of the first experimental studies was published by Beard in 1906 in the *British Medical Journal* wherein he showed that proteolytic enzymes significantly inhibited tumor growth in mice with implanted tumors,[58] and a year later in that same journal, Cutfield[59] reported tumor regression and other objective improvements in a patient treated with proteolytic enzymes. In the American research literature, anti-cancer effects of proteolytic enzymes were reported during this same time in the *Journal of the American Medical Association* in anecdotal case reports of patients with fibrosarcoma,[60] breast cancer,[61] and head and neck malignancy[62]—all of whom responded positively to the administration of proteolytic enzymes; no adverse effects were seen. Although nearly a century would pass before Beard's study and results were replicated with modern techniques,[63,64] by now it is well established that orally administered proteolytic enzymes are well absorbed from the gastrointestinal tract into the systemic circulation[65,66] and that the anti-tumor, anti-metastatic, anti-infectious, anti-inflammatory , analgesic, and anti-edematous actions result from synergism between a variety of mechanisms of action, including the dose-dependent stimulation of reactive oxygen species production and anti-cancer cytotoxicity in human neutrophils,[67] a pro-differentiative effect,[68]

reduction in PG-E2 production,[69] reduction in substance P production,[70] modulation of adhesion molecules and cytokine levels,[71] fibrinolytic effects and a anti-thrombotic effect mediated at least in part by a reduction in 2-series thromboxanes.[72] Unfortunately, enthusiasm for the enzyme treatment of cancer waned prematurely when trypsin was judged to not be a "miracle cure", when the mechanism of action could not be determined, and as enthusiasm surrounding drug and radiation treatments grabbed the attention of allopaths.[73] However, modern controlled clinical trials in cancer patients have established the value of enzyme therapy, which produces important clinical benefit (e.g., symptom reduction and prolonged survival) for little cost and with negligible adverse effects.[74,75,76] Research in other clinical applications for proteolytic enzymes has consistently shown benefit when properly formulated and manufactured preparations are administered appropriately in the treatment of cellulitis, diabetic ulcers, sinusitis, and bronchitis.[77] For example, in a double-blind placebo-controlled trial with 59 patients, Taub[78] documented that oral administration of bromelain significantly promoted the resolution of congestion, inflammation, and edema in patients with acute and chronic refractory sinusitis; no adverse effects were seen in any patient.

When not treating patients with cancer or infectious disease, chiropractic and naturopathic physicians today use these enzymes mostly for the treatment of inflammatory and injury-related disorders. Reporting from the Tulane University Health Service Center, Trickett[79] reported that a papain-containing preparation benefited 40 patients with various injuries (e.g., contusions, sprains, lacerations, strains, fracture, surgical repair, and muscle tears); no adverse effects were seen. In a recent open trial of patients with knee pain, Walker et al[80] found a dose-dependent reduction in pain and disability as well as a significant improvement in psychological well-being in patients consuming bromelain orally. Most of the studies reviewed by Brien et al[69] were suggestive of a positive benefit in patients with knee osteoarthritis, but inadequate dosing clearly prohibited the attainment of optimal results. Bromelain also attenuates experimental contraction-induced skeletal muscle injury,[81] reduces production of hyperalgesic PG-E2 and substance P, is generally effective in the amelioration of trauma-induced injury, edema, and inflammation, and is practically non-toxic.[70] Although bromelain may be used in isolation, enzyme therapy is generally delivered in the form of polyenzyme preparations containing pancreatin, bromelain, papain, trypsin and alpha-chymotrypsin.

Niacinamide: Niacinamide is a form of vitamin B3 that was first shown to be highly effective in the treatment of

osteoarthritis by Kaufman more than 50 years ago.[82] Furthermore, Kaufman's documentation of an "anti-aging" effect of vitamin supplementation in general and niacinamide therapy in particular[83] is consistent with recent experimental data demonstrating rapid reversion of aging phenotypes by niacinamide through possible modulation of histone acetylation.[84] A recent double-blind placebo-controlled repeat study found that niacinamide therapy improved joint mobility, reduced objective inflammation as assessed by ESR, reduced the impact of the arthritis on the activities of daily living, and allowed a reduction in medication use.[85] While the mechanism of action is probably multifaceted, inhibition of joint-destroying nitric oxide appears to be an important benefit.[86] The standard dose of 500 mg given orally 6 times per day is more effective than 1,000 mg 3 times per day. Hepatic dysfunction is rare when daily doses are kept below 3,000 mg per day, yet Gaby[87] suggests measurement of liver enzymes after 3 months of treatment and yearly thereafter. Antirheumatic benefit is generally significant following 2-6 weeks of treatment, and patients may also notice an anxiolytic benefit, which is probably due to the binding of niacinamide to GABA/benzodiazepine receptors.[88]

Boswellia (Boswellia serrata): Boswellia shows anti-inflammatory action via inhibition of 5-lipoxygenase with no apparent effect on cyclooxygenase. A recent clinical study showed that *Boswellia* was able to reduce pain and swelling while increasing joint flexion and walking distance in patients with osteoarthritis of the knee.[89] While reports from clinical trials published in English are relatively rare, a recent abstract from the German medical research[90] stated, "In clinical trials promising results were observed in patients with rheumatoid arthritis, chronic colitis, ulcerative colitis, Crohn's disease, bronchial asthma and peritumoral brains edemas." Additional recent studies have confirmed the effectiveness of Boswellia in the treatment of asthma[91] and ulcerative colitis.[92] Minor gastrointestinal upset has been reported. Products are generally standardized to contain 37.5–65% boswellic acids, which are currently considered the active constituents with clinical benefit. The target dose is approximately 150 mg of boswellic acids thrice daily; dose and number of capsules/tablets will vary depending upon the concentration found in differing products. Lower doses are effective when used as a part of a comprehensive, multicomponent treatment plan.

Devil's Claw (Harpagophytum procumbens): Harpagophytum has a long history of use in the treatment of musculoskeletal complaints, and recent clinical trials have substantiated its role as a moderately effective analgesic suitable for clinical utilization. At least 12 clinical trials have been published on the use of *Harpagophytum* in the treatment of musculoskeletal pain, and all trials have found the botanical to be clinically valuable and with adverse effects comparable to placebo.[93] *Harpagophytum's* clinical benefit appears to derive chiefly from its analgesic effect, since administration of the herb does not alter eicosanoid production in humans. In patients with osteoarthritis of the hip and knee, *Harpagophytum* is just as effective yet safer and better tolerated than the drug diacerhein.[94,95] In a study involving 183 patients with low-back pain, *Harpagophytum* was found to be safe and moderately effective in patients with "severe and unbearable pain" and radiating pain with neurologic deficit.[96] Most recently, *Harpagophytum* was studied in a head-to-head clinical trial with the formerly popular but dangerous selective cox-2 inhibitor Vioxx (rofecoxib); the data indicate that *Harpagophytum* was safer and at least as effective.[97] About 8% of patients may experience diarrhea or other mild gastrointestinal effects, and fewer patients may experience dizziness; *Harpagophytum* may potentiate anticoagulants. Treatment should be continued for at least 4 weeks, and many patients will continue to improve after 8 weeks from the initiation of treatment.[98] Products are generally standardized for the content of harpagosides, with a target dose of at least 30 and up to 60 mg harpagoside per day. However, the whole plant is considered to contain effective constituents, not only the iridoid glycosides. Chrubasik[99] noted that while *Harpagophytum* appears to be safe and moderately effective for the treatment musculoskeletal pain, different proprietary products show significant variances in potency and clinical effectiveness. Data suggest that *Harpagophytum* is better than placebo and at least as good as commonly used NSAIDs, suggesting that Harpagophytum should be clinically preferred over NSAIDs due to the lower cost and what appears to be greater safety.

Willow bark (Salix spp): In a double-blind placebo-controlled clinical trial in 210 patients with moderate/severe low-back pain (20% of patients had positive straight-leg raising test), extract of willow bark showed a dose-dependent analgesic effect with benefits beginning in the first week of treatment.[100] In a head-to-head study of 228 patients comparing willow bark (standardized for 240 mg salicin) with Vioxx (rofecoxib), treatments were equally effective yet willow bark was safer and 40% less expensive.[101] Actions of willow bark are manifold including anti-oxidative, anti-cytokine, along with cyclooxygenase- and lipoxygenase-inhibiting effects. A non-purified extract of the phytomedicinal is required for full clinical benefit. The daily dose should not exceed 240 mg of salicin, and products should include other components of the whole plant. Except for rare allergy, no adverse effects are known, yet use during pregnancy and with anti-coagulant medication is discouraged.

SPINAL MANIPULATION: MECHANISMS OF ACTION AND SYNERGISM WITH NUTRITIONAL/BOTANICAL INTERVENTIONS

Select nutritional interventions as surveyed in this paper may have enhanced effects and benefits when combined with spinal manipulative therapy. For example, enhanced respiratory burst clearly carries both antitumor and antimicrobial benefits, and this physiologic effect can be induced by oral consumption of proteolytic enzymes as well as by chiropractic spinal manipulative therapy.[102] Likewise, we would expect synergism between spinal manipulative therapy[103] and nutritional[104] and botanical (e.g., Boswellia) interventions in the treatment of asthma, particularly since these treatments are mediated primarily via different mechanisms—namely the neurophysiologic inhibition of neurogenic inflammation and the biochemical reduction in pro-inflammatory mediators such as leukotrienes, respectively. As a final example, synergism would be expected in the treatment of low-back pain when spinal manipulation, therapeutic exercise, proprioceptive retraining, oral vitamin D supplementation, and botanical medicines such as *Harpagophytum* and Willow Bark are used together in holistic, integrative, multicomponent treatment plans.[105] Taken together, these data form an integrative model that incorporates and mechanistically validates the chiropractic "triad of health" which appreciates the interconnectedness of physical, biochemical, and neurologic aspects of human physiology.[105]

CONCLUSIONS

The chiropractic profession continues to develop and mature over time and with advances in research that further our understanding of health and disease and the value of diet, nutrition, exercise, spinal manipulation and other natural therapeutics. In contrast to our allopathic counterparts, chiropractic and naturopathic physicians are the only healthcare providers trained to consider each patient as an integrated being and to give specific attention to the physiological and biochemical aspects of health and disease, including structural, spinal, musculoskeletal, neurological, vascular, nutritional, emotional and environmental relationships.[106] The anti-inflammatory and analgesic nutritional and botanical medicines described in this review are generally appropriate for the treatment of inflammatory and degenerative musculoskeletal conditions, and they comprise an attractive alternative to the too-often lethal effects of pharmacologic anti-inflammatory and anti-rheumatic drugs.

If we consider that medical/surgical interventions result in an excess of 110,000 – 225,000 iatrogenic American deaths each year,[107,108] we could reasonably conclude that undue restriction of chiropractic and naturopathic physicians to practice preventive healthcare and the discriminatory legal and financial barriers that inhibit patients from accessing alternatives to drugs and surgery ultimately deny patients' access to safe, effective, cost-effective, empowering, affordable healthcare by simultaneously restricting them to interventions that carry greater risk for harm and greater financial expense. With ever-increasing costs and ever-worsening health outcomes, the American healthcare system is destined for collapse unless we change the model upon which our healthcare system is founded—namely the belief that surgery and chemical drugs are the solutions to chronic diseases induced by nutritional deficiencies, oxidative stress, impaired detoxification, defects in fatty acid metabolism, altered gastrointestinal function, and neuromusculoskeletal dysfunction. We have reached an irrevocable impasse in which our current healthcare system dominated by drugs and surgery is no longer consistent with the balance of scientific research.[109] The time has come for patients and practitioners of natural healthcare to demand change and equitable access within the healthcare arena.

ABOUT THE AUTHOR:

Dr. Alex Vasquez is a licensed naturopathic physician in Washington and Oregon, and licensed chiropractor in Texas, where he maintains a private practice and is a member of the Research Team at Biotics Research Corporation. As former Adjunct Professor of Orthopedics and Rheumatology for the Naturopathic Medicine Program at Bastyr University, he is the author of more than 20 published articles and a recently published 486-page textbook for the chiropractic and naturopathic professions, "Integrative Orthopedics: The Art of Creating Wellness While Managing Acute and Chronic Musculoskeletal Disorders" available from OptimalHealthResearch.com.

ACKNOWLEDGEMENTS:

Pepper Grimm BA of Biotics Research Corporation reviewed the draft of this manuscript before submission.

REFERENCES:

1. Legorreta AP, Metz RD, Nelson CF, Ray S, Chernicoff HO, Dinubile NA. Comparative analysis of individuals with and without chiropractic coverage: patient characteristics, utilization, and costs. Arch Intern Med. 2004;164:1985-92

2. Bloomgarden ZT. Type 2 diabetes in the young: the evolving epidemic. Diabetes Care. 2004;27:998-1010

3. Nelson R. US infant mortality shows first rise in 40 years. Lancet. 2004;363(9409):626

4. Zack MM, Moriarty DG, Stroup DF, Ford ES, Mokdad AH. Worsening trends in adult health-related quality of life and self-rated health-United States, 1993-2001. Public Health Rep. 2004;119:493-505

5. Weir HK, Thun MJ, Hankey BF, Ries LA, Howe HL, Wingo PA, Jemal A, Ward E, Anderson RN, Edwards BK. Annual report to the nation on the status of cancer, 1975-2000, featuring the uses of surveillance data for cancer prevention and control. J Natl Cancer Inst. 2003;95(17):1276-99

6. US health care: a state lottery? Lancet. 2004 Nov 20;364(9448):1829-30

7. Legorreta AP, Metz RD, Nelson CF, Ray S, Chernicoff HO, Dinubile NA. Comparative analysis of individuals with and without chiropractic coverage: patient characteristics, utilization, and costs. Arch Intern Med. 2004;164:1985-92

8. Orme-Johnson DW, Herron RE. An innovative approach to reducing medical care utilization and expenditures. Am J Manag Care. 1997 Jan;3(1):135-44

9. Singh G. Recent considerations in nonsteroidal anti-inflammatory drug gastropathy. Am J Med. 1998;105(1B):31S-38S

10. Topol EJ. Failing the public health—rofecoxib, Merck, and the FDA. N Engl J Med. 2004 Oct 21;351(17):1707-9

11. Mukherjee D, Nissen SE, Topol EJ. Risk of cardiovascular events associated with selective COX-2 inhibitors. JAMA 2001; 286(8):954-9

12. Ray WA, Griffin MR, Stein CM. Cardiovascular toxicity of valdecoxib. N Engl J Med. 2004;351(26):2767

13. "Patients in the clinical trial taking 400 mg. of Celebrex twice daily had a 3.4 times greater risk of CV events compared to placebo. For patients in the trial taking 200 mg. of Celebrex twice daily, the risk was 2.5 times greater. The average duration of treatment in the trial was 33 months." FDA Statement on the Halting of a Clinical Trial of the Cox-2 Inhibitor Celebrex.http://www.fda.gov/bbs/topics /news/2004/NEW01144.html Available on January 4, 2005

14. "Preliminary information from the study showed some evidence of increased risk of cardiovascular events, when compared to placebo, to patients taking naproxen." FDA Statement on Naproxen. http://www.fda.gov/bbs/topics/news/2004/NEW01148.html Available on January 4, 2005

15. Monsanto, Pfizer celebrate Celebrex. St. Louis Business Journal. July 20, 1999

16. Markowitz GS, Falkowitz DC, Isom R, Zaki M, Imaizumi S, Appel GB, D'Agati VD. Membranous glomerulopathy and acute interstitial nephritis following treatment with celecoxib. Clin Nephrol. 2003;59(2):137-42

17. Grieco A, Miele L, Giorgi A, Civello IM, Gasbarrini G. Acute cholestatic hepatitis associated with celecoxib. Ann Pharmacother. 2002;36(12):1887-9

18. Berger P, Dwyer D, Corallo CE. Toxic epidermal necrolysis after celecoxib therapy. Pharmacotherapy. 2002 Sep;22(9): 1193-5

19. Lenzer J. Pfizer criticised over delay in admitting drug's problems. BMJ. 2004;329(7472):935

20. The Growth of Chiropractic and CAM: More Bad News for Medicine. Dynamic Chiropractic October 8, 2001, Volume 19, Issue 21 http://www.chiroweb.com/archives/19/21 /03.html accessed November 11, 2004

21. Kessler RC, Davis RB, Foster DF, Van Rompay MI, Walters EE, Wilkey SA, Kaptchuk TJ, Eisenberg DM. Long-term trends in the use of complementary and alternative medical therapies in the United States. Ann Intern Med. 2001 Aug 21;135(4):262-8

22. Segasothy M, Chin GL, Sia KK, Zulfiqar A, Samad SA. Chronic nephrotoxicity of anti-inflammatory drugs used in the treatment of arthritis. Br J Rheumatol. 1995 Feb; 34(2): 162-5

23. O'Connor N, Dargan PI, Jones AL. Hepatocellular damage from non-steroidal anti-inflammatory drugs. QJM. 2003 Nov;96(11): 787-91

24. Blower AL. Considerations for nonsteroidal anti-inflammatory drug therapy: safety. Scand J Rheumatol Suppl. 1996;105:13-24

25. Prathapkumar KR, Smith I, Attara GA. Indomethacin induced avascular necrosis of head of femur. Postgrad Med J. 2000 Sep; 76(899): 574-5

26. Newman NM, Ling RS. Acetabular bone destruction related to non-steroidal anti-inflammatory drugs. Lancet. 1985 Jul 6; 2(8445): 11-4

27. Brandt KD. Effects of nonsteroidal anti-inflammatory drugs on chondrocyte metabolism in vitro and in vivo. Am J Med. 1987; 83(5A): 29-34

28. "Systolic blood pressure increased significantly in 17% of rofecoxib- compared with 11% of celecoxib-treated patients (P = 0.032) at any study time point." Whelton A, Fort JG, Puma JA, Normandin D, Bello AE, Verburg KM; SUCCESS VI Study Group.Cyclooxygenase-2—specific inhibitors and cardiorenal function: a randomized, controlled trial of celecoxib and rofecoxib in older hypertensive osteoarthritis patients. Am J Ther 2001 Mar-Apr;8(2):85-95

29. Thie NM, Prasad NG, Major PW. Evaluation of glucosamine sulfate compared to ibuprofen for the treatment of temporomandibular joint osteoarthritis: a randomized double blind controlled 3 month clinical trial. J Rheumatol. 2001;28(6):1347-55

30. Braham R, Dawson B, Goodman C. The effect of glucosamine supplementation on people experiencing regular knee pain. Br J Sports Med. 2003;37(1):45-9

31. Matheson AJ, Perry CM. Glucosamine: a review of its use in the management of osteoarthritis. Drugs Aging. 2003; 20(14): 1041-60

32. Uebelhart D, et al. Intermittent treatment of knee osteoarthritis with oral chondroitin sulfate: a one-year, randomized, double-blind, multicenter study versus placebo. Osteoarthritis Cartilage. 2004;12:269-76

33. van Blitterswijk WJ, van de Nes JC, Wuisman PI. Glucosamine and chondroitin sulfate supplementation to treat symptomatic disc degeneration: biochemical rationale and case report. BMC Complement Altern Med. 2003;3(1):2

34. Morreale P, Manopulo R, Galati M, Boccanera L, Saponati G, Bocchi L. Comparison of the antiinflammatory efficacy of chondroitin sulfate and diclofenac sodium in patients with knee osteoarthritis. J Rheumatol. 1996;23(8):1385-91

35. Mazieres B, Combe B, Phan Van A, Tondut J, Grynfeltt M. Chondroitin sulfate in osteoarthritis of the knee: a prospective, double blind, placebo controlled multicenter clinical study. J Rheumatol. 2001;28(1):173-81

36. Reginster JY, Deroisy R, Rovati LC, Lee RL, Lejeune E, Bruyere O, Giacovelli G, Henrotin Y, Dacre JE, Gossett C. Long-term effects of glucosamine sulphate on osteoarthritis progression: a randomised, placebo-controlled clinical trial. Lancet. 2001;357(9252):251-6

37. Adams ME. Hype about glucosamine. Lancet. 1999;354(9176):353-4

38. Cumming A. Glucosamine in osteoarthritis. Lancet. 1999;354(9190):1640-1

39. Rovati LC, Annefeld M, Giacovelli G, Schmid K, Setnikar I. Glucosamine in osteoarthritis. Lancet. 1999;354(9190):1640

40. Scroggie DA, Albright A, Harris MD. The effect of glucosamine-chondroitin supplementation on glycosylated hemoglobin levels in patients with type 2 diabetes mellitus: a placebo-controlled, double-blinded, randomized clinical trial. Arch Intern Med. 2003;163(13):1587-9

41. Morrison LM. Treatment of coronary arteriosclerotic heart disease with chondroitin sulfate-A: preliminary report. J Am Geriatr Soc. 1968;16(7):779-85

42. Morrison LM, Branwood AW, Ershoff BH, Murata K, Quilligan JJ Jr, Schjeide OA, Patek P, Bernick S, Freeman L, Dunn OJ, Rucker P. The prevention of coronary arteriosclerotic heart disease with chondroitin sulfate A: preliminary report. Exp Med Surg. 1969;27(3):278-89

43. Morrison LM, Bajwa GS. Absence of naturally occurring coronary atherosclerosis in squirrel monkeys (Saimiri sciurea) treated with chondroitin sulfate A. Experientia. 1972 Dec 15;28(12):1410-1

44. Morrison LM, Enrick N. Coronary heart disease: reduction of death rate by chondroitin sulfate A. Angiology. 1973 May;24(5):269-87

45. Plotnikoff GA, Quigley JM. Prevalence of severe hypovitaminosis D in patients with persistent, nonspecific musculoskeletal pain. Mayo Clin Proc. 2003;78(12):1463-70

46. Masood H, Narang AP, Bhat IA, Shah GN. Persistent limb pain and raised serum alkaline phosphatase the earliest markers of subclinical hypovitaminosis D in Kashmir. Indian J Physiol Pharmacol. 1989;33:259-61

47. Al Faraj S, Al Mutairi K. Vitamin D deficiency and chronic low-back pain in Saudi Arabia. Spine. 2003;28:177-9

48. Holick MF. Vitamin D deficiency: what a pain it is. Mayo Clin Proc. 2003 Dec;78(12):1457-9

49. Timms PM, Mannan et al.. Circulating MMP9, vitamin D and variation in the TIMP-1 response with VDR genotype: mechanisms for inflammatory damage in chronic

disorders? QJM. 2002;95:787-96

50. Van den Berghe G, Van Roosbroeck D, Vanhove P, Wouters PJ, De Pourcq L, Bouillon R. Bone turnover in prolonged critical illness: effect of vitamin D. J Clin Endocrinol Metab. 2003;88(10):4623-32

51. Holick MF. Vitamin D: importance in the prevention of cancers, type 1 diabetes, heart disease, and osteoporosis. Am J Clin Nutr. 2004;79(3):362-71

52. Heaney RP. Vitamin D, nutritional deficiency, and the medical paradigm. J Clin Endocrinol Metab. 2003;88(11):5107-8

53. Hollis BW, Wagner CL. Assessment of dietary vitamin D requirements during pregnancy and lactation. Am J Clin Nutr. 2004;79(5):717-26

54. Heaney RP, Davies KM, Chen TC, Holick MF, Barger-Lux MJ. Human serum 25-hydroxycholecalciferol response to extended oral dosing with cholecalciferol. Am J Clin Nutr. 2003;77(1):204-10

55. Vasquez A, Manso G, Cannell J. The Clinical Importance of Vitamin D (Cholecalciferol): A Paradigm Shift with Implications for All Healthcare Providers. Alternative Therapies in Health and Medicine 2004; 10: 28-37

56. O'Leary JA, Klainer LM, Neuwirth RS. The management of hypoparathyroidism in pregnancy. Am J Obstet Gynecol. 1966;94(8):1103-7

57. Goodenday LS, Gordon GS. No risk from vitamin D in pregnancy. Ann Intern Med. 1971;75(5):807-8

58. Beard J. The action of trypsin upon the living cells of Jensen's mouse-tumour. Br Med J 1906; 4 (Jan 20): 140-1

59. Cutfield A. Trypsin Treatment in Malignant Disease. Br Med J. 1907; 5: 525

60. Wiggin FH. Case of Multiple Fibrosarcoma of the Tongue, With Remarks on the Use of Trypsin and Amylopsin in the Treatment of Malignant Disease." Journal of the American Medical Association 1906; 47: 2003-8

61. Goeth RA. Pancreatic treatment of cancer, with report of a cure. Journal of the American Medical Association 1907; (March 23) 48: 1030

62. Campbell JT. Trypsin Treatment of a Case of Malignant Disease. Journal of the American Medical Association 1907; 48: 225-226

63. Saruc M, Standop S, Standop J, Nozawa F, Itami A, Pandey KK, Batra SK, Gonzalez NJ, Guesry P, Pour PM. Pancreatic enzyme extract improves survival in murine pancreatic cancer. Pancreas. 2004;28(4):401-12

64. Batkin S, Taussig SJ, Szekerezes J. Antimetastatic effect of bromelain with or without its proteolytic and anticoagulant activity. J Cancer Res Clin Oncol. 1988;114(5):507-8

65. Gotze H, Rothman SS. Enteropancreatic circulation of digestive enzymes as a conservative mechanism. Nature 1975; 257(5527): 607-609

66. Liebow C, Rothman SS. Enteropancreatic Circulation of Digestive Enzymes. Science 1975; 189(4201): 472-474

67. Zavadova E, Desser L, Mohr T. Stimulation of reactive oxygen species production and cytotoxicity in human neutrophils in vitro and after oral administration of a polyenzyme preparation. Cancer Biother. 1995;10(2):147-52

68. Maurer HR, Hozumi M, Honma Y, Okabe-Kado J. Bromelain induces the differentiation of leukemic cells in vitro: an explanation for its cytostatic effects? Planta Med. 1988 Oct;54(5):377-81

69. Brien S, Lewith G, Walker A, Hicks SM, Middleton D. Bromelain as a Treatment for Osteoarthritis: a Review of Clinical Studies. Evidence-based Complementary and Alternative Medicine. 2004;1(3)251-257

70. Gaspani L, Limiroli E, Ferrario P, Bianchi M. In vivo and in vitro effects of bromelain on PGE(2) and SP concentrations in the inflammatory exudate in rats. Pharmacology. 2002;65(2):83-6

71. Leipner J, Saller R. Systemic enzyme therapy in oncology: effect and mode of action. Drugs. 2000 Apr;59(4):769-80

72. Vellini M, Desideri D, Milanese A, Omini C, Daffonchio L, Hernandez A, Brunelli G. Possible involvement of eicosanoids in the pharmacological action of bromelain. Arzneimittelforschung. 1986;36(1):110-2

73. The trypsin treatment of cancer. British Medical Journal 1907; March 2: 519-20

74. Gonzalez NJ, Isaacs LL. Evaluation of pancreatic proteolytic enzyme treatment of adenocarcinoma of the pancreas, with nutrition and detoxification support. Nutr Cancer. 1999;33(2):117-24

75. Sakalova A, Bock PR, Dedik L, Hanisch J, Schiess W, Gazova S, Chabronova I, Holomanova D, Mistrik M, Hrubisko M. Retrolective cohort study of an additive therapy with an oral enzyme preparation in patients with multiple myeloma. Cancer Chemother Pharmacol. 2001 Jul;47 Suppl:S38-44

76. Popiela T, Kulig J, Hanisch J, Bock PR. Influence of a complementary treatment with oral enzymes on patients with colorectal cancers—an epidemiological retrolective cohort study. Cancer Chemother Pharmacol. 2001;47 Suppl:S55-63

77. Taussig SJ, Yokoyama MM, Chinen A, Onari K, Yamakido M. Bromelain: a proteolytic enzyme and its clinical application. A review. Hiroshima J Med Sci. 1975;24(2-3):185-93

78. Taub SJ. The use of bromelains in sinusitis: a double-blind clinical evaluation. Eye Ear Nose Throat Mon. 1967 Mar;46(3):361-5

79. Trickett P. Proteolytic enzymes in treatment of athletic injuries. Appl Ther. 1964;30:647-52

80. Walker AF, Bundy R, Hicks SM, Middleton RW. Bromelain reduces mild acute knee pain and improves well-being in a dose-dependent fashion in an open study of otherwise healthy adults.Phytomedicine.2002;9:681-6

81. Walker JA, Cerny FJ, Cotter JR, Burton HW. Attenuation of contraction-induced skeletal muscle injury by bromelain. Med Sci Sports Exerc. 1992 Jan;24(1):20-5

82. Kaufman W. Niacinamide therapy for joint mobility. Therapeutic reversal of a common clinical manifestation of the "normal" aging process. Conn State Med J 1953;17:584-591

83. Kaufman W. The use of vitamin therapy to reverse cer-

tain concomitants of aging. J Am Geriatr Soc 1955;3:927-936

84. Matuoka K, Chen KY, Takenawa T. Rapid reversion of aging phenotypes by nicotinamide through possible modulation of histone acetylation. Cell Mol Life Sci. 2001;58(14):2108-16

85. Jonas WB, Rapoza CP, Blair WF. The effect of niacinamide on osteoarthritis: a pilot study. Inflamm Res 1996 Jul;45(7):330-4

86. McCarty MF, Russell AL. Niacinamide therapy for osteoarthritis—does it inhibit nitric oxide synthase induction by interleukin 1 in chondrocytes? Med Hypotheses. 1999;53(4):350-60

87. Gaby AR. Literature review and commentary: Niacinamide for osteoarthritis. Townsend Letter for Doctors and Patients. 2002: May; 32

88. Mohler H, Polc P, Cumin R, Pieri L, Kettler R. Nicotinamide is a brain constituent with benzodiazepine-like actions. Nature. 1979; 278(5704): 563-5

89. Kimmatkar N, Thawani V, Hingorani L, Khiyani R. Efficacy and tolerability of Boswellia serrata extract in treatment of osteoarthritis of knee—a randomized double blind placebo controlled trial. Phytomedicine. 2003 Jan;10(1):3-7

90. Ammon HP. [Boswellic acids (components of frankincense) as the active principle in treatment of chronic inflammatory diseases] [Article in German] Wien Med Wochenschr. 2002;152(15-16):373-8

91. Gupta I, Gupta V, Parihar A, Gupta S, Ludtke R, Safayhi H, Ammon HP. Effects of Boswellia serrata gum resin in patients with bronchial asthma: results of a double-blind, placebo-controlled, 6-week clinical study. Eur J Med Res. 1998 Nov 17;3(11):511-4

92. Gupta I, Parihar A, Malhotra P, Singh GB, Ludtke R, Safayhi H, Ammon HP. Effects of Boswellia serrata gum resin in patients with ulcerative colitis. Eur J Med Res. 1997 Jan;2(1):37-43

93. Gagnier JJ, Chrubasik S, Manheimer E. Harpgophytum procumbens for osteoarthritis and low-back pain: a systematic review. BMC Complement Altern Med. 2004 Sep 15;4(1):13

94. Chantre P, Cappelaere A, Leblan D, Guedon D, Vandermander J, Fournie B. Efficacy and tolerance of Harpagophytum procumbens versus diacerhein in treatment of osteoarthritis. Phytomedicine 2000;7(3):177-83

95. Leblan D, Chantre P, Fournie B. Harpagophytum procumbens in the treatment of knee and hip osteoarthritis. Four-month results of a prospective, multicenter, double-blind trial versus diacerhein. Joint Bone Spine 2000;67(5):462-7

96. Chrubasik S, Junck H, Breitschwerdt H, Conradt C, Zappe H. Effectiveness of Harpagophytum extract WS 1531 in the treatment of exacerbation of low-back pain: a randomized, placebo-controlled, double-blind study. Eur J Anaesthesiol 1999 Feb;16(2):118-29

97. Chrubasik S, Model A, Black A, Pollak S. A randomized double-blind pilot study comparing Doloteffin and Vioxx in the treatment of low-back pain. Rheumatology (Oxford). 2003 Jan;42(1):141-8 See www.WellBody-Book.com/articles.htm for the full-text of this article.

98. Chrubasik S, Thanner J, Kunzel O, Conradt C, Black A, Pollak S. Comparison of outcome measures during treatment with the proprietary Harpagophytum extract doloteffin in patients with pain in the lower back, knee or hip. Phytomedicine 2002 Apr;9(3):181-94

99. Chrubasik S, Conradt C, Roufogalis BD. Effectiveness of Harpagophytum extracts and clinical efficacy. Phytother Res. 2004 Feb;18(2):187-9

100. Chrubasik S, Eisenberg E, Balan E, Weinberger T, Luzzati R, Conradt C. Treatment of low-back pain exacerbations with willow bark extract: a randomized double-blind study. Am J Med. 2000;109:9-14

101. Chrubasik S, Kunzel O, Model A, Conradt C, Black A. Treatment of low-back pain with a herbal or synthetic anti-rheumatic: a randomized controlled study. Willow bark extract for low-back pain. Rheumatology (Oxford). 2001;40:1388-93

102. Brennan PC, Triano JJ, McGregor M, Kokjohn K, Hondras MA, Brennan DC. Enhanced neutrophil respiratory burst as a biological marker for manipulation forces: duration of the effect and association with substance P and tumor necrosis factor. J Manipulative Physiol Ther. 1992 Feb;15(2):83-9

103. Balon J, Aker PD, Crowther ER, Danielson C, Cox PG, O'Shaughnessy D, Walker C, Goldsmith CH, Duku E, Sears MR. A comparison of active and simulated chiropractic manipulation as adjunctive treatment for childhood asthma. N Engl J Med. 1998 Oct 8;339(15):1013-20

104. Vasquez A. Reducing Pain and Inflammation Naturally. Part 2: New Insights into Fatty Acid Supplementation and Its Effect on Eicosanoid Production and Genetic Expression. Nutr Perspect 2005; January: 5-16

105. Vasquez A. Integrative Orthopedics: The Art of Creating Wellness While Managing Acute and Chronic Musculoskeletal Disorders. Houston; Natural Health Consulting Corporation. (OptimalHealthResearch.com): 2004

106. American Chiropractic Association. What is Chiropractic? http://amerchiro.org/media/whatis/ Accessed January 9, 2005

107. Starfield B. Is US health really the best in the world? JAMA. 2000 Jul 26;284(4):483-5

108. Holland EG, Degruy FV. Drug-induced disorders. Am Fam Physician. 1997 Nov 1;56(7):1781-8, 1791-2

109. Hyman M. Paradigm shift: the end of "normal science" in medicine understanding function in nutrition, health, and disease. Altern Ther Health Med. 2004;10(5):10-5, 90-4

Reducing Pain and Inflammation Naturally - Part IV: Nutritional and Botanical Inhibition of NF-kappaB, the Major Intracellular Amplifier of the Inflammatory Cascade.

A Practical Clinical Strategy Exemplifying Anti-Inflammatory Nutrigenomics

Alex Vasquez, DC, ND

Abstract: Modulation of genetic expression by the skillful use of dietary, nutritional, and botanical interventions is clearly the leading edge of modern nutritional practice. Thus, familiarity with the concepts and implementation of "nutrigenomics" must become incorporated into the clinical skill set of chiropractic and naturopathic physicians. This article focuses on the nutritional and botanical inhibition of the primary "amplifier of inflammation" known as nuclear transcription factor kappaB (NF-kappaB). From both clinical and pharmacological standpoints, the safe and effective inhibition of NF-kappaB is considered a major therapeutic goal for the prevention and treatment of conditions associated with an upregulated inflammatory response, namely diabetes, arthritis, cancer, autoimmunity, and the aging process in general. This article introduces concepts and terminology that will facilitate the effective clinical implementation of a nutritional protocol aimed at relieving excess inflammation by inhibiting NF-kappaB.

INTRODUCTION

New research is showing that many diseases are associated with inappropriate activation of nuclear transcription factor kappaB, generally referred to as NF-kappaB. Inhibition of NF-kappaB is now a major therapeutic goal in the treatment and prevention of a wide range of illnesses, including cancer, arthritis, autoimmune diseases, and neurologic illnesses such as Alzheimer's and Parkinson's disease.[1] While the development and use of drugs that inhibit NF-kappaB will take several years of additional research and will likely be associated with numerous adverse effects and exorbitant expense, the nutritional and botanical inhibition of NF-kappaB is available to us immediately with proven safety and near-universal affordability. This paper will take readers beyond the benefits which can be obtained with the health-promoting diet[2], combination fatty acid therapy[3], and anti-inflammatory and analgesic nutrients and botanicals[4] that were described in the first three articles in this series.

THE BIOCHEMISTRY OF INFLAMMATION: FROM NF-KAPPAB TO EICOSANOIDS

The process of inflammation may be said to begin with the translation of an environmental trigger into a biochemical signal that initiates the inflammatory pathway. Proinflammatory environmental triggers can include injury, radiation, infection, oxidative stress, and certain foods, particularly those high in fat and those with a high glycemic index (ie, "simple sugars"), as well as vitamin D deficiency. Regardless of the original locus or etiology, each of these stimuli may lead to activation of the NF-kappaB cascade, which is a major pathway for the amplification of inflammatory processes.[5]

As a ubiquitous nuclear transcription factor that promotes the activation of genes that encode for inflammatory mediators and enzymes, NF-kappaB can be thought of as the major intracellular "amplifier" which ultimately increases the production of the direct mediators of inflammation such as cytokines, prostaglandins, leukotrienes, nitric oxide and other reactive oxygen species ("free radicals"). The process of inflammation begins when two subunit proteins—p50 and p65—merge in the cytoplasm to form NF-kappaB, which is kept in an inactive state by inhibitor kappaB (IkB). When triggered by any of the common stimuli listed above, IkB is phosphorylated and destroyed by inhibitor kappaB kinase (IKK). The destruction of IkB allows NF-kappaB to move into the nucleus of the cell where it binds with DNA and activates genes encoding for inflammatory responses. These genes then elaborate their inflammatory products such as interleukin-1 (IL-1), IL-6, tumor necrosis factor, and the proinflammatory destructive enzymes including inducible nitric oxide synthase (iNOS), cyclooxygenase-2 (COX-2), the lipoxygenases (LIPOX), and the matrix metalloproteinases (MMP) including collagenase and gelatinase, which destroy connective tissue. Nitric oxide synthase catalyses the formation of nitric oxide (NO-), which plays an important role in the development of peripheral osteoarthritis[6] and spinal disc degeneration[7] via oxidative destruction of articular tissues. Cyclooxygenase transforms arachidonic acid into prostaglandins and thromboxanes, which recruit leukocytes to the area of inflammation, exacerbate edema, sensitize peripheral neurons to increased pain perception, and ultimately facilitate the liberation of proteinases, such as matrix metaloproteinases, which destroy joint structures. Present in several isoforms, the lipoxygenase enzyme acts on arachidonic acid to produce leukotrienes that also increase inflammation, joint destruction, and production of MMP. Overall, this same inflammatory response contributes to the genesis and perpetuation of numerous inflammatory disorders, such as osteoarthritis, cancer, rheumatoid arthritis and other autoimmune diseases, and

**Figure 1.
The creation and activation of NF-kappaB—a crucial step in the amplification of proinflammatory gene expression.**
Adapted from Vasquez A. Integrative Orthopedics. (Optimal-HealthResearch.com): 2004

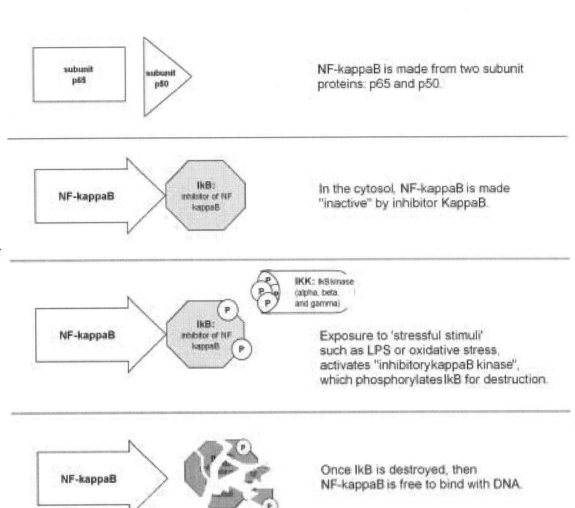

NF-kappaB is made from two subunit proteins: p65 and p50.

In the cytosol, NF-kappaB is made "inactive" by inhibitor KappaB.

Exposure to 'stressful stimuli' such as LPS or oxidative stress, activates "inhibitorykappaB kinase", which phosphorylates IkB for destruction.

Once IkB is destroyed, then NF-kappaB is free to bind with DNA.

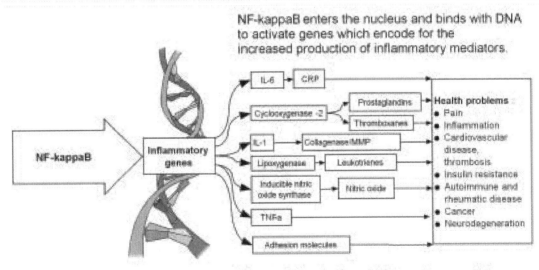

NF-kappaB enters the nucleus and binds with DNA to activate genes which encode for the increased production of inflammatory mediators.

Increased production of inflammatory mediators - such as cytokines, prostaglandins leukotrienes - promotes cellular dysfunction and tissue destruction.

Figure 2. Translation of environmental traumas into biochemical inflammation. Note the self-perpetuating "vicious cycle" where inflammatory mediators promote additional inflammation via activation of NF-kappaB. *Adapted from Vasquez A.* Integrative Orthopedics. *(OptimalHealthResearch.com): 2004*

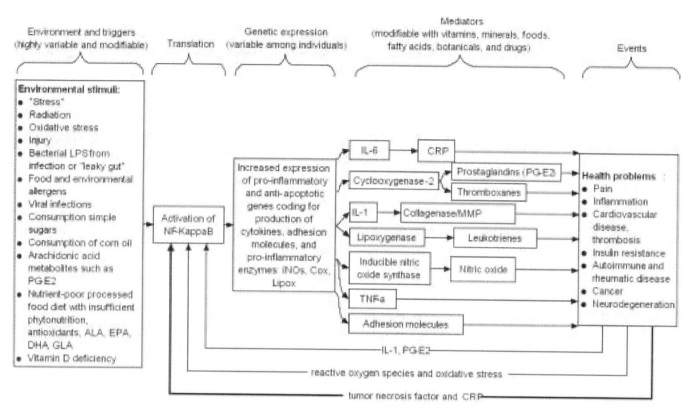

essentially all conditions associated with pain and inflammation. This process of NF-kappaB activation and modulation of genetic expression is illustrated in Figures 1 and 2.

FROM BIOCHEMICAL EFFECTS TO CLINICAL CONSEQUENCES

Activation of NF-kappaB leads to the elaboration of mediators that damage tissues and contribute to the clinical manifestations of poor health. IL-6 stimulates production of C-reactive protein (CRP), which is a sensitive serum marker of inflammation (such as in osteoarthritis and rheumatoid arthritis) and is associated with an increased risk of cardiovascular disease, progressively deteriorating health and "rapid biological aging" in men and women.[8,9] INOS increases production of the free radical nitric oxide which is elevated in degenerating joints[6] and spinal discs[7] and which contributes directly to joint destruction via oxidation of articular tissues.[10] COX-2 is responsible for the conversion of arachidonic acid to prostaglandins, several of which increase the perception of pain by sensitizing peripheral nociceptors[11] and by a central hyperalgesic effect[12] and by promoting destruction of articular structures by increasing

elaboration of proteolytic enzymes, variously named collagenases, gelatinases, and matrix metalloproteinases.[13] Similarly, LIPOX catalyzes the conversion of arachidonate to leukotrienes, which promote swelling, inflammation, chemotaxis, and tissue destruction via increased release of proteolytic enzymes. In their anti-inflammatory roles, LIPOX and COX act on GLA for the production of the anti-inflammatory 15-HETrE and prostaglandin E-1, respectively, as well as on EPA and DHA for the production of anti-inflammatory prostaglandins, leukotrienes, docosatrienes, and resolvins as discussed previously.[3] Our discussion of the mechanisms of anti-inflammatory nutritional interventions must also include the phytonutraceutical activation of peroxisome proliferator-activated receptors (PPARs), since fatty acids and selected botanical medicines exert their actions at least in part by activation of PPAR-alpha and PPAR-gamma, which then mediate health-promoting and clinically significant anti-inflammatory effects. As fatty acid receptors that influence genetic expression via suppression of NF-kappaB as well as via NF-kappaB-independent pathways, PPARs when moderately activated induce numerous beneficial physiologic responses, including direct and indirect anti-inflammatory, anti-cancer, and cardioprotective effects.[14-16]

NUTRIGENOMICS: MODULATION OF GENETIC EXPRESSION VIA INTERVENTIONAL NUTRITION

The study of how dietary components and nutritional supplements influence genetic expression is referred to as "nutrigenomics" or "nutritional genomics" and has been described as "the next frontier in the postgenomic era."[17] Various nutrients have been shown to modulate genetic expression and thus alter phenotypic manifestations of disease by upregulating or downregulating specific genes, interacting with nuclear receptors, altering hormone receptors, and modifying the influence of transcription factors, such as proinflammatory NF-kappaB and the anti-inflammatory peroxisome-proliferator activated receptors (PPARs). Indeed, the previous view that nutrients only interact with human physiology at the metabolic/post-transcriptional level must be updated in light of current research showing that nutrients can, in fact, modify human physiology and phenotype at the genetic/pre-transcriptional level.

Fatty acids and their end-products modulate genetic expression in several ways, as these examples will illustrate. In general, n-3 fatty acids decrease inflammation and promote health while n-6 fatty acids (except for GLA, which is generally health-promoting) increase inflammation, oxidative stress, and the manifestation of disease. Corn oil, probably as a result of its high LA content, rapidly activates NF-kappaB and thus promotes tumor development, atherosclerosis, and elaboration of pro-inflammatory mediators such as TNFa.[18-20] Similarly, arachidonic acid increases production of the free radical superoxide approximately 4-fold when added to isolated Kupffer cells *in vitro*. Prostaglandin-E2 is produced from arachidonic acid by cyclooxygenase and increases genetic expression of cyclooxygenase and IL-6; thus, inflammation manifested by an increase in PG-E2 leads to additive expression of cyclooxygenase, which further increases inflammation and elevates C-reactive protein.[21] Some of the unique health-promoting effects of GLA are nutrigenomically mediated via activation of PPAR-gamma, resultant inhibition of NF-kappaB, and impairment of estrogen receptor function.[22,23] Supplementation with ALA leads to a dramatic reduction of prostaglandin formation in humans[24], and this effect is probably mediated by downregulation of proinflammatory transcription, as evidenced by reductions in CRP, IL-6, and serum amyloid A.[25] EPA appears to exert much of its anti-inflammatory benefit by suppressing NF-kappaB activation and thus reducing elaboration of proinflammatory mediators.[26,27] EPA also indirectly modifies gene expression and cell growth by reducing intracellular calcium levels, thereby providing an anti-cancer benefit.[28] DHA is the precursor to docosatrienes and resolvins which downregulate gene expression for proinflammatory IL-1, inhibit of TNFa, and reduce neutrophil entry to sites of inflammation.[29] Oxidized EPA activates PPAR-alpha and thereby suppresses NF-kappaB and the activation of proinflammatory genes.[27,30] Therefore, we see that fatty acids (and other botanicals and nutrients, discussed below) directly affect gene expression by complex and multiple mechanisms, and the synergism and potency of these numerous anti-inflammatory nutraceuticals supports the rationale for the use of nutrition and select botanicals for the safe and effective treatment of inflammatory disorders.

NATURAL AND SYNERGISTIC INTERVENTIONS THAT INHIBIT NF-KAPPAB

This section efficiently reviews several of the more powerful nutritional and botanical treatments which have been shown to inhibit NF-kappaB. Using these treatments in combination provides additive and synergistic benefits compared to using one treatment at a time.

- *Vitamin D:* Vitamin D has potent anti-inflammatory and pain-relieving benefits in patients with musculoskeletal pain, as previously reviewed in this Journal[14] and elsewhere.[31,32] Impressively, vitamin D also modulates genetic transcription, as evidenced by its ability to reduce activation of NF-kappaB. Although 25-hydroxyvitamin D has limited biological activity, its more active metabolite, 1-alpha,25-dihydroxyvitamin D3 (1,25-(OH)2-D3) can inhibit NF-kappaB activity in human cells.[33,34] Thus, it is not surprising that clinical studies in patients with critical illness and multiple sclerosis have shown an anti-inflammatory benefit from vitamin D. Vitamin D supplementation can reduce inflammation by 23% as objectively assessed with C-reactive protein levels.[35]

- **Curcumin from *Curcuma longa* ("Turmeric"):** Turmeric is an ancient spice that has been used for thousands of years to add flavor and color to food. Although *in vitro* tests and animal studies have suggested that the active components related to curcumin may have potential as powerful agents against human diseases, most researchers and reporters have failed to realize that—in humans—curcumin is very poorly absorbed. Even when curcumin powder is administered in doses as high as 2,000 mg, there is no appreciable increase in serum levels in humans. However, when curcumin is coadministered with piperine, which increases intestinal absorption and reduces enterohepatic detoxification, serum levels of curcumin increase by 2,000% in humans.[36] Piperine is derived from *Piper nigrum,* also commonly known as black pepper, a spice found in nearly every kitchen in the world. Piperine enhances absorption and reduces clearance of some drugs such as theophylline (detoxified by CYP3A4 and CYP1A2) and propranolol (detoxified by CYP2D6); this combination of effects (e.g., enhanced absorption and reduced clearance) may require dosage modification for numerous drugs. No adverse reactions have been reported with doses of piperine up to 15 milligrams per day.[37] Pregnant women and nursing mothers should generally avoid piperine supplementation.

- **Lipoic acid:** As a fat-soluble and water-soluble antioxidant with clear biologic activity, it is not surprising that lipoic acid is also noted to inhibit NF-kappaB activity in a dose-dependent manner.[38]

- **Green tea extract:** Epigallocatechin gallate from green tea is an effective inhibitor of IKK activity. Thus, green tea extract inhibits activation of NF-kappaB. This may explain, at least in part, some of the reported anti-inflammatory and anticancer effects of green tea.[39]

- **Rosemary:** Carnosol in rosemary inhibits NF-kappaB activation, and this is a likely mechanism of its anti-inflammatory and chemopreventive action.[40]

- **Grape seed extract (GSE):** GSE is a potent antioxidant that has been shown to inhibit NF-kappaB.[41]

- **Propolis (a source of caffeic acid phenethyl ester):** Caffeic acid phenethyl ester (CAPE) is an anti-inflammatory component of propolis (honeybee resin) that is a specific inhibitor of NF-kappaB.[42] CAPE has shown clinical benefit in the treatment of asthma, which is the prototype of chronic airway inflammation.[43] As with all bee products, allergy to propolis has been reported and may be more common in patients with a history of allergy to honey or other bee products.

- **Resveratrol:** Resveratrol shows anticarcinogenic, anti-inflammatory, and growth-modulatory effects which are due in part to the inhibition of NF-kappaB.[44] In fact, according to recent *in vitro* research, resveratrol and quercetin inhibit NF-kappaB more powerfully than the glucocorticosteroid, dexamethasone.[45] Further support for an anti-inflammatory benefit from resveratrol comes from research showing that resveratrol pretreatment reduces elaboration of COX-2 following administration of the proinflammatory agent, phorbol ester.[46] This effect is almost certainly a reflection of the ability of resveratrol to inhibit NF-kappaB and thereby reduce transcription of proinflammatory genes.

- **Phytolens (a patented extract from legumes):** Phytolens is a patented polyphenolic extract from lentils. Published experimental research has documented the *in vivo* antioxidant activity of Phytolens against superoxide other reactive oxygen species.[47] Anecdotal reports have shown an anti-inflammatory benefit.

CONCLUSION AND CLINICAL IMPLEMENTATION

Inflammation is a destructive and self-perpetuating process wherein activation of NF-kappaB leads to the elaboration of proinflammatory mediators, several of which then lead to a cyclic, positive-feedback upregulation of NF-kappaB. In patients who require a rapid-onset anti-inflammatory benefit, or those who have not adequately responded to the dietary, fatty acid, and joint-supporting interventions described previously[2-4,32], intervention with the above-mentioned botanicals and nutrients can lead to efficient and objective reductions in inflammation. Using these natural treatments *in combination* helps to safely reduce activity of NF-kappaB and the resultant inflammation, thus promoting the restoration of homeostasis, the alleviation of pain, and a reduction in joint inflammation and degeneration.

Dr. Alex Vasquez is a licensed naturopathic physician in Washington and Oregon, and licensed chiropractor in Texas, where he maintains a private practice and is a member of the research team at Biotics Research Corporation. As former Adjunct Professor of Orthopedics and Rheumatology for the Naturopathic Medicine Program at Bastyr University, he is the author of more than 20 published articles and a recently published 486-page textbook for the chiropractic and naturopathic professions, "Integrative Orthopedics: The Art of Creating Wellness While Managing Acute and Chronic Musculoskeletal Disorders" available from OptimalHealthResearch.com.

ACKNOWLEDGEMENTS: Pepper Grimm BA of Biotics Research Corporation reviewed the final edition of this article before submission.

REFERENCES:

1. D'Acquisto F, May MJ, Ghosh S. Inhibition of Nuclear Factor Kappa B (NF-B): An Emerging Theme in Anti-Inflammatory Therapies. Mol Interv. 2002 Feb;2(1):22-35 http://molinterv.aspetjournals.org/ cgi/content/full/2/1/22
2. Vasquez A. Reducing Pain and Inflammation Naturally. Part 1: New Insights into Fatty Acid Biochemistry and the Influence of Diet. Nutritional Perspectives 2004; October: 5, 7-10, 12, 14
3. Vasquez A. Reducing Pain and Inflammation Naturally. Part 2: New Insights into Fatty Acid Supplementation and Its Effect on Eicosanoid Production and Genetic Expression. Nutritional Perspectives 2005; January: 5-16
4. Vasquez A. Reducing pain and inflammation naturally - Part 3: Improving overall health while safely and effectively treating musculoskeletal pain. Nutritional Perspectives 2005; 28: 34-38, 40-42
5. Tak PP, Firestein GS. NF-kappaB: a key role in inflammatory diseases. J Clin Invest. 2001;107(1):7-11
6. Pelletier JP, Martel-Pelletier J. Therapeutic targets in osteoarthritis: from today to tomorrow with new imaging technology. Ann Rheum Dis. 2003;62 Suppl 2:ii79-82

7. Kohyama K, Saura R, Doita M, Mizuno K. Intervertebral disc cell apoptosis by nitric oxide: biological understanding of intervertebral disc degeneration. Kobe J Med Sci. 2000;46(6):283-95

8. Kushner I. C-reactive protein elevation can be caused by conditions other than inflammation and may reflect biologic aging. Cleve Clin J Med. 2001 Jun;68(6):535-7

9. Black S, Kushner I, Samols D. C-reactive Protein. J Biol Chem. 2004 Nov 19;279(47):48487-90

10. Amin AR, Dave M, Attur M, Abramson SB. COX-2, NO, and cartilage damage and repair. Curr Rheumatol Rep. 2000;2:447-53

11. Schaible HG, Ebersberger A, Von Banchet GS. Mechanisms of pain in arthritis. Ann N Y Acad Sci. 2002;966:343-54

12. Grubb BD. Peripheral and central mechanisms of pain. Br J Anaesth. 1998 Jul;81(1):8-11

13. Mertz PM, DeWitt DL, Stetler-Stevenson WG, Wahl LM. Interleukin 10 suppression of monocyte prostaglandin H synthase-2. Mechanism of inhibition of prostaglandin-dependent matrix metalloproteinase production. J Biol Chem. 1994;269:21322-9

14. Vanden Heuvel JP. Peroxisome proliferator-activated receptors: a critical link among fatty acids, gene expression and carcinogenesis. J Nutr. 1999 Feb;129(2S Suppl):575S-580S

15. Chinetti G, Fruchart JC, Staels B. Peroxisome proliferator-activated receptors and inflammation: from basic science to clinical applications. Int J Obes Relat Metab Disord. 2003;27 Suppl 3:S41-5

16. Vamecq J, Latruffe N. Medical significance of peroxisome proliferator-activated receptors. Lancet. 1999;354(9173):141-8

17. Kaput J, Rodriguez RL. Nutritional genomics: the next frontier in the postgenomic era. Physiol Genomics. 2004 Jan 15;16(2):166-77

18. Rusyn I, Bradham CA, Cohn L, Schoonhoven R, Swenberg JA, Brenner DA, Thurman RG. Corn oil rapidly activates nuclear factor-kappaB in hepatic Kupffer cells by oxidant-dependent mechanisms. Carcinogenesis. 1999 Nov;20(11):2095-100

19. Rose DP, Hatala MA, Connolly JM, Rayburn J. Effect of diets containing different levels of linoleic acid on human breast cancer growth and lung metastasis in nude mice. Cancer Res. 1993 Oct 1;53(19):4686-90

20. Dichtl W, Ares MP, Jonson AN, Jovinge S, Pachinger O, Giachelli CM, Hamsten A, Eriksson P, Nilsson J. Linoleic acid-stimulated vascular adhesion molecule-1 expression in endothelial cells depends on nuclear factor-kappaB activation. Metabolism. 2002 Mar;51(3):327-33

21. Bagga D, Wang L, Farias-Eisner R, Glaspy JA, Reddy ST. Differential effects of prostaglandin derived from omega-6 and omega-3 polyunsaturated fatty acids on COX-2 expression and IL-6 secretion. Proc Natl Acad Sci U S A. 2003 Feb 18;100(4):1751-6. Available at http://www.pnas.org/cgi/reprint/100/4/1751.pdf

22. Menendez JA, Colomer R, Lupu R. Omega-6 polyunsaturated fatty acid gamma-linolenic acid (18:3n-6) is a selective estrogen-response modulator in human breast cancer cells: gamma-linolenic acid antagonizes estrogen receptor-dependent transcriptional activity, transcriptionally represses estrogen receptor expression and synergistically enhances tamoxifen and ICI 182,780 (Faslodex) efficacy in human breast cancer cells. Int J Cancer. 2004 May 10;109(6):949-54

23. Jiang WG, Redfern A, Bryce RP, Mansel RE. Peroxisome proliferator activated receptor-gamma (PPAR-gamma) mediates the action of gamma linolenic acid in breast cancer cells. Prostaglandins Leukot Essent Fatty Acids. 2000 Feb;62(2):119-27

24. Adam O, Wolfram G, Zollner N. Effect of alpha-linolenic acid in the human diet on linoleic acid metabolism and prostaglandin biosynthesis. J Lipid Res. 1986 Apr;27(4):421-6

25. Rallidis LS, Paschos G, Liakos GK, Velissaridou AH, Anastasiadis G, Zampelas A. Dietary alpha-linolenic acid decreases C-reactive protein, serum amyloid A and interleukin-6 in dyslipidaemic patients. Atherosclerosis. 2003 Apr;167(2):237-42

26. Zhao Y, Joshi-Barve S, Barve S, Chen LH. Eicosapentaenoic acid prevents LPS-induced TNF-alpha expression by preventing NF-kappaB activation. J Am Coll Nutr. 2004 Feb;23(1):71-8

27. Mishra A, Chaudhary A, Sethi S. Oxidized omega-3 fatty acids inhibit NF-kappaB activation via a PPARalpha-dependent pathway. Arterioscler Thromb Vasc Biol. 2004 Sep;24(9):1621-7

28. Palakurthi SS, Fluckiger R, Aktas H, Changolkar AK, Shahsafaei A, Harneit S, Kilic E, Halperin JA. Inhibition of translation initiation mediates the anti-cancer effect of the n-3 polyunsaturated fatty acid eicosapentaenoic acid. Cancer Res. 2000 Jun 1;60(11):2919-25

29. Hong S, Gronert K, Devchand PR, Moussignac RL, Serhan CN. Novel docosatrienes and 17S-resolvins generated from docosahexaenoic acid in murine brain, human blood, and glial cells. Autacoids in anti-inflammation. J Biol Chem. 2003 Apr 25;278(17):14677-87

30. Delerive P, Fruchart JC, Staels B. Peroxisome proliferator-activated receptors in inflammation control. J Endocrinol. 2001;169(3):453-9

31. Vasquez A, Manso G, Cannell J. The Clinical Importance of Vitamin D (Cholecalciferol): A Paradigm Shift with Implications for All Healthcare Providers. Alternative Therapies in Health and Medicine 2004; 10: 28-37

32. Vasquez A. Integrative Orthopedics: The Art of Creating Wellness While Managing Acute and Chronic Musculoskeletal Disorders. Houston; Natural Health Consulting Corporation. (www.OptimalHealth Research.com): 2004

33. Harant H, Wolff B, Lindley IJ. 1Alpha,25-dihydroxyvitamin D3 decreases DNA binding of nuclear factor-kappaB in human fibroblasts. FEBS Lett. 1998 Oct 9;436(3):329-34

34. D'Ambrosio D, Cippitelli M, Cocciolo MG, Mazzeo D, Di Lucia P, Lang R, Sinigaglia F, Panina-Bordignon P. Inhibition of IL-12 production by 1,25-dihydroxyvitamin D3. Involvement of NF-kappaB downregulation in transcriptional repression of the p40 gene. J Clin Invest. 1998 Jan 1;101(1):252-62

35. Timms PM, Mannan et al.. Circulating MMP9, vitamin D and variation in the TIMP-1 response with VDR genotype: mechanisms for inflammatory damage in chronic disorders? QJM. 2002;95:787-96

36. Shoba G, Joy D, Joseph T, Majeed M, Rajendran R, Srinivas PS. Influence of piperine on the pharmacokinetics of curcumin in animals and human volunteers. Planta Med. 1998 May;64(4):353-6

37. Piperine. Accessed at http://www.pdrhealth.com/drug_info/nmdrug-profiles/nutsupdrugs/pip_0322.shtml on April 7, 2005.

38. Lee HA, Hughes DA.Alpha-lipoic acid modulates NF-kappaB activity in human monocytic cells by direct interaction with DNA. Exp Gerontol. 2002 Jan-Mar;37(2-3):401-10

39. Yang F, Oz HS, Barve S, de Villiers WJ, McClain CJ, Varilek GW. The green tea polyphenol (-)-epigallocatechin-3-gallate blocks nuclear factor-kappa B activation by inhibiting I kappa B kinase activity in the intestinal epithelial cell line IEC-6. Mol Pharmacol. 2001 Sep;60(3):528-33

40. Lo AH, Liang YC, Lin-Shiau SY, Ho CT, Lin JK. Carnosol, an antioxidant in rosemary, suppresses inducible nitric oxide synthase through down-regulating nuclear factor-kappaB in mouse macrophages. Carcinogenesis. 2002 Jun;23(6):983-91

41. Dhanalakshmi S, Agarwal R, Agarwal C. Inhibition of NF-kappaB pathway in grape seed extract-induced apoptotic death of human prostate carcinoma DU145 cells. Int J Oncol. 2003 Sep;23(3):721-7

42. Fitzpatrick LR, Wang J, Le T. Caffeic acid phenethyl ester, an inhibitor of nuclear factor-kappaB, attenuates bacterial peptidoglycan polysaccharide-induced colitis in rats. J Pharmacol Exp Ther. 2001 Dec;299(3):915-20

43. Khayyal MT, el-Ghazaly MA, el-Khatib AS, Hatem AM, de Vries PJ, el-Shafei S, Khattab MM. A clinical pharmacological study of the potential beneficial effects of a propolis food product as an adjuvant in asthmatic patients. Fundam Clin Pharmacol. 2003 Feb;17(1):93-102

44. Manna SK, Mukhopadhyay A, Aggarwal BB. Resveratrol suppresses TNF-induced activation of nuclear transcription factors NF-kappa B, activator protein-1, and apoptosis: potential role of reactive oxygen intermediates and lipid peroxidation. J Immunol. 2000 Jun 15;164(12):6509-19

45. Donnelly LE, Newton R, Kennedy GE, Fenwick PS, Leung RH, Ito K, Russell RE, Barnes PJ. Anti-inflammatory Effects of Resveratrol in Lung Epithelial Cells: Molecular Mechanisms. Am J Physiol Lung Cell Mol Physiol. 2004 Jun 4 [Epub ahead of print]

46. Subbaramaiah K, Chung WJ, Michaluart P, Telang N, Tanabe T, Inoue H, Jang M, Pezzuto JM, Dannenberg AJ. Resveratrol inhibits cyclooxygenase-2 transcription and activity in phorbol ester-treated human mammary epithelial cells. J Biol Chem. 1998 Aug 21;273(34):21875-82

47. Sandoval M, Ronzio RA, Muanza DN, Clark DA, Miller MJ. Peroxynitrite-induced apoptosis in epithelial (T84) and macrophage (RAW 264.7) cell lines: effect of legume-derived polyphenols (phytolens). Nitric Oxide. 1997;1(6):476-83

Reducing Pain and Inflammation Naturally - Part V:
Improving Neuromusculoskeletal Health by Optimizing Immune Function and Reducing "Allergic" Reactions.
A Review of 16 Treatments and a 3-Step Clinical Approach

Alex Vasquez, DC, ND

Abstract: It is clear from experimental research and clinical experience that "allergic" reactions to foods and environmental toxicants can precipitate neuromusculoskeletal pain and inflammation. This is most obvious in patients with migraine headaches and inflammatory arthropathy such as "rheumatoid arthritis" – one of the most commonly overused diagnostic labels applied to patients with various types of idiopathic inflammatory arthropathy. Unfortunately, current treatments for the allergic diathesis have centered on either 1) symptom suppression, 2) identification and avoidance of the offending food/allergen, and/or 3) systemic immunosuppression with drugs. These approaches result in short-term and limited clinical improvement compared to what can be achieved with a more comprehensive approach that focuses on normalization of immune responsiveness. "Food allergies" are not the fault of the food; rather they are a manifestation of immune system hyper-responsiveness and dysfunction that must be treated comprehensively. This article focuses on techniques for reducing immune system hyper-responsiveness with the use of nutritional and botanical supplements, and the next article in this series (Part 6) will provide additional information on the optimization of gastrointestinal health by focusing on the eradication of immunodysregulatory microorganisms, particularly certain species of yeast, bacteria, amebas, and protozoa.

"Allergic disease is a manifestation of a fundamental distortion of the mechanism through which the individual adapts itself on a cellular level to a hostile environment."
Howard Rapaport, MD in *Journal of Asthma Research*[1]

INTRODUCTION:

Allergic disorders are common and their incidence appears to be increasing. These conditions are complex, multifactorial, and range in severity from asymptomatic, to moderately problematic, to life-threatening. Different names and ICD-9 codes are applied to different types of immunodysfunction within the genre of "allergy"; however, the underlying problem—immune dysfunction—is almost never addressed directly. Rather, symptom suppression via lifelong medicalization is the mainstay of treatment--a quagmire that leaves patients under-treated and dependent on endless cycles of prescription drugs that never offer the opportunity for cure. Furthermore, some conditions traditionally thought of as "allergic" may more accurately be ascribed as "microbial", "metabolic" or "deficiency-induced" as will be exemplified in the sections that follow. While it is true that some patients will require some form of long-term treatment, clinicians should consider addressing and correcting the underlying immune dysfunction before resorting to symptom suppression (ie, antihistamines) and immunosuppression (ie; corticosteroid drugs). Until proven otherwise, "allergic" patients should be assumed to have one or more treatable causes of their allergic disorder before it is conceded that their allergies are "genetic" or "idiopathic" and therefore treatable only with drugs.

The allergic phenomenon is complex, interconnected, and multifaceted. It goes far beyond the dogma that IgE binds with mast cells and results in the release of histamine, which then acts singly for the development of allergic manifestations.[2] The allergic response involves a wide range of cells including T-cells and epithelial cells, and the triggers and mediators of allergic pathophysiology extend beyond IgE and histamine to include corticotrophin-releasing hormone, IgG, cytokines, superoxide anion, IL-6, cyclooxygenase-2, lipoxygenase, NF-kappaB, and arachidonic acid metabolites, especially the leukotrienes. Evidence for the medical acceptance of the leukotriene theory of allergy is demonstrated by FDA approval and widespread use of montelukast, a leukotriene receptor type-1 blocker, marketed by the name of "Singulair" and FDA-approved for the treatment of asthma and allergic rhinitis.[3] As we would expect, NF-kappaB is upregulated in allergic tissues, and therefore the clinical utilization of NF-kappaB inhibitors is justified, as recently reviewed in this Journal.[4]

Allergies do not cause themselves, nor is the putative offending agent to blame. In a patient allergic to strawberries, are the strawberries guilty? Does a patient with allergies have an antihistamine drug deficiency? A more likely cause of the problem lies in subtle perturbations affecting numerous immunoregulatory mechanisms, and these disturbances may include genetic, nutritional, metabolic, and microbial aberrations—most of which can be modulated by appropriate clinical intervention for the attainment of improved clinical outcomes.

OVERVIEW: THE ORIGINS OF ALLERGY AND THE REALITY OF ALLERGY-INDUCED PAIN

Allergy-induced arthritis affects a small but significant

portion of patients with joint pain and inflammation.[5-11] Impressively, some patients with rheumatoid arthritis can have their "disease" literally cured by food allergy elimination, only to have the disease recur when allergens are again consumed.[12] Given this evidence, it is inappropriate that food allergy is ignored by medical textbooks and that chemotherapeutic drugs such as methotrexate are advocated as the medical "treatment of choice" for patients who do not respond to non-steroidal anti-inflammatory drugs (NSAIDs).[13] Advocated as "first line therapy" for the medical treatment of arthritis, NSAIDs are well-known to damage the intestinal mucosa (resulting in "leaky gut") and thereby allow increased absorption of food allergens which results in the exacerbation of allergic disease[14]—thus it is perfectly clear that medical treatment of arthritic patients with NSAIDs can lead to a worsening of their arthritis by amplifying the allergic reactions. Furthermore, it is also clear that NSAIDs promote joint destruction and bone necrosis.[15-18] I have discussed this in great detail elsewhere in support of the position that chiropractic physicians must gain prescription rights for the sake of managing the overpharmaceuticalization of patients treated medically.[19]

Migraine headaches are another example of allergy-induced pain. While any migraneur may be allergic to any particular food, the most common offenders are wheat (78%), orange (65%), eggs (45%), tea and coffee (40% each), chocolate and milk (37%) each), beef (35%), and corn, cane sugar, and yeast (33% each). It is not uncommon for patients to have to avoid up to 10 foods before attaining maximal improvement, and up to 85% of migraine patients can be cured of their headaches by the use of allergy avoidance alone.[20] While the allergen-avoidance approach to migraine treatment is highly efficacious and well documented in the biomedical research, patients and clinicians alike might wonder if a more convenient non-drug approach might be available that addresses the root of the problem. It is true that a dysfunctional immune system cannot react to an allergy-inducing food if the food is not eaten; however, the fact remains that the immune system is left in a state of dysfunction unless doctor and patient engage in the process of improving overall health. In contrast to a lifetime of allergen avoidance, improvement in immune function allows patients to consume a more normal diet and broader range of foods.

Patients with pain affecting the spine and peripheral joints may also respond to allergen avoidance or the immunomodulatory treatments described in this article. Doctors have an obligation to rule out common and serious diseases in patients with musculoskeletal pain, as I have described in extensive detail in my textbook *Integrative Orthopedics.*[21] Following the exclusion of conditions such as hemochromatosis[22], vitamin D deficiency[23], septic arthritis, and other systemic and urgent orthopedic conditions[21], both doctor and patient must engage in a process of therapeutic trial-and-error. This process is arduous and time-consuming unless the doctor uses a group of protocols such as those described herein which address the most common contributing factors to allergic problems. Here I describe a three-step process that has benefited many allergic patients in my clinical practice.

My clinical approach to improving immune function in patients with allergy begins with supplementation of vitamin E, CoQ-10, vitamin C, bioflavonoids, and fatty acids. We can also use honey, vitamin B-12, and glucosamine sulfate and purified chondroitin sulfate. In difficult cases, I look at hormones, particularly DHEA, progesterone, testosterone, and cortisol. I also look at diet and bowel health with respect to putrefaction and intestinal permeability. Although rarely powerful when used in isolation, these treatments when used in combinations tailored to the individual patient often result in an impressive reduction in allergic manifestations even when allergen avoidance is either not pursued or not feasible.

Step 1: From initial patient assessment to the first phase of treatment

In a patient with presumed "allergy" who is in otherwise good health, following a basic health assessment and exclusion of significant disease[21], I begin by correcting problems that are common to patients with allergy. Minor improvements in allergy symptoms as a result of a low-cost low-risk interventions can be multiplied with a specified group of interventions; we aim for a modest improvement with several treatments rather than a "silver bullet" miracle cure with a single intervention. For example, 10% improvement in symptoms may be insignificant in itself; however a 10% improvement from six interventions results in a 60% improvement and enhances patient confidence long enough for other interventions and assessments to be implemented, if necessary. The goal with the first step of treatment is to correct the most common and most likely problems, namely fatty acid imbalances, micronutrient deficiencies, phytonutrient insufficiencies, and dysbiosis. Basic treatments on the first visit generally include the following, in addition to multivitamin/multimineral supplementation with additional vitamin D:

1. **Avoidance of suspected food allergens:** The most common allergens are wheat, cow's milk, and eggs; however any patient can be allergic to any food. Food allergy avoidance for 1 month helps achieve symptomatic relief and allows the gut to heal and the immune system to recalibrate.

2. **Consumption of the Paleo-Mediterranean Diet:** The diet should emphasize consumption of lean

Figure 1. Allergic inflammation is the result of antigen exposure to a dysfunctional immune system.
From Vasquez A. Integrative Orthopedics. (OptimalHealthResearch.com): 2004

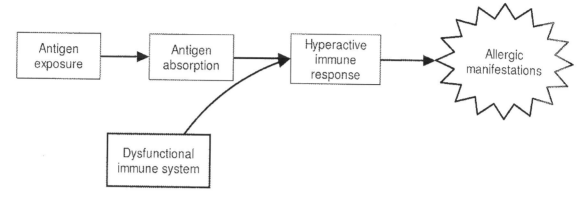

meats, fruits, vegetables, nuts, seeds, and berries to ensure a systemic anti-inflammatory effect and increased consumption of anti-inflammatory phytonutrients, especially flavonoids. High-glycemic foods are avoided as are "food additives" such as tartrazine, which is known to exacerbate allergic asthma. Details of this diet are provided on-line at OptimalHealthResearch.com/monograph05.

3. **Coenzyme Q-10:** CoQ-10 levels are low in approximately 40% of patients with allergies, according to a small study conducted by Folkers and Pfeiffer.[24] Asthmatics also have lower levels of CoQ-10 compared to healthy people.[25] In my experience, clinical improvement is commonly seen in allergic patients after supplementation with CoQ-10. I generally prescribe 100-200 mg per day of CoQ-10 for adults with allergy. Impressively, migraine headaches are known to be induced by consumption of allergenic foods[20], and migraine headaches can be powerfully prevented and alleviated with CoQ-10.[26]

4. **Vitamin C:** Vitamin C reduces blood levels of histamine by increasing urinary excretion and metabolic breakdown of histamine. Cathcart hypothesized that high doses of vitamin C (i.e., bowel tolerance) may impair the adsorption of IgE with allergens and thus retard the allergic cascade from being initiated.[27] Either of these two mechanisms, perhaps in addition to other mechanisms, may explain the anti-allergy effects of ascorbic acid.[28] A recent clinical trial showed that 2 grams per day of ascorbic acid reduced blood histamine levels by 38%.[29] Supplemental vitamin C improves the health of intervertebral discs and alleviates pain and reduces the need for surgery in patients with lumbar disc herniations.[30]

5. **Vitamin E:** Vitamin E has been shown to reduce IgE levels in humans and to reduce the manifestations of allergy-related disease.[31] Vitamin E has been shown to relieve joint pain.[32]

6. **Balanced fatty acid supplementation:** Balanced, combination fatty acid supplementation containing ALA, GLA, EPA, and DHA is the preferred method for fatty acid supplementation for reasons that I have detailed previously.[21,33] The combination of fish oil and borage oil is known to reduce formation of leukotrienes, which are among the primary mediators of allergic reactions and joint inflammation.[34] Fish oil supplementation helps correct the fatty acid abnormalities seen in allergic patients[35] and reduces production of prostaglandin-D2, which increases the release of histamine from mast cells.[36]

7. **Probiotics:** Supplementation with probiotics (beneficial strains of bacteria and yeast) appears to improve intestinal barrier function, promote microecological balance in the gastrointestinal tract, modulate immune function, and thus reduce manifestations of allergic disease.[37-39]

Step 2: Additional interventions for moderate or unresponsive allergies.

For patients who do not respond sufficiently to the first phase of treatment, the following interventions can be considered.

1. **Vitamin B-12:** Vitamin B-12 has been shown to reduce physiologic manifestations of allergy in ovalbumin-sensitized mice.[40] Since vitamin B-12 is safe, non-toxic, and bioavailable when administered orally in large doses to humans, I commonly prescribe 2,000-6,000 mcg per day for allergic patients. Although the benefit of vitamin B-12 in patients with sulfite-sensitive asthma is biochemically medi-

ated rather than immunologically mediated[41], this research adds tangential support to the use of high-dose vitamin B-12 in selected patients with allergy (particularly asthma), at least for a short-term clinical trial. It is impressive to note that vitamin B-12 has anti-allergy effects, and that a recent clinical trial showed that high-dose vitamin B-12 supplementation was effective in alleviating back pain even in patients who were not vitamin B-12 deficient.[42]

2. **Supplemental bioflavonoids/flavonoids:** Bioflavonoids stabilize mast cell membranes and thus reduce the liberation of histamine. Additionally, quercetin and catechin inhibit the action of histidine decarboxylase, which converts histidine into histamine. Many fruits, vegetables, and herbal teas are excellent sources of flavonoids such as quercetin, which can also be consumed in the form of tablets and capsules.

3. **Pancreatic and proteolytic enzymes:** Pancreatic enzymes have been shown to alleviate symptoms of food allergy in a controlled clinical trial.[43] Administration of enzyme preparations can alleviate intestinal and extra-intestinal manifestations of food allergy.[44] Proteolytic enzymes are safe and effective for the relief of musculoskeletal pain, as reviewed previously in this Journal.[45] When taken with food, pancreatic/proteolytic enzymes facilitate hydrolysis of proteins, fats, and carbohydrates and are then absorbed into the systemic circulation for an anti-inflammatory effect. Although individual enzymes may be used in isolation, enzyme therapy is generally delivered in the form of polyenzyme preparations containing pancreatin, bromelain, papain, amylase, lipase, trypsin and alpha-chymotrypsin.

4. **Honey:** Honey consumption has been shown to significantly reduce (-34%) serum IgE levels in humans.[46] The required dose is 1.2 g of honey per kg body weight. For a relatively large individual who weighs 220 lbs, the correct amount of honey to remain consistent with this study would be approximately 120 grams. Since one tablespoon of honey weighs 21 grams, the dose would be 5-6 tablespoons (one-third cup) of honey per day (for a person weighing 220 lbs). Since each tablespoon of honey contains 64 calories, six tablespoons of this powerful natural anti-inflammatory nutraceutical would add 384 calories to the daily diet. Honey should not be administered to infants because of the risk of botulism. Honey is a rich source of flavonoids, and many bee products contain caffeic

acid phenethyl ester, which is a potent inhibitor of NF-kappaB as I reviewed previously.[4,21]

5. **NF-kappa B inhibitors:** The clinical significance of NF-kappaB and its phytonutritional modulation was reviewed recently in this Journal.[4] Nutrients which can be used to downregulate inflammatory responses are vitamin D, curcumin (requires piperine for absorption), lipoic acid, green tea, rosemary, grape seed extract, propolis, and resveratrol.[21]

Step 3: Treatment for severe allergic disease

For some patients with severe allergies, we start with selected treatments from Step 2 or Step 3 on the first visit in addition to the treatments included in Step 1. Implementation can be customized based on history, examination, laboratory findings, and the doctor's experience and good judgment.

1. **Hormones:** Hormones such as DHEA, progesterone, testosterone, and cortisol tend to be lower in allergic/autoimmune individuals than in healthy controls.[47] I generally test with 24-hour urine samples before prescribing hormones, though I will empirically use progesterone in a woman or a 3-month trial of DHEA in a man with allergies if I find sufficient indications and no contraindications. Treatment is customized per patient based on clinical experience and lab tests.

2. **Calcium and magnesium butyrate:** Butyrate is a short-chain fatty acid which can be obtained from 1) a limited number of foods, namely butter, 2) intestinal fermentation of carbohydrates by probiotic bacteria, and 3) use of nutritional supplements. It is increasingly well-established that probiotic bacteria have immune-normalizing and "anti-allergy" effects, and this benefit is probably mediated at least in part by probiotic production of butyrate. The mechanisms of the anti-allergy effect of butyrate are manifold, and as a fatty acid butyrate activates peroxisome-proliferator activated receptor-alpha (PPAR-alpha) and thereby results in an immunomodulatory action and a suppressive effect on NF-kappaB.[48,49] Butyrate is also a primary fuel for enterocytes and may improve enterocyte metabolism for the normalization of intestinal permeability. In the treatment of patients with inflammatory bowel disease, 4 grams per day of orally administered butyrate salts safely improves the action of mesalamine[50] as does topical application of butyrate in distal ulcerative colitis.[51] As a normal dietary component and product of the gastrointestinal tract, supplemental calcium and magnesium salts of butyrate are safe and effective

for human consumption at doses of 1,000 – 4,500 mg butyrate per day for the alleviation of allergic diseases.[52,53]

3. **Purified Chondroitin Sulfate and Glucosamine Sulfate—underappreciated in the treatment of allergy:** Doctors and patients everywhere should know that chondroitin sulfate and glucosamine sulfate are safe and effective for the treatment of osteoarthritis.[45] There is also evidence that purified chondroitin sulfate is cardioprotective and that it helps to reduce the vessel occlusion characteristic of atherosclerosis.[54] Additionally, new experimental evidence shows that chondroitin sulfate and glucosamine sulfate can inhibit allergic reactions.[55] With this in mind, it is reasonable to speculate that many arthritic patients who respond to glucosamine and chondroitin may actually be responding to the anti-allergy benefits of chondroitin and glucosamine rather than or in addition to the "cartilage building" properties of these supplements. Furthermore, there is evidence that purified chondroitin sulfate can act as a "decoy" and reduce adhesion of harmful bacteria; the role of harmful gastrointestinal bacteria in the genesis and perpetuation of joint pain and inflammation will be discussed in the next article in this series. For now, it will suffice to say that occult gastrointestinal infections are a major contributor to the systemic pain and inflammation seen in conditions such as rheumatoid arthritis and ankylosing spondylitis.[21]

4. **Eradication of harmful intestinal yeast, bacteria, and other "parasites":** I have seen several patients become cured of their "allergies" once we eradicated the dysbiotic bacteria, yeast, amoebas, or other microorganisms from their gastrointestinal tract. Intestinal colonization with harmful bacteria/yeast/protozoa/amebas can cause mucosal injury and result in macromolecular absorption and thus promotes immune sensitization to dietary antigens; in these situations, correction of dysbiosis via eradication of harmful microorganisms can lead to an impressive reduction in food-associated allergic phenomena. Galland and Lee[56] reported that eradication of Giardia lamblia in patients with chronic digestive complaints lessened the severity of food intolerance/allergy in 54% of patients. The next article in this series will be completely dedicated to the topic of gastrointestinal flora assessment and modification, a supremely important topic.

CONCLUSIONS:

It is well established that musculoskeletal pain can result from "allergic" reactions to foods, and occasionally to allergens in the surrounding environment. Rather than suppress the entire immune system with drugs, we can modulate and improve immune function with nutritional and botanical interventions. Specific nutrients that have been shown to alleviate pain and allergy/inflammation include vitamin B-12, purified chondroitin sulfate, glucosamine sulfate, balanced fatty acid supplementation, CoQ10, vitamin E, flavonoids, vitamin C, vitamin D, and pancreatic/proteolytic enzymes. The next article in this series will detail assessment and treatment of gastrointestinal dysbiosis, a commonly overlooked cause of musculoskeletal pain and inflammation.

ABOUT THE AUTHOR:

Dr. Alex Vasquez is a licensed naturopathic physician in Washington and Oregon, and licensed chiropractor in Texas, where he maintains a private practice and is a member of the research team at Biotics Research Corporation. As former Adjunct Professor of Orthopedics and Rheumatology for the Naturopathic Medicine Program at Bastyr University, he is the author of "Integrative Orthopedics: The Art of Creating Wellness While Managing Acute and Chronic Musculoskeletal Disorders" available from OptimalHealthResearch.com. Dr. Vasquez has published research in nearly every major medical journal in the world, including The Lancet, Journal of the American Medical Association, British Medical Journal, and Arthritis & Rheumatism.

REFERENCES:

1. Rapaport HG. What to do about the growing problems of pediatric allergy. J Asthma Research 1967; 5: 21-7
2. Kita H, Kaneko M, Bartemes KR, Weiler DA, Schimming AW, Reed CE, Gleich GJ. Does IgE bind to and activate eosinophils from patients with allergy? J Immunol. 1999;162(11):6901-11
3. http://www.singulair.com   <http://www.singulair.com/> Accessed July 26, 2005
4. Vasquez A. Reducing pain and inflammation naturally - Part 4: Nutritional and Botanical Inhibition of NF-kappaB, the Major Intracellular Amplifier of the Inflammatory Cascade. A Practical Clinical Strategy Exemplifying Anti-Inflammatory Nutrigenomics. Nutritional Perspectives 2005: July: 5-12
5. Golding DN. Is there an allergic synovitis? J R Soc Med. 1990 May;83(5):312-4
6. Panush RS. Food induced ("allergic") arthritis: clinical and serologic studies. J Rheumatol. 1990 Mar;17(3):291-4
7. Pacor ML, Lunardi C, Di Lorenzo G, Biasi D, Corrocher R. Food allergy and seronegative arthritis: report of two cases. Clin Rheumatol. 2001;20(4):279-81
8. Schrander JJ, Marcelis C, de Vries MP, van Santen-Hoeufft HM. Does food intolerance play a role in juvenile chronic arthritis? Br J Rheumatol. 1997;36(8):905-8
9. van de Laar MA, van der Korst JK. Food intolerance in rheumatoid arthritis. I. A double blind, controlled trial of the clinical effects of elimination of milk allergens and azo dyes.

Ann Rheum Dis. 1992 Mar;51(3):298-302

10. Haugen MA, Kjeldsen-Kragh J, Forre O. A pilot study of the effect of an elemental diet in the management of rheumatoid arthritis. Clin Exp Rheumatol. 1994 May-Jun;12(3):275-9

11. van de Laar MA, Aalbers M, Bruins FG, van Dinther-Janssen AC, van der Korst JK, Meijer CJ. Food intolerance in rheumatoid arthritis. II. Clinical and histological aspects. Ann Rheum Dis. 1992 Mar;51(3):303-6

12. Panush RS, Stroud RM, Webster EM. Food-induced (allergic) arthritis. Inflammatory arthritis exacerbated by milk. Arthritis Rheum. 1986;29(2):220-6

13. Hellmann DB, Stone JH. Arthritis and musculoskeletal disorders. In: Tierney LM, McPhee SJ, Papadakis MA. Current medical diagosis and treatment. 44th edition. New York: Lange Medical Books; 2005: 805

14. Harada S, Horikawa T, Ashida M, Kamo T, Nishioka E, Ichihashi M. Aspirin enhances the induction of type I allergic symptoms when combined with food and exercise in patients with food-dependent exercise-induced anaphylaxis. Br J Dermatol. 2001 Aug;145(2):336-9

15. "At...concentrations comparable to those... in the synovial fluid of patients treated with the drug, several NSAIDs suppress proteoglycan synthesis... These NSAID-related effects on chondrocyte metabolism ... are much more profound in osteoarthritic cartilage than in normal cartilage, due to enhanced uptake of NSAIDs by the osteoarthritic cartilage." Brandt KD. Effects of nonsteroidal anti-inflammatory drugs on chondrocyte metabolism in vitro and in vivo. Am J Med. 1987 Nov 20; 83(5A): 29-34

16. "The case of a young healthy man, who developed avascular necrosis of head of femur after prolonged administration of indomethacin, is reported here." Prathapkumar KR, Smith I, Attara GA. Indomethacin induced avascular necrosis of head of femur. Postgrad Med J. 2000 Sep; 76(899): 574-5

17. "This highly significant association between NSAID use and acetabular destruction gives cause for concern, not least because of the difficulty in achieving satisfactory hip replacements in patients with severely damaged acetabula." Newman NM, Ling RS. Acetabular bone destruction related to non-steroidal anti-inflammatory drugs. Lancet. 1985 Jul 6; 2(8445): 11-4

18. Vidal y Plana RR, Bizzarri D, Rovati AL. Articular cartilage pharmacology: I. In vitro studies on glucosamine and non steroidal antiinflammatory drugs. Pharmacol Res Commun. 1978 Jun;10(6):557-69

19. Vasquez A. Chiropractic and Naturopathic Medicine for the Promotion of Optimal Health and Alleviation of Pain and Inflammation: A Detailed Review of Current "Daily Use" Research with Implications for Clinical Practice and Healthcare Policy. Updated August 16. 2005 http://www.OptimalHealthResearch.com/monograph05

20. Grant EC. Food allergies and migraine. Lancet. 1979 May 5;1(8123):966-9

21. Vasquez A. Integrative Orthopedics. Natural Health Consulting Corp:2004 Available at www.OptimalHealth Research.com <http://www.optimalhealth research.com/>

22. Vasquez A. Musculoskeletal disorders and iron overload disease: comment on the American College of Rheumatology guidelines for the initial evaluation of the adult patient with acute musculoskeletal symptoms. Arthritis Rheum. 1996 Oct;39(10):1767-8

23. Vasquez A. Manso G, Cannell J. The clinical importance of vitamin D (cholecalciferol): a paradigm shift with implications for all healthcare providers. Altern Ther Health Med. 2004 Sep-Oct;10(5):28-36 Available at http://www.bioticsresearch.com/ and http://optimalhealthresearch.com/major-monograph-04

24. Ye CQ, Folkers K, Tamagawa H, Pfeiffer C. A modified determination of coenzyme Q10 in human blood and CoQ10 blood levels in diverse patients with allergies. Biofactors. 1988 Dec;1(4):303-6

25. Gazdik F, Gvozdjakova A, Nadvornikova R, Repicka L, Jahnova E, Kucharska J, Pijak MR, Gazdikova K. Decreased levels of coenzyme Q(10) in patients with bronchial asthma. Allergy. 2002 Sep;57(9):811-4

26. Sandor PS, Di Clemente L, Coppola G, Saenger U, Fumal A, Magis D, Seidel L, Agosti RM, Schoenen J. Efficacy of coenzyme Q10 in migraine prophylaxis: a randomized controlled trial. Neurology. 2005 Feb 22;64(4):713-5

27. Cathcart RF 3rd. The vitamin C treatment of allergy and the normally unprimed state of antibodies. Med Hypotheses. 1986 Nov;21(3):307-21

28. Bucca C, Rolla G, Oliva A, Farina JC. Effect of vitamin C on histamine bronchial responsiveness of patients with allergic rhinitis. Ann Allergy. 1990 Oct;65(4):311-4

29. Johnston CS, Martin LJ, Cai X. Antihistamine effect of supplemental ascorbic acid and neutrophil chemotaxis. J Am Coll Nutr. 1992 Apr;11(2):172-6

30. Greenwood J Jr. Optimum vitamin C intake as a factor in the preservation of disc integrity: preliminary report. Med Ann Dist Columbia. 1964 Jun;33:274-6

31. Tsoureli-Nikita E, Hercogova J, Lotti T, Menchini G. Evaluation of dietary intake of vitamin E in the treatment of atopic dermatitis: a study of the clinical course and evaluation of the immunoglobulin E serum levels. Int J Dermatol. 2002 Mar;41(3):146-50

32. Edmonds SE, Winyard PG, Guo R, Kidd B, Merry P, Langrish-Smith A, Hansen C, Ramm S, Blake DR. Putative analgesic activity of repeated oral doses of vitamin E in the treatment of rheumatoid arthritis. Results of a prospective placebo controlled double blind trial. Ann Rheum Dis. 1997;56:649-55

33. Vasquez A. Reducing Pain and Inflammation Naturally. Part 2: New Insights into Fatty Acid Supplementation and Its Effect on Eicosanoid Production and Genetic Expression. Nutritional Perspectives 2005; January: 5-16

34. Surette ME, Koumenis IL, Edens MB, Tramposch KM. Clayton B, Bowton D, Chilton FH. Inhibition of leukotriene biosynthesis by a novel dietary fatty acid formulation in patients with atopic asthma: a randomized, placebo-controlled, parallel-group, prospective trial. Clin Ther. 2003 Mar;25(3):972-9

35. Yu G, Bjorksten B. Polyunsaturated fatty acids in school children in relation to allergy and serum IgE levels. Pediatr Allergy Immunol. 1998 Aug;9(3):133-8

36. Peters SP, Schleimer RP, Kagey-Sobotka A, Naclerio RM, MacGlashan DW Jr, Schulman ES, Adkinson NF Jr, Lichtenstein LM. The role of prostaglandin D2 in IgE-mediated reactions in man. Trans Assoc Am Physicians. 1982;95:221-8

37. Majamaa H, Isolauri E. Probiotics: a novel approach in the management of food allergy. J Allergy Clin Immunol 1997 Feb;99(2):179-85

38. von der Weid T, Ibnou-Zekri N, Pfeifer A. Novel probiotics for the management of allergic inflammation. Dig Liver Dis. 2002 Sep;34 Suppl 2:S25-8

39. Kirjavainen PV, Gibson GR. Healthy gut microflora and allergy: factors influencing development of the microbiota. Ann Med. 1999 Aug;31(4):288-92

40. "We infer that Cbl administration significantly reduced the IL-2 concentration, and secondarily the IL-4. IgE and histamine concentrations." Funada U, Wada M, Kawata T, Tanaka N, Tadokoro T, Maekawa A. Effect of cobalamin on the allergic

Continued on page 40

Type of Lung Cancer." U.S. Food and Drug Administration FDA News. November 19, 2004. <http://www.fda.gov/bbs/topics/NEWS/2004/NEW01139.html> March 16, 2005

13. "FDA Statement on Iressa." U.S. Food and Drug Administration. FDA News. December 17, 2004. <http://www.fda.gov/bbs/topics/news/2004/new01145.html > April 6, 2005

14. "FDA approves Erbitux for colorectal cancer." U.S. Food and Drug Administration. FDA news. February 12, 2004. <http://www.fda.gov/bbs/topics/NEWS/2004/NEW01024.html> April 14, 2005.

15. "Top health stories of 2004." Harvard Health Letter. December 2004.

16. "Clinical trial shows SU11248 benefits more than half of patients with gastrointestinal tumors resistant to Gleevec." Dana Farber Cancer Institute. June 8, 2004. <http://www.dfci.harvard.edu/abo/news/press/060804.asp> April 11, 2005.

BIBLIOGRAPHY

"Angiogenesis Inhibitors in the Treatment of Cancer." National Cancer Institute. May 20, 2002. <http://cis.nci.nih.gov/fact/7_42.htm> March 22, 2005

Tan, AR, Yang X, et al. "Evaluation of biologic end points and pharmacokinetics in patients with metastatic breast cancer after treatment with erlotinib, an epidermal growth factor receptor tyrosine kinase inhibitor." J Clin Oncol. 2004 Aug 1; 22(15):3080-90.

"Top ten scientific breakthroughs in 2003." Science. Dec 19 2003;302(5653):2038-2045.

REDUCING PAIN AND INFLAMMATION NATURALLY - PART V continued from page 35

response in mice. Biosci Biotechnol Biochem 2000 Oct;64(10):2053-8

41. Anibarro B, Caballero T, Garcia-Ara C, Diaz-Pena JM, Ojeda JA. Asthma with sulfite intolerance in children: a blocking study with cyanocobalamin. J Allergy Clin Immunol. 1992 Jul;90(1):103-9

42. Mauro GL, Martorana U, Cataldo P, Brancato G, Letizia G. Vitamin B12 in low back pain: a randomised, double-blind, placebo-controlled study. Eur Rev Med Pharmacol Sci. 2000 May-Jun;4(3):53-8

43. Raithel M, Weidenhiller M, Schwab D, Winterkamp S, Hahn EG. Pancreatic enzymes: a new group of antiallergic drugs? Inflamm Res. 2002 Apr;51 Suppl 1:S13-4

44. Gaby AR. Pancreatic enzymes block food allergy reactions. Townsend Letter for Doctors and Patients 2002; November http://www.townsendletter.com/Nov_2002/ gabyliteraturereview1102.htm Accesssed August 16, 2005

45. Vasquez A. Reducing pain and inflammation naturally - Part 3: Improving overall health while safely and effectively treating musculoskeletal pain. Nutritional Perspectives 2005; 28: 34-38, 40-42

46. Al-Waili NS. Effects of daily consumption of honey solution on hematological indices and blood levels of minerals and enzymes in normal individuals. J Med Food. 2003 Summer;6(2):135-40

47. Jefferies WM Mild adrenocortical deficiency, chronic allergies, autoimmune disorders and the chronic fatigue syndrome: a continuation of the cortisone story. Med Hypotheses. 1994 Mar;42(3):183-9

48. Zapolska-Downar D, Siennicka A, Kaczmarczyk M, Kolodziej B, Naruszewicz M. Butyrate inhibits cytokine-induced VCAM-1 and ICAM-1 expression in cultured endothelial cells: the role of NF-kappaB and PPARalpha. J Nutr Biochem. 2004 Apr;15(4):220-8

49. Luhrs H, Gerke T, Muller JG, Melcher R. Schauber J, Boxberge F, Scheppach W, Menzel T. Butyrate inhibits NF-kappaB activation in lamina propria macrophages of patients with ulcerative colitis. Scand J Gastroenterol. 2002 Apr;37(4):458-66

50. Vernia P, Monteleone G, Grandinetti G, Villotti G, Di Giulio E. Frieri G, Marcheggiano A, Pallone F, Caprilli R, Torsoli A. Combined oral sodium butyrate and mesalazine treatment compared to oral mesalazine alone in ulcerative colitis: randomized, double-blind, placebo-controlled pilot study. Dig Dis Sci. 2000 May;45(5):976-81

51. Vernia P, Annese V, Bresci G. d'Albasio G, D'Inca R, Giaccari S, Ingrosso M, Mansi C, Riegler G, Valpiani D, Caprilli R: Gruppo Italiano per lo Studio del Colon and del Retto. Topical butyrate improves efficacy of 5-ASA in refractory distal ulcerative colitis: results of a multicentre trial. Eur J Clin Invest. 2003 Mar;33(3):244-8

52. Neesby TE. Method for desensitizing the gastrointestinal tract from food allergies. United States Patent 4,721,716. January 26, 1988

53. Neesby TE. Method for desensitizing the gastrointestinal tract from food allergies. United States Patent 4,735,967. April 5, 1988

54. Morrison LM, Enrick N. Coronary heart disease: reduction of death rate by chondroitin sulfate A. Angiology. 1973 May;24(5):269-87

55. Theoharides TC, Bielory L. Mast cells and mast cell mediators as targets of dietary supplements. Ann Allergy Asthma Immunol. 2004 Aug;93(2 Suppl 1):S24-34

56. Galland L, Lee M. Abstract #170 High frequency of giardiasis in patients with chronic digestive complaints. Am J Gastroenterol 1989;84:1181

Reducing Pain and Inflammation Naturally.
Part 6: Nutritional and Botanical Treatments Against "Silent Infections" and Gastrointestinal Dysbiosis, Commonly Overlooked Causes of Neuromusculoskeletal Inflammation and Chronic Health Problems

Alex Vasquez, D.C., N.D.

Abstract: AT LEAST 56-70% OF PATIENTS WITH CHRONIC INFLAMMATORY ARTHRITIS ARE CARRIERS OF "SILENT INFECTIONS." Non-infectious microbiological causes of musculoskeletal pain are commonly overlooked, and many doctors are unfamiliar with appropriate assessments and treatments for these conditions. Many patients have musculoskeletal pain and systemic inflammation as a result of "occult infections", "silent infections", or "dysbiosis"—including several subcategories of harmful relationships between the human host and his/her microbial guests or neighbors. This article reviews basic and advanced concepts so that clinicians can gain the practical insight necessary for effective clinical intervention.

INTRODUCTION

Approximately 70% of patients with chronic arthritis are carriers of "silent infections", according to a 1992 article published in the peer-reviewed medical journal *Annals of the Rheumatic Diseases*.[1] A 2001 article in this same journal which focused exclusively on five bacteria showed that 56% of patients with idiopathic inflammatory arthritis had gastrointestinal or genitourinary dysbiosis.[2] Indeed, research evidence strongly indicates that bacteria, yeast/fungi, amebas, protozoa, and other "parasites" (rarely including helminths/worms) are an underappreciated cause of neuromusculoskeletal inflammation. This article will explain the mechanisms by which "silent infections" and "dysbiosis" can cause and perpetuate numerous health problems, and I will also discuss basic assessment and treatment measures that can be used clinically to help patients with microbe-induced musculoskeletal inflammation.

One of the problems that plagues many healthcare providers of all professions is that most doctors are still under the spell of the "Pasteurian paradigm of infectious disease", namely that pathogenic microorganisms cause disease by causing *infection.* Relatedly, Koch's Postulates first published in 1884 held that "the organism must be found in all animals suffering from the disease, but not in healthy animals" and "the cultured organism should cause disease when introduced into a healthy animal." The major problems with the models proposed by Pasteur and Koch are that both of these models fail to appreciate 1) adverse microbe-host interactions which may not result in nor result from a true "infection", and 2) the importance of the patient's biochemical individuality and genetic uniqueness which results in the observed phenomenon that not all patients exposed to a particular microbe will express the associated disease. Supported amply by the research reviewed herein, healthcare providers have an obligation to move beyond these primitive "pathogenic" and "infection-based" models of microorganism-induced disease to apprehend the more common "functional" disorders that can result from exposure to microbes.

PARADIGM SHIFT #1: MICROORGANISMS CAN CAUSE DISEASE EVEN WHEN NOT CAUSING "INFECTION"

We now recognize at least fourteen mechanisms by which microorganisms can cause immune dysfunction that promotes neuromusculoskeletal inflammation. Each of the following exemplifies a mechanism by which microbes can cause "disease" without causing an "infection." Mechanisms by which microorganisms can contribute to musculoskeletal inflammation without causing "infection" include but are not limited to the following:

1) Molecular mimicry: Several microbes have peptides and other structures that resemble or "mimic" the peptides and cell structures found in human tissues. Thus, when the immune system fights against the microbe, the antibodies and T-cells can "cross-react" with the tissues of the human host. In this way, the immune system begins attacking the human body, which is otherwise an innocent bystander—the victim of "friendly fire."[3]

2) Superantigens: Many viral, bacterial, and fungal microbes produce "superantigens", molecules which are capable of causing widespread, nonspecific, and unregulated pro-inflammatory immune activation. One of the hallmarks of superantigens is their ability to induce polyclonal T- and B-lymphocyte activation and the production of excessive levels of cytokines and other inflammatory effectors.[4] Obviously, when the body is in such a state of unregulated hyper-inflammation, inevitably some of this inflammation will affect the structures of the musculoskeletal system, especially since articular tissues are predisposed to immune attack. Several research groups have found evidence of superantigen involvement in the pathogenesis of rheumatoid arthritis.[5,6]

3) Peptidoglycans and exotoxins from gram-positive

bacteria: Peptidoglycans from gram-positive bacteria such as group-A streptococci can cause malaise, fever, dermatosis, tenosynovitis, cryoglobulinemia (immune complex disease), and arthritis.[7] Experimental arthritis can be induced in animals by exposing them to group-B streptococci isolated from the nasopharynx of human patients with rheumatoid arthritis.[8] *Staphylococcus aureus* is a gram-positive bacterium, certain strains of which produce the toxic shock syndrome toxin-1 (TSST-1) that causes scalded skin syndrome, toxic shock syndrome, and food poisoning; other strains of *Staph aureus* that do not produce TSST-1 are also capable of causing toxic shock syndrome from colonization of bone, vagina, wounds, or rectum.[9] Experimental evidence has shown that peptidoglycan-polysaccharide complexes from "good" and "normal" bacteria such as Bifidobacteria and *Lactobacillus casei* can also induce an inflammatory arthritis; this speaks against the "more is better" approach to probiotic supplementation and also demonstrates how bacterial overgrowth of the small bowel (detailed later) can induce joint pain even if the patient's stool test shows no pathogens.[10,11]

4) *Endotoxins (lipopolysaccharide) from gram-negative bacteria:* Many different species of gram-negative bacteria produce endotoxin, also known as bacterial lipopolysaccharide (LPS). Even in the absence of viable bacteria, the exposure of humans to endotoxin, say for example by intravenous administration for the purpose of experimentation, produces a wide range of adverse physiologic consequences, including 1) triggering an acute pro-inflammatory response resembling febrile illness or sepsis, 2) increasing intestinal permeability, causing "leaky gut"[12], 3) inhibiting hepatic detoxification[13], 4) disrupting the blood-brain barrier and promoting neurodegeneration via neuroinflammation.[14-16] Endotoxin/LPS often function similarly to superantigens, and their effects are synergistic, resulting in altered tissue function and widespread inflammation.

5) *Enhanced processing of autoantigens:* When the immune system perceives the presence of microbial molecules, processes are enhanced which facilitate the processing and presentation of preexistent antigens to the immune system, which then targets these antigens for destruction. Of course, this is beneficial when fighting a true infection; but there is mounting evidence that chronic silent infections can facilitate the processing and presentation of the body's own antigens (autoantigens) which are then attacked. Clinically, we see the immune system attacking the body, and we call this an "autoimmune disease" even though the original cause of the problem may have been an occult infection or exposure to specific microbial molecules.

6) *Bystander activation:* Evidence suggests that we all have immunocytes capable of attacking our body tissues, and thus we all have the potential to develop autoimmune disease. Normally, these autoreactive cells are kept anergic, dormant, quiescent, and otherwise inactive through various mechanisms that regulate the immune system; in this way, such autoreactive cells can be considered "bystanders" because they are not really doing anything and are basically "standing by." Bystander activation occurs when these cells are awakened by the cascade of inflammatory processes that occur as a result of superantigen exposure, molecular mimicry, immune complex deposition, or xenobiotic immunotoxicity. Bystander activation can contribute to the development of autoimmunity.

7) *Immune complex formation and deposition due to the activation of B-lymphocytes/plasma cells:* Chronic infection generally results in the increased production of immune complexes, which are polymeric antigen-antibody combinations. Antigen-antibody combinations are formed when the immune system is fighting against a virus, bacteria, yeast, or food allergen. Although essential for the destruction and clearance of pathogenic antigens, immune complexes pose a problem for the body due to 1) the difficulty in clearing them from the systemic circulation, and 2) their proclivity for deposition in the skin and joints.[17] Indeed, immune complexes are significant contributors to most "autoimmune" diseases; immune complex deposition is responsible for triggering joint inflammation in rheumatoid arthritis[18] and for the facial rash and other clinical manifestations which characterize systemic lupus erythematosus (SLE, lupus). Immune complex deposition directly contributes to the renal disease and vasculitis common in patients with autoimmune disease. Patients with autoimmune disease commonly have circulating IgM and IgA antibodies against bacteria from the gastrointestinal and genitourinary tracts[19] clearly indicating an active immune response against these bacteria and implying breaches in mucosal integrity. Research suggests that IgA immune complex diseases may be particularly amenable to treatment with physiotherapeutic treatments (colonics and enemas), nutritional supplementation (proteolytic enzymes), and botanical interventions ("liver herbs") as discussed later in this paper.

8) *Haptenization:* A nonantigenic microbial molecule may bind to a nonantigenic human molecule and result in the formation of a new hybridized or "haptenized" molecule which stimulates immunologic attack. Haptenization may be the underlying mechanism by which viruses induce autoimmunity[20] and appears to be a primary mechanism by which *Staphylococcus aureus* contributes to autoimmune vasculitis in Wegener's granulomatosis.[21] Indirectly, microbes—particularly bacteria—may induce xenobiotic-mediated haptenization by altering detoxification of pharmaceutical or pollutant chemicals, as discussed below.

Toxic metals and chemicals probably trigger autoimmunity via haptenization[22], and, in a recent animal study, exposure to bacterial endotoxin exacerbated metal-induced autoimmunity.[23] Thus, microbial exposure appears synergistic with toxic metal/chemical exposure for the incitement of autoimmunity.

9) *Damage to the intestinal mucosa:* One of the indirect ways by which gastrointestinal microbes can cause non-infectious disease is by damaging the intestinal mucosa, a situation which results in "leaky gut." The increased absorption of debris from the gut—"antigen overload" from otherwise benign yeast, bacteria, and foods—results in overstimulation of the immune system[24], resulting in enhanced autoantigen processing and bystander activation as discussed above. I have provided a detailed illustration of this complex phenomenon in *Integrative Orthopedics* and on-line at www.optimalhealthresearch.com/gastro. It is well-known that exacerbations and relapse of the autoimmune diseases ulcerative colitis and Crohn's disease are preceded by increases in intestinal permeability; this is direct evidence of "leaky gut" preceding clinical disease.[25] Evidence of "leaky gut" is seen in several systemic inflammatory disorders, including asthma[26], eczema[27], psoriasis[28], Behcet's disease[29], ankylosing spondylitis[30] and seronegative spondyloarthritis[31], and nearly all of the so-called "idiopathic" juvenile arthropathies" such as enteropathic spondyloarthropathy and oligoarticular juvenile idiopathic arthritis.[32] A "leaky gut" type of intestinal disease (protein-losing enteropathy) is also seen in some patients with lupus.[33]

10) *Inhibition of detoxification:* It is well-known that bioaccumulation of toxic chemicals can result in autoimmunity and systemic inflammation via immunodysregulation. Examples of this include 1) the increased autoimmunity seen in farmers exposed to pesticides[34], 2) the scleroderma-like disease that results from exposure to vinyl chloride[35], 3) the association of mercury and pesticide exposure with lupus[36], and 4) the well-recognized connection between drug and chemical exposure and various autoimmune syndromes such as drug-induced lupus.[37] Indeed, more than 40 pharmaceutical drugs are known to cause drug-induced lupus, and bystander activation appears to be one of the mechanisms involved.[38] Thus having established the general premise that "chemical exposure can promote autoimmune disease", it seems logical and probable that anything which would inhibit the body's ability to detoxify these chemicals would likewise increase the risk for autoimmunity. Stated differently, factors that inhibit detoxification and which therefore increase the body burden of immunotoxic xenobiotics would serve to indirectly contribute to immunodysfunction, including autoimmunity. Indeed, patients with lupus and systemic sclerosis show defects in detoxification[39], and it has been

reported that patients who undergo a comprehensive detoxification protocol commonly experience a normalization of their immune function and alleviation of their autoimmune diseases.[40,41] Dysbiotic bacterial overgrowth of the gastrointestinal tract directly impairs detoxification via the following four mechanisms: 1) Bacterial lipopolysaccharide (endotoxin) has been shown to dramatically impair Phase 1 of chemical detoxification.[42] 2) Bacterial overgrowth can lead to excess production of methane which causes constipation[43] and thus increases the "toxic load" in the colon which then increases the load on the liver via the portal circulation. 3) Several species of bacteria produce deconjugating enzymes (such as beta-glucuronidase) that cleave previously "detoxified" toxins from their water-soluble moieties thus allowing the toxin to be reabsorbed in a mechanism termed "enterohepatic recycling"[44] or "enterohepatic recirculation."[45] 4) Damage to the intestinal mucosa increases absorption of intraluminal contents and thus increase the toxic load placed on the detoxification mechanisms, which are mostly located in the liver; eventually these pathways become depleted, rendering the host susceptible to the consequences of nutritional depletion and impaired detoxification.[46] Taken together these enterometabolic mechanisms are consistent with the observance of increased risk for xenobiotic-associated diseases such as breast cancer[47,48] and Parkinson's disease[49,50] in patients with chronic constipation. Furthermore, we would expect that patients with endotoxin-producing bacterial overgrowth of the small intestine would be more susceptible to the chemical accumulation that leads to multiple chemical sensitivity syndrome (MCS) and the xenobiotic-induced immune dysfunction that may result. In my own clinical practice, I have seen many patients with chemical sensitivity respond very favorably to the eradication of their intestinal bacterial overgrowth, and I consider this treatment essential for all patients with autoimmune disease.

11) *Antimetabolites:* Yeast and bacteria can produce certain molecules which "jam up", "monkey wrench", or otherwise interfere with normal human cellular metabolism. The best example is D-lactic acid, which impairs human metabolic pathways that are designed to work with the "human" form of this metabolite: L-lactic acid. Commonly resulting in headache, fatigue, depression, and sometimes death, D-lactic acidosis is extensively well documented in the medical research literature and commonly occurs in association with bacterial overgrowth of the intestine, particularly following intestinal bypass surgery.[51] Other antimetabolites produced from (intestinal) microbes which are associated with human disease and dysfunction include ammonia, tryptamine, tyramine, octopamine, mercaptates, aldehydes, alcohol, tartaric acid, indolepropionic acid, indoleacetic acid, skatole, indole, putrescine, and cadaverine. Many of these metabolites are seen in higher amounts in patients with migraine, depression, weakness, confusion, schizophrenia, agitation, hepatic encephalopathy, chronic arthritis and rheumatoid arthritis. Gut-derived neurotoxins from bacteria and yeast may contribute to austistic symptomatology[52,53], and case reports have consistently demonstrated that excess absorption of bacterial metabolites can alter behavior in humans and result in acute neurocognitive decline and behavioral abnormalities in children.[54] Hydrogen sulfide, produced by intestinal bacteria such as *Citrobacter freundii*[55], is a mitochondrial poison[56] and is strongly associated with disease activity in ulcerative colitis.[57] Degradation of tryptophan by bacterial tryptophanase would predispose to a "functional tryptophan deficiency" with resultant insufficiency of serotonin which would contribute to hyperalgesia, depression, hypoadrenalism, and insomnia; indole and skatole, which are gut-derived bacterial degradation products of tryptophan, produce an inflammatory arthritis that is identical to rheumatoid arthritis in animal models.[58,59]

12) "Autointoxication", "hepatic encephalopathy" and "intestinal arthritis-dermatitis syndrome": The term "autointoxication" fell out of favor among American allopaths in the 1940s despite the recognition and objective documentation that systemically absorbed microbial metabolites from the colon could adversely affect systemic health, particularly neurocognitive function.[60] "Hepatic encephalopathy" seems to be one of the currently acceptable terms for this phenomenon, and it is probable that the condition exists among some outpatients to a milder degree than that which is classically seen in patients with fulminant liver failure. Recognition that excess or abnormal microbes in the gut could cause neuropsychiatric symptoms contributed to the rationale for the use of colonic irrigation in clinical practice which was fully endorsed by the American Medical Association in a position paper published in 1932.[61] Concurrently, an article published in the *New England Journal of Medicine*[62] in this same year documented the clinical benefits of colonic irrigation in patients with mental disease; the treatment was deemed effective against most cases of dementia, depression, neurosis and many cases of irritability, headaches, and hypertension. Enemas and colonics, which promote hepatobiliary detoxification[63] and cleanse the bowel of harmful microbes, were valued by clinicians as a cure or adjunctive treatment for numerous systemic diseases.[64] Although the term "autointoxication" has recently been eschewed as "unscientific", all medical professionals recognize that gastrointestinal dysbiosis can cause clinical condition characterized by inflammatory vasculitis, dermatitis, and arthritis; current terms for this condition include "bowel-associated dermatosis-**arthritis** syndrome"[65], "intestinal **arthritis**-dermatitis syndrome"[66], and "bypass disease"[67]—all of which are largely mediated by the

intraintestinal formation, mucosal resorption, and systemic deposition of immune complexes in skin, joints, kidneys, and vascular endothelium.

13) *Impairment of mucosal and systemic defenses:* Microbial colonization of mucosal surfaces can result in impaired local immunity by causing loss of protective secretory IgA or by causing direct tissue damage that results in increased absorption of microbial, dietary, or environmental antigens. Several microorganisms such as *Entamoeba histolytica*[68], *Streptococcus sanguis*[69], and *Candida albicans*[70] externalize a protein-digesting enzyme (proteinase) that "digests" defensive immunoglobulins, including secretory IgA and humoral immunoglobulins. The proteinases produced by *Candida* are capable of lysing not only sIgA but also keratin and collagen[71], obviously providing for a breach of protection from other infections and antigens. In this way, mucosal microbial colonization with yeast/bacteria that secrete proteases/proteinases can "open the door" to exposure to other microbes or antigens that promote resultant infection or "allergy", respectively. Furthermore, because IgA is destroyed by the protease, the infection is allowed to fester, resulting in on-going immune stimulation and its consequences such as bystander activation. This may explain why women with chronic vaginal candidiasis, which always implies chronic yeast overgrowth of the intestine[72], have nearly double the incidence of allergic rhinitis compared to patients without chronic yeast overgrowth.[73] Further supporting the link between yeast and allergy is another recent study showing that allergy/atopy is more common in patients with chronic yeast infections.[74] *Candida* produces an immunotoxin called "gliotoxin", which suppresses human immune function.[75] The combination of mucosal damage, destruction of sIgA, immunosuppression, and microbial overgrowth synergize to sensitize the systemic immune system toward allergic and pro-inflammatory disease.[76]

14) *Impairment of mucosal digestion by microbial proteases and inflammation:* Similar to the degradation of human IgA by microbial proteases/proteinases is the degradation of mucosal digestive enzymes such as the disaccharidases (sucrase, maltase, lactase, and isomaltase) and dipeptidases. First, impaired digestion of carbohydrates skews the intestinal milieu toward one favorable to bacterial/yeast overgrowth by increasing the levels of carbohydrate substrate upon which microbes feed. Impaired peptide breakdown promotes immune sensitization, protein malnutrition, and putrefaction. Second, inflammation resultant from intestinal dysbiosis further impairs carbohydrate digestion via downregulation of sucrase-isomaltase gene expression by inflammatory cytokines.[77] Third, destruction of microvilli exacerbates loss of mucosal enzymes and leads to additional malabsorption, maldigestion, and increased macromolecular absorption, such as seen in patients with intestinal giardiasis.[78] Impairment/reduction of disaccharidases and dipeptidases is also seen in patients with inflammatory bowel disease.[79] Fourth and finally, bacterial proteases work synergistically with biofilm formation to nullify immunologic attack (via immunosuppression and cytokine inactivation) and are important for the establishment of chronic mucosal colonization.[80]

In sum, this survey of the literature supports the concept that intestinal dysbiosis can contribute to systemic pain, inflammation, and immune activation by numerous mechanisms, and that many of these "silent infections" are self-perpetuating by various mechanisms. Clinical experience has shown us again and again that eradicating dysbiosis helps normalize immune function, alleviate autoimmunity and allergy, reduce inflammation, improve detoxification, and to help "cure" people of their previously "incurable" multiple chemical sensitivity and environmental illness.

PARADIGM SHIFT #2: ERADICATING HARMFUL MICROBES FROM THE INTERNAL/EXTERNAL ENVIRONMENT CAN HELP CURE OTHERWISE "INCURABLE DISEASE"

In the previous section, I described the biochemical/physiologic mechanisms by which microorganisms can contribute to disease (without causing a classic "infection") and promote systemic inflammation and human disease. Thus having developed the precept that "microorganisms can cause inflammatory disease by non-infectious means", I will state here that the cure of human disease by eradication of harmful microbes is not a requirement to prove the validity of this thesis. Inflammation and autoimmunity are self-perpetuating phenomena that can persist despite the effective eradication of the principle cause, and research has demonstrated that microbial antigens can remain present in synovial fluid for several years after the eradication of the primary infection. With that said, we are fortunate to observe that many patients with autoimmunity are indeed benefited and occasionally "cured" by removal of instigating microbes. I have seen this on numerous occasions in my clinical practice, and this phenomenon has also been documented in the research literature. Examples published in the research include the amelioration of one patient's scleroderma with the eradication of intestinal bacterial overgrowth[81], the amelioration of Wegener's granulomatosis with antimicrobial therapy against Staphylococcus aureus[82,83], and the alleviation of inflammatory arthritis following the use of antibiotics against genitourinary Chlamydia trachomatis and gastrointestinal Salmonella enteritidis, Yersinia enterocolitica, Shigella flexneri or Campylobacter jejuni.[84]

THE SIX MAIN LOCI OF DYSBIOSIS—FOCUS ON GASTROINTESTINAL DYSBIOSIS

For a microorganism to induce a systemic pro-inflammatory immunodysregulatory response in a human, the microbe or its metabolic products must be exposed to a susceptible host. Non-infectious microbial overgrowth can occur inside the body (gastrointestinal, sinus, genitourinary, or dental), on the surface of the body (dermal), or outside of the body (environmental). The adverse physiologic and clinical effects can be similar regardless of the location of the microorganism. The term "dysbiosis" is classically applied to harmful, non-infectious relationships between the human host and yeast, bacteria, protozoans, amoebas, or other "parasites" located specifically in the gastrointestinal tract, and "dysbiosis" is now an accepted term in the medical literature.[85] However, we must also appreciate that harmful, noninfectious microbe-host interactions can also occur when microbes are localized in the sinuses, oral cavity, genitourinary tract, skin, and in the external environment. I prefer to use a broad definition of dysbiosis that implies "a relationship of non-infectious host-microorganism interaction that adversely affects the human host" and then to specify the subtype based on the location: gastrointestinal, oral, sinus, genitourinary, dermatologic, or environmental. Gastrointestinal dysbiosis is clearly the prototype for understanding other types of dysbiosis; this is because it seems to be the most common form of dysbiosis, perhaps due to the large numbers and types of microbes in the gut and the extensive surface area of the gastrointestinal tract. For the sake of brevity, I will only emphasize gastrointestinal dysbiosis here and will provide an introduction to sinus, genitourinary, dental, cutaneous, and environmental dysbiosis, each of which is discussed in greater detail in my textbook Integrative Rheumatology.

Gastrointestinal dysbiosis: We all have bacteria and occasionally small quantities of yeast in our intestines, and this is normal and healthy. However, problems arise when these yeast/bacteria become imbalanced or when *harmful* yeast, bacteria, parasites take up residence within the gut. Particularly in the European research literature, this condition has been more widely researched and is referred to as "dysbacteriosis" or "dysbacterosis." These latter terms imply that the problem has a *bacterial* origin, which is potentially misleading since dysbiosis commonly involves bacteria and *yeast* (including but not limited to *Candida albicans*) and commonly other harmful non-bacterial microbes such as *Giardia lamblia, Blastocystis hominis, Endolimax nana, Entamoeba histolytica* and a cast of other malcontents that adversely affect the overall health of their human host.[86] "Candidiasis" and yeast-related problems have been described in the research literature and general press.[87] Dysbiosis is probably a major aspect of the phenomenon that was previously referred to in the medical literature as "autointoxication" and which was effectively treated with dietary modifications, nutritional supplementation, and colonic irrigation. Given that endotoxin/lipopolysaccharide is one of the major activators of nuclear factor Kappa-B (NF-kappaB)[88], and that NF-kappaB activation is a major rate-limiting step in the production of pro-inflammatory cytokines and in the induction of pro-inflammatory enzymes such as cyclooxygenase, lipoxygenase, and inducible nitric oxide synthase,[89] then the link between dysbiosis and systemic inflammation becomes clear: gastrointestinal bacterial overgrowth leads to excess production and absorption of endotoxin, which then initiates immune dysfunction and a systemic pro-inflammatory response. Thus, the sequelae of dysbiosis are mediated by alterations in human physiology rather than being directly caused by the microbe. Current research has linked several microbes with human autoimmune/inflammatory diseases, for example *Entamoeba histolytica* has been linked with Henoch Schonlein purpura[90], *Klebsiella pneumoniae* with ankylosing spondylitis[91], *Proteus mirabilis* with rheumatoid arthritis[92] and ankylosing spondylitis[93], *Pseudomonas aeruginosa* with multiple sclerosis[94], and *Helicobacter pylori* with reactive arthritis.[95] Building upon a previous system of categorization proposed by Galland[96], here I describe six different types of gastrointestinal dysbiosis:

1) Insufficiency dysbiosis: This results when there is an insufficient quantity of the "good bacteria." Absence of "good bacteria" such as *Bifidobacteria* and *Lactobacillus* leaves the gastrointestinal tract vulnerable to colonization with pathogens and is associated with increased risk for bacterial overgrowth and other intestinal diseases. Furthermore, good bacteria in the intestines normalize systemic immune response and promote proper digestion, elimination and nutrient absorption. Numerous scientific studies have documented the powerful benefits of supplementing with good bacteria (probiotics), supporting their growth with fermentable carbohydrates such as inulin and fructooligosaccharides (prebiotics), and by co-administering probiotics with prebiotics (synbiotics).

2) Bacterial overgrowth: This is a quantitative excess of yeast and bacteria in the gut. Bacterial overgrowth of the small bowel is a well-established medical problem that is particularly common in diabetics, the elderly, the immunosuppressed, and patients on "antacid" drugs.[97] This commonly results in gas, bloating, constipation and/or diarrhea as well as myalgias and systemic immune activation.[43] Animal studies have proven that it is possible to reactivate peripheral arthritis by inducing bacterial overgrowth of the small bowel; endotoxins and other microbial products stimulate a systemic pro-inflammatory state which re-activates inflammation of joints and periarticular structures.[98] Bac-

terial overgrowth of the small intestine is seen in 84% of patients with irritable bowel syndrome[43] and in 100% of patients with fibromyalgia.[99] Researchers recently demonstrated that endotoxins can lead to impairment of muscle function and a lowered lactate threshold[100], thereby explaining the link between intestinal dysbiosis and chronic musculoskeletal pain that is not responsive to drugs or manual therapies. In patients with lupus, gastrointestinal bacteria are abnormal (decreased colonization resistance[101]), and it is possible that gastrointestinal bacteria in these patients may translocate into the systemic circulation to induce formation of antibodies that cross-react with double-stranded DNA to produce the clinical manifestations of the disease.[101,102] Relatedly, Drs. Over and Bucknall[81] describe a patient with systemic sclerosis who achieved long-term remission of her disease following antibiotic treatment for intestinal bacterial overgrowth. Bacterial overgrowth generally leads to pathologically synergistic clinical effects mediated by fermentation, putrefaction, constipation, increased enterohepatic recycling, bile acid deconjugation, malabsorption (particularly fat-soluble nutrients and vitamin B-12), nutritional deficiencies, sugar cravings, increased intestinal permeability, immune complex formation, and induction of a systemic pro-inflammatory response which is particularly prone to manifest as vasculitis and arthritis.[43,103,104]

3) Immunosuppressive dysbiosis: Some microbes, particularly yeast, produce toxins that suppress immune function. The immunosuppressive mycotoxin produced by *Candia albicans* is called gliotoxin, and it is produced at the site of yeast overgrowth, thus suppressing local—and possibly, systemic—immune function.[105,106] Since secretory IgA is the first line of defense against allergens and infections in the gastrointestinal tract, its destruction by microbes such as *Candida albicans* and *Entamoeba histolytica* retards this immune barrier, and this can be considered a form of immunosuppression.

4) Hypersensitivity dysbiosis: Some people have an exaggerated immune response to otherwise "normal" yeast and bacteria. In this situation, we have to eradicate their "normal" yeast or bacteria in order to alleviate their hypersensitivity reaction. The best example of this is the severe intestinal inflammation that some patients develop in response to intestinal colonization with *Candida albicans,* which is generally considered "nonpathogenic" in small amounts. In susceptible patients *Candida* can induce a severe local inflammatory reaction, such as colitis, that only remits with antifungal treatment.[107] Gastrointestinal overgrowth of *Candida albicans* and *C. glabrata* caused near-fatal hypersensitivity alveolitis that remitted with eradication of gastrointestinal candidiasis.[108] It is clear that some women become "allergic" to their own vaginal *Can-*

dida albicans[109]; undoubtedly there are also men who are likewise allergic to their own intestinal yeast.

5) *Inflammatory dysbiosis and "reactive arthritis":* Some people with specific genotypes and HLA markers are susceptible to a pro-inflammatory "autoimmune" syndrome that occurs following a noninfectious exposure to specific microbial molecules that are structurally similar to human body tissues—a phenomenon previously described as molecular mimicry. The best-known example of systemic musculoskeletal inflammation caused by microbial exposure is "reactive arthritis" such as Reiter's syndrome, which is classically seen in patients with the genotype HLA-B27 following urogenital exposure to *Chlamydia trachomatis.*

6) *Amoebas, cysts, protozoans, and other "parasites":* In this case when we use the term "parasites'" we are not talking about worms, *per se,* although these are occasionally found with parasitology examinations. Certain microorganisms are not consistent with optimal health and should be eliminated even though the microbe is not classically identified as a "pathogen." Individual microorganisms are discussed later in this article.

Sinorespiratory dysbiosis: Patients with acute and chronic rhinosinusitis commonly display a rich mixture of bacteria and fungi in their sinuses. Regarding bacteria, both anaerobic and aerobic bacteria are seen, as are gram-positives such as *Staphylococcus aureus* and *Streptococcus* sp, and gram-negative (endotoxin-producing) species including *Klebsiella pneumoniae, Proteus mirabilis, Bacteroides, Haemophilus parainfluenzae, Haemophilus influenzae,* and Peptococcus/Peptostreptococcus.[110,111] In a landmark publication in *Mayo Clinic Proceedings*[112], the authors found that almost all patients with chronic sinus congestion had occult sinus infections, and they concluded, *"Fungal cultures of nasal secretions were positive in 202 (96%) of 210 consecutive chronic rhinosinusitis patients."* Perhaps the best current exemplification of the link between sinus infections and chronic inflammatory disease is seen in patients with Wegener's granulomatosis, who have a high incidence of sinus colonization with *Staphylococcus aureus.* Once considered "idiopathic", Wegener's granulomatosis is a systemic autoimmune disease characterized by vasculitis, respiratory complications, and renal failure; without treatment it is often fatal within 12 months of diagnosis. Recently, patients with Wegener's granulomatosis have been found to have subclinical sinus colonization with *Staphylococcus aureus.* In these patients, *Staphylococcus aureus* produces a superantigen as well as an antigenic acid phosphatase which induces autoimmune vasculitis, nephritis, the production of antineutrophil anticytoplasmic antibody (ANCA), and the formation of immune complexes. Antimicrobial treatment to eradicate

Staphylococcus aureus results in clinical remission of the "autoimmune" disease[82], thus proving the microbe-rheumatic link. Interestingly, 97% of patients severely infected with the gastrointestinal "parasite" *Entamoeba histolytica* develop self-destructive ANCA, leading to the possibility that this microbe can induce or sustain autoimmunity.[83]

Dental dysbiosis: The human oral cavity is heavily populated by microbes, and these microbes and their products such as endotoxin can enter the bloodstream to induce a pro-inflammatory response via "metastatic infection" and "metastatic inflammation", respectively.[113] The systemic inflammatory response triggered by mild oral/dental "infections" is now believed to exacerbate conditions associated with inflammation, such as cardiovascular disease and diabetes.[114] Patients with recalcitrant inflammation might be referred to a "biologic dentist" for evaluation and treatment of occult dental and mandibular infections.

Genitourinary dysbiosis: It is well-known that genitourinary infection with *Chlamydia trachomatis* can produce systemic inflammation—"reactive arthritis"—and result in the condition previously known as Reiter's syndrome.[84] Often fatal, toxic shock syndrome results from the absorption of toxins and superantigens from *Staphylococcus aureus* directly through the genitourinary mucosa. In a study of 234 patients with inflammatory arthritis, 44% of patients had a silent genitourinary infection, mostly due to *Chlamydia, Mycoplasma,* or *Ureaplasma.*[115] It is therefore clear that microbial contamination of the genitourinary tract may lead to a systemic pro-inflammatory response in susceptible individuals.

Cutaneous dysbiosis: Microorganisms from dermal infections such as acne can incite systemic inflammation either by dermal absorption of bacterial[116] and fungal[4] (super)antigens and by serving as loci for metastatic infections which produce septic arthritis.[117] Patients with the autoimmune vasculitic syndrome known as Behcet's disease are more likely to develop arthritis if their skin lesions are infected.[118] Thus, topical and/or systemic antimicrobial treatment along with immunonutrition (detailed later) may be necessary for complete treatment of patients with inflammatory autoimmunity caused by dermal infections.

Environmental dysbiosis: "Toxic mold syndrome" describes patients with systemic health problems resultant from exposure to fungal bioaeresols, classically associated with mold-contaminated buildings following water damage. Such individuals may develop neuromuscular autoimmunity that resembles multiple sclerosis and idiopathic inflammatory polyneuropathy mediated in part by antibodies against endogenous neuronal structures.[119] Additional evidence makes it clear that mold exposure can lead to pro-inflammatory immune activation and resultant multisystem autoimmunity.[120] This is yet another example of how microorganisms can cause human disease without causing "infection."

GASTROINTESTINAL DYSBIOSIS: IDENTIFICATION AND ERADICATION

Clinicians should suspect gastrointestinal dysbiosis in their patients with gas, bloating, alternating constipation/diarrhea, irritable bowel syndrome, fibromyalgia, chronic fatigue syndrome, multiple chemical sensitivity, severe allergies, and autoimmunity, especially Crohn's disease, ulcerative colitis, rheumatoid arthritis, and ankylosing spondylitis. Bacterial overgrowth of the small bowel can be objectively documented with measurement of post-carbohydrate hydrogen/methane, but I consider a history of postprandial gas and bloating to be sufficiently diagnostic. The single best test for the assessment of gastrointestinal dysbiosis is a comprehensive stool analysis and comprehensive parasitology examination performed by a specialty laboratory that provides bacterial culture, yeast culture, microscopic exam, and measurement of sIgA to assess mucosal immune response, along with markers of inflammation such as lactoferrin, calprotectin, and/or lysozyme. Additional markers can help put microbiological findings into the proper context.

CLINICAL AND LABORATORY ASSESSMENT OF GASTROINTESTINAL STATUS

Clinical assessment of gastrointestinal function begins with a thorough history. Frequent gas and bloating indicates excess gastrointestinal fermentation by yeast and/or overgrowth of aerobic bacteria. Abdominal pain, chronic constipation, and/or diarrhea are clear indications for stool testing; however clinicians must remember that some of the most heavily colonized patients will have no gastrointestinal symptoms. Thus, assessment and treatment for gastrointestinal dysbiosis is not unnecessary simply because the patient lacks gastrointestinal symptoms. The lactulose and mannitol assay evaluates paracellular (pathologic) and transcellular (physiologic) absorption, respectively; and an increased latulose:mannitol ratio is a non-specific finding that indicates gastrointestinal damage, generally due to 1) enterotoxin consumption such as with alcohol or NSAIDs, 2) malnutrition, 3) food allergy including celiac disease, 4) severe systemic illness, and/or 5) dysbiosis—excess/harmful yeast, bacteria, or parasites. Comprehensive stool analysis assesses digestion, absorption, inflammation, and comprehensive parasitology examinations (x3) assess for bacteria, yeast, and parasites. These tests should be performed by a specialty laboratory rather than a regular medical or hospital laboratory.

PROBLEMATIC BACTERIA, YEAST, AND PARASITES: A LISTING OF COMMONLY ENCOUNTERED MICROBES

With the single exception of *Dientamoeba fragilis*, all of the following yeast, bacteria, and "parasites" have been observed in various patients in my private practice of chiropractic and naturopathic medicine. Even though several of these are considered nonpathogenic by the outdated allopathic conceptualizations that are still hypnotized by Pasteur and Koch, their presence is generally inconsistent with optimal health and their eradication is rewarding for both doctor and patient. One of the benefits of specialized stool testing is that it allows the presence of microbes to be determined within a context that evaluates the patient's individualized response. For example, the finding of a mild degree of *Candida albicans* ("+1" on a 0-4 scale) might be considered insignificant; however if no other pathogens are identified, and the secretory IgA, lactoferrin, and lysozyme levels are highly elevated, then the clinician is justified in determining that the patient is having a hypersensitivity reaction to an otherwise "benign" yeast. Recently I worked with a patient with rheumatoid arthritis in whom we found mild *Citrobacter freundii* ("+1") which was barely enough to arouse my interest until I noted that he had an exaggerated mucosal inflammatory response; eradication of the bacteria lead to an immediate and profound reduction in his symptomatology and systemic inflammation (e.g., his C-reactive protein decreased from 124 to 7 mg/L within four weeks). Remember, we are not looking for classic "infection" here; we are looking to determine which underlying disruptions may be exacerbating inflammation and the patient's symptomatology.

Blastocystis hominis: Patients with *B. hominis* commonly have fatigue. Some patients will have abdominal pain, nausea, vomiting, diarrhea, weight loss as well as anorexia, flatus, and eosinophilia.[121-123] "Typical symptoms include diarrhea, crampy abdominal pain, nausea, vomiting, low-grade fever, gas, malaise, and chills. Fecal leukocytes are occasionally seen."[124] *B. hominis* can cause colitis.[125]

Candida albicans **and other yeasts:** Although normal in small amounts ("+1"), excess *Candida* in the intestines is never a sign of optimal health. Patients may have mild general symptoms such as fatigue and dyscognition ("brain fog"); gas and intestinal bloating following consumption of carbohydrates are common. *Candida* produces an immunosuppressive myotoxin called gliotoxin as well as an IgA-destroying protease and can cause watery diarrhea, particularly in elderly, ill, and immunosuppressed patients. It is always present in the gastrointestinal tract of women with recurrent yeast vaginitis.[72] Some people have an inflammatory hypersensitivity to *Candida*, as it can cause local allergic dermatitis/mucositis[109], colitis[107], and pulmonary inflammation (from gastrointestinal colonization).[108] Other yeasts such as *Candida parapsilosis* and *Geotrichum capitatum* are occasionally seen and should be eradicated.

Citrobacter freundii: Also known as C*itrobacter rodentium*, *Citrobacter freundii* is described as a gram-negative aerobe and facultative anaerobe; it may cause gastroenteritis in humans. Animal studies have shown that this bacterium can induce an intense inflammatory response in the gastrointestinal tract that resembles inflammatory bowel disease. Like several other intestinal bacteria, most strains of *Citrobacter freundii* produce hydrogen sulfide which interferes with mitochondrial function and energy production and appears to contribute to ulcerative colitis.[57]

Endolimax nana: *Endolimax nana* is a protozoa with world-wide distribution and is commonly considered an harmless commensal of the intestine. However, intestinal infection with *Endolimax nana* can cause a peripheral arthropathy that is clinically similar to rheumatoid arthritis and which remits with effective parasite eradication.[126] In my own clinical practice, I have seen several cases of intestinal colonization with *Endolimax nana* in patients who presented with chronic fatigue, myalgia, eczema, and especially refractory chronic vaginitis.

Entamoeba histolytica: *E histolytica* can induce tissue damage, amebic colitis, and liver abscess.[127] *E histolytica* was associated with Henoch Schonlein purpura in a single case report.[128] Amebic colitis may be misdiagnosed as ulcerative colitis.[86] Associated with induction of antineutrophil cytoplasmic antibodies, such as seen with the vasculitic disease Wegener's granulomatosis[83], *E histolytica* may produce manifestations similar to irritable bowel syndrome, rheumatoid arthritis, fibromyalgia, food allergy, or multiple chemical sensitivity and can exacerbate HIV infection.[86]

Giardia lamblia: Giardia is causatively associated with abdominal pain, diarrhea, constipation, bloating, chronic fatigue, and food allergy/intolerance, and can exacerbate irritable bowel syndrome, rheumatoid arthritis, food allergy, or multiple chemical sensitivity.[86,129] Some infections are relatively asymptomatic.

Klebsiella pneumoniae: Many cases of gastrointestinal colonization with this microorganism produce no acute gastrointestinal symptoms such as nausea, vomiting, constipation, or diarrhea. Patients may have mild general symptoms such as fatigue and dyscognition ("brain fog"). *Klebsiella* can cause diarrhea and acute gastroenteritis. It is associated with reactive arthritis such as ankylosing spondylitis.[91] Since it is a gram-negative bacteria, it produces an endotoxin that is capable of impairing cytochrome

p-450 and reducing clearance and excretion of drugs.[130]

Proteus mirabilis: *Proteus* is a gram-negative bacteria that produces endotoxin. Gastrointestinal and urinary tract colonization with *Proteus* is associated with rheumatoid arthritis[92] and ankylosing spondylitis.[93] In one of my patients, his response to gastrointestinal *Proteus* caused an "idiopathic inflammatory polyneuropathy" that disappeared within one month of parasite eradication; this patient had previously been assessed by several neurologists with MRI, CT, CSF analysis, and neuroconductive tests, none of which lead to diagnosis or effective treatment.

Pseudomonas aeruginosa: Many cases of gastrointestinal colonization with this microorganism produce no acute gastrointestinal symptoms such as nausea, vomiting, constipation, or diarrhea. Patients may have mild general symptoms such as fatigue and dyscognition ("brain fog"). *Pseudomonas aeruginosa* is a gram-negative bacteria, produces endotoxin and can cause antibiotic-associated diarrhea. Patients with multiple sclerosis show evidence of a heightened immune response against *Pseudomonas aerugeniosa*, suggesting the possibility of immune cross-reactivity.[94]

Helicobacter pylori: *H. pylori* is a gram-negative endotoxin-producing rod that causes stomach ulcers and appears to cause reactive arthritis in some patients.[95]

Group A streptococci, Streptococcus pyogenes: Intestinal overgrowth of this bacterium, which produces peptidoglycans, can cause dermatosis, polyarthritis, tenosynovitis, malaise, fever, and cryoglobulinemia.[7] Non-infectious manifestations precipitated by infection with *S. pyogenes* include autoimmune neuropsychiatric disorders (including obsessive-compulsive disorder and Sydenham's chorea), dystonia, glomerulonephritis, and reactive arthritis.[131] Certain strains of *S. pyogenes* produce an exotoxin that can cause toxic shock syndrome.[132]

"Gamma strep" and Enterococcus: "Gamma strep", *Enterococcus faecalis*, and S*treptococcus faecalis* are somewhat interchangeable terms. These terms refer to gram-positive Enterococcus species such as *Enterococcus faecalis*, which cause urinary tract infections, bacteremia, intra-abdominal infections, and endocarditis. Enterococci produce lipoteichoic acid which is pro-inflammatory in a manner similar to endotoxin from gram-negative bacteria, and these gram-positive bacteria also appear to produce a superantigen.[133] "Gamma strep" is commonly identified in stool tests of patients with chronic unwellness and fatigue.

Staphylococcus aureus: Gastrointestinal colonization with *Staph aureus* should be eradicated immediately due to the well-known inflammatory consequences of the toxins and superantigens this bacterium produces. *Staphylococcus aureus* is a gram-positive bacterium, certain strains of which produce the toxic shock syndrome toxin-1 (TSST-1) that produces scalded skin syndrome, toxic shock syndrome, and food poisoning; other strains of *Staph aureus* that do not produce TSST-1 are also capable of causing toxic shock syndrome from colonization of bone, vagina, wounds, or rectum.[134] Gastrointestinal colonization with *Staph aureus* is a known cause of acute colitis[135], and nasal carriage of this bacterium appears to trigger autoimmunity in patients with Wegener's granulomatosis.[82]

Aeromonas hydrophila: *Aeromonas hydrophila* can cause colitis and should be eradicated immediately upon detection.[136]

Dientamoeba fragilis: *Dientamoeba fragilis* is a flagellate protozoan that can cause diarrhea, abdominal pain, nausea, vomiting, fatigue, malaise, eosinophilia, urticaria, pruritus and/or weight loss. It is commonly associated with pinworm infection and may produce a clinical picture that mimics food allergy, colitis, or eosinophilic enteritis.[137]

NATURAL TREATMENTS FOR THE ERADICATION OF GI DYSBIOSIS AND RELATED IMMUNE-COMPLEX DISEASES

Although antimicrobial drugs may be used, these are not universally curative and are not necessarily "more powerful" or "more effective" than natural treatments. Even when treating dysbiosis caused by microorganisms, we must look "beyond the bugs" and ensure that treatment is comprehensive, as well as effective.

Diet modifications *("starve the microbes"):* The diet plan should ensure avoidance of sugar, grains, soluble fiber, gums, prebiotics, and dairy products since these contain fermentable carbohydrates that promote overgrowth of bacteria and other microorganisms in the gut. Short-term fasting starves intestinal microbes, temporarily eliminates dietary antigens, alleviates "autointoxication", and stimulates the humoral immune system in the gut to more effectively destroy local microbes.[138,139] Thus, implementation of the "specific carbohydrate diet" popularized by Gotschall[140] along with periodic fasting, which has obvious anti-inflammatory benefits[141], can be used therapeutically in patients with conditions associated with dysbiosis-induced inflammation. Plant-based low-carbohydrate diets can lead to favorable changes in the quality and quantity of intestinal microflora. Hypoallergenic diets are proven beneficial for the treatment of the immune complex disease mixed cryoglobulinemia.[142,143]

Antimicrobial treatments *("poison the microbes, not the patient"):* Anti-microbial herbs can be used which directly kill or strongly inhibit the intestinal microbes. The

most commonly used and well-documented botanicals in this regard are listed in the section below. Antimicrobial treatment is frequently continued for 1-3 months, and co-administration of drugs can be utilized when appropriate. Sometimes antimicrobial drugs are necessary, especially for acute and severe infections; often nutritional and botanical interventions are safer and more effective. Although these herbs are generally taken orally, some of them can also be applied topically (in a cream or lotion), and nasally (in a water lavage). Botanical medicines are generally used in combination, and lower doses of each can be used when used in combination compared to the doses that are necessary when the herbs are used in isolation.

Oregano oil in an emulsified and time-released tablet: Botanical oils that are not emulsified do not attain maximal dispersion in the gastrointestinal tract; products that are not time-released may be absorbed before reaching the colon in sufficient concentrations. Emulsified oil of oregano in a time-released tablet is proven effective in the eradication of harmful gastrointestinal microbes, including *Blastocystis hominis*, *Entamoeba hartmanni*, and *Endolimax nana*.[144] An in vitro study[145] and clinical experience support the use of emulsified oregano against *Candida albicans*. The common dose is 600 mg per day in divided doses.

Berberine: Berberine is an alkaloid extracted from plant such as *Berberis vulgaris*, and *Hydrastis canadensis*, and it shows effectiveness against *Giardia*, *Candida*, and *Streptococcus* in addition to its direct anti-inflammatory and antidiarrheal actions. Oral dose of 400 mg per day is common for adults.[146]

Artemisia species: Artemisinin has been safely used for centuries in Asia for the treatment of malaria, and it also has effectiveness against anaerobic bacteria due to the pro-oxidative sesquiterpene endoperoxide.[147] In a recent study treating patients with malaria, "the adult artemisinin dose was 500 mg; children aged < 15 years received 10 mg/kg per dose" and thus the dose for an 80-lb child would be 363 mg per day by these criteria.[148] I commonly use artemisinin at 200 mg per day in divided doses for adults with dysbiosis. One of the main benefits of artemisinin is its systemic bioavailability.

St. John's Wort (*Hypericum perforatum*): Best known for its antidepressant action, hyperforin from *Hypericum perforatum* also shows impressive antibacterial action, particularly against gram-positive bacteria such as *Staphylococcus aureus*, *Streptococcus pyogenes* and *Streptococcus agalactiae*. According to in vitro studies, the lowest effective hyperforin concentration is 0.1 mcg/mL against *Corynebacterium diphtheriae* with increasing effectiveness against multiresistant *Staphylococcus aureus* at higher concentrations of 100 mcg/mL.[149] Since oral dosing with hyperforin can result in serum levels of 500 nanogram /mL (equivalent to 0.5 microgram/mL) then it is possible that high-dose hyperforin will have systemic antibacterial action. Regardless of its possible systemic antibacterial effectiveness, hyperforin should clearly have antibacterial action when applied "topically" such as when it is taken orally against gastric and upper intestinal colonization. Extracts from St. John's Wort hold particular promise against multidrug-resistant *Staphylococcus aureus*[150], and there is also evidence for its effectiveness against *Helicobacter pylori*.[151]

Myrrh (*Commiphora molmol*): Myrrh is remarkably effective against parasitic infections.[152] A recent clinical trial against schistosomiasis showed "The parasitological cure rate after three months was 97.4% and 96.2% for *S. haematobium* and *S. mansoni* cases with the marvelous clinical cure without any side-effects."[153]

Bismuth: Bismuth is commonly used in the empiric treatment of diarrhea and is commonly combined with other antimicrobial agents to reduce drug resistance and increase antibiotic effectiveness.

Peppermint (*Mentha piperita*): Peppermint shows antimicrobial and antispasmodic actions and has demonstrated clinical effectiveness in patients with bacterial overgrowth of the small bowel.

Uva Ursi: Uva ursi can be used against gastrointestinal pathogens on a limited basis per culture and sensitivity findings; its primary historical and modern use is as a urinary antiseptic which is effective only when the urine pH is alkaline.[154] Components of uva ursi potentiate antibiotics. This herb has some ocular and neurologic toxicity and should be used with professional supervision for low-dose and/or short-term administration only.[155]

Cranberry: Cranberry is particularly effective for the prevention and adjunctive treatment of urinary tract infections, mostly by inhibiting adherence of *E. coli* to epithelial cells.[156]

Thyme (*Thymus vulgaris*): Thyme extracts have direct antimicrobial actions and also potentiate the effectiveness of tetracycline against drug-resistant *Staphylococcus aureus*.[157] Thyme also appears effective against *Aeromonas hydrophila*.[158]

Clove (*Syzygium species*): Clove's eugenol has been show in animal studies to have a potent antifungal effect.[159]

Anise: Although it has weak antibacterial action when used alone, anise does show in vitro activity against molds.[160]

Buchu/betulina: Buchu has a long history of use against urinary tract infections and systemic infections.[161]

Caprylic acid: Caprylic acid is a medium chain fatty acid that is commonly used in patients with dysbiosis, particularly that which has a fungal/yeast component. Beside empiric use, caprylic acid may be indicated by culture-sensitivity results provided with comprehensive parasitology.

Dill (*Anethum graveolens*): Dill shows activity against several types of mold and yeast.[162]

Brucea javanica: Extract from *Brucea javanica* fruit shows *in vitro* activity against *Babesia gibsoni*, *Plasmodium falciparum*[163], *Entamoeba histolytica*,[164] and *Blastocystis hominis*.[165,166]

Acacia catechu: *Acacia catechu* shows moderate in vitro activity against *Salmonella typhi*.[167]

Oral administration of proteolytic enzymes: The use of polyenzyme therapy in patients with dysbioic inflammation is justified for at least four reasons. First, orally administered proteolytic enzymes are efficiently absorbed by the gastrointestinal tract into the systemic circulation[168] to then provide a clinically significant anti-inflammatory benefit as I reviewed recently.[169] Second and more specifically, oral administration of proteolytic enzymes is generally believed to effect a reduction in immune complexes and their clinical consequences[170], and immune complexes are probably a major mechanism of dysbiosis-induced disease and are pathogenic in rheumatoid arthritis[171] and many other autoimmune diseases such as systemic lupus erythematosus, dermatomyositis, Sjogren's syndrome, and polyarteritis nodosa.[172] Third, proteolytic enzymes have been shown to stimulate immune function[173] and may thereby promote clearance of occult infections. Fourth, proteolytic enzymes degrade microbial biofilms and increase immune penetration and the effectiveness of antimicrobial therapeutics.[174]

Probiotic supplementation (*"crowd out the bad with the good"*): Given that "healthy" intestinal bacteria can alleviate disease and promote normal immune function[175], then it is conversely true that a condition of harmful or suboptimal intestinal bacteria could promote disease and lead to immune dysfunction. For patients with gastrointestinal and genitourinary dysbiosis, supplementation with *Bifidobacteria, Lactobacillus,* and perhaps *Saccharomyces* and other beneficial strains is mandatory. The wide-ranging and well-documented benefits seen with probiotic supplementation provide direct and indirect support for the importance of microbial balance in health and disease. Supplementation with probiotics (live bacteria) is the best option, however prebiotics (such as fructooligosaccharides), and synbiotics (probiotics + prebiotics) may also be used. Synbiotic supplementation has been shown to reduce endotoxinemia and clinical symptoms in 50% of patients with minimal hepatic encephalopathy[176], and probiotic supplementation safely ameliorated the adverse effects of bacterial overgrowth in a clinical study of patients with renal failure.[177]

Immunonutrition: Obviously the diet should be nutritious and free of sugars and other "junk foods" that promote inflammation and suppress immune function.[178] Especially in patients with gastrointestinal dysbiosis, vitamin and mineral supplementation should be used to counteract the effects of malabsorption, maldigestion, and hypermetabolism that accompany immune activation. Additionally, oral glutamine in doses of six grams three times daily can help normalize intestinal permeability, enhance immune function, and improve clinical outcomes in severely ill patients.[179] Zinc and vitamin A supplementation are each well-known to support immune function against infection. Selenium has anti-inflammatory, antioxidant, and antiviral actions.[180] Vitamin D supplementation reduces inflammation, protects against autoimmunity, and promotes immunity against viral and bacterial infections.[181] Supplementation with IgG from bovine colostrum can also provide benefit against chronic and acute infections.[182,183] Extracts from bovine thymus are safe for clinical use in humans and have shown anti-infective and anti-inflammatory benefits[184] as well as antirheumatic/anti-inflammatory benefits in patients with autoimmune diseases[185-187]; in an animal study of experimental dental disease, administration of thymus extract was shown to normalize immune function and reduce orodental dysbiosis.[188]

Hepatobiliary stimulation for IgA-complex removal: The binding of immunoglobuin A (IgA) with antigen creates IgA immune complexes that contribute to tissue destruction by complement activation (alternate pathway) and other pathomechanisms in IgA nephropathy[189], Henoch-Schonlein purpura[190], rheumatoid vasculitis[191], lupus[192], and Sjogren's syndrome.[193] Autoreactive IgA antibodies are a characteristic of lupus and Sjogren's syndrome[193] and correlate strongly with disease activity in rheumatoid arthritis.[194] Immune complexes containing secretory IgA that has been reabsorbed from mucosal surfaces mediate many of the clinical phenomenon of dysbiosis-related disease[17], and these same IgA-containing immune complexes are eliminated from the systemic circulation via the liver and biliary system[195,196], thus providing the rationale for the use of botanicals and physiotherapeutics that promote liver function and bile flow in the treatment of IgA-mediated inflammatory disorders. Numerous experimental studies in animals have shown that circulating IgA immune complexes are taken up by hepatocytes and then secreted into the bile for elimination.[197,198] The fact that bile duct obstruction retards systemic clearance of IgA immune complexes and that normalization/optimization of bile flow reduces serum IgA levels by enhancing biliary excretion in animals[199-200] and humans[201] proves the importance of ensuring optimal hepatobiliary function and supports the use of botanical and physiological therapeutics that facilitate bile flow. A 1929 clinical study with human patients published in *Archives of Internal Medicine* provided irrefutable radiographic documentation that therapeutic enemas safely and effectively stimulate bile flow for 45-60 minutes following administration[63], and this finding, along with the obvious quantitative reduction in intestinal microbes induced by such "cleansing", helps explain the reported benefits of colonics/enemas in patients with systemic illness[40,61,62,64] and other immune-complex associated diseases such as cancer.[202] Validation of this concept is demonstrated by the significant efficacy of immunoadsorption[203] and plasmapheresis[204,205] (techniques for removing immune complexes) in patients with lupus. Furthermore, this directly supports the naturopathic concept of "treating the liver" in patients with systemic disease by the use of dietary and botanical therapeutics that stimulate bile flow, such as beets, ginger[206], curcumin/turmeric[207], *Picrorhiza*[208], milk thistle[209], *Andrographis paniculata*[210], and *Boerhaavia diffusa*.[211]

Ensure generous bowel movements and consider therapeutic purgatives *(purge: to free from impurities):* Dysbiotic patients should consume a low-fermentation fiber-rich diet that allows for 1-2 very generous bowel movements per day. Constipation must absolutely be eliminated; there is no place for constipation in patients being treated for dysbiosis of any type. Patients with severe or recalcitrant dysbiosis can start the day with a laxative dose of ascorbic acid (e.g., 20 grams with 4 cups of water) and should expect liquid diarrhea within 30-60 minutes. The goal here is purgative physical removal of enteric microbes; in high concentrations, ascorbic acid has a direct antibacterial effect. Magnesium in elemental doses of 500-1,200 mg also helps soften stool and promote laxation.

SUMMARY AND CONCLUSIONS

Microbes contribute to noninfectious human diseases by numerous and complex direct and indirect mechanisms. Patients may have several types of dysbiosis at the same time, as we see in patients with Behcet's syndrome characterized by pulmonary infection with *Chlamydia pneumonia*[212], cutaneous infection with *Staphylococcus aureus*[213], and orodental infection with *Streptococcus sanguis*.[69] Add in a few genetic traits and some nutritional deficiencies, and it becomes easy to see why rheumatic diseases are generally still considered "idiopathic" when reviewed from a reductionistic medical paradigm that fails to appreciate the interconnected and "holistic" web of influences that synergize to produce systemic inflammation. For the majority of patients in outpatient clinical practice, the location of their dysbiosis is the gut, which is easily assessed with specialized stool testing and parasitology examinations, and which is easily treated with oral botanical antimicrobials and dietary modification. In my own clinical practice, I consider stool testing extremely valuable and estimate that 80% of parasitology examinations return with at least one clinically-relevant abnormality. Testing for and treating dysbiosis is an absolutely essential consideration in patients with gas, bloating, alternating constipation/diarrhea, irritable bowel syndrome, fibromyalgia, chronic fatigue syndrome, multiple chemical sensitivity, severe allergies, arthritis, and autoimmunity. In addition to hundreds to thousands of years of traditional use, many botanical medicines have modern peer-reviewed clinical and experimental research supporting their role in the eradication of acute and chronic infections. Beyond the use of antimicrobial herbs, other treatments such as diet therapy, immunonutrition, hepatobiliary stimulation, probiotics, and proteolytic enzymes clearly have a role in the treatment of patients with musculoskeletal inflammation secondary to dysbiosis. With their superior knowledge of natural anti-inflammatory therapeutics including diet[214], balanced broad-spectrum fatty acid supplementation[215], botanical and nutritional antiinflammatories[216] (including high-dose vitamin D)[181], NF-kappaB inhibitors[217], and anti-allergy treatments[218], chiropractic and naturopathic physicians have the power to safely and effectively aid the vast majority of patients with degenerative and inflammatory musculoskeletal disorders. Additional details for testing and treatment of all major autoimmune disorders are provided in *Integrative Rheumatology*.[219]

ABOUT THE AUTHOR:

Dr. Alex Vasquez is a licensed naturopathic physician in Washington and Oregon, and licensed chiropractor in Texas, where he maintains a private practice and is a member of the research team at Biotics Research Corporation. As the author of *"Integrative Orthopedics: The Art of Creating Wellness While Managing Acute and Chronic Musculoskeletal Disorders"* available from OptimalHealthResearch.com, Dr. Vasquez has published articles in many major medical journals, including *The Lancet, Journal of the American Medical Association (JAMA), British Medical Journal (BMJ), Annals of Pharmacotherapy, Journal of Manipulative and Physiological Therapeutics (JMPT),* and *Arthritis & Rheumatism.*

ACKNOWLEDGEMENTS:

Rachel Olivier, Nilima Trivedi, and Barb Berta critiqued portions of this paper prior to publication.

REFERENCES (ABBREVIATED):

References for this article are available on-line at http://www.optimalhealthresearch.com/part6 or by calling the Council Office.

16601812R00146

Made in the USA
Lexington, KY
03 August 2012